Progress in Parkinson's Disease Research—2

Edited by

Franz Hefti, Ph.D.

Professor of Gerontology, University of Southern California,
National Parkinson Foundation Research Scholar,
Los Angeles, California

and

William J. Weiner, M.D.

Professor of Neurology,
Director of the Movement Disorders Center,
University of Miami School of Medicine,
National Parkinson Foundation Clinical Research Scholar,
Miami, Florida

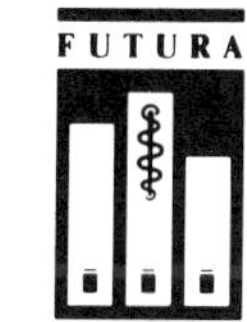

**Futura Publishing
Company, Inc.**
Mount Kisco, NY

Library of Congress Cataloging-in-Publication Data

Progress in Parkinson's disease research—2 / editors, Franz Hefti and
  William J. Weiner
     p. cm.
    Includes bibliographical references and index.
    ISBN 0-87993-530-8
    1. Parkinsonism. I. Hefti, Franz. II. Weiner, William J.
[DNLM: 1. Dopamine—physiology—congresses. 2. Parkinson
Disease—physiopathology—congresses. 3. Receptors, Dopa-
mine—physiology—congresses. 4. 1-Methyl-4-phenyl-1,2,3,6,-
tetrahydropyridine—metabolism—congresses. WL 359 P9632]
RC3.82.P74   1992
616.8'33—dc20
DNLM/DLC
for Library of Congress   92-9895
                                                              CIP

Published by
Futura Publishing Company, Inc.
2 Bedford Ridge Road
Mount Kisco, New York 10549

LC: 92-9895
ISBN: 0-87993-530-8

Contributors

Ralph F. Alderson, Ph.D. Regeneron Pharmaceuticals, Inc., Tarrytown, New York

Per Almqvist, M.D., Ph.D. Department of Geriatrics, Karolinska Center, Stockholm, Sweden

Norman Arnheim Molecular Biology Section, University of Southern California, Los Angeles, California

Klaus Dieter Beck, M.D. University of Southern California, Andrus Gerontology Center and Department of Biological Sciences, Los Angeles, California

Debra A. Bergstrom, Ph.D. Pharmacologist, Neurophysiological Pharmacology Section, Experimental Therapeutics Branch, National Institutes of Health, National Institute of Neurological Disorders and Stroke, Bethesda, Maryland

Anders Björklund, M.D., Ph.D. Professor of Medical Cell Research, Institutionen för Medicinsk Cellforskning, Neurobiologiska Avdelningen, Lunds Universitet, Lund, Sweden

Alan A. Boulton, B.Sc., Ph.D., D.Sc. Professor of Psychiatry and Director of the Neuropsychiatric Research Unit, University of Saskatchewan, Saskatoon, Saskatchewan, Canada

George R. Breese, Ph.D. Professor, Psychiatry & Pharmacology, University of North Carolina at Chapel Hill, Chapel Hill, North Carolina

Robert E. Breeze, M.D. Assistant Professor of Surgery, Division of Neurosurgery, University of Colorado Health Sciences Center, Denver, Colorado

Patrik Brundin, M.D., Ph.D. Assistant Professor of Medical Cell Research, Institutionen för Medicinsk Cellforskning, Neurobiologiska Avdelningen, Lunds Universitet, Lund, Sweden

James R. Bunzow, M.S. Senior Research Associate, Vollum Institute for Advanced Biomedical Research, Oregon Health Sciences University, Portland, Oregon

Carolyn Burkhardt, M.D. Instructor, Department of Neurology, University of Colorado School of Medicine, Denver, Colorado

Louis E. Burton, Ph.D. Genentech Inc., Developmental Biology Department, South San Francisco, California

Marc Bygdeman, M.D., Ph.D. Department of Obstetrics and Gynecology, Karolinska Institute, Stockholm, Sweden

Donald B. Calne, D.M. Professor and Director, Neurodegenerative Disorders Centre, University of British Columbia, British Columbia

Heng-Wei Cheng, M.D., Ph.D. Research Associate, Andrus Gerontology Center, University of Southern California, Los Angeles, California

Hyung Choi, Ph.D. Research Associate, Department of Pharmacological and Physiological Sciences, The University of Chicago, Chicago, Illinois

Olivier Civelli, Ph.D. Scientist, Vollum Institute for Advanced Biomedical Research, Oregon Health Sciences University, Portland, Oregon

Gino A. Cortopassi, Ph.D. Assistant Professor of Molecular Pharmacology and Toxicology, Institute for Toxicology, University of Southern California, Los Angeles, California

Hugh E. Criswell, Ph.D. Research Associate Professor, University of North Carolina at Chapel Hill, Chapel Hill, North Carolina

Bruce A. Davis, B.Sc., Ph.D. Adjunct Professor of Psychiatry and Research Scientist, Neuropsychiatric Research Unit, University of Saskatchewan, Saskatoon, Saskatchewan, Canada

Ariel Y. Deutch, Ph.D. Departments of Psychiatry and Pharmacology, Yale University School of Medicine, Connecticut Mental Health Center, New Haven, Connecticut

Guy Doucet, Ph.D. Assistant Professor of Pathology, Centre du recherche en sciences neurologiques, Département de pathologie, Université de Montréal, Montréal, Québec, Canada

Gary E. Duncan, Ph.D. Research Associate Professor, University of North Carolina at Chapel Hill, Chapel Hill, North Carolina

David A. Durden, B.Sc., Ph.D. Adjunct Professor of Psychiatry and Research Scientist Neuropsychiatric Research Unit, University of Saskatchewan, Saskatoon, Saskatchewan, Canada

Roger C. Duvoisin, M.D. Professor and Chairman, Department of Neurology, University of Medicine & Dentistry of New Jersey-Robert Wood Johnson Medical School, New Brunswick, New Jersey

Curt R. Freed, M.D. Professor of Medicine and Pharmacology, University of Colorado Health Sciences Center, Denver, Colorado

Beth Friedman, Ph.D. Regeneron Pharmaceuticals, Inc., Tarrytown, New York

Mark E. Furth, Ph.D. Regeneron Pharmaceuticals, Inc., Tarrytown, New York

Charles R. Gerfen, Ph.D. Laboratory of Cell Biology, National Institute of Mental Health, National Institutes of Health, Bethesda, Maryland

Greg Gerhardt, Ph.D. Departments of Pharmacology and Psychiatry, University of Colorado Health Sciences Center, Denver, Colorado

Bernardino Ghetti, M.D. Professor of Pathology (Neuropathology), Psychiatry and Medical & Molecular Genetics, Laboratory of Cellular and Molecular Neuropathology, Department of Pathology, Departments of Psychiatry and Medical & Molecular Genetics, and Program in Medical Neurobiology, Indiana University School of Medicine, Indianapolis, Indiana

Jean-Antoine Girault, M.D., Ph.D. Charge de Recherche, INSERM U 114, Chaire de Neuropharmacologie, College de France, Paris, France and Member of the Adjunct Faculty, Laboratory of Molecular and Cellular Neuroscience, The Rockefeller University, New York, New York

Menek Goldstein, Ph.D. Professor of Neurochemistry, New York University Medical Center, Neurochemistry Research Laboratories, New York, New York

David K. Grandy, Ph.D. Senior Research Associate, Vollum Institute for Advanced Biomedical Research, Oregon Health Sciences University, Portland, Oregon

Franz F. Hefti, Ph.D. University of Southern California, Andrus Gerontology Center and Department of Biological Sciences, Los Angeles, California

Richard E. Heikkila, Ph.D.* Professor of Neurology, University of Medicine & Dentistry of New Jersey-Robert Wood Johnson Medical School, Piscataway, New Jersey

Alfred Heller, Ph.D., M.D. Professor of Pharmacology, Department of Pharmacological and Physiological Sciences, The Committee on Neurobiology, The University of Chicago, Chicago, Illinois

Barry Hoffer, M.D., Ph.D. Department of Pharmacology, University of Colorado Health Sciences Center, Denver, Colorado

Philip C. Hoffman, Ph.D. Professor of Pharmacology, Department of Pharmacological and Physiological Sciences, The Committee on Neurobiology, The University of Chicago, Chicago, Illinois

Kai-Xing Huang, Ph.D. Guest Researcher, Neurophysiological Pharmacology Section, Experimental Therapeutics Branch, National Institutes of Health, National Institute of Neurological Disorders and Stroke, Bethesda, Maryland

Carolyn Hyman, Ph.D. Regeneron Pharmaceuticals, Inc., Tarrytown, New York

Nancy Y. Ip, Ph.D. Regeneron Pharmaceuticals, Inc., Tarrytown, New York

Peter Jenner, B.Pharm., Ph.D., D.Sc., MRPharmS. Professor of Pharmacology & Head of Department, Pharmacology Group, Biomedical Sciences Division, King's College London, Chelsea Campus, London, England

Karl F. Jensen, Ph.D. Environmental Health Scientist, Environmental Protection Agency, Research Triangle Park, North Carolina

Kevin B. Johnson, B.S. Research Fellow, University of North Carolina at Chapel Hill, Chapel Hill, North Carolina

---

*deceased

Augusto V. Juorio, B.S.P., B.Sc., Ph.D. Adjunct Professor of Psychiatry and Senior Research Scientist, Neuropsychiatric Research Unit, University of Saskatchewan, Saskatoon, Saskatchewan, Canada

Mark D. Kelland, Ph.D. Senior Staff Fellow, Neurophysiological Pharmacology Section, Experimental Therapeutics Branch, National Institutes of Health, National Institute of Neurological Disorders and Stroke, Bethesda, Maryland

Beat Knüsel, Ph.D. University of Southern California, Andrus Gerontology Center, Los Angeles, California

Irwin J. Kopin, M.D. Director Intramural Research Program, National Institute of Neurological Diseases and Stroke, Bethesda, Maryland

John F. Kurtzke, M.D. Professor of Neurology & Professor of Community and Family Medicine, Georgetown University School of Medicine, Washington, D.C. and Chief, Neurology Service & Chief, Neuroepidemiology Research Program, VA Medical Center, Washington, D.C.

Robert M. Lindsay, Ph.D. Program Director, Neurobiology, Regeneron Pharmaceuticals, Inc., Tarrytown, New York

Walter C. Low, Ph.D. Associate Professor of Neurosurgery, Physiology, and Neuroscience, Departments of Neurosurgery and Physiology, and Program in Neuroscience, University of Minnesota Medical School, Minneapolis, Minnesota

Lawrence C. Mahan, Ph.D. Laboratory of Cell Biology, National Institute of Mental Health, National Institutes of Health, Bethesda, Maryland

Peter C. Maisonpierre, Ph.D. Regeneron Pharmaceuticals, Inc., Tarrytown, New York

Ann M. Marini, M.D., Ph.D. Clinical Neuroscience Branch, National Institute of Mental Health, Bethesda, Maryland

Deborah C. Mash, Ph.D. Associate Professor of Neurology and Cellular and Molecular Pharmacology, Director, University of Miami Brain Endowment Bank, University of Miami School of Medicine, Miami, Florida

Thomas H. McNeill, Ph.D. Associate Professor of Neurogerontology/Neurobiology, Andrus Gerontology Center and Department of Biological Sciences, University of Southern California, Los Angeles, California

Frederick J. Monsma, Jr., Ph.D. Experimental Therapeutics Branch, National Institutes of Health, National Institute of Neurological Disorders and Stroke, Bethesda, Maryland

Nozomu Mori, Ph.D. Research Assistant Professor, Andrus Gerontology Center, University of Southern California, Los Angeles, California

Robert A. Mueller, M.D. Professor of Anesthesiology, University of North Carolina at Chapel Hill, Chapel Hill, North Carolina

William J. Nicklas, Ph.D. Professor of Neurology, University of Medicine & Dentistry of New Jersey-Robert Wood Johnson Medical School, Piscataway, New Jersey

Karoly Nikolics, Ph.D. Genentech Inc., Developmental Biology Department, South San Francisco, California

James O'Callaghan, Ph.D. Environmental Health Scientist, Environmental Protections Agency, Research Triangle Park, North Carolina

Anne-Marie O'Carroll, B.A., Ph.D. Laboratory of Cell Biology, National Institutes of Mental Health, Bethesda, Maryland

Lars Olson, Ph.D. Department of Histology and Neurobiology, Karolinska Institute, Stockholm, Sweden

W. Davis Parker, Jr., M.D. Associate Professor, Departments of Neurology and Pediatrics, University of Colorado School of Medicine, Denver, Colorado

Giulio Pasinetti Andrus Gerontology Center, University of Southern California, Los Angeles, California

I. Alick Paterson, B.Sc., Ph.D. Assistant Professor of Psychiatry and Research Scientist, Neuropsychiatric Research Unit, University of Saskatchewan, Saskatoon, Saskatchewan, Canada

Alexia E. Pollack, Ph.D. Postdoctural Fellow, Laboratory of Molecular Neurobiology, Massachusetts General Hospital East, Charlestown, Massachusetts

Berton Pressman, Ph.D. Professor of Cellular and Molecular Pharmacology, University of Miami School of Medicine, Miami, Florida

José A. Rafols, Ph.D. Professor of Anatomy and Cell Biology, Department of Anatomy and Cell Biology, Wayne State University, Detroit, Michigan

Luis Reynoso, M.D. Research Associate, Department of Cellular and Molecular Pharmacology, University of Miami School of Medicine, Miami, Florida

Suzanne Roffler-Tarlov, Ph.D. Associate Professor of Neurology and Anatomy, Program in Neurosciences, Tufts University School of Medicine, Boston, Massachusetts

Neil L. Rosenberg, M.D. Medical Director, Center for Occupational Neurology and Neurotoxicology, Colorado Neurologic Institute, Denver, Colorado

Juan Sanchez-Ramos, Ph.D., M.D. Associate Professor of Neurology, University of Miami School of Medicine, Miami, Florida

Michael Saporito, Ph.D. Cephalon, Inc., West Chester, Pennsylvania, formerly with University of Medicine & Dentistry of New Jersey-Robert Wood Johnson Medical School, Department of Neurology, Piscataway, New Jersey

Stuart A. Schneck, M.D. Professor of Neurology and Neuropathology, University of Colorado Health Sciences Center, Denver, Colorado

David R. Sibley, Ph.D. Experimental Therapeutics Branch, National Institutes of Health, National Institute of Neurological Disorders and Stroke, Bethesda, Maryland

Peter E. Simson, Ph.D. Research Assistant Professor, University of North Carolina at Chapel Hill, Chapel Hill, North Carolina

Carlos Singer, M.D. Assistant Professor of Neurology, University of Miami School of Medicine, Miami, Florida

Ann C. Smith Departments of Psychiatry and Pharmacology, Yale University School of Medicine, New Haven, Connecticut

Stephen P. Squinto, Ph.D. Regeneron Pharmaceuticals, Inc., Tarrytown, New York

Ingrid Strömberg, Ph.D. Department of Histology and Neurobiology, Karolinska Institute, Stockholm, Sweden

James P. Sullivan, B.A., Ph.D. Abbott Laboratories, Abbott Park, Illinois

Keith Francis Tipton, M.A., Ph.D. Professor, Head of Biochemistry Department, University of Dublin, Trinity College, Dublin, Ireland

Lazaros C. Triarhou, M.D., Ph.D. Assistant Professor of Pathology (Neuropathology) and Neurobiology, Laboratory of Cellular and Molecular Neuropathology, Department of Pathology, and Program in Medical Neurobiology, Indiana University School of Medicine, Indianapolis, Indiana

Joseph Tsui, M.D. Assistant Professor of Neurology, Division of Neurology, University of British Columbia, British Columbia

Craig van Horne, M.D., Ph.D. Department of Pharmacology, University of Colorado Health Sciences Center, Denver, Colorado

Hubert H.M. Van Tol, Ph.D. Assistant Professor, Department of Pharmacology, University of Toronto, Toronto, Canada

Bruce H. Wainer, M.D., Ph.D. Professor of Pathology & Pharmacology, Chief, Section of Pharmacology, Departments of Pharmacological and Physiological Sciences, Pediatrics and Pathology, and the Committees on Neurobiology and Immunology, The University of Chicago, Chicago, Illinois

Judith R. Walters, Ph.D. Chief, Neurophysiological Pharmacology Section, Experimental Therapeutics Branch, National Institutes of Health, National Institute of Neurological Disorders and Stroke, Bethesda, Maryland

William J. Weiner, M.D. Director of the Movement Disorders Center, Professor of Neurology, University of Miami School of Medicine, Miami, Florida

John W. Winslow, Ph.D. Genentech Inc., Developmental Biology Department, South San Francisco, California

Erik Ch. Wolters, M.D. Professor of Neurologie, Vrije Uniersiteit, Amsterdam, The Netherlands

Lisa A. Won, Ph.D. Instructor (Research Associate) of Pharmacology, Department of Pharmacological and Physiological Sciences, The University of Chicago, Chicago, Illinois

G. Frederick Wooten, M.D. Mary Anderson Harrison Professor and Chair of Neurology, Department of Neurology, University of Virginia Health Sciences Center, Charlottesville, Virginia

George D. Yancopoulos, M.D., Ph.D. Regeneron Pharmaceuticals, Inc., Tarrytown, New York

Peter H. Yu, B.Sc., M.Sc., Ph.D Adjunct Professor of Psychiatry and Senior Research Scientist, Neuropsychiatric Research Unit, University of Saskatchewan, Saskatoon, Saskatchewan, Canada

Qun-Yong Zhou, M.S. Graduate Student, Department of Biochemistry and Molecular Biology, Vollum Institute for Advanced Biomedical Research, Oregon Health Sciences University, Portland, Oregon

Preface

This book evolved from the Second International Conference on Parkinson Research, sponsored and hosted by the National Parkinson Foundation, Inc., which was held in January, 1991, in Miami Beach, Florida. The meeting brought together scientists actively engaged in research relevant to Parkinson's disease. Since loss of dopaminergic neurons is the hallmark of Parkinson's disease, many of the contributions focused on these cells. Rapid progress has been made in recent years in Parkinson research and answers to many of the questions raised during a "first" similar meeting sponsored by the National Parkinson Foundation 3 years earlier were evident. Since that initial meeting, receptors for dopamine have been cloned, and significant initial steps have been taken to understand the molecular nature of the interaction between dopamine and mediation of its actions in the brain. The mechanisms of action of MPTP, a toxin producing parkinsonism in humans and animals, has been further elucidated and is now largely understood. Rapid advances have been made in the cell biology of dopaminergic neurons and the discovery of growth factors acting on these cells has been reported. Transplantation remains an uncertain but forceful approach to the replacement of lost dopaminergic neurons. Despite this progress, the cause of Parkinson's disease remains an enigma. While just a few years ago the discovery of MPTP's dopaminergic toxicity resulted in wide acceptance of the theory that the disease might be caused by an environmental toxic agent, causative agents present in the environment remain elusive and other, conflicting findings have appeared. Families have been reported with clear hereditary transmission of Parkinson's disease. A genetic influence in dopaminergic cell death is also suggested by the weaver mutant mouse in which the development of these cells is selectively impaired. These conflicting findings have renewed interest in epidemiological studies, an interest reflected at the conference and in this volume.

Although much has been accomplished, an enormous amount of work remains to be done in the search for a better understanding of the etiology and biology of Parkinson's disease. We hope that the publication of the proceedings of the conference serves to accelerate current research efforts in the field.

We thank the National Parkinson Foundation for making the conference possible and for its help with the publication of this volume. We also thank Sandoz Pharmaceuticals for a grant that has partially underwritten the publication of this book. Finally, we thank the staff of the National Parkinson Foundation for excellent organization and planning of the meeting.

Franz Hefti, Ph.D.
National Parkinson Foundation
Research Scholar

William J. Weiner, M.D.
National Parkinson Foundation
Clinical Research Scholar

Dedication

It is with great sadness that we at the National Parkinson Foundation note the death of Dr. Richard Heikkila and his wife, Dawn. Dr. Heikkila was a leader in neuropharmacologic research and specialized in the field of neurotoxicology. His work in this field led to improved understanding of how specific chemical toxins can cause the death of neurons in the brain. His work with MPTP was particularly valuable in understanding how this toxin affected dopaminergic neurons in the brain. This work helped establish new therapeutic approaches to the treatment of Parkinson's disease and in particular was extremely useful in designing the DATATOP study that may have laid the foundation for preventative treatment in Parkinson's disease. Dr. Heikkila collaborated with many of the scientists who are supported by the National Parkinson Foundation and these collaborations were always fruitful and useful in helping to advance the fight against Parkinson's disease. He was recognized across our country and in the international community as well as a leading research scientist in this particular field.

Only days before he died, Dr. Heikkila attended the Second International Conference on Parkinson Research. His presentation at that meeting was articulate and pertinent to the subject of advancing our knowledge concerning the causes of Parkinson's disease. As always, in addition to presenting his scientific knowledge, he was a warm and generous individual. This book represents the work of that symposium and all who participated in the proceedings join in dedicating this book to the memory of Dr. Heikkila.

Dr. Heikkila received his bachelor's degree and his Ph.D. from Ohio State University. From 1973 to 1979 he was a researcher at Mount Sinai School of Medicine and in 1979 he joined the faculty of UMDNJ-RWJMS as an associate professor of neurology. In 1985 he was promoted to professor in the department of neurology at the same medical school. During his life he published numerous articles in the scientific literature.

All of us at the National Parkinson Foundation will miss Dr. Heikkila's astute mind and the help that he provided in helping to search for the cause of Parkinson's disease. Also and without question, we will miss him as a friend.

Contents

1

Neurotoxins

Chapter 1

Role of Astrocytes in MPTP Toxicity

Ann M. Marini and Irwin J. Kopin

The discovery that systemic administration of 1-methyl-4-phenyl-1,2,5,6-tetrahydropyridine (MPTP) produces in humans and other primates a typical parkinsonian syndrome has spawned a host of investigations into the mechanisms involved in its toxicity.[1,2] In monkeys, the toxin destroys mainly nigrostriatal dopaminergic neurons, but in mice, which require higher doses of the toxin, the effects are less specific and involve noradrenergic, as well as other dopaminergic neurons. After entry into peripheral tissues or the brain, MPTP is converted by monoamine oxidase B (MAO-B) to a toxic metabolite, 1-methyl-4-phenyl-pyridinium (MPP$^+$) via 1-methyl-4-phenyl-2,3-dihydropyridinium (MPDP$^+$). In brain, this conversion appears to occur mainly in astrocytes, the major site of localization of MAO-B, but the toxic metabolite, MPP$^+$, which is a substrate for the catecholamine uptake system, accumulates in dopaminergic neurons. Uptake of MPP$^+$ by dopaminergic neurons appears to account, at least in part, for the specificity of the toxic effects of MPTP. Further concentration of MPP$^+$ into mitochondria and consequent inhibition of mitochondrial respiration is thought to be an important factor in MPP$^+$ cytotoxicity.

Since systemically administered MPP$^+$ (or MPP$^+$ formed in peripheral tissues) does not pass the blood–brain barrier, initial

From Hefti F, and Weiner WJ, (eds.) *Progress in Parkinson's Disease Research—2.* Mount Kisco NY, Futura Publishing Co., Inc., © 1992.

entry of MPTP is clearly important for its pharmacologic and toxic effects in the brain. Riachi et al.[3] found that [³H]MPTP was extracted almost totally during a single passage of blood through the brain, with almost uniform distribution of tritium among the various areas examined. [¹⁴C]Butanol was also almost totally removed from blood during a single passage, but was rapidly washed out of the brain, whereas levels of tritium from [³H]MPTP declined much more slowly. Since the decline in brain tritium concentration was unaltered by inhibition of MAO, retention of the radioisotope was not due to formation of [³H]MPP$^+$. After its intravenous administration, blood MPTP levels fall rapidly and most MPTP that enters the brain appears to do so during the first passage of blood through the brain. Presumably MPTP would be less toxic if it were removed from the brain as rapidly as is butanol.

Unilateral intracarotid infusion of MPTP into the carotid artery of monkeys produces a hemiparkinsonian syndrome on the opposite side.[4] On the side administered MPTP, there is striking depletion of dopamine in the basal ganglia and almost total obliteration of the nigrostriatal neurons. The unilateral effects are consistent with almost complete extraction of MPTP from blood into brain during the first passage and rapid clearance of MPTP from the circulation. Prompt removal of MPTP from blood protects the opposite side from exposure to the toxin, whereas its retention in the exposed hemisphere allows formation of the toxic metabolite, MPP$^+$. Herkenham et al.[5] found that at 1, 3, or 10 days after administration of [¹⁴C]MPTP to hemiparkinsonian monkeys (1 year after they had received a toxic dose of MPTP into one carotid artery), striatal levels of [¹⁴C]MPP$^+$ were markedly lower on the MPTP-lesioned side, consistent with accumulation of MPP$^+$ in the dopaminergic nerve terminals, but the reverse was found in the substantia nigra; levels of MPP$^+$ were higher on the MPTP-treated side. This can be explained by the increased glia in the damaged substantia nigra; MPTP is captured more efficiently and within 1 day converted to MPP$^+$ which is then slowly cleared. These observations strongly suggest that retention of MPTP in brain contributes importantly to the efficacy of brain MPP$^+$ formation and to MPTP toxicity.

Although Riachi et al.[3] attributed relative retention of MPTP to its higher octanol–water partition coefficient (15.6 vs 7.0 for butanol), this twofold difference does not appear to be sufficient to account for the greater than 15-fold difference in washout rate constants for MPTP and butanol (0.09/min and 1.37/min, respectively). An alternative explanation for MPTP retention might be related to its amine moiety, which at physiological pH is almost totally protonated. Since binding of cationic MPTP to acidic intracellular sites could contribute to its retention and conversion to MPP^+, we examined the uptake and disposition of MPTP in cultured astrocytes.

Methods

Astrocytes obtained from the cerebellum of 8-day-old rats (15–19 g) were seeded on plastic culture dishes at a density of 10,000 cells/cm^2 and incubated at 37°C in a humidified atmosphere of 95% air–5% CO_2 in basal Eagle medium containing fetal calf serum (10%), glutamine (2 mM), and gentamicin (100 ug/ml). The medium was changed at 3-day intervals and the studies were performed after incubation for 14–28 days, at which time more than 95% of the cultured cells were GFAP positive.

Uptake studies were performed in modified Locke's solution containing NaCl (154 mM), KCl (5.6 mM), $CaCl_2$ (2.3 mM), $MgCl_2$ (1.0 mM), glucose (5.6 mM), and HEPES (8.6 mM) at pH 7.4. After washing the cells twice with this solution, 0.9 ml of the solution was added to each plate and the culture plates were transferred to a water bath at the appropriate temperature (3, 24, or 37°C). At various times after addition of 100 μl of the modified Locke's solution containing either [^{3}H]MPTP (25 nM, 82.3 Ci/mM) or [^{3}H]MPP$^+$ (25 nM, 88.4 Ci/mM) with or without appropriate amounts (indicated in results) of unlabeled carrier, the incubation medium was aspirated and the cells washed twice with Locke's solution. The cells were then solubilized by addition of 1.0 ml 0.2 N NaOH and aliquots removed for assay of protein and of total tritium. Results are expressed as picomoles/amine per milligram protein.

In some studies, to inhibit MAO, the cultured astrocytes were preincubated with pargyline (100 μM) for 15 minutes before the cells were washed with Locke's solution. To examine the possible role of pH gradients, particularly that associated with lysosomes, in other experiments, the acidity of the medium was adjusted to pH 6.4 or pH 8.4 and incubations carried out for 15 minutes with or without chloroquine (100 μM) or NH_4Cl (10 mM). In another study, the effects of varying concentrations of monensin, a sodium ionophore that acts as a sodium–hydrogen ion antiporter, on the uptake of [^{3}H]MPTP were examined.

To determine if more MPTP was accumulated than could be accounted for by its amine properties and by differences in intra- and extracellular pH, the ratios of concentrations of methylamine and of MPTP in the cells and medium were compared using a technique in which a weak nonbinding amine (methylamine) is used to measure the difference between external and internal pH of lipid-bound membrane vesicular structures of cells.[6] In these experiments, in which the concentrations of MPTP or of methylamine in cells relative to that in media were to be determined, astrocytes were first detached from the incubation dishes. After 8 days in culture, the medium was aspirated and 5 ml of modified Locke's solution without calcium and containing EGTA (10 mM) was added to each of two dishes. After continued incubation for 5 minutes at 37°C, the medium was decanted; the cells were then detached by gently striking the plates on a flat surface and suspended in 5 ml modified Locke's solution with Ca^{2+} and without EGTA. The suspension was centrifuged for 5 minutes at low speed (890g), the supernatant discarded, and the cells suspended in 10 ml Locke's solution and their density determined in a Coulter counter. The cell suspension was then centrifuged at low speed again, the supernatant discarded, and the cells taken up in a volume (about 3.2 ml) to yield a suspension of 8 × 10^6 cells/ml. Only about 10% of the cells were found to be dead, as determined by trypan blue exclusion.

Aliquots (1 ml) of the cell suspension were transferred to Eppendorf tubes (1.5 ml), each of which contained 5 µl Locke's buffer with: (1) [^{14}C]polydextran sulfate (0.5 µCi, 1.24 mCi/g) and 1.25 µCi ^{3}H$_2$O or (2) [^{14}C]methylamine (0.5 µCi, 46 mCi/mmol) and 1.25 µCi ^{3}H$_2$O or (3) [^{3}H]MPTP (0.2 µCi, 82.3 Ci/mmol) and [^{14}C]polydextran sulfate (0.5 µCi, 1.24 mCi/g). After incubation at room temperature (25°C) for 10 minutes, the tubes were centrifuged (Eppendorf Microfuge) for 5 minutes. An aliquot (100 µl) of the supernatant was removed and added to 200 µl 14% perchloric acid. The remainder of the supernatant was decanted, the walls of the centrifuge tubes wiped with cotton swabs, and 300 µl perchloric acid (14%) added to the pellet. After standing overnight, the perchloric acid solutions were centrifuged and aliquots (250 µl) of the supernatants added to 10 ml Aquasol in scintillation vials and assayed for ^{3}H and ^{14}C by liquid scintillation spectrometry.

The ratio of [^{14}C]polydextran (which is confined to the extracellular space) to ^{3}H$_2$O in the pellet (after centrifugation) divided by that ratio in the medium (supernatant after centrifugation) represents the fraction (x) of extracellular label included in the radioactivity in the pellet. This fraction was calculated from the results obtained in (1) above. Similarly, the ratio of [^{14}C]methylamine to ^{3}H$_2$O in the pellet of cells divided by this ratio in the medium yields a fraction (R) that must be greater than that obtained with polydextran because at least some of the [^{14}C]methylamine enters the cells. This ratio, R, was calculated from the data obtained with (2) above. The ratio of the concentration of the amine in the cells (C_{in}) to the concentration of the amine in the medium (C_{out}) is given by:

$$C_{in}/C_{out} = (R - x)/(1 - x)$$

In the experiment in which [^{14}C]polydextran and [^{3}H]MPTP were used, (3) above, [^{14}C]polydextran in the pellet provided a marker for the extracellular space. The ratio of [^{3}H]MPTP to [^{14}C]polydextran in the pellet to that in the supernatant yields a fraction (T), >1, which is the inverse of the proportion of total MPTP in the pellet that is extracellular. The ratio of MPTP concentrations inside (C_{in}) and outside (C_{out}) of the cells is given by:

$$C_{in}/C_{out} = x\cdot(T - 1)/(1 - x)$$

Because there appeared to be so little MPP$^+$ formed in 20 minutes, metabolic conversion of MPTP to MPP$^+$ in the cultures was examined over an interval of 3 days. After 2 weeks in culture, rat cerebellar astrocytes were exposed to 2.5 pmol[^{3}H]MPTP in 1 ml incubation medium and the amounts of [^{3}H]MPTP and MPP$^+$ in the medium and in the cells were determined after various intervals indicated in Results. MPTP was separated from MPP$^+$ by addition of 10 μl 50% NaOH and extraction into an equal volume of hexane. Aliquots of the organic and aqueous phases were assayed for tritium associated with MPTP and MPP$^+$, respectively. The validity of the assumption that there is almost complete separation of MPTP from MPP$^+$ by extraction into hexane at alkaline pH was confirmed by HPLC.

Results

Tritium from [^{3}H]MPTP was accumulated rapidly from the incubation medium into the cultured rat cerebellar astrocytes and reached a plateau of about 1.6 pmol/mg protein within about 10 minutes, whereas almost no tritium from [^{3}H]MPP$^+$ appeared to have been taken up during the 20-minute incubation interval. If the protein concentration in the cells is about 10% (100 mg/ml), then the concentration of MPTP in the cells was about 160 pmol/ml or over 60-fold greater than that in the medium. The initial rate of uptake of [^{3}H]MPTP appeared to be as rapid at 25°C as at 37°C, but was slightly slower at 3°C. Preincubation with pargyline had no significant effect on the astrocytic accumulation of tritium, indicating that metabolism to MPP$^+$ was not necessary for retention of the radioactivity. The amount of MPTP that accumulates in the cultured astrocytes appears to be directly proportional to its concentration in the medium over a wide range of concentrations up to 10 mM, indicating the absence of a saturable carrier mediating uptake of MPTP.

Concentration of MPTP by astrocytes was far greater than that of methylamine. The cell medium concentration ratio for methylamine, determined as described in Methods, was about 2.7, indicating that the net intracellular hydrogen ion concentration was higher than in the incubation medium. The apparent difference in hydrogen ion concentration was equivalent to about 0.44 pH units. The cell-to-medium ratio for MPTP, however, was calculated to be about 52.

MPTP accumulation by cultured astrocytes was clearly affected by changes in the pH of the incubation medium. At pH 6.4, MPTP uptake was reduced markedly from that found at pH 7.4, whereas at pH 8.4, MPTP accumulation was over threefold greater than at pH 7.4 (Table 1). Addition of chloroquine significantly reduced the accumulation of MPTP; this effect was most marked at pH 8.4 and least at pH 6.4. Addition of ammonium chloride (10 mM) almost completely abolished MPTP accumulation at pH 7.4 (data not shown). Furthermore, monensin diminished, in a dose-dependent manner, MPTP uptake by cultured astrocytes.

During a 3-day interval in culture, almost all [^{3}H]MPTP was converted to MPP$^+$, most of which was found in the incubation medium. Conversion of MPTP to MPP$^+$ in the astrocyte cultures proceeded at a much slower pace than did astrocyte accumulation of MPTP. After about 8 hours, half of the total MPTP that had been

Table 1.
Effects of pH and Chloroquine on MPTP Uptake into Cultured Astrocytes[a]

pH of medium	MPTP uptake (fmol/dish)	Inhibition by chloroquine (%)
6.4	20	15
7.4	160	57
8.4	525	93

[a]Astrocytes were cultured as described in Methods and incubated with [3H]MPTP, with or without chloroquine (100μM) for 15 minutes in medium adjusted to the indicated pH. After washing, the cells were solubilized in 1 ml 0.2 N NaOH and the total tritium remaining in the cells determined by liquid scintillation spectrometry and expressed as fem to moles MPTP per dish.

added to the astrocyte cultures had been converted to MPP$^+$, and by 48 hours, the conversion was almost complete. Although only a small fraction (10–15%) of the MPP$^+$ was retained in the cultured astrocytes (considering the relative volumes of the cells and incubation medium (the protein contents were 250–300 μg/dish), the total volume of cells, assuming a protein concentration of about 100 mg/ml, was less than 3.0 μl in 1.0 ml of medium), the concentration of MPP$^+$ in the cells was well over an order of magnitude greater than in the medium.

Discussion

The results of this study support the view that retention of MPTP in brain appears to be a consequence of its sequestration in acidic binding sites, possibly lysosomes, in astrocytes. Many physiologically and pharmacologically active substances contain a hydrophobic ring structure and side chain with an amine group. These compounds, which are protonated at physiological pH, have both hydrophilic and lipophilic moieties. Their amphophilic properties result in complex interactions with phospholipids and phospholipid-containing membranes and affect their distribution and disposition. Such compounds accumulate selectively in tissues, such as lung, brain, and liver, which contain high concentrations of phospholipids (see, e.g., Kodavanti and Mehendale[7]). Their ability to be retained in specific cells and to produce pathological changes is related to their physical properties and to their metabolism. MPTP may be considered to be included in this class of compounds; it is the special properties of its metabolite, MPP^+, which confers specific toxicity involving catecholaminergic neurons in most species and particularly nigrostriatal neurons in primates.

In vitro, concentration by cells or organelles of amines from surrounding medium results, at least in part, from differences in hydrogen ion concentration; in fact differences in methylamine concentration have been used to estimate differences in pH between medium and chromaffin granules, lysosomes, chloroplasts, bacteria, etc. (see Johnson et al.[6]). It is assumed that only the unpronated form of the methylamine can diffuse freely across the lipid cell membrane, that the concentration of the unprotonated amine in the lipid membrane-bounded compartment is identical to that in the medium, and that there is no significant binding of this simple amine. From the Henderson-Hasselbach equation it follows that the ratio of the concentrations of unprotonated methylamine in the organelle and in the medium are directly proportional to the ratio of the hydrogen ion concentrations. Since at physiological pH almost all of a weak base is in the pronated form, total amine concentrations closely approximate the concentrations of the amine cations. The difference between the pH in the medium and that in the organelles is equal to log C_{in}/C_{out}. Since the pH of the medium is known, the intraorganelle pH can be determined. When intact cells are used, if there are intracellular organelles, only an apparent pH, based on the net H^+ concentration in the cell, can be obtained. The ratio, C_{in}/C_{out}, can, however, provide a valid estimate of methylamine accumulation based on differences in pH between the medium and various intracellular compartments.

In the present study, the intracellular concentration of methylamine was found to be about 2.7-fold greater than that in the medium, whereas when MPTP was used, the intracellular concentration appeared to be about 50-fold greater than in the medium. Differences in net hydrogen ion concentration account for only a small portion of MPTP accumulation, since at pH 7.4 methylamine was concentrated only 2.7-fold. MPTP accumulation was, however, pH dependent. When the pH of the medium was reduced, the ratio of concentrations of MPTP in the cells to that in the medium was markedly diminished and when the pH of the medium was increased, the ratio of those concentrations was increased. The amphophilic nature of MPTP is consistent with binding to intracellular acidic compounds, such as phospholipids, which are present in high concentration in brain. Cationic amphophilic drugs generally accumulate in lysosomes (are lysosomotropic) and at other intracellular acidic binding sites. Such organelles or acidic binding sites in astrocytes may serve as a reservoir of accumulated MPTP, which is sequestered until metabolized by MAO-B to MPDP$^+$ or MPP$^+$. Consistent with this hypothesis, MPTP accumulation in cultured astrocytes was pH dependent. Furthermore, chloroquine, which is highly lysosomotropic, diminished MPTP accumulation in the cultured astrocytes. This effect of chloroquine was also, as expected, dependent upon pH; chloroquine was much more effective in preventing MPTP accumulation at pH 8.4 than at pH 6.4. Similarly, ammonium ions markedly reduced MPTP accumulation by the astrocytes. Furthermore, monensin, a carboxylic ionophore that acts as an antiporter for sodium–hydrogen exchange[8] and disrupts pH gradients, diminished in a dose-dependent manner MPTP uptake by cultured astrocytes. These results indicate that MPTP accumulation in astrocytes is pH dependent and suggest that intracellular anionic binding sites, probably mostly in lysosomes, are important in the retention of MPTP in brain.

The relatively slow appearance of MPP$^+$ in the cultured astrocytes and surrounding medium is consistent with the view that the bound, sequestered stores of MPTP provide a reservoir for cytoplasmic MPTP during its MAO-B-mediated, relatively slow, oxidation to MPDP$^+$ and MPP$^+$. Reinhard et al.[9] using molecular orbital calculations, showed that the positive charge of MPP$^+$ is highly delocalized throughout the pyridinium ring, making the compound less polar, and suggested that this could confer some ability to diffuse through lipid membranes. However, persistence of high intracellular levels of MPP$^+$ formed in the cultured astrocytes, in contrast to its low penetration into cells when added directly into the medium, suggests that MPP$^+$ does not readily equilibrate across the lipid membrane of cultured astrocytes. Furthermore, MPP$^+$ is toxic to hepatocytes in culture only after a long lag period, presumably reflecting poor penetration through the cell membrane and very slow intracellular accumulation.[10] MPP$^+$ in the medium might, however, be formed from MPDP$^+$. In vitro, during MAO-B-catalyzed oxidation of MPTP, MPDP$^+$ formation is more rapid than its oxidation to MPP$^+$,[11] and until its formation is limited by depletion of MPTP, MPDP$^+$

concentration is higher than that of MPP^+. In isolated hepatocytes, $MPDP^+$ is readily converted to intracellular MPP^+; when added directly to the medium, MPDP is more toxic than MPP^+ or MPTP.[12] These results suggest that $MPDP^+$ enters the cells more rapidly than MPP^+. Unlike MPP^+, $MPDP^+$ can form a free base that is able to diffuse readily from the medium into the cytoplasm. Similarly, because of its rapid formation from MPTP and lipid-soluble properties, MPDP might be expected to diffuse from the cytoplasm into the medium more rapidly than it is oxidized to MPP^+. At physiological pH, $MPDP^+$ readily disproportionates to MPTP and MPP^+.[13] In isolated hepatocytes, intracellular accumulation of MPP^+ after addition of $MPDP^+$ to the culture medium is unaffected by pretreatment with the MAO inhibitor, pargyline[14] suggesting that intracellular disproportionation may be important in generating MPP^+ from $MPDP^+$. If MPDP diffuses out of the astrocytes, extracellular disproportionation might also account in part for appearance of MPP^+ in the medium.

In summary, the results of the present study show that astrocytes in culture concentrate MPTP about 50-fold from the culture medium by a pH-dependent process that appears to involve intracellular binding to acidic (possibly phospholipid) membranes, acidic proteins, or acidic organelles (e.g., lysosomes). These binding sites might serve as a reservoir from which cytoplasmic levels of MPTP are maintained during its MAO-B-mediated conversion to $MPDP^+$ and MPP^+. Diffusion of MPDP into the medium and subsequent disproportionation to MPP^+ and MPTP may provide a source for at least some of extracellular MPP^+. These mechanisms may be important for retention in brain of MPTP cleared from the blood and for its conversion to MPP^+ at a site (extracellular) where it is available for uptake by dopaminergic neurons.

References

1. Singer TP, Ramsay RR. 1990. Mechanism of the neurotoxicity of MPTP. An update. FEBS Lett 274:1–8.
2. Sayre LM. 1989. Biochemical mechanism of action of the dopaminergic neurotoxin 1-methyl-4-phenyl-1,2,3,6-tetrahydropyridine (MPTP). Toxicol Lett 4:121–149.
3. Riachi NJ, LaManna JC, Harik SI. 1989. Entry of 1-methyl-4-phenyl-1,2,3,6-tetrahydropyridine into the rat brain. J Pharmacol Exp Ther 249:744–748.

4. Bankiewicz KS, Oldfield EH, Chiueh CC, Doppman JL, Jacobowitz DM, Kopin IJ. 1986. Hemiparkinsonism in monkeys after unilateral internal carotid artery infusion of 1-methyl-4-phenyl-1,2,3,6-tetrahydropyridine (MPTP). Life Sci 39:7–16.
5. Herkenham M, Little MD, Bankiewicz K, Yang S-C, Markey SP, Johannessen JN. 1991. Selective retention of MPP$^+$ within the monoaminergic systems of the primate brain following MPTP administration; an *in vivo* autoradiographic study. Neuroscience 40:133–158.
6. Johnson RG, Carlson NJ, Scarpa A. 1978. ΔpH and catecholamine distribution in isolated chromaffin granules. J Biol Chem 253:1512–1521.
7. Kodavanti UP, Mehendale HM. 1990. Cationic amphiphilic drugs and phospholipid storage disorders. Pharmacol Rev 42:327–354.
8. Pressman BC. 1968. Ionophorous antibiotics as models for biological transport. Fed Proc 27:1283–1288.
9. Reinhard JF Jr, Daniels AJ, Painter GR. 1990. Carrier-independent entry of 1-methyl-4-phenylpyridinium (MPP$^+$) into adrenal chromaffin cells as a consequence of charge delocalization. Biochem Biophys Res Commun 168:1143–1148.
10. DiMonte D, Ekstrom G, Shinka T, Smith MT, Trevor AJ, Castagnoli N Jr. 1987. Role of 1-methyl-4-phenylpyridinium ion formation and accumulation in 1-methyl-4-phenyl-1,2,3,6-tetrahydropyridine toxicity to isolated hepatocytes. Chem Biol Interact 62:105–116.
11. Trevor AJ, Chiba K, Yu EY, Caldera PS, Castagnoli KP, Castagnoli N, Peterson LA, Salach JI, Singer TP. 1986. Metabolism of MPTP *in vitro*: The intermediate role of 2,3-MPDP$^+$ and studies on its chemical and biochemical reactivity. *In* MPTP: A Neurotoxin Producing a Parkinsonian Syndrome. SP Markey, N Castagnoli Jr, AJ Trevor, IJ Kopin (eds). Academic Press, Orlando, Florida.
12. Ekstrom G, DiMonte D, Sandy MS, Smith MT. 1987. Comparative toxicity and antioxidant activity of 1-methyl-4-phenyl-1,2,3,6-tetrahydropyridine and its monoamine oxidase B-generated metabolites in isolated hepatocytes and liver microsomes. Arch Biochem Biophys 255:14–18.
13. Castagnoli N Jr, Chiba K, Trevor AJ. 1985. Potential bioactivation pathways for the neurotoxin 1-methyl-4-phenyl-1,2,3,6-tetrahydropyridine (MPTP). Life Sci 36:225–230.
14. DiMonte D, Shinka T, Sandy MS, Castagnoli N Jr, Smith MT. 1988. Quantitative analysis of 1-methyl-4-phenyl-1,2,3,6-tetrahydropyridine metabolism in isolated rat hepatocytes. Drug Metab Dispos 16:250–255.

Chapter 2

MPTP-Induced Parkinsonism:
Recovery, Species Differences, and Relevance to Parkinson's Disease

Peter Jenner

The cause of Parkinson's disease remains unknown, and there have been few clues as to the nature of the toxic mechanism involved. Recent epidemiological studies have suggested an association with industrialization and the use of agrochemicals, but no specific agent has been identified.[1] It has also been suggested that such substances might only be active in susceptible individuals less able to metabolize the toxic species or to inactivate oxygen radicals produced by its action.[2,3] However, the only major clue that has emerged to a possible toxic cause of Parkinson's disease stems from the discovery of the ability of 1-methyl-4-phenyl-1,2,3,6-tetrahydropyridine (MPTP) to selectively destroy the dopamine-containing cells in substantia nigra and to induce parkinsonism in man and other primate species.[4-8] Indeed, MPTP may provide vital clues to the cause of Parkinson's disease through, first, providing the most effective model of the illness so far available and, second, by revealing the mechanism by which dopamine cells are vulnerable to toxin action.

The administration of MPTP to primates produces the majority of the cardinal motor symptoms of the illness with the possible

This study was supported by the Parkinson's Disease Society and the Medical Research Council.
From Hefti F, and Weiner WJ, (eds.) *Progress in Parkinson's Disease Research—2*. Mount Kisco NY, Futura Publishing Co., Inc., © 1992.

exception of tremor.[6–10] The syndrome produced responds to known antiparkinsonian drugs when subsequently administered to man. Animals repeatedly treated with L-dopa develop most of the long-term complications associated with chronic therapy in Parkinson's disease.[11,12] However, MPTP does not produce a precise mimic of the illness since overall the pathological and biochemical changes are more limited than occurs in Parkinson's disease.[13] MPTP exhibits a high degree of specificity for destroying nigral dopamine-containing neurons and induces corresponding decreases in caudate-putamen dopamine content. There is, however, one aspect of the syndrome that differs markedly from what occurs in Parkinson's disease, namely primates treated with MPTP show initial gross parkinsonism but then over a period of months may recover a considerable portion of normal mobility.[14–16] Why this occurs will be considered in a following section.

The mechanism of action of MPTP has been extensively researched. The critical steps appear to be the metabolism by MAO-B in glial cells to produce MPDP$^+$ and then the pyridinium species MPP$^+$.[17–20] MPP$^+$ is actively accumulated within dopamine neurons,[21,22] but its primary mechanism of toxicity is due to active uptake into mitochondria[23,24] and the inhibition of complex I of the respiratory chain.[25,26] Precisely how this inhibition occurs is not understood, but there is some evidence for the involvement of oxygen radical formation (see later). The significance of this sequence of events depends on the relevance to mechanisms occurring in brain in Parkinson's disease and this issue will be discussed later.

Recovery from MPTP-Induced Parkinsonism

Initially, following acute MPTP administration, most primates exhibit profound parkinsonism consisting of gross akinesia, rigidity, postural abnormalities, a loss of vocalization and impaired ability to eat and to drink.[6–8] In our hands, common marmosets treated with MPTP in this manner then exhibit a slow and progressive recovery during which gross akinesia disappears, although the animals remain static for long periods and spontaneous movement is slow; however, when challenged such animals move rapidly.[14,15] All animals exhibit clumsy and poorly coordinated movements when undertaking complex tasks. This situation might appear akin to a stable compensated form of

Parkinson's disease. Similar behavioral recovery has been reported in macaque monkeys following MPTP treatment, although this occurred over a relatively short period and appeared to be complete in some animals.[15] There are also numerous, but largely unpublished, anecdotal reports by others of similar events.

In the short term following MPTP administration, marmosets exhibit marked losses of caudate-putamen dopamine content and [^{3}H]dopamine uptake, corresponding to the initial marked parkinsonism.[8,27] However, by some 4–6 weeks following treatment, and at a time when some behavioral recovery has already occurred, dopamine levels in the caudate-putamen are still markedly reduced (Table 1). However, at this time there is an apparent increase in caudate-putamen dopamine turnover as indicated by dopamine–metabolite ratios. Thus, some of the initial recovery may be due, at least in part, to a compensatory increase in dopamine turnover as is thought to occur in the early stages of Parkinson's disease itself. However, the large losses of dopamine occurring equally in both the caudate nucleus and putamen in MPTP-treated primates more closely mimics what occurs in postencephalitic parkinsonism[28] than the greater loss in putamen compared to caudate occurring in idiopathic Parkinson's disease.[29]

At this time there is also a large decrease in dopamine levels in the nucleus accumbens, which is disparate to the relatively small and variable degree of cell loss that occurs in the ventral tegmental area (VTA) (Table 1). However, by 3–4 months following MPTP treatment, and at a time when the compensatory increase in dopamine turnover in the caudate-putamen is no longer apparent, there is a recovery to 80% of normal levels of dopamine in the nucleus accumbens.[30] This recovery of mesolimbic dopamine content parallels more closely the behavioral recovery than any obvious alteration within the caudate-putamen.

Others have reported on differences in dopamine losses in brain between symptomatic and asymptomatic individuals following MPTP treatment of primates, and this may have relevance to the mechanisms underlying recovery. In vervet monkeys there were dramatic decreases in dopamine levels in caudate-putamen in both symptomatic and asymptomatic animals following MPTP treatment.[31] However, overall, the losses in asymptomatic animals (75–99%) were less than those in symptomatic individuals (95–99%), and there were subtle but distinct regional differences in dopamine loss between the two groups. There may also be regional differences in the susceptibility of dopamine cells to MPTP treat-

Table 1.
Alteration in Neurochemical Parameters in Caudate Nucleus and Nucleus Accumbens at (A) 10 Days and 4–6 Weeks, and (B) 10 Days and 3–4 Months following Treatment of Common Marmosets with MPTP[a]

A.	Control	10 Days	4–6 Weeks
Caudate nucleus			
Dopamine	8.86 ± 0.60	0.35 ± 0.20[b]	0.89 ± 0.32[b]
DOPAC	5.17 ± 0.53	0.27 ± 0.08[b]	0.87 ± 0.17[b,c]
HVA	5.66 ± 0.61	0.26 ± 0.02[b]	1.39 ± 0.41[b,c]
Ratio (HVA + DOPAC/DA)	1.27 ± 0.14	2.60 ± 0.51[b]	3.88 ± 0.85[b]
Nucleus accumbens			
Dopamine	3.50 ± 1.12	0.84 ± 0.46	0.66 ± 0.29
DOPAC	2.94 ± 0.84	0.49 ± 0.20	0.97 ± 0.23
HVA	4.31 ± 1.26	0.29 ± 0.06[b]	0.71 ± 0.23[b]
Ratio (HVA + DOPAC/DA)	3.66 ± 0.86	1.33 ± 0.36	5.88 ± 2.68

B.	10 Days		3–4 Months	
	Control	MPTP	Control	MPTP
Caudate nucleus				
Dopamine	14.17 ± 1.30	0.22 ± 0.09[b]	16.75 ± 2.55	1.79 ± 0.86[b,c]
DOPAC	1.84 ± 0.25	0.18 ± 0.02[b]	1.06 ± 0.22	0.20 ± 0.08[b]
HVA	8.10 ± 1.06	0.01 ± 0.00[b]	10.01 ± 1.78	2.20 ± 0.90[b,c]
Ratio (HVA + DOPAC/DA)	0.70 ± 0.05	1.87 ± 0.63	0.67 ± 0.09	1.24 ± 0.35
Nucleus accumbens				
Dopamine	10.37 ± 1.12	1.82 ± 0.40[b]	10.14 ± 0.80	7.36 ± 0.83[b,c]
DOPAC	1.41 ± 0.23	0.04 ± 0.03[b]	2.26 ± 0.32	1.21 ± 0.23[b,c]
HVA	9.71 ± 2.12	0.17 ± 0.12[b]	8.32 ± 0.44	4.56 ± 1.46[c]
Ratio (HVA + DOPAC/DA)	1.09 ± 0.15	0.21 ± 0.12[b]	1.14 ± 0.13	0.74 ± 0.12[c]

[a]Values given as mean ± 1 SEM in μg/g tissue. n = 4–9 individual animals. Analysis of variance followed by Student's t test. Data taken from refs. 27 and 30.
[b]$P < 0.05$ compared to control values.
[c]$P < 0.05$ compared to values obtained at 10 days following MPTP treatment.

ment. Thus, in asymptomatic vervet monkeys dopamine losses occurred in the central substantia nigra and dorsomedial VTA, whereas in symptomatic individuals dopamine depletion affected all regions of substantia nigra and both dorsomedial and ventromedial VTA.[32]

Extrastriatal dopamine levels may also be differentially affected in symptomatic and asymptomatic primates. Dopamine concentrations in the supplementary motor area and cingulate cortex are markedly decreased in symptomatic, but not asymptomatic, vervet monkeys.[33] Similarly, in MPTP-treated rhesus monkeys there was no loss of dopamine in the nucleus accumbens, nucleus of the stria terminalis, VTA, globus pallidus, and cingulate gyrus in asymptomatic animals, but all these regions were affected in animals exhibiting motor symptoms.[34] There were, however, dopamine losses in the somatosensory, motor, and cerebellar cortex of asymptomatic monkeys. Again, the overall loss in caudate-putamen dopamine levels was extensive in both groups but more marked in symptomatic animals.

These data would support our own concept that the recovery of nucleus accumbens dopamine content is an important event in the production of recovery from MPTP-induced parkinsonism. It is interesting to note that it is the reversal of akinesia that is the most marked component of behavioral recovery and that, at least in lower species, the nucleus accumbens is concerned primarily with locomotion. Studies of the reasons why some animals recover from MPTP parkinsonism and others remain asymptomatic following treatment may reveal important relationships between the losses of dopamine content in differing areas of the brain and the production of individual disease symptoms. Indeed, much effort has been concentrated on the losses of dopamine in the caudate-putamen in Parkinson's disease and until now the smaller decreases occurring in other dopamine systems have not generally been thought to be involved in the production of the motor deficits characterizing the illness.

The studies described so far largely deal with changes occurring in a few weeks or months following MPTP treatment. A further possibility is that in the long term there is a recovery of dopamine function based on sprouting or regrowth of remaining nigrostriatal neurons. This possibility has been examined in animals treated 1 year previously with MPTP and who have exhibited an almost complete recovery in gross motor behavior, although remaining obviously affected when undertaking more complex tasks.[16] At this time there is a maintained >90% loss of caudate-putamen dopamine content, indicating that the neurotoxic actions of MPTP have not been reversed over this period (Table 2). However, no alteration in nucleus accumbens dopamine content was obvious compared to the levels found in age-matched control animals. The use of [³H]mazindol binding to identify dopamine reuptake sites indicated a profound loss (>80%) of specific binding in the caudate-putamen with the relative preservation (60%) of uptake sites in the nucleus accumbens. These studies would indicate that there is no obvious recovery of dopamine function in the caudate-putamen indicative of a regeneration of the nigrostriatal fibers. Interestingly, there was a disparity between the number of remaining dopamine cells in the substantia nigra as identified by tyrosine hydroxylase immunocytochemistry, which indicated some 40% of control levels compared to the more dramatic loss of [³H]mazindol binding in the caudate-putamen (>80%). The lack of correlation between these parameters might

Table 2.
Content of Dopamine (DA), DOPAC, and HVA of Caudate, Putamen, and Nucleus Accumbens after Administration of MPTP, 12–18 Months to Common Marmosets[a]

		Tissue (ng/mg)		Ratio
	DA	DOPAC	HVA	(DOPAC + HVA)/DA
Caudate				
Control	13.2 ± 0.7	4.5 ± 0.1	7.1 ± 0.6	0.89 ± 0.05
MPTP	0.7 ± 0.2**	0.6 ± 0.1**	1.1 ± 0.4*	2.45 ± 0.40*
Putamen				
Control	13.4 ± 2.2	5.9 ± 0.2	12.3 ± 1.5	1.52 ± 0.22
MPTP	1.0 ± 0.6**	1.6 ± 0.6**	2.0 ± 1.0**	6.86 ± 3.78
Nucleus ac- cumbens				
Control	5.2 ± 0.2	4.6 ± 0.5	5.8 ± 0.5	2.02 ± 0.50
MPTP	4.5 ± 1.5	3.8 ± 1.0	4.4 ± 1.2	1.89 ± 0.20

[a]The results are shown as the mean ± 1 SEM of groups of three or four animals. **$P < 0.001$, *$P < 0.05$ compared to control; one way analysis of variance (ANOVA) followed by Dunnet's test. Data taken from ref. 16.

indicate an action of MPTP to strip dopamine neurons of their terminal network. This might explain why such animals are difficult to render parkinsonian on the subsequent administration of MPTP since uptake of MPP[+] would be limited.[16]

Recovery of motor function may not be reflected in alterations in presynaptic dopamine levels alone. An alternative concept is that the postsynaptic dopamine receptor sensitivity is altered to compensate for decreased dopaminergic tone following MPTP treatment. Our own studies of specific [3H]spiperone binding to D-2 sites in striatal homogenates have failed to show any alteration in MPTP-treated common marmosets.[8,27] However, in cynomolgus monkeys others have found both decreases and increases in [3H]spiperone binding and shown that at least 90% dopamine depletion is required to produce an increase in D-2 deceptor density.[11,35,36] In a single baboon treated with MPTP, PET examination using [76Br]bromo-spiperone showed a reduction in striatal binding that was confirmed by subsequent in vitro measurement of specific [3H]spiperone binding.[37] However, there was only an 80% loss of neuronal cell bodies in substantia nigra. The precise extent of dopamine loss induced by MPTP and the effect on postsynaptic receptor density may also determine whether recovery occurs, and this may differ from species to species. The alterations in D-2 receptor density appear to be regionally localized in the caudate-putamen as judged by autoradiographic analysis of [3H]spiperone binding to tissue slices. Similarly in cynomolgus monkeys with a unilateral MPTP lesion, autoradiographic studies have shown an increase in D-2, but not D-1, receptor density as judged by the specific binding of [3H]sulpiride and [3H]SCH 23390, respectively.[38,39]

Another important factor that may govern the extent to which behavioral recovery is observed relates to the age of the animals being used.[40–43] In a comparison of the effects of MPTP on juvenile, adult, and aged marmosets, the extent to which behavioral recovery occurred in animals treated with MPTP titrated to an identical degree of parkinsonism was less marked in aged animals than it was in the younger age groups. Interestingly, the induction of parkinsonism in the older animals was associated with a smaller degree of cell loss and reduction in caudate-putamen dopamine content, perhaps suggesting a lesser degree of plasticity of the aged dopamine systems.[44] Interestingly, in older animals it has been suggested that the pathology produced by MPTP spreads to involve other areas and is also associated with the presence of Lewy bodies.[45,46] It may be that in these animals there is a more permanent deficit in mesolimbic–mesocortical dopamine content than occurs in younger animals, so resulting in a more marked persistence of MPTP-induced parkinsonism but this remains to be investigated.

Functional Evidence for Dopaminergic Recovery in MPTP-Treated Animals

Terguride (transdihydrolisuride) is a partial dopamine agonist having mixed agonist and antagonist actions on brain dopamine receptors.[47,48] In normal common marmosets the administration of terguride produces an inhibition of locomotor activity in agreement with its action of rats.[49] In animals treated with MPTP 2 months previously and exhibiting marked parkinsonism, the administration of terguride produced a stimulation of locomotion and restoration of normal motor behaviour (Figure 1). This effect was most marked at the lowest dose tested (4.0 mg/kg), since at higher doses (8.0 and 12.0 mg/kg) marked stereotyped movements were also evident. The effect of terguride was modest in the first 3 hours following administration but more marked in the following hours. These results are consistent with the contralateral rotation induced by terguride in cynomolgus monkeys with a unilateral MPTP lesion placed at least 2 months previously.[50] In contrast, at 6 months following MPTP treatment, at a time when the animals had shown a degree of behavioral recovery, the administration of terguride no longer resulted in a stimulation of motor responses and stereotyped movements were not observed (Figure 1).[49]

This evidence suggests that at a time when dopamine levels are severely depleted (particularly in the nucleus accumbens), terguride acts as an agonist, but at a time when dopamine function in the nucleus accumbens is restored, terguride no longer produces its agonist activity but rather acts as a dopamine antagonist. The different effects of terguride at various time points following MPTP administration may have important consequences for both the testing of other partial agonist compounds in this model of Parkinson's disease including those that may be effective on the D-1 system such as SKF 38393[51] or CY 208-243.[52]

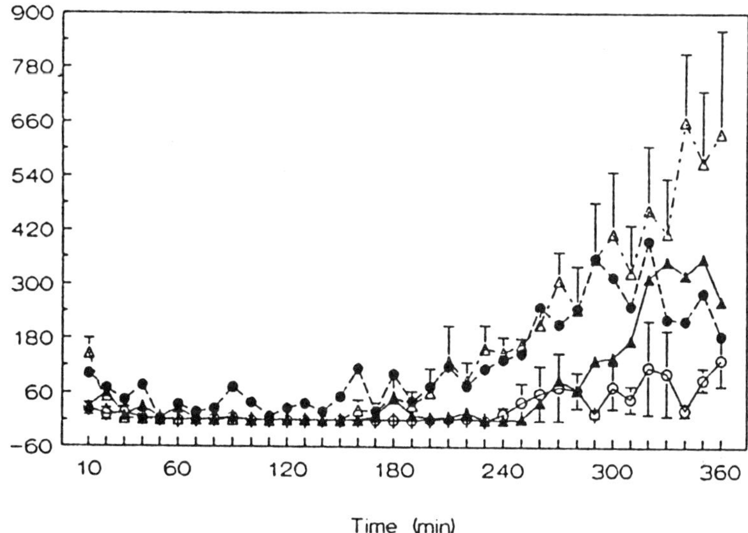

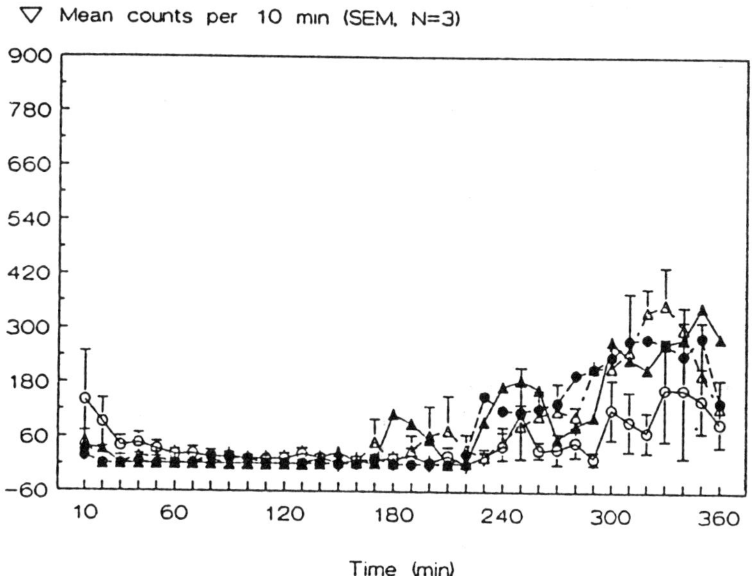

Figure 1. Mean locomotor activity counts (± SEM, $N = 3$) accumulated in 10-min intervals for 360 min for common marmosets pretreated with MPTP (top) 2 months and (bottom) 10 months prior to the administration of vehicle —○— or 4.0 (—●—), 8.0 (—△—) and 12.0 mg/kg (—▲—) of terguride, respectively. Error bars for the higher doses are left out for clarity, but were within the same range of those shown for 8.0 mg/kg or vehicle *IP*. Taken from ref. 49.

Species Variation in Actions of MPTP and Its Analogs

The administration of MPTP to man and other primate species produces varying degrees of cell loss and motor deficits. However, its effects are more marked than in other species of animals. Most rodent species, with the exception of some mouse strains, are relatively resistant to the effects of peripheral administration of MPTP. In particular, there have been extensive studies by Heikkila and colleagues on the use of black C57 mice as a model of the neurotoxic actions of MPTP.[53-60] There is some evidence that cats and dogs treated with MPTP also show nigral cell loss and develop transient motor abnormalities.[61-64] Indeed, one would expect a high degree of species variation for a toxin that mimics Parkinson's disease since the idiopathic syndrome appears peculiar to man. However, it is most unlikely that MPTP itself represents a cause of Parkinson's disease as it is not commonly found in the environment. There are, however, many analogs of MPTP (and MPP$^+$) that have been described in the literature, many of which are also neurotoxic.[65-69] Indeed, there may also be endogenous molecules that contain the MPTP moiety within their molecule such as beta-carbolines and tetrahydroisoquinolines and that have neurotoxic actions and represent endogenous toxic moieties.[70-73]

Heikklia and colleagues and other groups have undertaken important structure–activity studies aimed at determining the extent to which the MPTP molecule may be modified while retaining its neurotoxic activity.[74-76] These have identified substances that are equal to or greater in toxic activity than MPTP in susceptible mouse strains.[77] The relevance of these to parkinsonism in man remains to be determined. However, an important discovery made by Heikkila and colleagues was the demonstration that not only MAO-B but also MAO-A may be involved in the activation of these compounds to toxic pyridinium species.[78-81] In particular, it was shown that 2'-methyl MPTP was metabolized in a complex manner by both MAO-A and -B and on administration to black C57 mice was 6–8 times more toxic than MPTP itself.[77] Another interesting analog is the 2'-methyl derivative, since this is metabolized mainly by MAO-A and it also appears to be more toxic than MPTP on administration to mice.[81] However, the relative toxicity of these compounds on administration to other species including primates is only now being evaluated.

We administered 2'-methyl MPTP to common marmosets in comparison to an identical group of animals receiving MPTP treatment.[82] The dosage regime used initially was lower than that employed for MPTP itself since greater toxicity had been experienced in mice. However, at this dosage level little behavioral effect was observed, and so the dosage level was increased to be equivalent to that for MPTP. However, even at these doses 2'-methyl MPTP produced a smaller effect on motor behavior than MPTP itself, and this was confirmed by the smaller nonsignificant decreases in striatal dopamine content and the lack of evidence for histological damage to substantia nigra (Figure 2). Thus, in the marmoset 2'-methyl MPTP is not more toxic than MPTP itself in contrast to what happens in mice. Species variations exist for analogs of MPTP that are in the opposite direction to those occurring for MPTP itself.

More recently we have also examined the effects of 2'-ethyl MPTP compared to MPTP in common marmosets.[83] The administration of equivalent doses of these compounds showed that while MPTP, as expected, induced profound motor deficits, the administration of 2'-ethyl MPTP did not produce any sustainable abnormalities (Figure 3). Subsequently, administration of MPTP to the animals previously treated with 2'-ethyl MPTP precipitated these common marmosets into obvious parkinsonism (Figure 3).

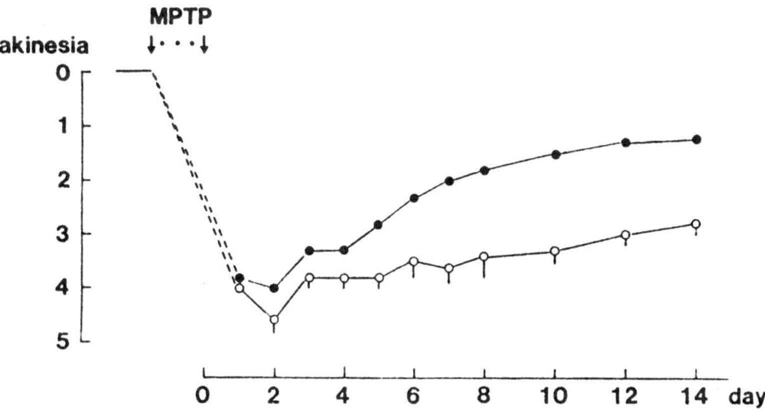

Figure 2.   Akinesia scores for common marmosets in the 14-day period following administration of MPTP (6.9–9.2 mg/kg) (N = 4–8) (—O—) or 2'-methyl-MPTP (11.0–11.6 mg/kg) (N = 2) (—●—). Values are expressed as mean ± 1 SEM.

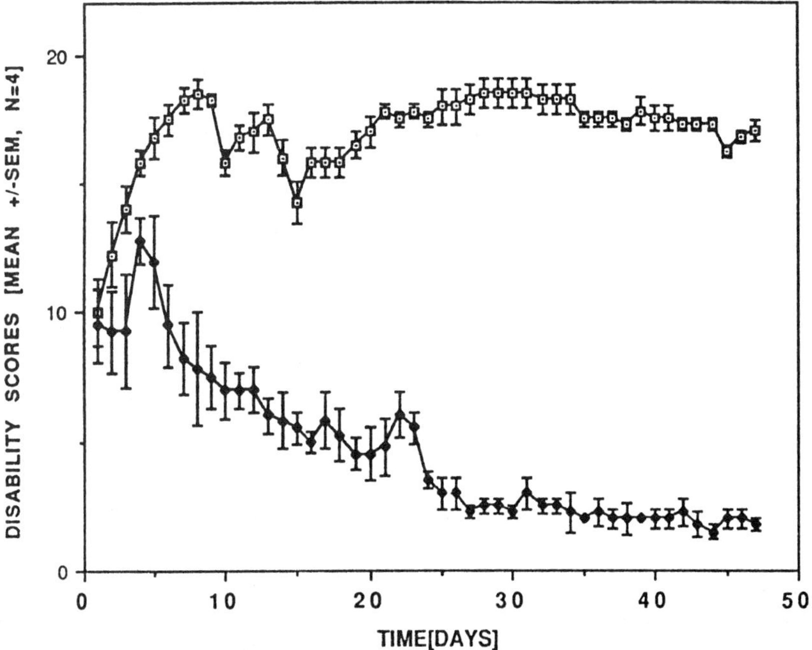

Figure 3. Disability scores for common marmosets in the 48-day period following administration of MPTP (—□—) or 2'-ethyl-MPTP (—◆—) 2 mg/kg IP for 5 days. N = 4. Values are expressed as mean ± 1 SEM.

The discrepancy between species may relate to differences in the formation of the corresponding pyridinium ions in brain.[81] This in turn may be due to the relative involvement of MAO-A and -B in the metabolism of 2'-methyl and 2'-ethyl MPTP. The relatively greater involvement of MAO-B in the metabolism of dopamine in primates compared to the increased importance of MAO-A in rodents suggests that compounds such as 2'-methyl and 2'-ethyl MPTP may not be so toxic in higher species.

Clearly, however, there is a need for further structure–activity studies, but these involve the testing of MPTP analogs not only in rodent species but also in primates to determine the relevance of their toxicity to man and the production of idiopathic Parkinson's disease.

Relevance of Mechanism of Action of MPTP to Parkinson's Disease in Man

The current concept of the action of MPTP is that it acts by one of two mechanisms. Initially it was proposed that MPP^+ underwent redox cycling to generate oxygen radical species which then initiated cell death, but the chemical stability of MPP^+ makes this unlikely.[84] More recently it has been suggested that a redox reaction might take place between MPP^+ and the other metabolite $MPDP^+$ to generate superoxide radicals,[85] but so far this has not been shown to be involved in the final steps of MPTP toxicity. However, others have suggested that MPTP and its metabolites may interact with NADH reductase or with NADPH cytochrome P-450 reductase to generate toxic oxygen radicals.[86] This may represent another pathway by which MPTP is neurotoxic. However, it is generally thought that the final step in MPTP toxicity is the accumulation of MPP^+ within mitochondria and the subsequent inhibition of complex I of the mitochondrial respiratory chain.[25,26] This mechanism might also give rise to the generation of oxygen radicals as an overspill from the respiratory chain following complex I inhibition. However, the importance of the mechanism of action of MPTP depends on whether similar mechanisms can be found to be operative in Parkinson's disease itself.

The available evidence from studies of postmortem tissues in Parkinson's disease suggests that oxidative stress may be operative. This is based on the detection of a decrease in levels of reduced glutathione or total glutathione content of substantia nigra,[87–89] an increase in nigral lipid peroxidation as judged by levels of malondialdehyde or lipid hydroperoxides,[90,91] and increased mitochondrial superoxide dismutase activity.[92] Indeed, a toxic process appears to be continuing up to the time of death in Parkinson's disease since a reactive microgliosis can be demonstrated in postmortem nigral tissue.[93] However, the important question is whether inhibition of mitochondrial function occurs in Parkinson's disease itself.

Examination of the enzymes of the mitochondrial respiratory chain in substantia nigra from patients dying with Parkinson's disease showed a decrease in the activity of NADH cytochrome *c* reductase but not of succinate cytochrome *c* reductase or citrate synthase (Table 3).[94,95] This would appear to indicate a selective

Table 3.
Complex I Activity in Substantia Nigra and Other Brain Areas from Patients with Parkinson's Disease or Multiple System Atrophy (MSA) and from Control Subjects[a]

	NADH CoQ₁ reductase activity (rotenone sensitive) (nmol/min/mg total protein)		
	Control	Parkinson's disease	MSA
Substantia nigra	3.45 ± 0.45	1.99 ± 0.90*	2.81 ± 0.98
Caudate nucleus	3.20 ± 0.93	3.69 ± 1.51	3.03 ± 0.98
Globus pallidus (medial)	5.41 ± 2.28	4.78 ± 1.31	
Globus pallidus (lateral)	5.18 ± 1.24	4.26 ± 1.66	
Cerebral cortex	5.69 ± 1.48	6.51 ± 2.59	
Cerebellum	4.77 ± 1.49	4.30 ± 1.69	

[a]Results are expressed as the mean ± SD for samples from N = 4–7 patients. *$P < 0.005$ Mann-Whitney U test. Data from ref. 95.

inhibition of complex I, which was confirmed by the detection of low levels of activity of NADPH coenzyme Q (CoQ) reductase. The anatomical and disease specificity of these findings was shown by the lack of change in NADH CoQ reductase in areas of brain other than substantia nigra and by the failure to find differences in NADH CoQ reductase in substantia nigra or other brain regions in another degenerative disease of basal ganglia, namely multiple system atrophy.[95]

Others have reported that similar changes may occur in platelets[96] and muscle,[97] but the findings in platelets need replication and the changes in muscle appear due to aging rather than to Parkinson's disease. Alterations in some subunits of complex I have been suggested to account for the overall enzyme inhibition, but these were detected in the striatum and not in substantia nigra and in a region where no pathology occurs and where no overall change in NADH CoQ reductase could be detected.[98] The same group of authors suggested that there may be a common mitochondrial deletion in the striatum and cortical regions in Parkinson's disease and that, although this occurred in normal aging, it is present in greater amounts in Parkinson's disease.[99] In contrast, studies by two other groups have failed to find any deletions that would account for the complex I inhibition.[100,101]

There thus appears to be a common link between the mechanism of action of MPTP and the cause of cell death in Parkinson's disease in man. However, it is not known whether alterations in mitochondrial function are a primary cause of nigral cell death or whether these are secondary effects occurring once the disease process has been initiated. Relatively few brains from patients with the early stages of the disease are available for biochemical analysis, so it is difficult to determine at which stage mitochondrial defects can be detected. However, in brain material from apparently normal individuals, approximately 10% show cell loss in substantia nigra, the presence of free melanin and Lewy bodies (incidental Lewy body disease). These individuals are presumably in an early stable stage of the illness and so can be considered as having presymptomatic Parkinson's disease. We have been able to examine brains from a group of such subjects, but no alterations in NADH CoQ reductase activity could be detected in this group.[102]

There are two possible interpretations of these data. First, the degree of cell loss at this stage of the illness may be sufficiently small for us not to be able to detect an overall change in complex I activity. Second, it may be that the changes in complex I activity are not a primary cause of Parkinson's disease but are only apparent once the disease process has been initiated and, as such, might act as an accelerator of neuronal cell loss. However, there is a need to establish why complex I activity is inhibited in Parkinson's disease since this might either refute or support the concept of toxin involvement as a cause of the illness.

Concluding Remarks

The study of MPTP toxicity may have provided vital clues to the cause and mechanism underlying nigral cell death in Parkinson's disease. Certainly, MPTP has provided the best model of the disorder so far available and one that can be used to evaluate the cause of individual symptoms of the illness as well as providing a viable means of establishing the effect of age on the susceptibility to develop Parkinson's disease. In addition, the model is an excellent test bed for examining the properties of new potential antiparkinsonian therapies and for investigating the underlying cause of the long-term complications associated with chronic L-dopa therapy in man.

It may be that the anomalies between the MPTP model of parkinsonism and idiopathic Parkinson's disease will throw more light onto specific issues related to the illness than the ability of the toxin to kill nigral dopamine cells. Thus, understanding the reasons why some species of monkey recover from MPTP toxicity may provide vital information on the mechanisms that compensate or, indeed, control motor function and that become vulnerable in Parkinson's disease.

The search for a specific toxin to which individuals might be generally exposed continues by studying MPTP analogs. It has become clear, however, that one must consider the role of both MAO-A and -B in the activation of these molecules and the relative role that this enzyme plays in the metabolism of dopamine in different species. Since Parkinson's disease is restricted to man, it would be expected that any toxin causing the illness would also show marked species variations in its effects. However, to date, analogs of MPTP that appear more toxic than MPTP itself in mice appear to be less toxic to primate species. It is essential that structure-activity relationships should take this species variation into account, since in most studies of this kind the analogs synthesized are tested in rodents rather than in primates. It may be that compounds that are potentially highly toxic to primate substantia nigra will be weak or inactive in mouse models.

The whole story of MPTP toxicity has stimulated considerable research into the mechanisms by which it produces parkinsonism and the relevance of such mechanisms to the cause of nigral cell death in the illness itself. The finding that in Parkinson's disease there is a selective inhibition of complex I in substantia nigra may have provided a vital clue to the cause of the illness. If no genetic cause of this mitochondrial deficit can be demonstrated, then it may be due to some endogenous or environmental toxin that is able to inhibit complex I in susceptible individuals.

Had it not been for the chance discovery of the neurotoxic properties of MPTP, many of these avenues of research would never have been opened up and the advances that are currently being made would not have been possible today. We must be thankful for those individuals who have contributed so markedly to this field, and one must give thanks for the work and efforts of the late Dick Heikkila, who stimulated many of us to strive to understand more about the cause of Parkinson's disease.

References

1. Tanner CM. 1989. The role of environmental toxins in the etiology of Parkinson's disease. TINS 12:49–54.
2. Steventon GB, Heafield MTE, Waring RH, Williams AC. 1989. Xenobiotic metabolism in Parkinson's disease. Neurology 39:883–887.
3. Waring RH, Sturman SG, Smith MCG, Steventon GB, Heafield MTE, Williams AC. 1989. S-methylation in motor neuron disease and Parkinson's disease. Lancet 2:355–356.
4. Davis GC, Williams AC, Markey SP, Ebert MH, Caine ED, Reichert CM, Kopin IJ. 1979. Chronic parkinsonism secondary to intravenous injection of meperidine analogues. Psychiatr Res 1:249–254.
5. Langston JW, Ballard P, Tetrud JW, Irwin I. 1983. Chronic parkinsonism in humans due to a product of meperidine-analog synthesis. Science 219:979–980.
6. Burns RS, Chiueh CC, Markey SP, Ebert MH, Jacobowitz DM, Kopin IJ. 1983. A primate model of parkinsonism: Selective destruction of dopaminergic neurons in the pars compacta of the substantia nigra by N-methyl-4-phenyl-1,2,3,6-tetrahydropyridine. Proc Natl Acad Sci USA 80:4546–4550.
7. Langston JW, Forno LS, Rebert CS, Irwin I. 1984. Selective nigral toxicity after systemic administration of 1-methyl-4-phenyl-1,2,5,6-tetrahydropyridine (MPTP) in the squirrel monkey. Brain Res 292:390–394.
8. Jenner P, Rupniak NMY, Rose S, Kelly E, Kilpatrick G, Lees A, Marsden CD. 1984. 1-Methyl-4-phenyl-1,2,3,6-tetrahydropyridine-induced parkinsonism in the common marmoset. Neurosci Lett 50:85–90.
9. Kitt CA, Cork LC, Eidelburg F, Joh TH, Price DL. 1986. Injury of nigral neurons exposed to 1-methyl-4-phenyl-1,2,3,6-tetrahydropyridine: A tyrosine hydroxylase immunocytochemical study in monkey. Neuroscience 17:1089–1103.
10. German DC, Dubach M, Askari S, Speciale SG, Bowden DM. 1988. 1-Methyl-4-phenyl-1,2,3,6-tetrahydropyridine-induced parkinsonian syndrome in macaca fascicularis: Which midbrain dopaminergic neurons are lost? Neuroscience 24:161–174.
11. Bedard PJ, Di Paolo T, Falardeau P, Boucher R. 1986. Chronic treatment with L-dopa, but not bromocriptine induces dyskinesia in MPTP-parkinsonian monkeys. Correlation with [^{3}H]spiperone binding. Brain Res 379:294–299.
12. Crossman AR. 1987. Primate models of dyskinesia: The experimental approach to the study of basal ganglia-related involuntary movement disorders. Neuroscience 21:1–40.
13. Jenner P. 1990. Parkinson's disease: Clues to the cause of cell death in substantia nigra. Semin Neurosci 2:117–126.
14. Jenner PG, Marsden CD, Costall B, Marsden CD. 1986. MPTP and MPP$^+$ induced toxicity in rodents and the common marmoset as experimental models for investigating Parkinson's disease. *In* MPTP: A Neurotoxin

Producing a Parkinsonian Syndrome. SP Markey, N Castagnoli, AJ Trevor, IJ Kopin, (eds). Academic Press, New York, pp 45–68.

15. Eidelberg E, Brooks BA, Morgan WW, Walden JG, Kokemoor RH. 1986. Variability and functional recovery in the N-methyl-4-phenyl-1,2,3,6-tetrahydropyridine model of parkinsonism in monkeys. Neuroscience 18:817–822.

16. Ueki A, Chong PN, Albanese A, Rose S, Chivers JK, Jenner P, Marsden CD. 1989. Further treatment with MPTP does not produce parkinsonism in marmosets showing behavioural recovery from motor deficits induced by an earlier exposure to the toxin. Neuropharmacology 28:1089–1097.

17. Chiba K, Trevor A, Castagnoli N Jr. 1984. Metabolism of the neurotoxic tertiary amine, MPTP, by brain monoamine oxidase. Biochem Biophys Res Commun 120:574–578.

18. Salach JI, Singer TP, Castagnoli N Jr, Trevor A. 1984. Oxidation of the neurotoxic amine 1-methyl-4-phenyl-1,2,3,6-tetrahydropyridine (MPTP) by monoamine oxidases A and B and suicide inactivation of the enzymes by MPTP. Biochem Biophys Res Commun 125:831–835.

19. Heikkila RE, Manzino L, Cabbat FS, Duvoisin RC. 1985. Studies on the oxidation of the dopaminergic neurotoxin 1-methyl-4-phenyl-1,2,3,6-tetrahydropyridine by monoamine oxidase B. J Neurochem 45:1049–1054.

20. Peterson LA, Caldera PS, Trevor A, Chiba K, Castagnoli N Jr. 1985. Studies on the 1-methyl-4-phenyl-1,2,3-dihydropyridinium species 2,3-MPDP$^+$, the monoamine oxidase catalyzed oxidation product of the nigrostriatal toxin 1-methyl-4-phenyl-1,2,3,6-tetrahydropyridine (MPTP). J Med Chem 28:1432–1436.

21. Javitch JA, D'Amato RJ, Strittmatter SM, Snyder SH. 1985. Parkinsonism-inducing neurotoxin, N-methyl-4-phenyl-1,2,3,6-tetrahydropiridine: Uptake of the metabolite N-methyl-4-phenylpyridine by dopamine neurons explains selective toxicity. Proc Natl Acad Sci USA 82:2173–2177.

22. Mayer RA, Kindt MV, Heikkila RE. 1986. Prevention of the nigrostriatal toxicity of 1-methyl-4-phenyl-1,2,3,6-tetrahydropyridine by inhibitors of 3,4-dihydroxyphenylethylamine transport. J Neurochem 47:1073–1079.

23. Ramsay RR, Singer TP. 1986. Energy-dependent uptake of N-methylphenylpyridinium, the neurotoxic metabolite of 1-methyl-4-phenyl-1,2,3,6-tetrahydropyridine, by mitochondria. J Biol Chem 261:7585–7587.

24. Ramsay RR, Salach JI, Singer TP. 1986. Uptake of the neurotoxin 1-methyl-4-phenylpyridine (MPP$^+$) by mitochondria and its relation to the inhibition of the mitochondrial oxidation of NAD$^+$-linked substrates by MPP$^+$. Biochem Biophys Res Commun 134:743–748.

25. Nicklas WJ, Vyas I, Heikkila RE. 1985. Inhibition of NADH-linked oxidation in brain mitochondria by 1-methyl-4-phenylpyridine, a metabolite of the neurotoxin, 1-methyl-4-phenyl-1,2,3,6-tetrahydropyridine. Life Sci 36:2503–2508.

26. Vyas I, Heikkila RE, Nicklas WJ. 1986. Studies on the neurotoxity of

1-methyl-4-phenyl-1,2,3,6-tetrahydropyridine: Inhibition of NAD-linked substrate oxidation by its metabolite, 1-methyl-4-phenylpyridinium. J Neurochem 46:1501–1507.

27. Rose S, Nomoto M, Kelly E, Kilpatrick G, Jenner P, Marsden CD. 1989. Increased caudate dopamine turnover may contribute to the recovery of motor function in marmosets treated with the dopaminergic neurotoxin MPTP. Neurosci Lett 101:305–310.

28. Pifl Ch, Schingnitz G, Hornykiewicz O. 1988. The neurotoxin MPTP does not reproduce in the rhesus monkey the interregional pattern of striatal dopamine loss typical of human idiopathic Parkinson's disease. Neurosci Lett 92:228–233.

29. Bernheimer H, Birkmeyer W, Horneykiewicz O, Jellinger K, Setelberger F. 1973. Brain dopamine and the syndrome of Parkinson and Huntington. J Neurol Sci 20:415–455.

30. Rose S, Nomoto M, Jenner P, Marsden CD. 1989. Transient depletion of nucleus accumbens dopamine content may contribute to initial akinesia induced by MPTP in common marmosets. Biochem Pharmacol 38:3677–3681.

31. Elsworth JD, Deutch AY, Redmond DE, Taylor JR, Sladek JR, Roth RH. 1989. Symptomatic and asymptomatic 1-methyl-4-phenyl-1,2,3,6-tetrahydropyridine-treated primates: Biochemical changes in striatal regions. Neuroscience 33:323–331.

32. Elsworth JD, Deutch AY, Redmond DE Jr, Sladek JR Jr, Roth RH. 1990. MPTP-induced parkinsonism: Relative changes in dopamine concentration in subregions of substantia nigra, ventral tegmental area and retrorubral field of symptomatic and asymptomatic vervet monkeys. Brain Res 513:320–324.

33. Elsworth JC, Deutch AY, Redmond DE Jr, Sladek JR Jr, Roth RH. 1990. MPTP reduces dopamine and norepinephrine concentrations in the supplementary motor area and cingulate cortex of the primate. Neurosci Lett 114:316–322.

34. Pifl C, Bertel O, Schingnitz G, Hornykiewicz O. 1990. Extrastriatal dopamine in symptomatic and asymptomatic rhesus monkeys treated with 1-methyl-4-phenyl-1,2,3,6-tetrahydropyridine (MPTP). Neurochem Int 17:263–270.

35. Falardeau P, Bouchard S, Bedard PJ, Boucher R, Di Paolo T. 1988. Behavioural and biochemical effect of chronic treatment with D-1 and/or D-2 dopamine agonists in MPTP monkeys. Eur J Pharmacol 150:59–66.

36. Falardeau P, Bedard PJ, Di Paolo T. 1988. Relation between brain dopamine loss and D-2 dopamine receptor density in MPTP monkeys. Neurosci Lett 86:225–229.

37. Hantraye P, Loc'h C, Tacke U, Riche D, Stulzafit O, Doudet D, Guibert B, Naquet R, Maziere B, Maziere M. 1986. "In vivo" visualization by position emission tomography of the progressive striatal dopamine receptor damage occurring in MPTP-intoxicated non-human primates. Life Sci 39:1375–1382.

38. Joyce JN, Marshall JF, Bankiewicz KS, Kopin IJ, Jacobowitz DM. 1985. Hemiparkinsonism in a monkey after unilateral internal carotid artery

infusion of 1-methyl-4-phenyl-1,2,3,6-tetrahydropyridine (MPTP) is associated with regional ipsilateral changes in striatal dopamine D-2 receptor density. Brain Res 382:360–364.

39. Graham WC, Clarke CE, Boyce S, Sambrook MA, Crossman AR, Woodruff GN. 1990. Autoradiographic studies in animal models of hemi-parkinsonism reveal dopamine D-2 but not D-1 receptor supersensitivity. II. Unilateral intra-carotid infusion of MPTP in the monkey. Brain Res 514:103–110.

40. Jarvis MF, Wagner GC. 1985. Age-dependent effects of 1-methyl-4-phenyl-1,2,5,6-tetrahydropyridine (MPTP). Neuropharmacology 24:581–583.

41. Gupta M, Gupta BK, Thomas R, Bruemmer V, Sladek JR Jr, Felten DL. 1986. Aged mice are more sensitive to 1-methyl-4-phenyl-1,2,3,6-tetrahydropyridine treatment than young adults. Neurosci Lett 70:326–331.

42. Saitoh T, Niijima K, Mizuno Y. 1987. Long-term effect of 1-methyl-4-phenyl-1,2,3,6-tetrahydropyridine (MPTP) on striatal dopamine content in young and mature mice. J Neurol Sci 77:229–235.

43. Ricaurte GA, Irwin I, Forno LS, DeLanney LE, Langston E, Langston JW. 1987. Aging and 1-methyl-4-phenyl-1,2,3,6-tetrahydropyridine-induced degeneration of dopaminergic neurons in the substantia nigra. Brain Res 403:43–51.

44. Rose S, Nomoto M, Jackson EA, Gibb WRG, Jenner P, Marsden CD. 1990. The age-related effects of 1-methyl-4-phenyl-1,2,3,6-tetrahydropyridine treatment of the common marmoset. Eur J Pharmacol 181(1–2):97–103.

45. Forno LS, Langston JW, DeLanney LE, Irwin I, Ricaurte GA. 1986. Locus ceruleus lesions and eosinophilic inclusions in MPTP-treated monkeys. Ann Neurol 20:449–455.

46. Forno LS, Langston JW, DeLanney LE, Irwin I. 1988. An electron microscopic study of MPTP-induced inclusion bodies in an old monkey. Brain Res 448:150–157.

47. Wachtel H, Dorow R. 1983. Dual action on central dopamine function of transdihydrolisuride, a 9,10-dihydrogenated analogue of the ergot dopamine agonist lisuride. Life Sci 32:421.

48. Loschmann P-A, Rettig KJ, Horowski R, Wachtel H, Lange KW, Jenner P, Marsden CD. 1991. Terguride, a dopamine partial agonist for the treatment of Parkinson's disease. *In* Basic Clinical and Therapeutic Aspects of Alzheimer's and Parkinson's Disease, Vol. 2. T Nagatsu, A Fisher, M Yoshida (eds). Plenum Publishing Corporation, New York, pp. 569–572.

49. Lange KW, Loschmann P-A, Wachtel H, Jahnig P, Jenner P, Marsden CD. 1991. The dopamine partial agonist terguride stimulates locomotor activity in common marmosets at 2 months but *not* 6 months following MPTP treatment. Eur J Pharmacol (submitted).

50. Brucke T, Bankiewicz K, Harvey-White J, Kopin I. 1988. The partial dopamine receptor agonist terguride in the MPTP-induced hemiparkinsonian monkey model. Eur J Pharmacol 148:445–448.

51. Nomoto J, Jenner P, Marsden CD. 1988. The D-1 agonist SKF 38393 inhibits the antiparkinsonian activity of the D-2 agonist LY 171555 in the MPTP-treated marmoset. Neurosci Lett 93:275–280.
52. Temlett JA, Chong PN, Oertel WH, Jenner P, Marsden CD. 1988. The D-1 dopamine receptor partial agonist, CY 208-243, exhibits antiparkinsonian activity in the MPTP-treated marmoset. Eur J Pharmacol 156:197–206.
53. Heikkila RE, Sieber B-E, Manzino L, Sonsalla PK. 1989. Some features of the nibrostriatal dopaminergic neurotoxin 1-methyl-4-phenyl-1,2,3,6-tetrahydropyridine (MPTP) in the mouse. Mol Chem Neuropathol 10:171–183.
54. Heikkila RE, Cabbat FS, Manzino L, Duvoisin RC. 1984. Effects of 1-methyl-4-phenyl-1,2,5,6-tetrahydropyridine on neostriatal dopamine in mice. Neuropharmacology 23:711–713.
55. Heikkila RE. 1985. Differential neurotoxicity of 1-methyl-4-phenyl-1,2,3,6-tetrahydropyridine (MPTP) in Swiss-Webster mice from different sources. Eur J Pharmacol 117:131–133.
56. Heikkila RE, Hess A, Duvoisin RC. 1984. Dopaminergic neurotoxicity of 1-methyl-4-phenyl-1,2,5,6-tetrahydropyridine (MPTP) in mice. Science 224:1451–1453.
57. Heikkila RE, Manzino L, Cabbat FS, Duvoisin RC. 1984. Protection against the dopaminergic neurotoxicity of 1-methyl-4-phenyl-1,2,5,6-tetrahydropyridine by monoamine oxidase inhibitors. Nature 311:467–469.
58. Mayer RA, Walters AS, Heikkila RE. 1986. 1-Methyl-4-phenyl-1,2,3,6-tetrahydropyridine (MPTP) administration to C57 black mice leads to parallel decrements in neostriatal dopamine content and tyrosine hydroxylase activity. Eur J Pharmacol 120:375–377.
59. Sonsalla PK, Heikkila RE. 1986. The influence of dose and dosing interval on MPTP-induced dopaminergic neurotoxity in mice. Eur J Pharmacol 129:339–345.
60. Sonsalla PK, Youngster SK, Kindt MV, Heikkila RE. 1987. Characteristics of 1-methyl-4-(2'-methylphenyl)-1,2,3,6-tetrahydropyridine-induced neurotoxicity in the mouse. J Pharmacol Exp Ther 242:850–857.
61. Williams JL, Schneider JS. 1989. MPTP-induced ventral mesencephalic cell loss in the cat. Neurosci Lett 101:258–262.
62. Schneider JS, Markham CH. 1986. Neurotoxic effects of N-methyl-4-phenyl-1,2,3,6-tetrahydropyridine (MPTP) in the cat. Tyrosine hydroxylase immunohistochemistry. Brain Res 373:258–267.
63. Parisi JE, Burns RS. 1986. The neuropathology of MPTP-induced parkinsonism in man and experimental animals. In MPTP: A Neurotoxin Producing a Parkinsonian Syndrome. SP Markey, N Castagnoli Jr, AJ Trevor, IJ Kopin (eds). Academic Press, Orlando, pp. 141–148.
64. Johannessen JN, Chiueh CC, Bacon JP, Garrick NA, Burns RS, Weise VK, Kopin IJ, Parisi JE, Markey SP. 1989. Effects of 1-methyl-4-phenyl-1,2,3,6-tetrahydropyridine in the dog. Effect of pargyline pretreatment. J Neurochem 53:582–589.

65. Hoppel CL, Greenblatt D, Kowk H-C, Arora PK, Singh MP, Sayre LM. 1987. Inhibition of mitochondrial respiration by analogs of 4-phenylpyridine and 1-methyl-4-phenylpyridinium cation (MPP$^+$). The neurotoxic metabolite of MPTP. Biochem Biophys Res Commun 148:684–693.

66. Heikkila RE, Youngster SK, Panek DU, Giovanni A, Sonsalla PK. 1988. Studies with the neurotoxicant 1-methyl-4-phenyl-1,2,3,6-tetrahydropyridine (MPTP) and several of its analogs. Toxicology 49:493–501.

67. Booth RG, Trevor A, Singer TP, Castagnoli N Jr. 1989. Studies on semirigid tricyclic analogues of the nigrostriatal toxin 1-methyl-4-phenyl-1,2,3,6-tetrahydropyridine. J Med Chem 32:473–477.

68. Johnson EA, Wu EY, Rollema H, Booth RG, Trevor AJ, Castagnoli N Jr. 1989. 1-Methyl-4-phenylpyridinium (MPP$^+$) analogs: In vivo neurotoxicity and inhibition of striatal synaptosomal dopamine uptake. Eur J Pharmacol 166:65–74.

69. Arora PK, Riachi NJ, Fiedler GC, Singh MP, Abdallah F, Harik SI, Sayre LM. 1990. Structure–neurotoxicity trends of analogues of 1-methyl-4-phenylpyridinium (MPP$^+$), the cytotoxic metabolite of the dopaminergic neurotoxin MPTP. Life Sci 46:379–390.

70. Collins MA, Neafsey EJ. 1985. β-Carboline analogues of N-methyl-4-phenyl-1,2,5,6-tetrahydropyridine (MPTP): Endogenous factors underlying idiopathic parkinsonism. Neurosci Lett 55:179–184.

71. Albores R, Neafsey EJ, Drucker G, Fields JZ, Collins MA. 1990. Mitochondrial respiratory inhibition by N-methylated β-carboline derivatives structurally resembling N-methyl-4-phenylpyridine. Proc Natl Acad Sci USA 87:9368–9372.

72. Nagatsu T, Yoshida M. 1988. An endogenous substance of the brain, tetrahydroisoquinoline, produces parkinsonism in primates with decreased dopamine, tyrosine hydroxylase and biopterin in the nigrostriatal regions. Neurosci Lett 87:178–182.

73. Ogawa M, Araki M, Natatsu I, Nagatsu T, Yoshida M. 1989. The effect of 1,2,3,4-tetrahydroisoquinoline (TIQ) on mesencephalic dopaminergic neurons in C57BL/6J mice: Immunohistochemical studies—tyrosine hydroxylase. Biogenic Amines 6:427–436.

74. Youngster SK, Sonsalla PK, Heikkila RE. 1987. Evaluation of the biological activity of several analogs of the dopaminergic neurotoxin 1-methyl-4-phenyl-1,2,3,6-tetrahydropyridine. J Neurochem 48:929–934.

75. Youngster SK, Sonsalla PK, Sieber B-A, Heikkila RE. 1989. Structure-activity study of the mechanism of 1-methyl-4-phenyl-1,2,3,6-tetrahydropyridine (MPTP)-induced neurotoxicity. I. Evaluation of the biological activity of the MPTP analogs. J Pharmacol Exp Ther 249:820–828.

76. Youngster SK, Nicklas WJ, Heikkila RE. 1989. Structure–activity study of the mechanism of 1-methyl-4-phenyl-1,2,3,6-tetrahydropyridine (MPTP)-induced neurotoxicity. II. Evaluation of the biological activity of the pyridinium metabolites formed from the monoamine oxidase-

catalyzed oxidation of MPTP analogs. J Pharmacol Exp Ther 249:829–835.

77. Youngster SK, Cuvoisin RC, Hess A, Sonsalla PK, Kindt MV, Heikkila RE. 1986. 1-Methyl-4-(2'-methylphenyl)-1,2,3,6-tetrahydropyridine (2'-CH$_3$-MPTP) is a more potent dopaminergic neurotoxin than MPTP in mice. Eur J Pharmacol 122:283–287.

78. Sonsalla PK, Youngster SK, Kindt MV, Heikkila RE. 1987. Characteristics of 1-methyl-4-(2'-methylphenyl)-1,2,3,6-tetrahydropyridine-induced neurotoxicity in the mouse. J Pharmacol Exp Ther 242:850–857.

79. Kindt MV, Heikkila RE, Nicklas WJ. 1987. Mitochondrial and metabolic toxicity of 1-methyl-4-(2'-methylphenyl)-1,2,3,6-tetrahydropyridine. J Pharmacol Exp Ther 242:858–863.

80. Kindt MV, Youngster SK, Sonsalla PK, Douvisin RC, Heikkila RE. 1988. Role for monoamine oxidase-A (MAO-A) in the bioactivation and nigrostriatal dopaminergic neurotoxicity of the MPTP analog, 2'-Me-MPTP. Eur J Pharmacol 146:313–318.

81. Heikkila RE, Kindt MV, Sonsalla PK, Giovanni A, Youngster SK, McKeown KA, Singer TP. 1988. Importance of monoamine oxidase A in the bioactivation of neurotoxic analogs of 1-methyl-4-phenyl-1,2,3,6-tetrahydropyridine. Proc Natl Acad Sci USA 85:6172–6176.

82. Rose S, Nomoto M, Jackson EA, Gibb WRG, Jenner P, Marsden CD. 1990. 1-Methyl-4-(2'-methylphenyl)-1,2,3,6-tetrahydropyridine (2'-methyl-MPTP) is less neurotoxic than MPTP in the common marmoset. Eur J Pharmacol 181:97–103.

83. Smith LA, Jenner P, Marsden CD. 1991. Lack of neurotoxicity of 2'-ethyl-MPTP in the common marmoset. Mov Disord (submitted).

84. Frank DM, Arora PK, Blumer JL, Sayre LM. 1987. Model study on the bioreduction of paraquat, MPP$^+$, and analogs. Evidence against a "redox cycling" mechanism in MPTP neurotoxicity. Biochem Biophys Res Commun 147:1095–1104.

85. Rossetti ZL, Sotgiu A, Sharp DE, Hadjiconstantinou M, Neff NH. 1988. 1-Methyl-4-phenyl-1,2,3,6-tetrahydropyridine (MPTP) and free radicals *in vitro*. Biochem Pharmacol 37:4573–4574.

86. Adams JD Jr, Odunze IN. 1991. Biochemical mechanisms of 1-methyl-4-phenyl-1,2,3,6-tetrahydropyridine toxicity. Biochem Pharmacol 41:1099–1105.

87. Perry TL, Godin DV, Hansen S. 1982. Parkinson's disease: A disorder due to nigral glutathione deficiency? Neurosci Lett 33:305–310.

88. Perry TL, Yong VW. 1986. Idiopathic Parkinson's disease, progressive supranuclear palsy and glutathione metabolism in the substantia nigra of patients. Neurosci Lett 67:269–274.

89. Riederer P, Sofic E, Rausch W-D, Schmidt B, Reynolds GP, Jellinger K, Youdim MBH. 1989. Transition metals, ferritin, glutathione, and ascorbic acid in parkinsonian brains. J Neurochem 52:515–520.

90. Dexter DT, Carter CJ, Wells FR, Javoy-Agid F, Agid Y, Lees A, Jenner P, Marsden CD. 1989. Basal lipid peroxidation in substantia nigra is increased in Parkinson's disease. J Neurochem 52:381–389.

91. Dexter DT, Holley AE, Flitter WD, Slater TF, Wells FR, Daniel SE, Lees AJ, Jenner P, Marsden CD. 1991. Increased levels of lipid hydroperoxides but no evidence for increased free radical formation in the parkinsonian substantia nigral. J Neurochem (submitted).

92. Saggu H, Cooksey J, Dexter D, Wells FR, Lees A, Jenner P, Marsden CD. 1989. A selective increase in particulate superoxide dismutase activity in parkinsonian substantia nigra. J Neurochem 53:692–697.

93. McGeer PL, Itagaki S, Akiyama H, McGeer EG. 1989. Comparison of neuronal loss in Parkinson's disease and aging. *In* Parkinsonism and Aging. DB Calne, D Crippa, M Trabucchi, C Comi, R Horowski (eds). Raven Press, New York, pp. 25–34.

94. Schapira AHV, Holt IJ, Sweeney M, Harding AE, Jenner P, Marsden CD. 1990. Mitochondrial DNA analysis in Parkinson's disease. Mov Disord 5:294–297.

95. Schapira AHV, Mann VM, Cooper JM, Dexter D, Daniel SE, Jenner P, Clark JB, Marsden CD. 1990. Anatomic and disease specificity on NADH CoQ$_1$ reductase (complex I) deficiency in Parkinson's disease. J Neurochem 55:2142–2145.

96. Parker WD, Boyson SJ, Parks JK. 1989. Abnormalities of the electron transport chain idioipathic Parkinson's disease. Ann Neurol 26:719–723.

97. Bindoff LA, Birch-Machin M, Cartilage NEF, Parker WD, Turnbull DM. 1989. Mitochondrial function in Parkinson's disease. Lancet 2:49.

98. Mizuno Y, Ohta S, Tanaka M, Takamiya S, Suzuk K, Sato T, Oya H, Ozawa T, Kagawa Y. 1989. Deficiencies in complex I subunits of the respiratory chain in Parkinson's disease. Biochem Biophys Res Commun 163:1450–1455.

99. Ikebe S-I, Tanaka M, Ohno K, Sato W, Hattori K, Kondon T, Mizuno Y, Ozawa T. 1990. Increase of deleted mitochondrial DNA in the striatum in Parkinson's disease and senescence. Biochem Biophys Res Commun 170:1044–1048.

100. Schapira AHV, Cooper JM, Dexter D, Clark JB, Jenner P, Marsden CD. 1990. Mitochondrial complex I deficiency in Parkinson's disease. J Neurochem 54:823–827.

101. Lestienne P, Nelson J, Riederer P, Jellinger K, Reichmann H. 1990. Normal mitochondrial genome in brain from patients with Parkinson's disease and complex I defect. J Neurochem 55:1810–1812.

102. Dexter DT, Schapira AHV, Fearnley J, Lees A, Daniel SE, Wells FR, Jenner P, Marsden CD. 1991. No alteration in iron, ferritin or mitochondrial respiratory chain enzymes in substantia nigra in incidential Lewy body disease. Ann Neurol (submitted).

Chapter 3

Platelet Membrane Fluidity in Parkinson's Disease

Juan R. Sanchez-Ramos, Luis Reynoso, Carlos Singer, William J. Weiner, and Burton Pressman

Recent studies have demonstrated mitochondrial abnormalities in striatum or substantia nigra from brains of patients dying with Parkinson's disease (PD).[1-3] Interestingly, decreases in complex I activity (NADH: ubiquinone oxidoreductase) have also been reported in mitochondria isolated from platelets of PD patients.[4] The finding of a platelet abnormality suggests that PD may be a more generalized disease in which the brunt of the illness is borne by the vulnerable nigrostriatal dopaminergic system. The possibility that the underlying basic pathology of PD is not restricted to the CNS prompted the study of platelet membrane fluidity as a potential peripheral marker or indicator of the disease.

The rationale for studying platelet membrane "fluidity" as a marker for PD is based on the following observations. The defect observed in platelet mitochondria is similar to that induced by the neurotoxin 1-methyl-1,2,3,6-tetrahydropyridine (MPTP). MPP$^+$, the active metabolite of MPTP, inhibits mitochondrial electron transport at complex I resulting in decreased ATP production, accumulation of

Supported by grants from NPF-Allied Signal and a Clinical Investigator Development Award (K08-NS01142) to J.S-R.
From Hefti F, and Weiner WJ, (eds.) *Progress in Parkinson's Disease Research—2.* Mount Kisco NY, Futura Publishing Co., Inc., © 1992.

lactate, and decreased oxygen consumption.[5-7] Another critical consequence of complex I inhibition produced by MPP[+] or rotenone is induction of NADH-dependent superoxide formation and lipid peroxidation of mitochondrial membranes.[8] Since oxygen-derived free radicals are known to alter membrane fluidity,[9] we proposed to test the hypothesis that the putative complex I abnormality in PD platelets is associated with an alteration in platelet membrane "fluidity."

Methods

Patients with a diagnosis of Parkinson's disease were recruited from the Movement Disorder Clinic of the University of Miami to participate in the study ($N = 38$). Healthy spouses were also invited to contribute a sample of blood to serve as age-matched control subjects ($N = 30$). Informed consent was obtained, and the research protocol was approved by the University of Miami Investigational Review Board.

Ten milliliters of whole blood samples, drawn (9 AM until noon) from the antecubital vein into purple-top anticoagulated tubes (EDTA) was centrifuged $150g$ for 10 minutes. The platelet-rich plasma was removed and centrifuged at $650g$ for 6 minutes. The cleared plasma was removed and the sedimented platelets were suspended in 2 ml of Tyrode's solution. A 100-μl aliquot of the suspension was diluted to a volume which yields an absorbance of 0.06 at 546 nm. To this suspension, 5 μl of diphenylhexatriene (DPH) in DMSO was added to yield a final concentration of 2 nm. The suspension was incubated for 1 hour with gentle shaking at 32–34°C. Fluorescence anisotropy was determined by exciting with vertically polarized light (360–375 nm) and measuring the intensity of emitted fluorescence in parallel ($F_{\parallel}$) and perpendicular ($F_{\perp}$) planes in an L-shaped configuration fluorescence spectrometer. Fluorescence anisotropy (r_s) is calculated by the equation:

$$r_s = \frac{F_{\parallel} - F_{\perp}}{F_{\parallel} + 2\,F_{\perp}}$$

and compared to a standard of DPH in mineral oil.

The term r_s is conventionally regarded as a measure of "membrane fluidity," or reciprocal viscosity, but this is not strictly accurate; r_s is a fundamental measure of the rotational diffusion of the DPH probe, which, in a true biological membrane (containing a large proportion of protein), is controlled by the orientation of the phospholipid fatty acid hydrocarbon chains or "membrane order." Much of the membrane lipid is strongly influenced by the intramembranous proteins, hence r_s is an empirical function of the integrated membrane organization. Any gross abnormality of membrane composition, whether it be in the phospholipids, their degree of stiffening by intramembranous sterols, the structure of the intramembranous proteins, or even an imbalance in the proportions of otherwise normal constituents, can produce abnormal r_s values.

Statistics

Analysis of data was performed using RS1 Statistical software (BNN Software, Cambridge, MA). Comparison of mean values between groups was performed using two-tailed t tests. Relationships among continuous variables were explored using regression analysis.

Results

The mean age of the PD group and spouses was 65.1 and 64.9 years, respectively; 57% of the PD group and 37% of the control group were male. The mean r_s of the platelets in the PD group was not different from the r_s of the spouses' platelets (Table 1). Mean r_s of the

Table 1.

Fluorescence Anisotropy (r_s) of Blood Elements in PD Patients and Controls

	PD	Control	P
N	38	30	
M/F	21/16 (57%)	11/19 (37%M)	
Age (yr)	65.6	64.9	ns
(Range)	41–87	44–85	
Disease duration (yr)	4.6	—	
Platelet r_s	0.1576	0.1557	ns
SEM	0.0039	0.0047	
WBC r_s	0.1520	0.1533	ns
SEM	0.0042	0.0037	
RBC r_s	0.1769	0.1803	ns
SEM	0.0040	0.0045	

monocytes and erythrocyte ghosts were also not significantly different in the two groups.

Sorting the platelet r_s as a function of age in both PD and healthy spouses demonstrated a tendancy towards increasing r_s with age (Figure 1). Regression analysis, however, did not support a significant relationship between age and platelet r_s in either group. Regression analysis of the relationship between platelet r_s and duration of disease in the PD group also showed no significant relationship between these two parameters (Figure 2).

Monocyte r_s and erythrocyte ghost r_s were also sorted as a function of age in PD subjects and spouses (data not shown). Similar to the platelet r_s, there was no significant relationship between age and membrane r_s of the monocytes or erythrocytes.

The PD group was further analyzed for possible effects of L-dopa, deprenyl, and tocopherol on membrane r_s. There was no significant relationship between platelet r_s and the use of L-dopa (Figure 3), deprenyl, or tocopherol (Figure 4).

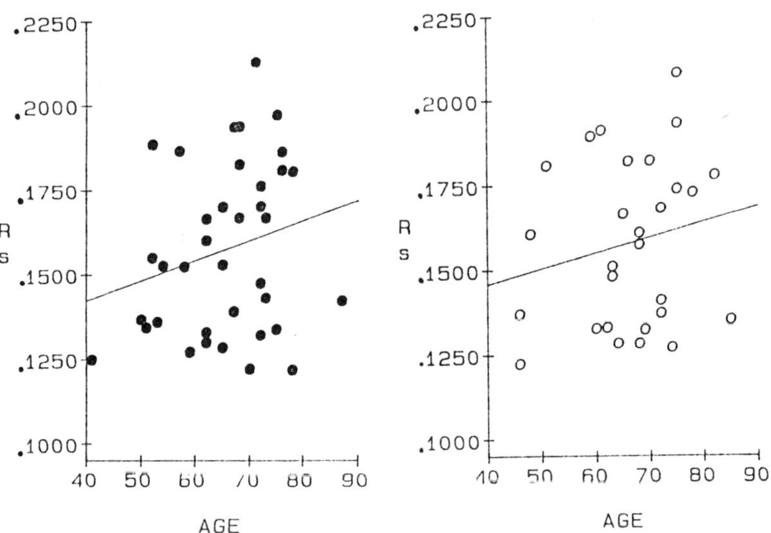

Figure 1.   Distribution of platelet r_s as a function of age in PD patients (left panel) (correlation coefficient = 0.228; coefficient of determination r^2 = 0.051) and controls (right panel) (correlation coefficient = 0.271; coefficient of determination r^2 = 0.073).

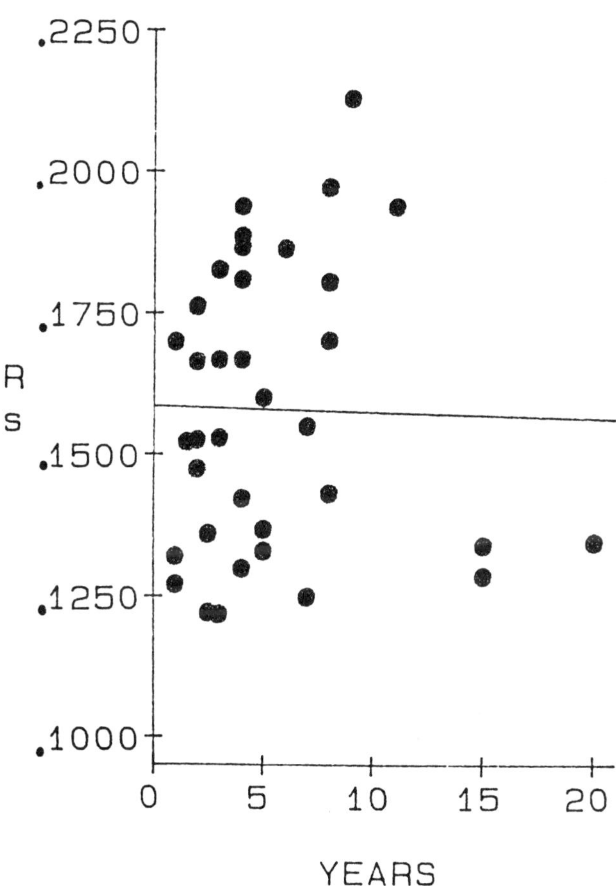

Figure 2. Distribution of platelet r_S as a function of duration of disease (correlation coefficient = −0.020; coefficient of determination r^2 = 0.004).

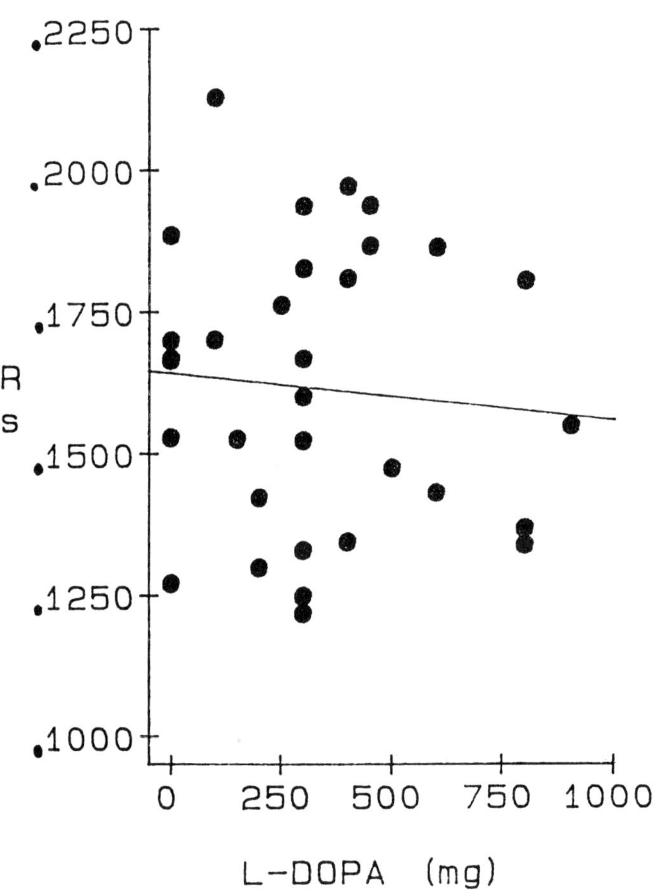

Figure 3. Distribution of platelet r_s as a function of L-dopa dose (correlation coefficient = 0.087; coefficient of determination r^2 = 0.007).

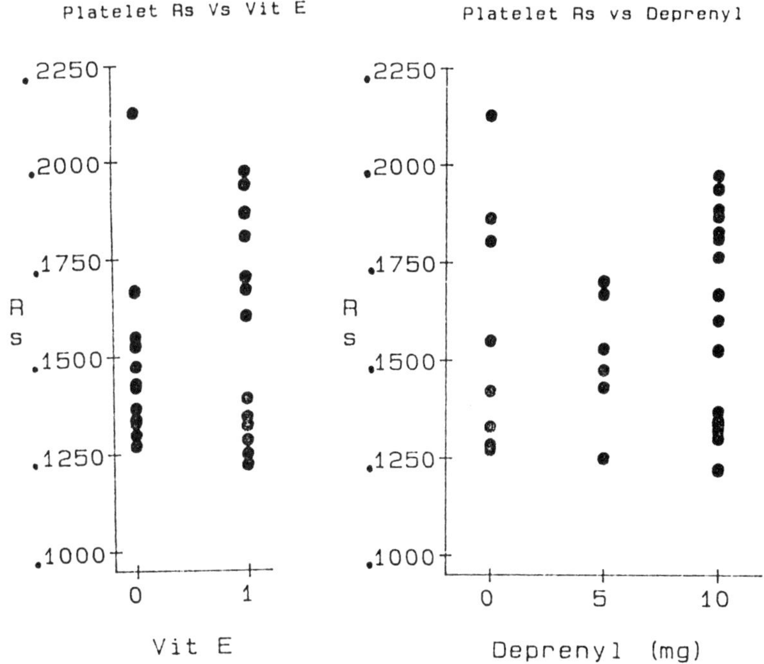

Figure 4. Distribution of platelet r_S as a function of vitamin E use and dose of deprenyl.

Discussion

Studies of membrane fluidity of platelets, monocytes, and erythrocytes from PD patients failed to demonstrate alterations in r_s when compared to normal age-matched controls. A tendency of the r_s to increase with normal aging was noted in both groups. A similar increase with age in membrane DPH fluorescence polarization was reported in a population of normal individuals ranging in age from 17 to 86 years.[10]

There was no relationship between platelet r_s and duration of disease, nor were medication effects noted. L-Dopa, deprenyl, and tocopherol ingestion appeared to have no systematic effect on platelet r_s.

In contrast to these negative results, similar studies of membrane fluidity in Alzheimer's disease showed a sigificant increase in fluidity in patients with the disease compared to aged-matched controls.[11] The explanation for the increased fluidity (decrease in DPH fluorescence anisotropy) in the platelet membrane was related, in part, to the proliferation of internal membranes in the Alzheimer's samples.[12] Interestingly, when DPH fluorescence anisotropy was determined in intact platelets rather than in platelet membrane preparations, there was no difference in Alzheimer's versus the age-matched control group.[12] Since the results presented here were based on studies of intact platelets, it is possible that further studies of membrane biophysical properties will be detected if membrane preparations are used for analysis.

It should be emphasized that the impetus for investigating the platelet membrane properties in this study was triggered by the report of a mitochondrial deficit at complex I in platelets as well as in substantia nigra and striatum of PD patients.[1–4] The inhibition of mitochondrial electron transport at complex I can produce cellular damage by two apparent mechanisms that are not mutually exclusive: (1) inhibition of biological energy production (ATP), which inhibits cellular function including cellular repair; and (2) increased production of H_2O_2, hydroxyl radical, and superoxide anion,[8] which oxidize membrane lipids to debris difficult to degrade and damage structural and catalytic proteins. The remarkable finding that mitochondria isolated from peripheral tissue (platelets) of PD patients exhibit this defect in complex I leads to the speculation that PD may be a more generalized disease than previously recognized, with the burden of the disease localized to the CNS because DA neurons are more susceptible to oxidant stresses. The hypothesis that abnormalities in platelet mitochondria result in alteration of membrane fluidity has not been supported by the results presented here. However, these results do not disprove the finding by Parker et al.[4] that a complex I deficiency is present in platelet mitochondria. It may be that the reported 50% reduction of complex I activity is insufficient to promote superoxide generation to levels which can cause measurable changes in membrane order. In addition, the mitochondrial deficit may result only in mitochondrial membrane changes and the plasma membrane may be uninjured. Future studies will assess mitochondrial membrane fluidity using fluorescent probes selective for mitochondrial membranes.

References

1. Mizuno Y, Ohta S, Tanaka M, Takamiya S, Suzuki K, Sato T, Oya H, Ozawa T, Kagawa Y. 1989. Deficiencies in complex I subunits of the respiratory chain in Parkinson's disease. Biochem Biophys Res Commun 163:1450–1455.
2. Schapira AHV, Cooper JM, Dexter D, Jenner P, Clark JB, Marsden CD. 1989. Mitochondrial complex I deficiency in Parkinson's disease. Lancet 1:1269.
3. Schapira AHV, Cooper JM, Dexter D, Clark JB, Jenner P, Marsden CD. 1990. Mitochondrial complex I deficiency in Parkinson's disease. J Neurochem 54:823–827.
4. Parker WD, Boyson SJ, Parks JK. 1989. Abnormalities of the electron transport chain in idiopathic Parkinson's disease. Ann Neurol 26:719–723.
5. Nicklas WJ, Vyas I, Heikkila RE. 1985. Inhibition of NADH-linked oxidation in brain mitochondria by 1-methyl-4-phenyl pyridinium, a metabolite of the neurotoxin, 1-methyl-1,2,5,6-tetrahydropyridine. Life Sci 36:2503–2508.
6. Vyas I, Heikkila RE, Nicklas WJ. 1986. Studies on the neurotoxicity of MPTP inhibition of NAD-linked substrate oxidation by its metabolite MPP$^+$. J Neurochem 46:1501–1507.
7. Sanchez-Ramos J, Hollinden G, Sick T, Rosenthal M. 1988. MPP$^+$ increases oxidation of cytochrome b in rat striatal slices. Brain Res 443:183–189.
8. Hawegawa E, Takeshige K, Oishi T, Murai Y, Minakami S. 1990. 1-Methyl-4-phenylpyridinium (MPP$^+$) induces NADH-dependent superoxide formation and enhances NADH-dependent lipid peroxidation in bovine heart sub-mitochondrial particles. Biochem Biophys Res Commun 170:1049–1055.
9. Watanabe H, Kobayashi A, Yamamoto T, Suzuki S, Hayashi H, Yamazaki N. 1990. Alterations of human erythrocyte membrane fluidity by oxygen-derived free radicals and calcium. Free Radio Biol Med 9:507–514.
10. Cohen BM, Zubenko GS. 1985. Aging and the biophysical properties of cell membranes. Life Sci 37:1403–1409.
11. Zubenko Gs, Cohen BM, Boller F, Malinakova I, Keefe N, Chojnacki B. 1987. Platelet membrane abnormality in Alzheimer's disease. Ann Neurol 22:237–244.
12. Zubenko GS, Malinakova I, Chojnacki B. 1987. Proliferation of internal membranes in platelets from patients with Alzheimer's disease. J Neuropathol Exp Neurol 46:407–418.

Chapter 4

Interactions of Dopaminergic Neurotoxin MPTP with Monoamine Oxidase in Human Brain Synaptosomes

Keith F. Tipton, Anne-Marie O'Carroll, and James P. Sullivan

1-Methyl-4-phenyl-1,2,3,6-tetrahydropyridine (MPTP) causes a condition resembling idiopathic Parkinson's disease in humans and some animals (for reviews see references 1–4). MPTP toxicity is prevented by pretreatment with inhibitors of monoamine oxidase-B (MAO-B). That enzyme has been shown to catalyze the oxidation of MPTP to the dihydropyridine derivative (1-methyl-4-phenyl-1,2-dihydropyridine; MPDP). This compound can then be further oxidized, either by the action of MAO-B[3] or nonenzymically[5,6] to form the 1-methyl-4-phenyl-pyridinium ion (MPP$^+$), which is the effective neurotoxin.

MPP$^+$ is actively taken up by dopaminergic nerve terminals,[7] and the administration of inhibitors of the presynaptic dopamine uptake system protect against the neurotoxic effects of MPTP and MPP$^+$.[8–10] The results suggest that MPTP is converted to MPP$^+$ outside the dopaminergic nerves and that its selectivity as a neurotoxin arises from the pyridinium ion being a selective substrate for the neuronal dopamine uptake system.

We are grateful to the Eolas Ireland for support.
From Hefti F, and Weiner WJ, (eds.) *Progress in Parkinson's Disease Research—2.* Mount Kisco NY, Futura Publishing Co., Inc., © 1992.

MPP$^+$ is an inhibitor of mitochondrial oxidation of NADH-linked substrates[11,12] and, at the high concentrations present in the dopaminergic nerve terminals, the resulting depletion of ATP appears to be sufficient to result in degeneration.

This simple model of the neurotoxicity of MPTP, which is summarized in Figure 1, has led to speculation that there might be a naturally occurring toxic compound, acting in a similar way, which causes the idiopathic condition. Such ideas have been given some impetus by the reports that the selective MAO-B inhibitor l-deprenyl (selegiline) has a protective effect in those suffering from the disease.[13,14] However, it should be borne in mind that the involvement of MAO-B may be merely fortuitous, since other neurotoxic analogs of MPTP are converted to the toxic pyridinium species by the action of MAO-A.[15]

Although much of the experimental work on the mechanisms of MPTP toxicity has involved rodents, these are considerably less sensitive to the neurotoxicity of this compound than primates.[16] Furthermore the neurotoxic effects of MPTP in rodents appears to be at least partly reversible,[17] whereas there is no evidence for such reversibility in the human. Clearly, any understanding of the actions of this neurotoxin and its possible relevance to Parkinson's disease must involve studies in the human brain and must also take account of the considerable species differences that exist. In the present work we report the results of some studies of the interactions of human brain MAO with MPTP.

Materials and Methods

Homogenates were prepared from postmortem human brain samples, which were obtained 15 ± 3 hours after death. Synaptosomal preparations were prepared from samples that had been stored at −70°C after slow freezing and thawed rapidly before use by the procedure of Hardy et al.[18] Details of these procedures as applied in our laboratory have been published elsewhere.[19,20] The integrity of the synaptosomal preparations was assessed by measurement of occluded lactate dehydrogenase,[21] and an example of the results of such a determination is shown in Figure 2. The increase in detectable lactate dehydrogenase activity by a factor of 2.15 that occurred on lysis of the synaptosomes is in good agreement with values reported

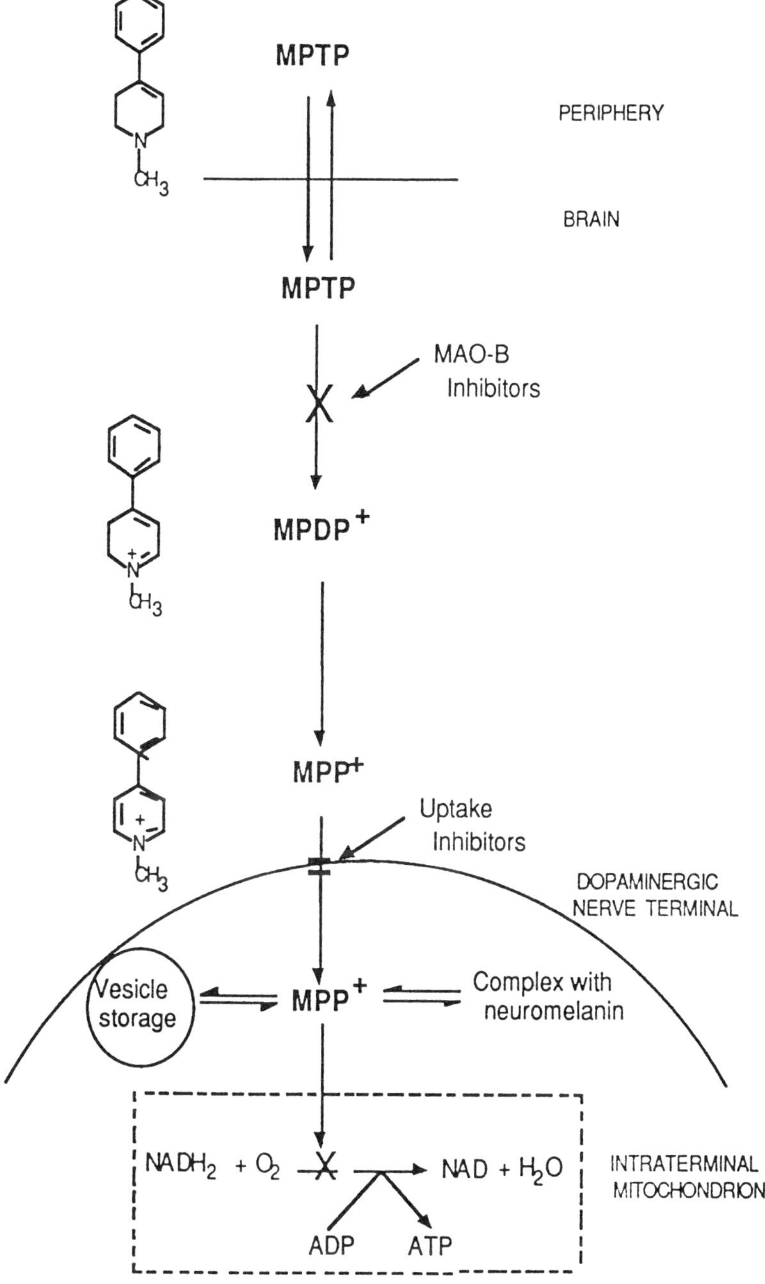

Figure 1. A simple mechanism for the neurotoxic effects of MPTP. Further discussion of the mechanisms involved may be found in refs. 2–4.

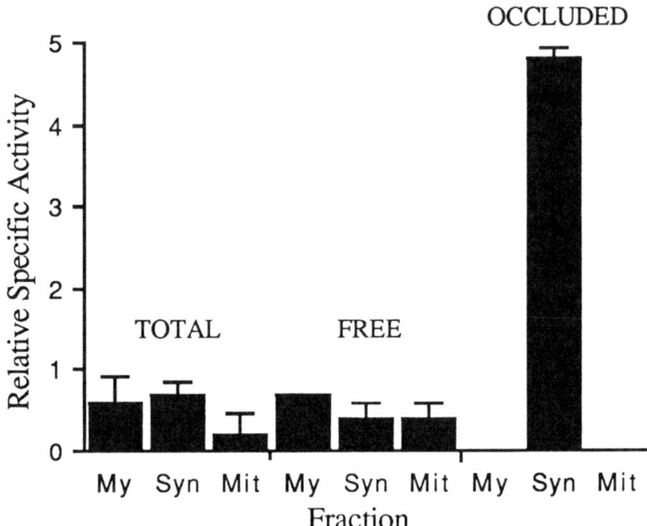

Figure 2. Lactate dehydrogenase activities in human brain fractions. Human brain homogenates were treated and fractionated, and the lactate dehydrogenase activities were determined as described in the text; each value is the mean ± SEM from three separate determinations. The fractions obtained from gradient centrifugation were: myelin (my), synaptosomes (syn), and mitochondria (mit). The protein content of the synaptosomal fraction was approximately twice that in each of the other two.

for such preparations from fresh brain samples.[21] Synaptosomes prepared by the sucrose-gradient procedure of Gray and Whittaker[22] could be incubated for up to 90 minutes at 37°C under the conditions used in the present work without any significant change in the occluded lactate dehydrogenase values, but there was an increase in the accessibility of this enzyme, with a corresponding decrease in the occluded activity over longer incubation periods. However, when the more rapid fractionation procedure of Dodd et al.[23] was used, the occluded lactate dehydrogenase levels were stable over incubation periods of up to 240 minutes, and hence this procedure was used for preparations that were to be subjected to extended periods of incubation.

MAO activities were determined radiochemically. The procedure described by Tipton[24] was used when dopamine (DA), 5-hydroxytryptamine (5-HT), or 2-phenylethylamine (PEA) were used as substrates, whereas an alternative procedure[25] was used with noradrenaline (NA) as substrate. In experiments with synaptosomal preparations, low substrate concentrations (0.25 μM DA, 0.1 μM 5-HT, and 0.25 μM NA) were used so that the metabolism of amines actively transported into the nerve terminals would predominate.[19] In all experiments, unless otherwise stated, the concentration of PEA, which readily penetrates membranes, was 5 μM, unless otherwise stated. In all cases incubation times were chosen to be in the region where product formation was linear with time and the initial velocity of the reaction was proportional to the enzyme concentration.

Results

By using selective MAO and uptake inhibitors in preparations of synaptosomes from human brain we had previously shown that MAO-B activity was essentially absent from caudatal dopaminergic nerve terminals.[19] This result, which was consistent with data obtained immunologically,[26,27] provided an explanation for the protection afforded against MPTP toxicity by dopamine uptake inhibitors, since it established that the site of oxidation of this compound to MPP$^+$ had to be extraneuronal. In contrast, the noradrenergic nerve terminals from human hypothalamus were found to contain both forms of the enzyme, as shown in Figure 3. The serotoninergic nerves from human brain were also found to contain significant activities of MAO-B in immunological studies.[26,27] However this approach failed to detect any MAO-A in these neurons, whereas significant activity of that was detected in our studies with intact synaptosomal preparations from human hypothalamus.[19] Although these results provide a plausible explanation for the extraneuronal formation of MPP$^+$ in the caudatal dopaminergic system, they do not explain why significant noradrenergic and dopaminergic neurotoxicity does not arise from the conversion of MPTP to MPP$^+$ by the MAO-B within those nerve terminals. The relatively nonpolar nature of MPTP might lead one to expect that it would quite readily cross the synaptosomal membrane to reach intraneuronal MAO.

MPTP is a time-dependent inhibitor of MAO-B in human brain synaptosomes, as has previously been shown to be the case with

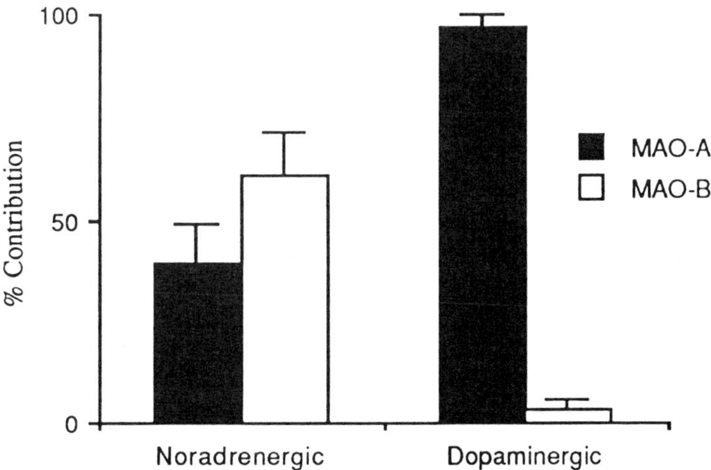

Figure 3. Monoamine oxidases in human brain synaptosomes. The contributions of the two forms of monoamine oxidase to the intrasynaptosomal metabolism of dopamine and noradrenaline were determined in synaptosomes prepared from human caudatus and hypothalamus, respectively, by the use of selective amine uptake inhibitors and MAO inhibitors. (Taken from the data in ref. 19.) Each value is the mean ± SEM from three to five separate determinations.

preparations of this enzyme from other sources (for review see Kinemuchi et al.[2]) and this is shown by the data in Figure 4, which also shows that the inhibition of MAO-A showed no significant time dependence. In contrast, Salach et al.[28] reported that the time course for the inhibition of human placental MAO-A by MPTP was complex, with an initial phase of activation being followed by one of inhibition. Kinemuchi et al.,[29] who did not observe any activating phase with the enzyme from liver, attributed the time-dependent inhibition of MAO-A to the formation of MPP$^+$, which is a more potent inhibitor of MAO-A than MPTP. Since the inhibition of MAO by MPP$^+$ is reversible and competitive,[29] no time-dependent inhibitory effects would be expected if the experiments are conducted with sufficient care to exclude reversible inhibition by dilution and the use of adequately high assay substrate concentrations.

These results would suggest that, as with the enzyme from rat and ox liver, MPTP is a mechanism-based irreversible inhibitor of MAO-B,[30,31] whereas the interaction with MAO-A is noncovalent. The reversibility of the inhibition was assessed by repeatedly

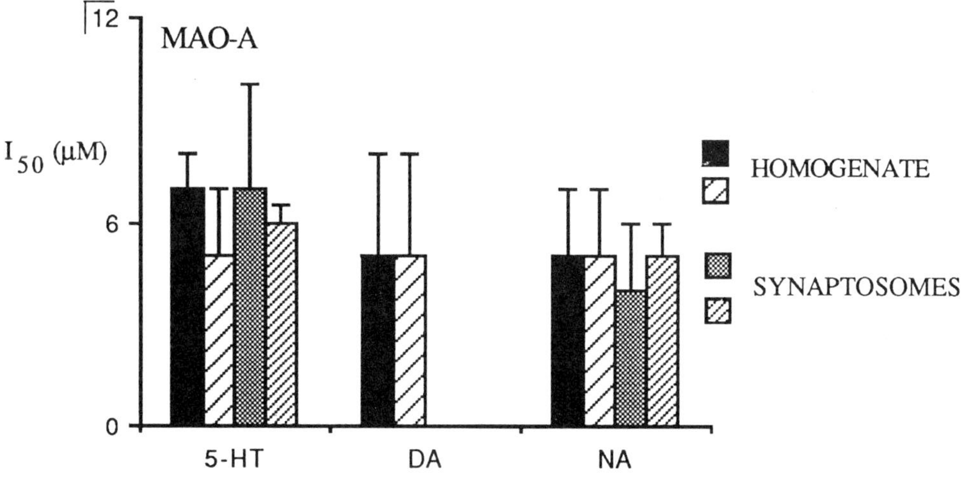

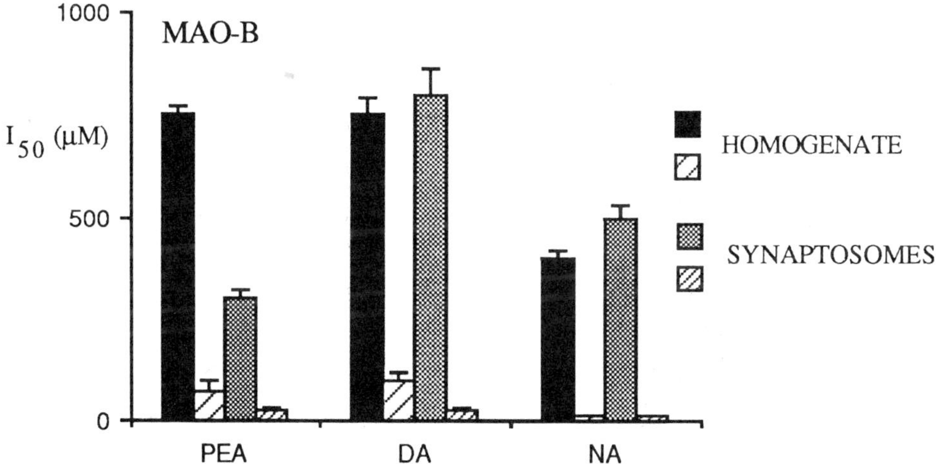

Figure 4. Inhibition of human brain MAO by MPTP. The activities of MAO-A (upper panel) and MAO-B (lower panel) were determined in homogenates and synaptosomes. These were prepared from caudatus for the studies with dopamine and from hypothalamus for the studies with all other substrates. Activities were assayed immediately after addition of MPTP (solid bars) or after preincubating the preparation with MPTP for 60 minutes at 37°C before addition of substrate (hatched bars). Activities were determined as described in the text and each value is the mean ± SEM from triplicate determinations. The substrate concentrations used for the determinations in homogenates were dopamine (DA) 50 μM, 5-HT 100 μM, (−)-noradrenaline (NA) 500 μM, and 2-phenylethylamine (PEA) 20 μM. In the experiments with intact synaptosomes, the substrate concentrations were DA 0.25 μM, 5-HT 0.1 μM, NA 0.25 μM, and PEA 20 μM.

washing and by centrifugation and resuspension[32] of tissue samples that had been preincubated with MPTP for 1 hour at 37°C. Homogenates of hypothalamus and caudatus were used for studies on the reversibility of the inhibition of MAO-A and -B, respectively, and synaptosomes from the former region were also used to assess the interactions with MAO-A. Because of the essential absence of MAO-B activity from human caudatal dopaminergic nerve terminals, no reversibility studies were attempted for that enzyme in such synaptosomal preparations. The results of these studies, summarized in Figure 5, indicate a substantial irreversible component to the inhibition of MAO-B by MPTP, whereas that of MAO-A was reversed to a considerable extent. Reversibility was also assessed by dilution (see Waldmeier et al.[32] for a description of the procedure) of samples that had been preincubated with MPTP for 1 hour at 37°C. The results (not shown) confirmed MPTP to be an irreversible

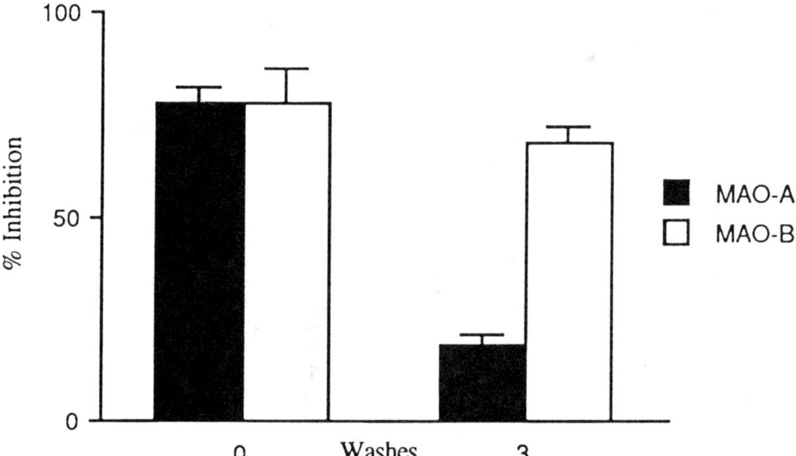

Figure 5. Effects of repeated washing on the inhibition of human brain MAO by MPTP. Synaptosomes from human caudatus were incubated for 60 minutes at 37°C with 20 μM or 1 mM MPTP, for determinations of MAO-A and -B, respectively, and the activity remaining, with respect to controls in which the inhibitor was omitted, was determined (0 wash). Samples and controls were then washed three times, centrifuged and resuspended in Krebs-Henseleit buffer, pH 7.2, and the activity remaining was again determined (3 washes). MAO-A and -B activities were determined with 0.1 μM 5-HT and 5 μM 2-phenylethylamine, respectively. Each value is the mean ± SER from triplicate determinations.

inhibitor of MAO-B but a reversible inhibitor of MAO-A in homogenates from human caudatus and hypothalamus, respectively.

The initial interaction of MPTP with MAO (without preincubation) would be expected to occur at the active site of the enzyme since it is a substrate for both forms of MAO,[30,31] as well as being a time-dependent irreversible inhibitor of MAO-B. That the inhibition arises solely through interactions with the active site of the enzymes is indicated by the nature of the reversible component of the reaction. Inhibition was found to be strictly competitive with both enzymes, as shown for MAO-B in Figure 6. Fuller and Hemrick-Leucke[33] also found the inhibition of human brain MAO-A by MPTP to be competitive. However, they reported that the inhibition of MAO-B was noncompetitive. This may have been a result of their having failed to determine the truly reversible component of the inhibition, since the occurrence of any time-dependent irreversible inhibition in their studies would give rise to the appearance of apparently noncompetitive behavior.

The inhibitor constants (K_i values) determined from the kinetic plots were 11 ± 1 and 120 ± 5 μM for MAO-A and -B, respectively.

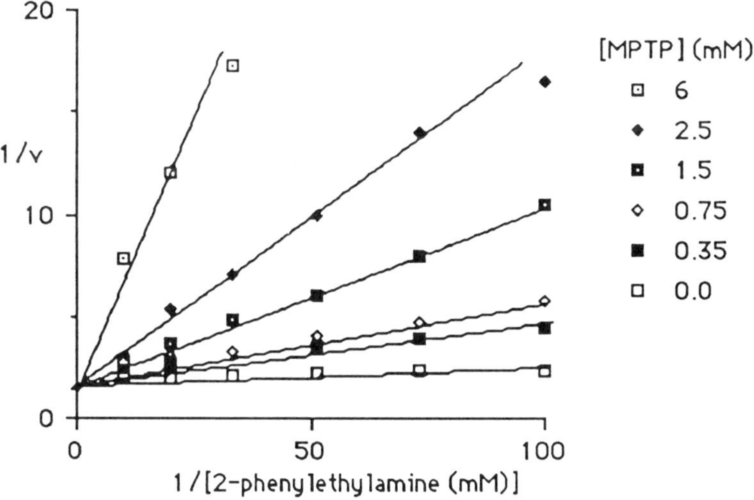

Figure 6. Reversible-phase inhibition of human brain MAO-B by MPTP. Human caudatal homogenates were incubated for 60 minutes at 37°C with 0.1 μM clorgyline, to inhibit MAO-A, before initial rates were determined.

Unlike the I_{50} values determined without enzyme-inhibitor preincubation, which are shown in Figure 4, the K_i values are independent of the relative substrate concentration. Both sets of data indicate that the noncovalent binding of MPTP is much tighter to MAO-A than it is to MAO-B, despite the fact that it is a much better substrate for the latter enzyme.[28–30] These K_i values for the human brain enzyme are also quite similar to the K_m values determined for MPTP as a substrate for the two enzyme forms from rat liver.[30]

Since MPTP is a reversible inhibitor of MAO-A, it is possible to assess its ability to penetrate intact synaptosomes by determining the extent of inhibition of that enzyme. In these experiments low concentrations of substrates were used so that the active presynaptic uptake system would be an important factor in determining the apparent oxidative activity,[19] and samples were preincubated at 37°C for 60 minutes with 5μM 1-deprenyl to inhibit the MAO-B activity. Under these conditions inhibition of MAO-B activity was found to be essentially complete, whereas there was no significant inhibition of MAO-A (results not shown). Since deprenyl has been shown to be an inhibitor of presynaptic dopamine uptake,[34,35] the free inhibitor was subsequently removed by washing three times and by centrifugation and resuspension before the effects of MPTP were studied.

Figure 7 shows the inhibition of MAO activity towards dopamine in synaptosomes from human caudatus resulting from incubation with different concentrations of MPTP for 60 minutes at 37°C. The majority of the MAO-A activity towards this substrate was apparently insensitive to inhibition by MPTP. If, however, the synaptosomes were disrupted by treatment with the detergent Triton X-100 or by sonication, the total MAO-A was sensitive to inhibition by MPTP (Figure 7). Thus, only some 20% of the MAO-A activity in the intact human caudatal synaptosomal preparation was sensitive to inhibition by MPTP at concentrations as high as 1 μM, but total inhibition was obtained if disrupted synaptosomes were used. These results would suggest that the smaller sensitive pool represents MAO-A activity associated with any extrasynaptosomal material present together with that in broken synaptosomes. Such a value for the "nonsynaptosomal" component of such preparations would be consistent with that estimated in our earlier studies.[19] That would indicate that the intrasynaptosomal pool of MAO-A was not accessible to MPTP unless the synaptosomes were disrupted. Time courses and incubation periods longer than the 60 minutes used here might

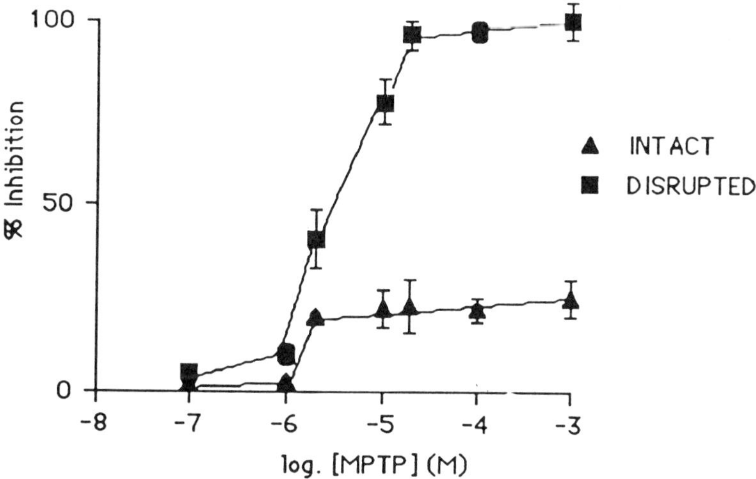

Figure 7.   Inhibition of MAO-A activity in human brain synaptosomes by MPTP. Synaptosomal preparations from human caudatus were pretreated for 60 minutes at 37°C with 5 μM 1-deprenyl, to inhibit MAO-B, prior to incubation for a further 60 minutes at 37°C with the indicated concentrations of MPTP, followed by assay in the presence of 0.25 μM dopamine. Each point is the mean ± SER of triplicate determinations. Either intact synaptosomes or preparations that had been disrupted by treatment with 1% Triton were used as indicated.

indicate whether the compound did slowly penetrate the synaptosomal membrane, but the results presented here suggest that MPTP does not readily penetrate the nerve terminal membrane. In similar experiments (not shown) with synaptosomes prepared from human hypothalamus and with noradrenaline as the substrate, it was found that a smaller pool of MAO-A, about 20%, was only accessible to inhibition by MPTP if the synaptosomes were disrupted. These results would also be consistent with the intraneuronal MAO pool being inaccessible to MPTP.

Discussion

MPTP is a time-dependent irreversible inhibitor of MAO-B in the human brain that interacts initially with the active site of the enzyme. In contrast, MPTP is a simple competitive inhibitor of the A form of the enzyme, and the inhibition is reversible and shows no time dependence. The use of intact synaptosomal preparations that had been pretreated with deprenyl to inhibit the MAO-B revealed that the pool of MAO-A within the synaptosomes was not accessible to MPTP but became so when the synaptosomes were disrupted.

These results would provide an explanation for the apparent lack of sensitivity of noradrenergic and serotoninergic neurons to the neurotoxic effects of MPTP. The sensitivity of the dopaminergic neurons to MPTP has been shown to result from the active transport of extraneuronally produced MPP$^+$ into them by the presynaptic dopamine carrier. However, although dopaminergic nerve terminals from human caudatus lack significant MAO-B activity, that enzyme is present in the noradrenergic and serotoninergic terminals from human hypothalamus. Thus, it might appear likely that MPTP entering these synaptosomes would be converted to MPP$^+$ by the MAO-B present there. Such MPP$^+$ formed *in situ* might be expected to be trapped in the nerve terminal because of its positive charge and thus accumulate to an extent sufficient to cause neurotoxicity. The fact that external MPTP does not readily reach the sites of intrasynaptosomal MAO, therefore, offers an explanation for the relative insensitivity of these MAO-B-containing nerves.

The mechanisms underlying this inability of MPTP to reach the presynaptic compartment containing the MAO are still to be fully resolved. The simplest explanation might be that, despite its relatively hydrophobic nature, MPTP does not readily penetrate the nerve-terminal membrane. However, the possibility that the compound is sequestered either by binding to components of the synaptosome or by active accumulation cannot yet be excluded. The nature of any such processes, which would have to be prevented by the procedures used to disrupt the synaptosomes, is obscure. It has been shown that the presynaptic adrenergic storage vesicles can accumulate MPP$^+$,[36] but there has been no suggestion that the uncharged MPTP might also be accumulated by the vesicles.

Although these results may help to clarify aspects of the neurotoxicity of MPTP, the possible relevance of this compound to idiopathic Parkinson's disease remains unclear. The evidence that MPTP itself or a compound with very similar behavior is unlikely to be involved in the etiology of the idiopathic condition has been reviewed elsewhere,[4] however, an environmental factor contributing, in some way, to the genesis or progress of the condition remains a possibility. Much has been made of the parallel between the ability of deprenyl to protect against the neurotoxicity of MPTP and its apparent beneficial actions in the therapy of Parkinson's disease. However, it may be that the parallel with MPTP may be purely fortuitous, since it is now known that with some analogs of this compound inhibitors of MAO-B do not provide protection against neurotoxicity and that it is necessary to inhibit MAO-A or both forms of the enzyme to prevent the formation of the neurotoxic pyridinium derivative.[15]

Although several possibilities have been advanced for a naturally occurring toxin that might cause parkinsonism by a mechanism similar, at least in part, to that involved with MPTP toxicity, none has yet been convincingly established. If an MAO-B substrate is not involved in the idiopathic disease, the apparent beneficial effects of l-deprenyl might be due to other facets of its activity. These might involve inhibition of the oxidation of amine substrates leading to a decrease in the formation of the potentially toxic products hydrogen peroxide, ammonia, and an aldehyde. Alternatively, the effects of deprenyl on neurotransmitter uptake might contribute to its beneficial properties. Since dopamine is a substrate for both forms of MAO in human brain,[37] but the dopaminergic nerve terminals contain essentially only the A form of the enzyme, any direct effects of deprenyl would be limited to dopamine oxidation occurring outside these terminals, presumably in glial cells.

The earlier data suggesting that deprenyl treatment might prolong the effective life-span of parkinsonian patients[38] have only limited relevance to the situation, since in those retrospective studies the drug was coadministered with L-dopa and any interpretation of the behavior might be complicated by possible toxic effects of that compound or the formation of relatively high concentrations of dopamine in the brain. If the present DATATOP studies[13,14] confirm that there is a beneficial effect of deprenyl treatment, the mechanisms must be understood in terms of the effects of that drug alone. Clearly it is not possible, at this stage, to exclude the inhibition of an endogenously formed or environmental protoxin that is converted to the active species by the action of MAO-B. Therefore, a closer understanding of the mode of action of the selective dopaminergic toxin MPTP may well prove to be more than an academic problem.

References

1. Snyder SH, D'Amato RJ. 1986. MPTP: A neurotoxin relevant to the pathophysiology of Parkinson's disease. Neurology 36:250–258.
2. Kinemuchi H, Fowler CJ, Tipton KF. 1987. The neurotoxicity of 1-methyl-4-phenyl-1,2,3,6-tetrahydropyridine (MPTP) and its relevance to Parkinson's disease. Neurochem Int 11:359–373.
3. Singer TP, Castagnoli N, Ramsay RR, Trevor AJ. 1987. Biochemical events in the development of Parkinson's disease induced by 1-methyl-4-phenyl-1,2,3,6-tetrahydropyridine. J Neurochem 49:1–8.
4. McCrodden JM, Tipton KF, Sullivan JP. 1990. The neurotoxicity of MPTP and the relevance to Parkinson's disease. Pharmacol. Toxicol. 67:8–13.
5. Trevor AJ, Chiba K, Yu EY, Caldera PN, Castagnoli KP, Peterson I, Salach JI, Singer TP. 1986. Metabolism of MPTP *in vitro*. The intermediate role of 2,3-MPDP$^+$ and studies on its chemical and biochemical reactivity. *In* MPTP: A Neurotoxin Producing a Parkinsonian Syndrome. SP Markey, N Castagnoli, AJ Trevor, IJ Kopin (eds). Academic Press, New York, pp. 161–172.
6. Castagnoli N, Chiba K, Trevor AJ. 1985. Potential bioactivation pathways for the neurotoxin 1-methyl-4-phenyl-1,2,3,6-tetrahydropyridine (MPTP). Life Sci 36:225–230.
7. Javitch JA, D'Amato RJ, Strittmater SM, Snyder SH. 1985. Parkinsonism-inducing neurotoxin N-methyl-4-phenyl-1,2,3,6-tetrahydropyridine: Uptake of the metabolite N-methyl-4-phenylpyridine by dopamine neurons explains selective toxicity. Proc Natl Acad Sci USA 82:2173–2177.
8. Sundström E, Jonsson G. 1986. Differential time course of protection by monoamine oxidase inhibition and uptake inhibition against MPTP neurotoxicity on central catecholamine neurons in mice. Eur J Pharmacol 122:275–278.
9. Pileblad E, Carlsson A. 1985. Catecholamine uptake inhibitors prevent the neurotoxicity of 1-methyl-4-phenyltetrahydropyridine (MPTP) in mouse brain. Neuropsychopharmacol 24:689–692.
10. Melamed E, Rosenthal J, Cohen O, Globus M, Uzzan A. 1985. Dopamine but not norepinephrine or serotonin uptake inhibitors protect mice against neurotoxicity of MPTP. Eur J Pharmacol 116:179–181.
11. Nicklas WJ, Vyas I, Heikkila RE. 1985. Inhibition of NADH-linked oxidation in human brain mitochondria by 1-methyl-4-phenyl-1,2,3,6-tetrahydropyridine. Life Sci 36:2503–2508.
12. Ramsay RR, Dadgar JI, Trevor A, Singer TP. 1986. Energy-driven uptake of N-methyl-4-phenylpyridinium by brain mitochondria mediates the neurotoxicity. Life Sci 39:581–588.
13. Tetrud JW, Langston VW. 1989. The effect of deprenyl on the natural history of Parkinson's disease. Science 245:519–522.
14. Parkinson Study Group. 1989. Effect of deprenyl on the progression of disability in early Parkinson's disease. N Engl J Med 321:1364–1371.

15. Heikkila RE, Kindt MV, Sonsalla PK, Giovani A, Youngster SK, McKeown KA, Singer TP. 1988. The importance of MAO-A in the bioactivation of neurotoxic MPTP analogs. Proc Natl Acad Sci USA 85:6172–6176.

16. Heikkila RE, Hess A, Duvoisin R. 1984. Dopaminergic neurotoxicity of 1-methyl-4-phenyl-1,2,3,6-tetrahydropyridine in mice. Science 224: 1451–1453.

17. Chiueh CC, Johannessen JN, Sun JL, Bacon JP, Markey SP. 1986. Reversible neurotoxicity of MPTP in the nigrostriatal dopaminergic system in mice. In MPTP: A Neurotoxin Producing a Parkinsonian Syndrome. SP Markey, N Castagnoli, AJ Trevor, IJ Kopin (eds). Academic Press, New York, pp. 473–479.

18. Hardy JA, Dodd PR, Oakley AE, Perry RH, Edwardson JA, Kidd AM. 1983. Metabolically active synaptosomes can be prepared from frozen rat and human brain. J Neurochem 40:608–614.

19. O'Carroll AM, Tipton KF, Sullivan JP, Fowler CJ, Ross SB. 1987. Intra and extraneuronal deamination of dopamine and noradrenaline by the two forms of human brain monoamine oxidase. Implications for the neurotoxicity of N-methyl-4-phenyl-1,2,3,6-tetrahydropyridine in man. Biogenic Amines 4:165–178.

20. Sullivan JP, Tipton KF. 1988. Interactions of monoamine oxidase and MPTP in human brain. In Neurotoxins in Neurochemistry. JO Dolly (ed). Ellis Horwood, Chichester, pp. 125–131.

21. Johnson MR, Whittaker VP. 1963. Lactate dehydrogenase as a cytoplasmic marker in brain. Biochem J 88:404–409.

22. Gray EG, Whittaker VP. 1962. Isolation of nerve endings from brain. An electron microscope study of cell fragments derived from homogenization and centrifugation. J Anat 96:79–88.

23. Dodd PR, Hardy JA, Oakley AE, Edwardson JA, Perry EK, Delaunoy JP. 1981. A rapid method for preparing synaptosomes: Comparison with alternative procedures. Brain Res 226:107–118.

24. Tipton KF. 1985. Determination of monoamine oxidase. Meth Find Exp Clin Pharmacol 7:361–367.

25. O'Carroll AM, Bardsley ME, Tipton KF. 1986. The oxidation of adrenaline and noradrenaline by the two forms of monoamine oxidase from human and rat brain. Neurochem Int 8:493–500.

26. Thorpe LW, Westlund KN, Kochersperger LM, Abell CW, Denney RM. 1987. Immunocytochemical localisation of monoamine oxidase A and B in human peripheral tissue and brain. J Histochem Cytochem 35:23–32.

27. Westlund KM, Denney RM, Kochersperger LM, Rose RM, Abell CW. 1985. Distinct MAO A and B populations in primate brain. Science 230:180–182.

28. Salach JP, Singer TP, Castagnoli N, Trevor AJ. 1984. Oxidation of the neurotoxic amine 1-methyl-4-phenyl-1,2,3,6-tetrahydropyridine (MPTP) by monoamine oxidases A and B and suicide inactivation of the enzymes by MPTP. Biochem Biophys Res Commun 125:831–835.

29. Kinemuchi H, Arai Y, Toyoshima Y. 1985. Participation of brain monoamine oxidase B form in neurotoxicity of 1-methyl-4-phenyl-

1,2,3,6-tetrahydropyridine: Relationship between the enzyme inhibition and the neurotoxicity. Neurosci Lett 58:195–200.

30. Tipton KF, McCrodden JM, Youdim MBH. 1986. Oxidation and enzyme-activated irreversible inhibition of rat liver monoamine oxidase-B by 1-methyl-4-phenyl-1,2,3,6-tetrahydropyridine (MPTP). Biochem J 240:379–383.

31. Kreuger MJ, McKeown K, Ramsay RR, Youngster S, Singer TP. 1990. Mechanism-based inactivation of monoamine oxidase A and B by tetrahydropyridines and dihydropyridines. Biochem J 268:219–224.

32. Waldmeier PC, Felner AE, Tipton KF. 1983. The monoamine oxidase inhibiting properties of CGP 11305A. Eur J Pharmacol 94:73–83.

33. Fuller RW, Hemrick-Luecke SK. 1985. Inhibition of types A and B monoamine oxidase by 1-methyl-4-phenyl-1,2,3,6-tetrahydropyridine. J Pharmacol Exp Ther 232:696–701.

34. Harsing LG, Magyar K, Tekes K, Vizi ES, Knoll J. 1979. Inhibition by deprenyl of dopamine uptake in rat striatum: A possible correlation between dopamine uptake and acetylcholine release inhibition. Pol J Pharmacol Pharm 31:297–307.

35. Lai JCK, Leung TKS, Guest JF, Lim L, Davison AN. 1980. The monoamine oxidase inhibitors clorgyline and l-deprenyl also affect the uptake of dopamine, noradrenaline and serotonin by rat brain. Biochem Pharmacol 29:2763–2767.

36. Daniels AJ, Reinhard JF, Painter GR. 1988. Reversible neurotoxicity of MPTP in the nigrostriatal dopaminergic system in mice. Biochem Biophys Res Commun 156:1243–1249.

37. O'Carroll AM, Fowler CJ, Phillips JP, Tobbia I, Tipton KF. 1983. The deamination of dopamine by human brain monoamine oxidase: Specificity for the two enzyme forms in seven brain regions. Naunyn-Schmiedeberg's Arch Pharmacol 322:198–202.

38. Birkmeyer W, Knoll J, Riederer P, Youdim MBH, Hars V, Marton J. 1985. Increased life expectancy resulting from addition of L-deprenyl to Madopar treatment in Parkinson's disease: A long term study. J Neural Transm 64:113–127.

Chapter 5

Phenylethylamine:
A Trace Amine and Modulator of Catecholaminergic Neurotransmission—Possible Role in Parkinsonism

*Alan A. Boulton, Bruce A. Davis,
David A. Durden, Augusto V. Juorio,
I. Alick Paterson, and Peter H. Yu*

Phenylethylamine (PE) is the simplest of the endogenous arylal-kylamines; it is present in minute quantities in all tissues including the brain,[1-3] hence its rubric "trace amine."[4] Evidence that will be reviewed very briefly in this chapter, implicates it, or phenylacetic acid (PAA), its principle oxidative deaminated product, in several neuropsychiatric disorders. As a biogenic amine PE is heterogeneously distributed across the brain; it is synthesized by aromatic L-amino acid decarboxylase (AADC, Ec 4.1.1.28) and degraded very rapidly by monoamine oxidase (MAO type B),[5-10] and it seems to act primarily as a neuromodulator.[3,11,12] Because it is the favored endogenous MAO-B substrate,[9,10] because it amplifies dopaminergic (and noradrenergic) neurotransmission,[3,13-16,51] and because its tissue levels are rapidly and selectively increased following treatment

From Hefti F, and Weiner WJ, (eds.) *Progress in Parkinson's Disease Research—2.* Mount Kisco NY, Futura Publishing Co., Inc., © 1992.

with small, therapeutically effective, doses of deprenyl,[17,18,51] we postulate that it might be involved in the mechanism of action of deprenyl and in the etiology of Parkinson's disease[3,18,19] and perhaps other neuropsychiatric and neurodegenerative disorders.

Identification, Distribution, Metabolism, and Excretion of Phenylethylamine

Early attempts to quantitate PE yielded erroneously high values; it was only after the application of mass spectrometric (MS) techniques that benchmark values were obtained. These procedures include the TLC–high-resolution MS–electron impact method of Durden and coworkers,[1,20,21] GC-MS by Willner et al.[22] and Syzmanski et al.,[23] GC-MS-negative chemical ionization by Durden and coworkers,[24–26] and GC-MS-positive chemical ionization by Lauber and Waldmeier[27] and Edwards and Blau.[28] Using these values, established by mass spectrometry, it subsequently proved possible to develop and apply alternative highly sensitive techniques such as HPLC-ED, fluorimetry, and GC-ECD (see ref. 21 for further details). Tables 1 and 2 list PE levels in the central nervous system (CNS) and regions of the brain of various species.

PE is formed from phenylalanine by the action of AADC and this can be considered the rate-limiting step in its synthesis (although this is not the case for other biogenic amines that also involve AADC). PE's accumulation is a remarkable 1.5 nmol/g/hr making it comparable to the synthesis of dopamine (DA) and much greater than that of noradrenalin (NA).[3,8] Since the concentration of PE is so low (less than 10^{-3} that of DA), it is apparent that it is also catabolized at a similarly fast rate by MAO-B to produce its oxidatively deaminated product, PAA (see Figure 1 for an outline of the synthesis and metabolism of PE).

PAA is present in brain and cerebrospinal fluid (CSF) (about 30 ng/g), although it exists in blood at a higher level (130 ng/ml) and in urine in very large quantities (about 150 mg/24 hr) (see ref. 29 for tables of PE and PAA in body fluids of normal, psychiatric, and neurologically disordered individuals). Although the turnover rate for PE in brain is very fast (half-life 0.4 min), it cannot be assumed that all of the PAA arises from PE. The relative magnitudes of the deamination (from PE) and transamination (from phenylalanine) reactions have not been reported.

Table 1.
PE in CNS of Various Species[a]

Rat (whole brain)	1.8
Mouse (whole brain)	1.0
Human (caudate nucleus)	1.5
Rabbit (whole brain)	0.4
Fowl (whole brain)	0.7
Octopus (optic lobe)	3.0
Snail (circumoesophageal ganglia)	0.6
Lobster (whole CNS)	1.2
Starfish (arm nerve)	4.4

[a]Concentrations in ng/g. See ref. 3 for source references.

Table 2.
PE in Different Brain Regions of Various Species[a]

	Mouse	Rat	Sheep	Human
Caudate nucleus	3.3	1.3	1.9	1.5
Putamen	—	—	2.3	0.9
Globus pallidus	—	3.6	0.8	1.7
Olfactory tubercles	3.4	5.3	—	—
Nucleus accumbens	—	4.8	—	—
Thalamus	—	—	0.9	0.9
Hypothalamus	1.7	2.1	1.3	—
Cerebellum	<0.5	—	1.1	1.1
Brain stem	0.5	—	1.6	—
Spinal cord	1.1	—	1.0	—

[a]Concentrations in ng/g. See ref. 3 for source references.

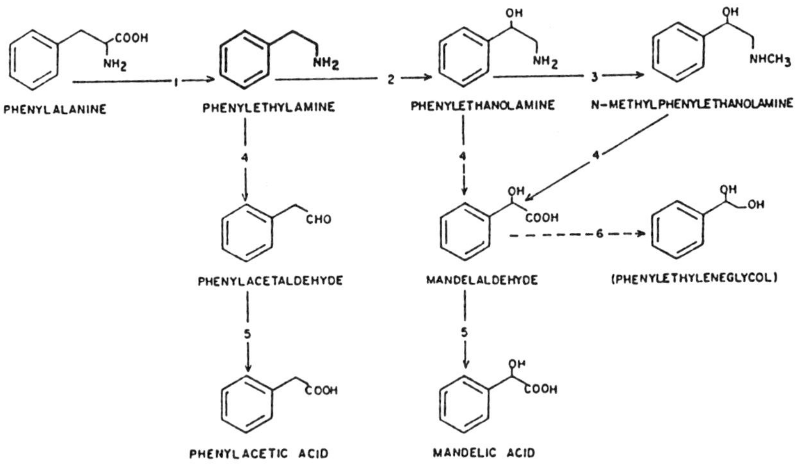

Figure 1. Metabolism of phenylethylamine. 1. AADC; 2. dopamine-β-hydroxylase; 3. *N*-methyltransferase; 4. monoamine oxidase; 5. aldehyde oxidase; 6. alcohol dehydrogenase.

Phenylacetic acid is reduced in blood plasma and urine of depressed patients, and it has been claimed to be a state marker[30–34] in this condition, although others have failed to confirm this. In schizophrenia circulating blood levels of PE have been claimed to be increased,[26] although Szymanski et al.[23] claimed it to be reduced from control levels in the paranoid subgroup. In urine several groups,[35–37] but not all,[38] have also claimed it to be increased, and in blood and CSF it has variously been claimed to be either increased, decreased, or not changed (see refs. 29 and 39 for review). In aggressive psychopaths, incarcerated in a maximum security prison, three studies based on: (1) the court record[40]; (2) the court record and institutional ratings and assessments[41]; and (3) longitudinal studies on selected aggressive patients[42] all showed that blood PAA levels were reduced in comparison with matched controls from the same institutions. From all this it does seem that PE and/or PAA levels are abnormal in some neuropsychiatric conditions; whether this means that they are markers for those particular conditions or rather whether it reflects a more general role as a marker of catecholaminergic dysfunction remains to be elucidated.

Table 3.
Effect of Some MAOIs on PE Levels in Rat Striatum[a]

Drug	Dose (mg/kg)	PE (ng/g)
Control		2.2
Deprenyl	1	7.7
Clorgyline	10	2.0
Pargyline	75	213
Phenelzine	10	2.9
	100	33.3
Tranylcypromazine	1	11.9
Iproniazid	100	227

[a]Data taken from ref. 43.

Effect of Drugs

Table 3 illustrates the effects of various MAO inhibitors on PE levels in the rat striatum.[43,44] It can be seen that the MAO-A inhibitor clorgyline is without effect on PE levels while deprenyl increases them. The other monoamine oxidase inhibitors (MAOIs, Ec 1.4.3.4), which block both type A and B MAO, all caused substantial increases in the levels of PE.

The importance of deprenyl in the treatment of parkinsonism,[45,46] its claimed neuroprotective properties,[47] its demonstrated ability to prolong the life-span of rats,[48,49] and the ability of PE to amplify the effects of DA when it is applied iontophoretically have caused us to begin to investigate the effects of acute and chronic doses of deprenyl on PE and DA and their metabolism in the striatum of the rat (see Figures 2–4 and refs. 50 and 51).

Figure 2 shows the time course and Figure 3 the effect of deprenyl in the rat caudate nucleus at doses up to 8 mg/kg. As can be seen, deprenyl increases striatal PE levels, but it is without effect on DA. It was similarly without effect on 3,4-dehydroxyphenylacetic acid (DOPAC) and homovanillic acid (HVA) except at the higher dose (Figure 4).

In order to assess whether or not the usual pharmacologic and lesion manipulations affected PE in the same way as is the case for the more conventional biogenic amines such as DA, NA, and

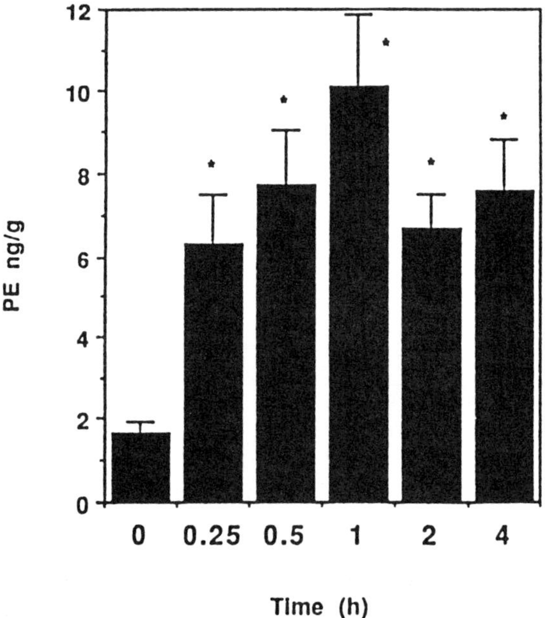

Figure 2.   Time course of deprenyl treatment of PE in rat caudate nucleus. See ref. 51 for further details.

5-hydroxytryptamine (5-HT), it is first necessary, because of PE's tiny endogenous concentration, to increase its level to a point where decreases can be observed. This is done by first treating the animal with low doses of deprenyl so as to increase, moderately, its striatal levels. When this had been achieved, it became possible to demonstrate decreases in PE levels following lesions to the substantia nigra (SN) (Table 4) and electrical stimulation of the SN (Figure 5). The increases following treatment with reserpine (Table 5) and after treatment with antipsychotic drugs (Table 6) were, of course, easier to observe.

Treatment with the specific DA receptor blockers SCH 23390 and pimozide led to increases in AADC (see Figure 6 and ref. 52). These findings that PE is not stored, is not released,[59] is increased by DA receptor blockers, and is intimately associated with the nigrastriatal dopaminergic pathway all support the neuromodulator model presented in Figure 12 later in this chapter.

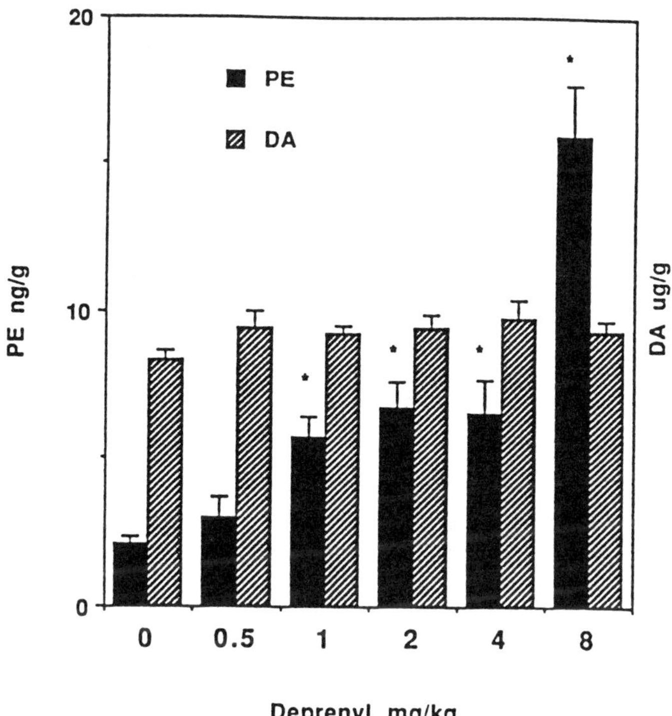

Figure 3.   Effect of different doses of deprenyl on PE and DA levels in rat caudate nucleus. See ref. 51 for further details.

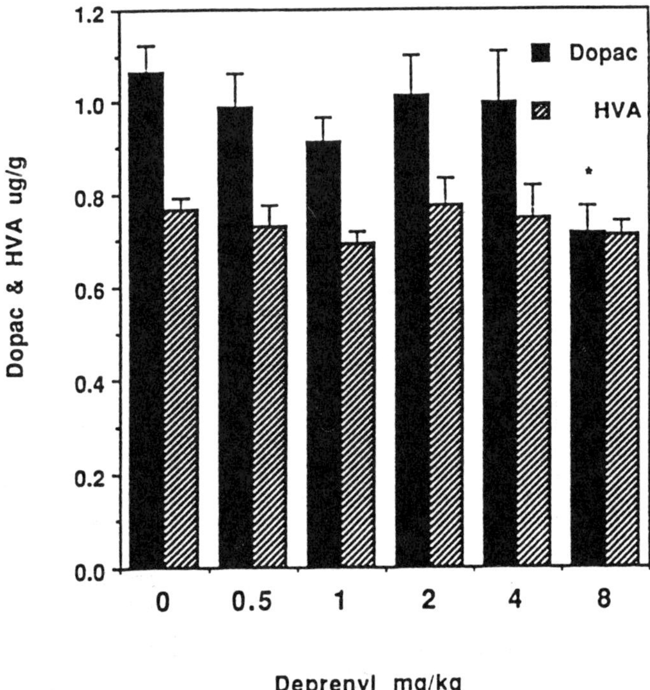

Figure 4. Effect of different doses of deprenyl on DOPAC and HVA in rat caudate nucleus. See ref. 51 for further details.

Table 4.
Effect of Unilateral Lesions of Substantia Nigra on Rat Striatal PE and DA in Deprenyl Treated Rats[a]

	PE (ng/g)	DA (mg/g)
6-OHDA lesion		
Control	14.9	10.4
Lesion	8.2[b]	3.1[b]
Electrolytic lesion		
Control	11.6	9.3
Lesion	7.3[b]	3.0[b]

[a]Data taken from ref. 55.
[b]Significantly different from control.

Table 5.
Effect of Reserpine on Striatal PE and DA Levels in Rat[a]

	Dopamine (% control)	Phenylethylamine (% control)
Reserpine		
1 mg/kg, 2 hr	43[b]	127
10 mg/kg, 2 hr	2.2[b]	80
Deprenyl, 2mg/kg, 4 hr + 1 mg/kg, 2 hr	37.8[b]	130.3[b]
+		
Reserpine, 2 mg/kg, 4hr + 10 mg/kg, 2hr	2.1[b]	196.7[b]

[a]Taken from ref. 56.
[b]Values significantly different from appropriate controls.

Table 6.
Effect of Some Antipsychotic Drugs on Striatal PE Levels in MAOI-Treated Mice[a]

	Phenylethylamine (% control)
Pargyline (2 mg/kg, 4 hr)	100
Pargyline (low) + chlorpromazine (2 mg/kg, 4 hr; 2 mg/kg, 2 hr)	140[b]
Pargyline (high) + chlorpromazine (200 mg/kg, 4 hr; 2 mg/kg, 2 hr)	151[b]
Pargyline + fluphenazine (2 mg/kg, 4 hr, 0.2 mg/kg, 2 hr)	150[b]
Pargyline + spirerone (2 mg/kg, 4 hr; 2 mg/kg, 2 hr)	157[b]
Deprenyl (2 mg/kg, 4 hr)	100
Deprenyl + chlorpromazine (2 mg/kg, 4 hr; 2 mg/kg, 2 hr)	156[b]

[a]Taken from ref. 57.
[b]Significantly increased over the MAOI control value.

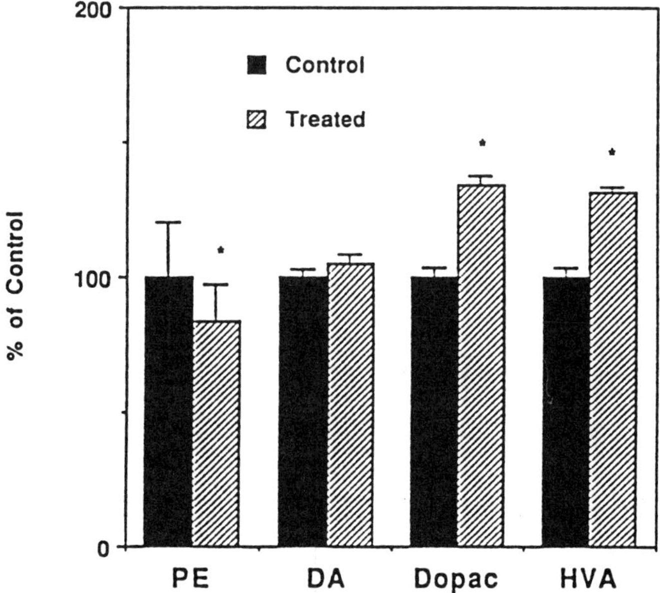

Figure 5. Effect of unilateral SN stimulation on rat striatal PE, DA, DOPAC, and HVA levels. Data taken from ref. 58.

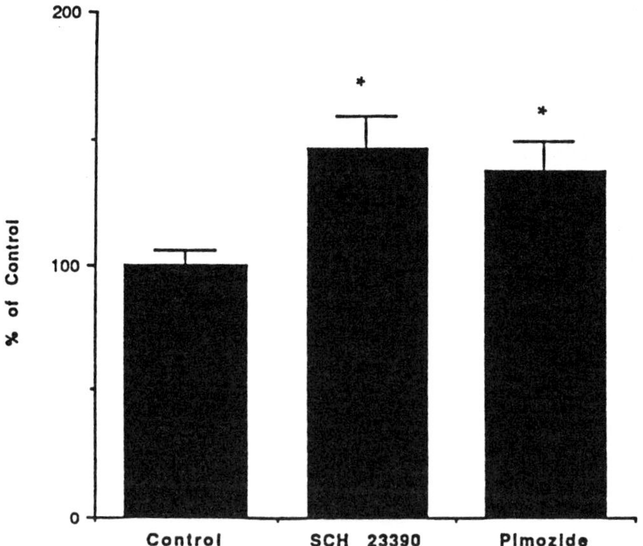

Figure 6. Effect of DA receptor blockers on AAAD activity in the rat striatum. See ref. 52 for further details.

Electrophysiological Effects

Although PE can exhibit conventional inhibitory effects, similar to those of DA and NA, when iontophoresed onto cortical neurons,[53] it is its neuromodulatory effects that seem important and significant. When PE is iontophoresed onto cortical or striatal neurons in amounts that do not by themselves cause any significant effects on spontaneous activity, they do cause substantial potentiation of the effects of simultaneous iontophoresis of the catecholamines (Figures 7 and 8). When the SN is stimulated, iontophoretic or intracarotid injections of PE cause a potentiation (Figures 9 and 10) that is mimicked by deprenyl.[54] PE and deprenyl are similarly effective in potentiating the inhibiting effects of the DA agonists apomorphine and 2-(N-phenethyl-N-propyl)amino-5-hydroxytetralin hydrochloride (PPHT) when they are iontophoresed (Figure 11),[51,54] an effect that is eliminated after treatment with NSD-1015, which blocks the synthesis of PE.

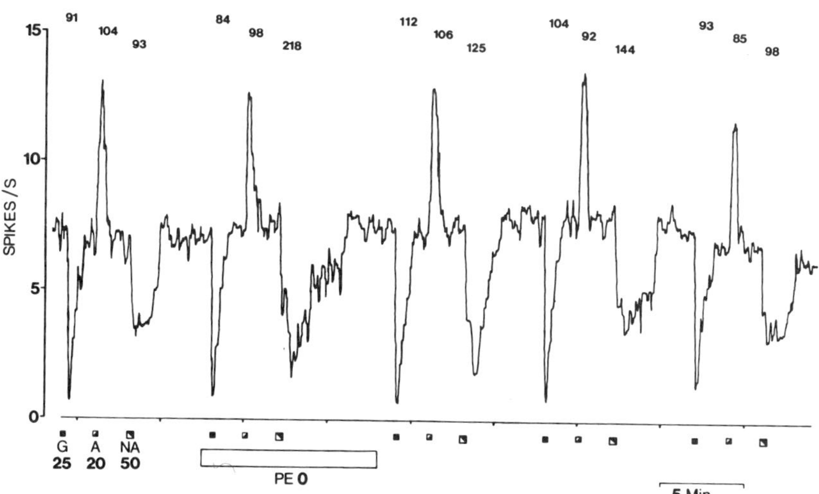

Figure 7. Modulating effect of PE on NA but not GABA or acetylcholine on a cortical cell.

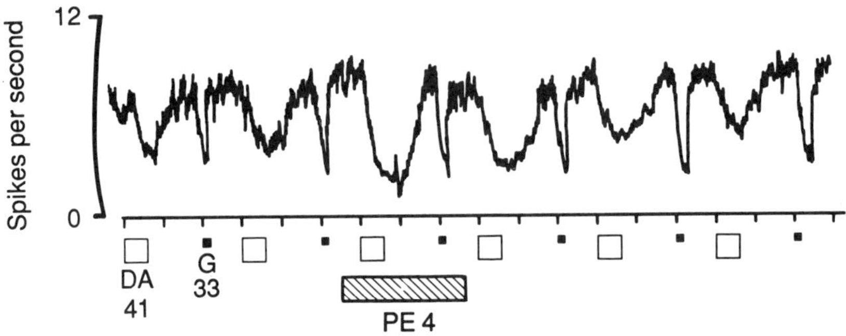

Figure 8.   Modulatory effect of PE to DA but not GABA on a caudate neuron.

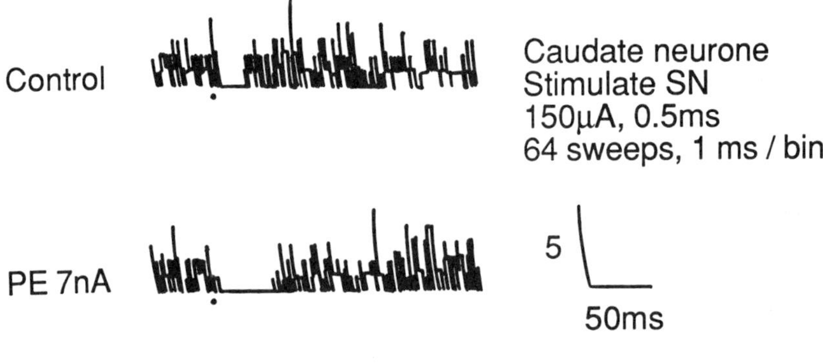

Figure 9.   Peristimulus time histograms of caudate neuron responses to electrical stimulation of substantia nigra.

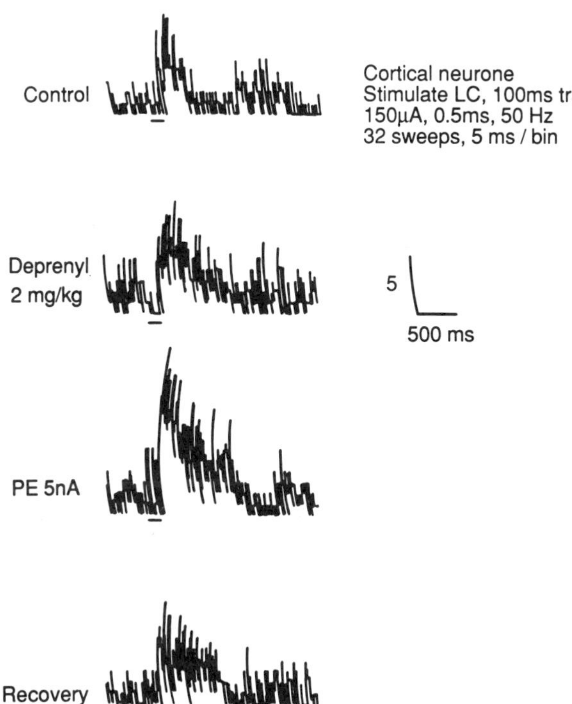

Figure 10.   Effects of deprenyl and PE on peristimulus time histograms of cortical neuron responses to electrical stimulation of locus ceruleus.

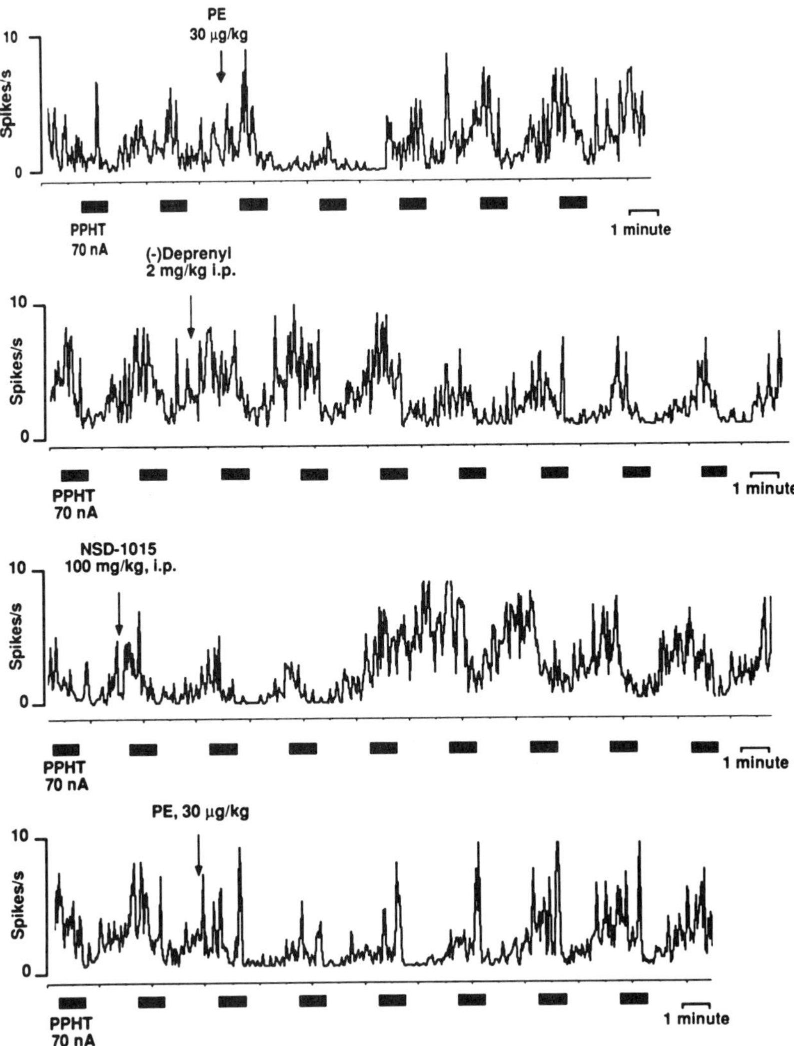

Figure 11. Modulatory effects of PE, deprenyl, and NSD-1015 to PPHT on a caudate neuron. See refs. 51 and 54 for further details.

Hypothesis

Figure 12 illustrates the way in which we think PE acts as a neuromodulator of dopaminergic transmission. Briefly DA is synthesized, stored, and released from the nerve terminal in a Ca^{2+}-dependent manner and in the synaptic cleft acts on pre- and postsynaptic receptors in the usual way. PE is synthesized from phenylalanine by the action of AADC; it is not stored and diffuses out of the terminal into the synaptic cleft; it is metabolized to PAA by the action of MAO-B, which exists only in the glia. In the synaptic gap PE potentiates, probably at the postsynaptic site, the actions of DA but in a way that we do not yet understand. It is also suggested that the extent of activation of the presynaptic DA receptor controls the synthesis of PE so that when DA levels decrease, as in Parkinson's disease or during DA receptor blockade, L-AADC is activated, thus increasing the synthesis and level of PE in the terminal and synaptic

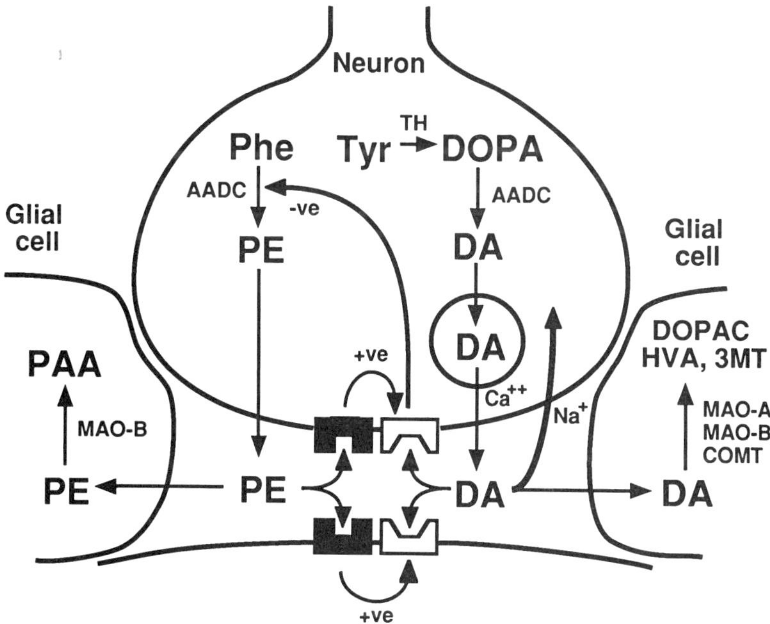

Figure 12. Schematic representation of the neuromodulatory actions of PE on DA transmission.

gap. It is clear that the MAO-B blocker deprenyl will similarly increase PE levels by preventing its breakdown, thus amplifying the synaptic actions of DA. Clearly further studies will be required before these neuromodulatory actions of PE are understood and, additionally, it will be important to establish whether chronic deprenyl treatment acts as does an acute dose.

Acknowledgments: We thank the *Journal of Neurochemistry* for permission to reproduce Tables 1 and 2 and Figures 8 and 12, Pergamon Press for Figures 9–11, and Saskatchewan Health and the Canadian Medical Research Council for continuing financial support.

References

1. Durden DA, Philips SR, Boulton AA. 1973. Identification and distribution of β-phenylethylamine in the rat. Can J Biochem 51:995–1003.
2. Boulton AA, Juorio AV. 1982. Brain trace amines. *In* Handbook of Neurochemistry I. A Lajtha (ed). Plenum Press, New York, pp 189–222.
3. Paterson IA, Juorio AV, Boulton AA. 1990. 2-Phenylethylamine: A modulator of catecholamine transmission in the mammalian central nervous system? J Neurochem 55:1827–1837.
4. Usdin E, Sandler M (eds). 1976. Trace Amines and the Brain. Marcel Dekker Inc., New York.
5. Saavedra JM. 1974. Enzymatic isotopic assay for the presence of β-phenylethylamine in brain. J Neurochem 26:1359–1365.
6. Wu PH, Boulton AA. 1975. Metabolism, distribution and disappearance of injected β-phenylethylamine in the rat. Can J Biochem 53:42–50.
7. Dyck LE. 1983. Release of monoamines from striatal slices by phenelzine and β-phenylethylamine. Prog Neuropsychopharmacol Biol Psychiatr 7:797–800.
8. Durden DA, Philips SR. 1980. Kinetic measurements of the turnover rates of phenylethylamine and tryptamine in vivo in rat brain. J Neurochem 34:1725–1732.
9. Yang H-YT, Neff NH. 1973. β-Phenylethylamine: A specific substrate for type B monoamine oxidase of brain. J Pharmacol Exp Ther 187:365–371.
10. Yu PH. 1986. Monoamine oxidase. *In* Neuromethods, Vol. 5: Neurotransmitter Enzymes. AA Boulton, GB Baker, PH Yu (eds). Humana Press, New Jersey, pp. 235–272.
11. Boulton AA. 1974. Amines and theories in psychiatry. Lancet 2:7871.
12. Boulton AA. 1976. Cerebral aryl alkyl aminergic mechanisms. *In* Trace Amines and the Brain, Vol. I. E Usdin, M Sandler (eds). Marcel Dekker Inc., New York, pp. 22–29.
13. Jones RSG, Boulton AA. 1980. Interactions between *p*-tyramine, *m*-tyramine or β-phenylethylamine and dopamine on single neurones in the cortex and caudate nucleus of the rat. Can J Physiol Pharmacol 58:222–227.

14. Paterson IA, Boulton AA. 1988. β-Phenylethylamine enhances single cortical neurone responses to noradrenaline in the rat. Brain Res Bull 20:173–177.

15. Paterson IA. 1988. An interaction between β-phenylethylamine and noradrenaline: An iontophoretic study in the rat cerebral cortex. *In* Trace Amines. Comparative and Clinical Neurobiology. AA Boulton, AV Juorio, RGH Downer (eds). Human Press, New Jersey, pp. 201–212.

16. Paterson IA. 1988. The potentiation of cortical neurone responses to noradrenaline by β-phenylethylamine: Effects of lesions of the locus coeruleus. Neurosci Lett 87:139–144.

17. Juorio AV, Paterson IA, Boulton AA. 1991. The effect of MAO-type B inhibition on rat striatal dopamine and 2-phenylethylamine. Canadian College of Neuropsychopharmacology Meeting, p. 37, Hamilton, Ontario.

18. Boulton AA. 1991. Phenylethylaminergic modulation of catecholaminergic neurotransmission. Prog Neuro-psychopharmacol Biol Psychiatr 15:139–156.

19. Paterson IA, Juorio AV, Boulton AA. 1990. Possible mechanism of action of deprenyl in parkinsonism. Lancet 2:183.

20. Durden DA, Boulton AA. 1982. Mass spectrometric analysis of some neurotransmitters and their precursors and metabolites. *In* Handbook of Neurochemistry, Vol. 2. A Lajtha (ed). Plenum Press, New York, pp. 397–428.

21. Durden DA, Davis BA. 1991. Analytical methods for the quantitation of trace amines in physiological fluids and neurological tissues. *In* Methods in Biogenic Amine Research. M Naoi, T Nagatsu, H Parvez (eds). Elsevier Publishers, Amsterdam (in press).

22. Willner J, LeFevre HF, Costa E. 1974. Assay by multiple ion detection of phenylethylamine and phenylethanolamine in rat brain. J Neurochem 23:857–859.

23. Szymanski HV, Naylor EW, Karoum F. 1987. Plasma phenylethylamine and phenylethylamine in chronic schizophrenic patients. Biol Psychiatry 22:194–198.

24. Durden DA. 1991. An evaluation of the negative ion mass spectra of electron capturing derivatives of the biogenic trace amines: I. Phenylethylamine. Biol Mass Spec 20:367–374.

25. Durden DA, Davis BA, Boulton AA. 1991. Quantification of plasma phenylethylamine by electron capture negative ion gas chromatography-mass spectrometry of the *N*-acetyl-*N*-pentafluorobenzoyl derivative. Biol Mass Spec 20:375–381.

26. O'Reilly R, Davis BA, Durden DA, Thorpe L, Machnee H, Boulton AA. 1991. Plasma phenylethylamine in schizophrenic patients. Biol Psychiat 30:145–150.

27. Lauber J, Waldmeier PC. 1984. Determination of 2-phenylethylamine in rat brain after MAO inhibition and in human csf and urine by capillary column GC and chemical ionization MS. J Neural Transm 60:247–264.

28. Edwards DJ, Blau K. 1972. Analysis of phenylethylamines in biological

tissues by gas-liquid chromatography with electron capture detection. Anal Biochem 45:387–402.

29. Davis BA. 1990. Biogenic Monoamines and their Metabolites in the Urine, Plasma and Cerebrospinal Fluid of Normal, Psychiatric and Neurological Subjects. CRC Press, Boca Raton, Florida, pp. 1–444.

30. Sabelli HC, Fawcett J, Gusovsky F, Javaid J, Edwards J, Jeffriess H. 1983. Urinary phenylacetate: A diagnostic test for depression. Science 220:1187–1188.

31. De Lisi LE, Murphy DL, Karoum F, Mueller E, Targum S, Wyatt RJ. 1984. Phenylethylamine excretion in depression. Psychiatry Res 13:193–201.

32. Gonzalez-Sastre F, Mora J, Guillamat R, Queralto JM, Alvarez E, Udina C, Massana J. 1988. Urinary phenylacetic acid excretion in depressive patients. Acta Psychiatr Scand 78:208–210.

33. Davis BA, Boulton AA, Yu PH, Durden DA, Keegan DL, Bowen RC, Blackshaw S, D'Arcy C, Remillard AJ, Dayal N, Shrikhande S, Saleh S, Stegeman GH, Paterson IA. 1991. Longitudinal effect of amitriptyline and fluoxetine treatment plasma phenylacetic acid concentrations in depression. Biol Psychiat 30:600–608.

34. Yu PH, Bowen RC, Davis BA, Boulton AA. 1983. Platelet monoamine oxidase activity and trace acid levels in plasma of agoraphobic patients. Acta Psychiatr Scand 67:188–194.

35. Potkin SG, Karoum F, Chuang L-W, Cannon-Spoor HE, Philips I, Wyatt RJ. 1979. Phenylethylamine in paranoid chronic schizophrenia. Science 206:470–471.

36. Jeste DV, Poongaji DR, Panjwani D, Datta M, Potkin SG, Karoum F, Thatte S, Sheth AS, Apte JS, Wyatt RJ. 1980. Cross-cultural study of a biochemical abnormality in paranoid schizophrenia. Psychiatry Res 3:341–352.

37. Yoshimoto S, Kaku H, Shimogawa S, Watanabe A, Nakagawara M, Takahashi R. 1987. Urinary trace amine excretion and platelet MAO activity in schizophrenia. Psychiatry Res 21:229–236.

38. Beckman H, Reynolds GP, Sandler M, Waldmeier P, Lauber J, Riederer P, Gattaz WF. 1982. Phenylethylamine and phenylacetic acid in csf of schizophrenic and healthy controls. Arch Psychiatr Nervenkr 232:463–471.

39. Davis BA. 1989. Biogenic amines and their metabolites in body fluids of normal, psychiatric and neurological subjects. J Chromatogr 466:89–218.

40. Boulton AA, Davis BA, Yu PH, Wormith JS, Addington D. 1983. Trace acid levels in the plasma and MAO activity in the platelets of violent offenders. Psychiatry Res 8:19–23.

41. Yu PH, Davis BA, Gordon A, Reid DM, Green C, Boulton AA. 1986. Biochemical links to aggressive psychopathy. *In* Biological Psychiatry 1985. C Shagrass, WH Bridger, D Stoff, R Josiassen, K Weiss, GM Simpson (eds). Elsevier Science Publishing, New York, pp 341–343.

42. Davis BA, Yu PH, Pease K, Green C, Menzies R, Gordon A, Durden DA,

Templeman R, Boulton AA. 1991. Longitudinal study of inmates of a prison for the psychiatrically disturbed: Plasma concentrations of biogenic amine metabolites and amino acids. Psychiatry Res 36:85–97.

43. Philips SR, Boulton AA. 1979. The effect of monoamine oxidase inhibitors on some arylalkylamines in rat striatum. J Neurochem 33:159–167.

44. Dyck LE, Juorio AV, Durden DA, Boulton AA. 1988. Effect of chronic deuterated and non-deuterated phenelzine on rat brain monoamines and MAO. NS Arch Pharmacol 337:279–283.

45. The Parkinson Study Group. 1989. Effect of deprenyl on the progression of disability in early Parkinson's disease (DATATOP) N Engl J Med 321:1364–1371.

46. Tetrud JW, Langston JW. 1989. The effect of deprenyl (Selegiline) on the natural history of Parkinson's disease. Science 245:519–522.

47. Tatton W. 1991. Modulation of nigrostriatal abiotrophy. 3rd Canadian Conference on Neurodegenerative Diseases, Montreal, 1991.

48. Knoll J, Dallo J, Yen TT. 1989. Striatal dopamine sexual activity and lifespan longevity of rats treated with (−)-deprenyl. Life Sci 45:525–531.

49. Milgram NW, Racine RJ, Nellis P, Mendonca A, Ivy GO. 1990. Maintenance on L-deprenyl prolongs life in aged male rats. Life Sci 47:415–420.

50. Juorio AV, Paterson IA, Boulton AA. 1991. The effect of MAO-type B inhibition on rat striatal DA and PE. Canadian College of Neuropsychopharmacology Meeting, p 37.

51. Paterson IA, Juorio AV, Berry MD, Zhu MY. 1992. Inhibition of monoamine oxidase-B by (−)-deprenyl potentiates neuronal responses to dopamine agonists but does not inhibit dopamine catabolism in the rat striatum. J Pharmacol Exp Ther (in press).

52. Zhu MY, Juorio AV, Paterson IA, Boulton AA. 1992. The regulation of aromatic L-amino acid decarboxylase by dopamine receptors in the rat brain. J Neurochem 58:636–641.

53. Henwood RW, Boulton AA, Phillis JW. 1979. Iontophoretic studies of some trace amines in the mammalian CNS. Brain Res 164:347–351.

54. Berry MD, Paterson IA. 1990. Deprenyl and PE potentiate neuronal responses to a D2 agonist. Canadian College of Neuropsychopharmacology Meeting, Banff Alberta, 1990, p. 59.

55. Greenshaw AJ, Juorio AV, Nguyen T-V. 1986. Depletion of striatal β-phenylethylamine following dopamine but not 5-HT denervation. Brain Res Bull 17:477–484.

56. Juorio AV, Greenshaw AJ, Wishart TB. 1988. Reciprocal changes in striatal dopamine and β-phenylethylamine induced by reserpine in the presence of monoamine oxidase inhibitors. Naunyn-Schmiedeberg's Arch Pharmacol 338:644–648.

57. Juorio AV, Greenshaw AJ, Zhu M-Y, Paterson IA. 1991. The effects of some neuroleptics and d-amphetamine in striatal 2-phenylethylamine in the mouse. Gen Pharmacol 22(2):407–413.

58. Juorio AV, Paterson IA, Zhu MY, Matte G. 1990. Electrical stimulation of the substantia nigra and changes in 2-PE synthesis in the rat striatum. J Neurochem 56:213–220.
59. Dyck LE. 1989. Release of some endogenous trace amines from rat striatal slices in the presence and absence of MAOIs. Life Sci 44:1149–1156.

Chapter 6

MPTP, Mitochondrial Inhibition, and Parkinson's Disease

William J. Nicklas, Michael Saporito, and Richard E. Heikkila

The neurotoxicant, 1-methyl-4-phenyl-1,2,3,6-tetrahydropyridine (MPTP), causes a parkinsonian syndrome in humans[1,2] and a relatively selective destruction of nigrostriatal dopaminergic neurons in monkeys[3–5] and in other animal species including mice.[6–8] The mechanism(s) by which this toxicity is engendered has been elaborated by studies in laboratories throughout the world. Our laboratories, as well as others, have suggested that MPTP-induced cell death is associated ultimately with the ability of the pyridinium, 1-methyl-4-phenylpyridinium (MPP$^+$), formed from MPTP by the action of MAO-B, to inhibit the electron transport system of mitochondria at complex I within dopaminergic neurons of the nigrostriatal pathway.[9–15] Thus, this inhibition of mitochondrial oxidation results in depletion of ATP within affected cells, thereby directly contributing to cell death. It is the purpose of this chapter to review the status of these studies and place them in the context of current studies on the possible involvement of mitochondrial pathology in Parkinson's disease (PD).

From Hefti F, and Weiner WJ, (eds.) *Progress in Parkinson's Disease Research—2.* Mount Kisco NY, Futura Publishing Co., Inc., © 1992.

MPTP is a Protoxin: MPP$^+$ is the True Toxic Species

Soon after the discovery that MPTP caused a parkinsonian syndrome in humans and experimental animals, the question was raised whether MPTP was the actual toxic agent. It was shown that the MPP$^+$ species was the major metabolite of MPTP found in brains of experimental animals and that the enzyme MAO-B was responsible for this transformation.[16,17] The formation of MPP$^+$ from MPTP occurred in two steps, an initial MAO catalyzed oxidation to a dihydropyridinium intermediate and subsequent oxidation to MPP$^+$. MPTP-induced neurotoxicity was prevented and MPP$^+$ formation was decreased substantially in experimental animals by inhibitors of MAO-B, suggesting that the enzyme-catalyzed oxidation of MPTP is a necessary step in the neurotoxic process.[18,19] Studies in our and other laboratories with many analogs of MPTP have shown conclusively that this bioactivation by MAO is necessary for toxicity and has produced several potent MPTP analogs that utilize MAO-A rather than MAO-B.[20] Moreover, small amounts of MPP$^+$ stereotaxically injected into rat brain cause a profound lesion, indicating its potent toxicity.[21] MPP$^+$ and its analogs are also potent toxins in a variety of tissue culture model systems.[22] Thus there is an overwhelming consensus that the pyridiniums formed from MAO-catalyzed oxidation of the tetrahydropyridines are the true neurotoxic agents.

Selectivity of MPTP for Dopaminergic Neurons is Partly Determined by Affinity of MPP$^+$ for Dopaminergic Carrier

An explanation for the relative specificity of MPTP for the nigrostriatal dopaminergic system remains somewhat controversial, but there seems to be a major role for the uptake of MPP$^+$ by the dopaminergic carrier system. MPP$^+$ has been shown to be a substrate for the dopamine carrier,[23] and inhibitors of this uptake system prevent the neurotoxicity of MPTP (see ref. 20 for discussion). Moreover, only those tetrahydropyridines whose pyridiniums are good substrates for the dopamine carrier have dopaminergic neurotoxicity.[20] Problems remain with the relative specificity for the nigrostriatal system. For example, it is not completely clear why the dopaminergic neurons of the limbic system are not similarly affected.

It may be that the absolute number of uptake sites are different in the two areas, but this remains to be explored more completely. It may also be that the nigrostriatal neurons are more susceptible to the mechanism of toxicity of MPP$^+$ and its analogs than are some other neurons. Certainly from the tissue culture models it is apparent that the metabolic requirements of the neurons (i.e., glycolytic or aerobic oxidation) may play a major role (see refs. 22 and 28). The latter may also have implications for the current findings that mitochondria might be implicated in the pathology of PD (see below).

Evidence that Mitochondrial Inhibition is the Ultimate Cause of Cell Death

The necessity for bioactivation of MPTP and its toxic analogs via MAO and the accumulation of resulting pyridiniums via the dopaminergic carrier now seems well supported by relevant experiments. However, early on it was not very clear how these pyridiniums might cause cell death. One theory proposed was that of oxidative stress but consistent correlative evidence for this hypothesis has remained elusive. Since MAO isozymes are known to be localized to the outer mitochondrial membrane, we hypothesized that MPTP or its metabolic products might exert some negative effects on mitochondrial function. In subsequent experiments, it was found that MPP$^+$, but not MPTP, inhibited ADP-stimulated respiration.[13] Moreover, only respiration linked to substrates such as pyruvate, glutamate, or β-hydroxybutyrate were affected. This suggested that complex I (NADH dehydrogenase) activity was selectively inhibited. The oxidation of substrates for complexes further down the electron transport chain such as succinate or TMPD plus ascorbate[13] were unaffected by concentrations of MPP$^+$ that completely inhibited NADH-linked oxidation. The inhibition was both time and concentration dependent. MPP$^+$ worked as an inhibitor in both brain and liver mitochondria with similar potency, suggesting that it was a general inhibitor of NADH dehydrogenase similar to the classical inhibitor, rotenone. However, rotenone acts instantaneously when incubated with mitochondria and is several orders of magnitude more inhibitory than MPP$^+$. In vivo studies showed that rotenone, like MPP$^+$ produces lesions when injected stereotaxically into rat brain, demonstrating that inhibition of complex I is sufficient to cause toxicity.[21] The concentrations of MPP[+] needed to inhibit complex I activity were rather high (e.g., 200 μM MPP[+] inhibits by 50% with an incubation time of 4 minutes). Most probably for the latter reason, these results were not immediately accepted. The demonstration by Javitch et al.[23] that MPP[+] could be accumulated by the dopamine transporter gave a rationale for the ability of a dopaminergic cell to accumulate sufficient pyridinium to inhibit the mitochondria. Furthermore, the elegant studies of Ramsay, Singer, and their colleagues showed that MPP[+] was actively accumulated by mitochondria (see ref. 24 for review). Thus, mitochondria in dopaminergic cells potentially could accumulate large concentrations of MPP[+], sufficient to inhibit mitochondrial respiration. Other laboratories have also contributed greatly to our knowledge of the mitochondrial inhibition by MPP[+] and its analogs.[9,11,12] It should also be noted that this mitochondrial focus does not rule out some role for oxidative stress, because inhibition of respiration in this way can itself increase the formation of oxygen radicals by the mitochondrial electron transport chain.

It was important to demonstrate that this effect of MPP[+] on mitochondria was not simply an artifact of this in vitro system, which had nothing to do with the effects of MPTP on intact brain tissue. Therefore, we also developed the striatal tissue slice model of MPTP toxicity.[10,25,26] The reasoning was as follows: if NADH dehydrogenase is inhibited by MPP[+], mitochondrial and cytoplasmic pools of NADH should become reduced, glycolysis increased to produce more ATP, both phenomena resulting in an increase in lactate production. Using the striatal slice one should be able to examine MPTP-induced metabolic inhibition, bypassing the possible artifacts of looking at mitochondria alone. This indeed proved to be the case; MPP[+] and certain of its analogs induced increased lactate production by striatal slices. Moreover, MPTP and certain analogs were effective in inducing lactate formation in mouse striatal slices at concentrations similar to that found in brain after in vivo administration. That this effect in inducing lactate formation occurs via MPP[+] is shown by the inhibition of this phenomenon in slices prepared from animals that were predosed with the MAO-B inhibitor, deprenyl. Using this preparation we have also been able to approach answering the critical question of whether metabolic inhibition actually occurs in the dopaminergic nerve endings of the striatum when presented with MPTP.[26] Dopamine uptake blockers attenuated the increased lactate production caused by MPTP or other analogs of MPTP. At low concentrations of the more potent analog, 2'-Me-MPTP (<5 μM), increased lactate was inhibited completely by dopamine uptake blockers. These data suggested that at low concentrations of MPTP, comparable to that found in brain after peripheral MPTP administration, the increased lactate accumulation was associated primarily with dopaminergic nerve terminals. Selective doses of norepinephrine or serotonin uptake blockers did not attenuate this lactate accumulation. Lactate formation promoted by low concentrations of 2'-Me-MPTP was also significantly attenuated in neostriatal tissue slices prepared from mice or rats with a lesion of the nigrostriatal pathway. All of these results are consistent with the hypothesis that tetrahydropyridine-promoted inhibition of mitochondrial respiration does indeed occur within dopaminergic nerve terminals. Moreover, this system seems to be selectively affected when the slices are incubated with low concentrations of the tetrahydropyridines.

The proposition that inhibition of mitochondrial metabolism is responsible for the cell death has also been confirmed using the potentiation caused by a novel agent, tetraphenylboron anion (TPB) (see ref. 27 for details and background references). TPB can potentiate the inhibitory actions on isolated mitochondria of MPP^+ and its analogs 50- to 1000-fold (Table 1). Indeed analogs that are

Table 1.
MPP^+ Analogs as Mitochondrial Inhibitors: Potentiation by Tetrahydropyridine Anion (TPB)[a]

	IC_{50} value (μM)		Potentiation by TPB
Compound	−TPB	+TPB	
MPP^+	193	2.6	75
4'-Fluoro-MPP^+	415	5.5	75
4'-Methyl-MPP^+	62	1.3	50
N-Methyl-(4-t-butyl)pyridinium	7400	7.0	1000
N,N-dimethyl-$MPTP^+$	>20,000	67	>300

[a]Mouse liver mitochondria were incubated with 2.5 mM glutamate-malate for 2 minutes, then MPP^+ analogs added for 1 minute, followed by 10 μM TPB. After 5 minutes of further incubation, ADP was added to initiate state 3.

essentially impotent in producing inhibition [e.g., N-methyl-(4-t-butyl)pyridinium on N,N-dimethyl-MPTP$^+$] even at mM concentration, in the presence of TPB, become potent in the low μM range. Part of this potentiation is due to an enhancement of the mitochondrial accumulation of the organic cations, but this does not fully account for the tremendous potentiation. The interaction of these analogs with the inhibitory site within the mitochondria is somehow directly enhanced by TPB. This lipophilic anion also increased the amount of lactate formed during the incubation of neostriatal tissue slices with MPTP and other tetrahydropyridines.[27] In addition, TPB enhanced the toxic effect of MPTP analogs on cultured PC12 cells as well as the dopaminergic neurotoxicity of MPTP in mice.[27] Again, all of these observations, taken together, support the hypothesis that the inhibition of mitochondrial metabolism by MPP$^+$ underlies the neurotoxicity of MPTP.

Dopaminergic Toxicity of MPP$^+$ Analogs in Cultured Neurons

To further understand the relative roles of the dopaminergic uptake system and the inhibition of mitochondrial respiration in mediating the specificity and potency of toxicity, a variety of structural analogs of MPP$^+$ have been tested using a cultured mesencephalic neuronal model. Several laboratories, including our own, have previously shown that MPP$^+$ and its analogs, as well as MPTP analogs, are potent and selective neurotoxins in this model system.[28,29] In Table 2 the potencies of several examples of these analogs to inhibit mitochondrial respiration and to act as substrates for the dopamine uptake system are given. The potency of each of these compounds is compared in this table to that of MPP$^+$ itself. Other studies have indicated that the ability of these compounds to release preloaded radioactive dopamine is a carrier-mediated process and therefore correlates with the relative potency of these compounds as substrates for the dopamine transporter. As can be seen from Table 2, some compounds are equipotent with MPP$^+$ in both properties (e.g., 2'-Me-MPP$^+$), some are less potent than MPP$^+$ as substrates for the carrier but equipotent or more potent than MPP$^+$ as mitochondrial inhibitors (e.g., 2'-fluoro-MPP$^+$ and 3'-Me-MPP$^+$), some are not substrates for the carrier at all but are very potent

Table 2.
Potencies of MPP⁺ Analogs in Causing Release of [³H]Dopamine from Neostriatal Synaptosomes and as Inhibitors of Mitochondrial Respiration

Compound	Relative Release Capacity[a]	Relative Inhibitory Activity[b]
MPP⁺	100	100
2'-Methyl-MPP⁺	172	98
2'-Fluoro-MPP⁺	55	111
3'-Methyl-MPP⁺	29	238
4'-Propyl-MPP⁺	<8	2800
MPPyrim	39	<0.01
M(4tBu)P⁺	<8	<0.04

[a]Mouse striatal synaptosomes were loaded with [³H]dopamine for 10 minutes. The preloaded synaptosomes were preincubated for 5 minutes and then MPP⁺ or analogs added at 0.1–10 μM. After 10 minutes of incubation, the synaptosomes were filtered and radioactivity remaining on filter measured. MPPyrim is N-methyl-(4-phenyl)-pyrimidinium species and M(4tBu)P⁺ is N-methyl-(4-tert-butyl)pyridinium species. Values given are percentages of the EC_{50} for MPP⁺, which was 0.81 $\pm$ 0.16 μM.
[b]Mouse liver mitochondria were preincubated for 6 minutes with 5 mM glutamate-malate with or without MPP⁺ or its analogs. ADP was then added, and state 3 oxygen uptake measured. The relative activity is calculated as a percentage of the IC_{50} for MPP⁺, which was 112 $\pm$ 5 μM in this series of studies.

mitochondrial inhibitors (e.g., 4'-propyl-MPP⁺), and, finally, some are weak or impotent in both properties [e.g., N-methyl-(4-phenyl)-pyrimidinium and N-methyl-(4-t-butyl)pyridinium]. These compounds produce a neurotoxic pattern in mesencephalic cultures consistent with these disparate properties (Table 3). Analogs that are similar to MPP⁺ as both dopamine releasing agents and mitochondrial inhibitors (2'Me-MPP⁺), or are somewhat weaker as dopamine releasing agents, but potent as mitochondrial blockers (2'-fluoro-MPP⁺ and 3'-Me-MPP⁺), are, like MPP⁺, potent and selective dopaminergic toxins; the GABAergic system is unaffected at concentrations of pyridiniums that are toxic to the dopamine cells. Analogs that are very poor as dopamine releasing agents but very potent as mitochondrial inhibitors (e.g., 4'-propyl-MPP⁺) are potent but nonselective neurotoxins. Compounds that are not mitochondrial inhibitors and are either weak [N-methyl-(4-phenyl)-pyrimidinium] or impotent [N-methyl-(4-t-butyl)pyridinium] as dopamine releas-

Table 3.
Neurotoxic Potency of MPP$^+$ and Analogs in Cultured Dopaminergic and GABAergic Neurons[a]

Compound	$LD_{50}^{DA}(\mu M)$	Relative DA Toxicity	$LD_{50}^{GABA}(\mu M)$	$LD_{50}^{GABA}/LD_{50}^{DA}$
MPP$^+$	0.6	100	>30	>49
2'-Methyl-MPP$^+$	0.2	370	>30	>182
2'-Fluoro-MPP$^+$	1.6	30	>30	>16
3'-Methyl-MPP$^+$	1.6	40	>30	>19
4'-Propyl-MPP$^+$	1.6	40	7.3	4.7
MPPyrim	>100	<1	>100	
M(4tBu)P$^+$	>30	<2	>30	

[a]Mesencephalic cultures were exposed to various concentrations of MPP$^+$ or analogs in culture medium for 24 hours prior to assessing damage by measuring simultaneous uptake of [^{3}H]dopamine and [^{14}C]GABA. LD_{50} values were obtained from plots of percent loss of uptake vs analog concentration. Values are expressed as mean of three to four experiments. Abbreviations are as in Table 2.

ing agents are not neurotoxins at all. These data support the hypothesis that affinity for the dopaminergic carrier is necessary for MPP$^+$ analogs to be selective dopaminergic neurotoxins. These studies offer strong support for the hypothesis that the critical event in neuronal death caused by MPP$^+$ and its analogs is the inhibition of mitochondrial respiration.

MPTP, Mitochondria, and Parkinson's Disease

Although MPTP has proven to be a fruitful experimental tool in animal studies as a model of PD, the relevance of the findings with MPTP to furnishing an etiology for human PD has been questionable. The recent DATATOP study using the MAO-B inhibitor, deprenyl, was based in part on the proposition that an MPTP-like substance might be involved in PD,[30] but its utility could also be due to its dopamine sparing properties. In any case, as we have demonstrated, compounds have been developed that are bioactivated by MAO-A and are as toxic as MPTP, if not more so, in animal studies. However, great excitement has been engendered by recent reports that suggest that PD patients have altered activities of the electron transport system, especially in complex I. Schapira et al.[31] reported activities of various respiratory chain components in homogenates of autopsied substantia nigra. Compared to control patients, in PD they found a substantial decrease in the activities of rotenone sensitive NADH CoQ reductase but not of succinate cytochrome c reductase, clearly suggesting an alteration of complex I. Others have reported decreases in specific polypeptides of complex I in PD.[32] Decreases in complex I activity have even been reported in platelet mitochondria from idiopathic PD patients.[33] These results are extremely provocative. The specificity of these changes and whether they are primary to the disease or secondary to the degenerative processes remain to be demonstrated. If these data prove reproducible and relatively specific to PD, they indicate a new direction to take in examining the possible etiology of PD. It may be that these are genetic factors predisposing to PD or, indeed, endogenous MPP^+-like compounds may be overexpressed in PD brain.[34]

Acknowledgments: This contribution is also dedicated to the memory of our late friend and colleague, Dick Heikkila, who was a major contributor to much of what is discussed in this chapter.

References

1. Davis GC, Williams AC, Markey SP, Ebert MH, Caine CD, Reichert CM, Kopin IJ. 1979. Chronic parkinsonism secondary to intravenous injection of meperidine analogues. Psychiatry Res 1:249–254.
2. Langston JW, Ballard P, Tetrud JW, Irwin I. 1983. Chronic parkinsonism in humans due to a product of meperidine analog synthesis. Science 219:979–980.
3. Burns RS, Chiueh CC, Markey SP, Ebert MH, Jacobowitz DM, Kopin IJ. 1983. A primate model of parkinsonism: Selective destruction of dopaminergic neurons in the pars compacta of the substantia nigra by *N*-methyl-4-phenyl-1,2,3,6-tetrahydropyridine. Proc Natl Acad Sci USA 80:4546–4550.
4. Elsworth JD, Deutch AY, Redmond DE Jr, Sladek JR, Roth RH. 1987. Effects of 1-methyl-4-phenyl-1,2,3,6-tetrahydropyridine (MPTP) on catecholamines and metabolites in primate brain and CSF. Brain Res 415:293–299.
5. German DC, Dubach M, Askari S, Speciale SG, Bowden DM. 1988. 1-Methyl-4-phenyl-1,2,3,6-tetrahydropyridine-induced parkinsonian syndrome in *Macaca fascicularis:* Which midbrain dopaminergic neurons are lost. Neuroscience 24:161–174.

6. Fuller RW, Hemrick Luecke SK, Perry SK. 1988. Deprenyl antagonizes acute lethality of 1-methyl-4-phenyl-1,2,3,6-tetrahydropyridine in mice. J Pharmacol Exp Ther 247:531–535.

7. Heikkila RE, Hess A, Duvoisin RC. 1984. Dopaminergic neurotoxicity of 1-methyl-4-phenyl-1,2,3,6-tetrahydropyridine in mice. Science 224:1451–1453.

8. Sundstrom E, Stromberg I, Tsutsumi T, Olson L, Jonsson G. 1987. Studies on the effect of 1-methyl-4-phenyl-1,2,3,6-tetrahydropyridine (MPTP) on central catecholamine neurons in C57BL/6 mice. Comparison with three other strains of mice. Brain Res 405:26–38.

9. Hoppel CL, Grinblatt D, Kwok HC, Arora PK, Singh MP, Sayre LM, Greenblatt D. 1987. Inhibition of mitochondrial respiration by analogs of 4-phenylpyridine and 1-methyl-4-phenylpyridinium cation (MPP$^+$), the neurotoxic metabolite of MPTP [published erratum appears in Biochem Biophys Res Commun, Dec 31 1987; 149(3):1220]. Biochem Biophys Res Commun 148:684–693.

10. Kindt MV, Heikkila RE, Nicklas WJ. 1987. Mitochondrial and metabolic toxicity of 1-methyl-4-(2'-methylphenyl)-1,2,3,6-tetrahydropyridine. J Pharmacol Exp Ther 242:858–863.

11. Mizuno Y, Sone N, Saitoh T. 1987. Effects of 1-methyl-4-phenyl-1,2,3,6-tetrahydropyridine and 1-methyl-4-phenylpyridinium ion on activities of the enzymes in the electron transport system in mouse brain. J Neurochem 48:1787–1793.

12. Mizuno Y, Sone N, Suzuki K, Saitoh T. 1988. Studies on the toxicity of 1-methyl-4-phenylpyridinium ion (MPP$^+$) against mitochondria of mouse brain. J Neurol Sci 86:97–110.

13. Nicklas WJ, Vyas I, Heikkila RE. 1985. Inhibition of NADH-linked oxidation in brain mitochondria by 1-methyl-4-phenylpyridine, a metabolite of the neurotoxin, 1-methyl-4-phenyl-1,2,5,6-tetrahydropyridine. Life Sci 36:2503–2508.

14. Ramsay RR, Salach JI, Dadgar J, Singer TP. 1986. Inhibition of mitochondrial NADH dehydrogenase by pyridine derivatives and its possible relation to experimental and idiopathic parkinsonism. Biochem Biophys Res Commun 135:269–275.

15. Ramsay RR, Singer TP. 1986. Energy-dependent uptake of N-methyl-4-phenylpyridinium, the neurotoxic metabolite of 1-methyl-4-phenyl-1,2,3,6-tetrahydropyridine, by mitochondria. J Biol Chem 261:7585–7587.

16. Castagnoli N Jr, Chiba K, Trevor AJ. 1985. Potential bioactivation pathways for the neurotoxin 1-methyl-4-phenyl-1,2,3,6-tetrahydropyridine (MPTP). Life Sci 36:225–230.

17. Chiba K, Trevor AJ, Castagnoli N Jr. 1984. Metabolism of the neurotoxic tertiary amine, MPTP, by brain monoamine oxidase. Biochem Biophys Res Commun 120:574–578.

18. Heikkila RE, Manzino L, Cabbat FS, Duvoisin RC. 1984. Protection against the dopaminergic neurotoxicity of 1-methyl-4-phenyl-1,2,5,6-tetrahydropyridine by monoamine oxidase inhibitors. Nature 311:467–469.

19. Langston JW, Irwin I, Langston EB, Forno LS. 1984. Pargyline prevents MPTP-induced parkinsonism in primates. Science 225:1480–1482.
20. Youngster SK, Nicklas WJ, Heikkila RE. 1989. Structure–activity study of the mechanism of 1-methyl-4-phenyl-1,2,3,6-tetrahydropyridine (MPTP)-induced neurotoxicity II. Evaluation of the biological activity of the pyridinium metabolites formed from the monoamine oxidase-catalyzed oxidation of MPTP analogs. J Pharmacol Exp Ther 249:829–835.
21. Heikkila RE, Nicklas WJ, Vyas I, Duvoisin RC. 1985. Dopaminergic toxicity of rotenone and the 1-methyl-4-phenylpyridinium ion after their stereotaxic administration to rats: Implication for the mechanism of 1-methyl-4-phenyl-1,2,3,6-tetrahydropyridine toxicity. Neurosci Lett 62:389–394.
22. Basma AN, Heikkila RE, Nicklas WJ, Giovanni A, Geller HM. 1990. 1-Methyl-4-(2'-ethylphenyl)-1,2,3,6-tetrahydropyridine-induced toxicity in PC12 cells: Role of monoamine oxidase A. J Neurochem 55:870–877.
23. Javitch JA, D'Amato RJ, Strittmatter SM, Snyder SH. 1985. Parkinsonism-inducing neurotoxin, N-methyl-4-phenyl-1,2,3,6-tetrahydropyridine: Uptake of the metabolite N-methyl-4-phenylpyridine by dopamine neurons explains selective toxicity. Proc Natl Acad Sci USA 82:2173–2177.
24. Ramsay RR, Youngster SK, Nicklas WJ, McKeown KA, Jin YZ, Heikkila RE, Singer TP. 1989. Inhibition of NADH-linked oxidation in brain mitochondria by 1-methyl-4-phenylpyridine, a metabolite of the neurotoxin, 1-methyl-4-phenyl-1,2,5,6-tetrahydropyridine. Proc Natl Acad Sci USA 86:9168–9172.
25. Vyas I, Heikkila RE, Nicklas WJ. 1986. Studies on the neurotoxicity of 1-methyl-4-phenyl-1,2,3,6-tetrahydropyridine: Inhibition of NAD-linked substrate oxidation by its metabolite, 1-methyl-4-phenyl-pyridinium. J Neurochem 46:1501–1507.
26. Ofori S, Heikkila RE, Nicklas WJ. 1989. Attenuation by dopamine uptake blockers of the inhibitory effects of 1-methyl-4-phenyl-1,2,3,6-tetrahydropyridine and some of its analogs on NADH-linked metabolism in mouse neostriatal slices. J Pharmacol Exp Ther 251:258–266.
27. Heikkila RE, Hwang J, Ofori S, Geller HM, Nicklas WJ. 1990. Potentiation by the tetraphenylboron anion of the effects of MPTP and its pyridinium metabolite. J Neurochem 54:743–750.
28. Danias P, Nicklas WJ, Ofori S, Shen J, Mytilineou C. 1989. Mesencephalic dopamine neurons become less sensitive to 1-methyl-4-phenyl-1,2,3,6-tetrahydropyridine toxicity during development in vitro. J Neurochem 53:1149–1155.
29. Michel PP, Dandapani BK, Knusel B, Sanchez-Ramos J, Hefti F. 1990. Toxicity of 1-methyl-4-phenyl pyridinium for rat dopaminergic neurons in culture: Selectivity and irreversibility. J Neurochem 54:1102–1109.
30. The Parkinson Study Group. 1989. Effect of deprenyl on the progression of disability in early Parkinson's disease. N Engl J Med 321:1364–1371.

31. Schapira AHV, Cooper JM, Dexter D, Jenner P, Clark JB, Marsden CD. 1989. Mitochondrial complex I deficiency in Parkinson's disease. Lancet 1:1269–1269.
32. Mizuno Y, Ohta S, Tanaka M, Takamiya S, Suzuki K, Sato T, Oya H, Ozawa T, Kagawa Y. 1989. Deficiencies in complex I subunits of the respiratory chain in Parkinson's disease. Biochem Biophys Res Commun 163:1450–1455.
33. Parker WD Jr, Boysen SJ, Parks JK. 1989. Abnormalities of the electron transport chain in idiopathic Parkinson's disease. Ann Neurol 26:719–723.
34. Albores RA, Neafsey EJ, Drucker G, Fields JZ, Collins MA. 1990. Mitochondrial respiratory inhibition by N-methylated β-carboline derivatives structurally resembling N-methyl-4-phenylpyridine. Proc Natl Acad Sci USA 87:9368–9372.

Chapter 7

Complex I and the Etiology of Parkinsonism

Carolyn Burkhardt and W. Davis Parker

The etiology of Parkinson's disease (PD) is a subject under intensive investigation at the present time. Previous theories have implicated toxins, genetic inheritance, genetic mutation, oxidative stress, and accelerated aging. Recent developments in studies of energy metabolism in PD suggest that a deficiency of complex I of the electron transport chain (NADH:ubiquinone oxidoreductase) may play a role in the pathogenesis of PD. How this deficiency interacts with the above theories remains unclear, but proponents of all of the above theories have found complex I deficiency supportive to their arguments.

Complex I of the electron transport chain (ETC) is a large enzyme complex embedded in the inner mitochondrial membrane, composed of approximately 26 polypeptides and including seven nonheme iron sulfur centers and a flavin mononucleotide. Most of the polypeptides are encoded by the nuclear genome, but seven are encoded by mitochondrial DNA. Mitochondrial DNA also encodes for the rRNA and tRNA required to construct these subunits. The ETC is responsible for processing over 90% of the oxygen taken up by aerobic animal cells. By virtue of its role as a conductor of electrons among various redox centers, the ETC is a major potential source of free radicals, particularly when normal electron flow is impaired by dysfunction in

From Hefti F, and Weiner WJ, (eds.) *Progress in Parkinson's Disease Research—2*. Mount Kisco NY, Futura Publishing Co., Inc., © 1992.

one of the complexes. Complex I, as the first enzyme complex in the ETC, is responsible for receiving the highest energy electrons that are handled by the ETC and passing them from NADH to ubiquinone (coenzyme Q). The ETC allows the production of 32 of the 36 molecules of ATP from one molecule of glucose through oxidative phosphorylation of ADP to ATP. Energy metabolism is a fundamental and crucial process in all human cells, yet generalized defects in ETC function are known to produce extremely focal disease. For instance, Leber's hereditary optic neuropathy patients have a systemic point mutation in a mitochondrial gene encoding a complex I subunit and deficient activity of that enzyme. Why a generalized bioenergetic defect might produce such focal neurological involvement is unclear.

The link between complex I and parkinsonism initially came about because of the neurotoxin MPTP (1-methyl-4-phenyl-1,2,3,6-tetrahydropyridine). In the early 1980s, MPTP was identified as the toxin responsible for an irreversible condition remarkably similar to PD developed by a group of drug abusers.[1] MPTP becomes toxic after oxidation by MAO (monoamine oxidase) B to the lipophilic pyridinium ion, MPP$^+$,[2–4] which is taken up by dopaminergic neurons,[5,6] and concentrated in the mitochondria.[7] MPP$^+$ appears to cause cell death by interfering with cellular respiration via selective inhibition of complex I.[5,8] Subsequently, several studies have implicated deficiency of ETC enzymes, especially complex I, in PD.

Parker et al.[9] found that complex I activity measured in mitochondria isolated from the platelets of 10 patients with PD was less than half of that found in eight comparably aged controls, while succinate:cytochrome c reductase activity (representing complexes II and III) was slightly, but not significantly lower, and cytochrome oxidase (complex IV) activity was normal.[9] Two studies by Mizuno et al.[10,11] reported ETC deficiencies. Complex I subunits were found deficient in PD brain samples through immunoblot studies, while complexes III and IV studied in the same manner showed no abnormalities.[10] They also measured the activities of complexes I–IV in mitochondria isolated from the striata of five PD patients and five controls; they found all activities to be lower in PD patients than controls, but this was statistically significant only for complex III.[11] Schapira et al.[12] measured complex I activity in homogenized tissue from the substantia nigra of nine PD patients and nine controls and found it was decreased to approximately 60% of control activity in the PD brains. Reichmann et al.[13] reported both complex I and III to be decreased in homogenates from the substantia nigra but not other brain regions taken from eight PD patients and controls. Bindhoff et al.[14] evaluated complexes I, II, and IV in mitochondrial fractions from skeletal muscle biopsies taken from five PD patients and four controls and found all to be reduced in PD. Shoffner et al.[15] measured the activity of ETC complexes in mitochondria isolated from muscle biopsy in six PD patients and found complex I to be deficient in four, and complex IV deficient in one of the patients. Neither Dagani et al.[16] nor Ferrante et al.[17] were able to demonstrate significant evidence of decreased ETC enzyme activity in whole platelets taken from PD patients, although both were able to demonstrate other abnormalities in oxygen consumption in at least some PD patients.

The majority of these studies were able to demonstrate abnormalities in complex I and less so in other ETC enzymes. The fact that a number of different tissues are reportedly involved, such as platelets and skeletal muscle, implies a systemic problem. At least part of the reason for the inconsistencies reported is the fact that some groups used isolated mitochondria to measure ETC enzyme activities (the most sensitive and specific manner), while others used homogenized whole tissue.

Furthering the connection between complex I and parkinsonism, we have recently investigated another class of parkinsonism-inducing drugs, neuroleptics, and found them to be toxic to complex I in add-back experiments using disrupted rat brain mitochondria, as well as in intact rat brain mitochondria studied with polarographic assays. We also found patients taking neuroleptic medications to have decreased complex I activity in mitochondria isolated from their platelets, similar to that seen in PD. We hypothesize that this underlies the drugs' tendencies to cause extrapyramidal dysfunction.

The fact that complex I has also been found to be deficient in other diseases does not necessarily speak against it being pathogenic in PD. Complex I abnormalities have been reported in Leber's hereditary optic neuropathy,[18] Huntington's disease,[19] MELAS syndrome,[20,21] and other myopathies.[22] Studies of patients with genetically determined primary complex I deficiency indicate that defects affecting different subunits can produce different phenotypes.[23] It has also been reported that the levels of complex I subunits can vary from tissue to tissue in parallel with complex I activity, seeming to explain the apparently tissue specific manifestation of symptoms in complex I deficiency.[18,19]

The underlying cause of complex I deficiency in PD is unknown. Possible theories include all the traditional ones proposed for the pathogenesis of PD. Proponents of the theory that an environmental toxin causes PD have received a great amount of support by the discovery of the effects of MPTP, a toxin causing a syndrome remarkably similar to PD. The differences that do exist between MPTP-induced parkinsonism and PD could possibly all be explained by the difference between intravenous administration and another more chronic form of exposure to a similar environmental toxin. PD has also been shown to progress more slowly in patients taking deprenyl,[24,25] which inhibits MAO-B. Since MAO-B is needed to convert MPTP from a protoxin to its toxic metabolite, MPP^+, this has been considered supporting evidence for the theory that PD may be caused by an environmental toxin similar to MPP^+. Other mechanisms of action of deprenyl could also be responsible for the findings, which have themselves been disputed.[26] Many compounds related structurally to MPP^+ have been demonstrated to have the same action of toxicity;[27] however, as yet no such environmental toxin has clearly been identified.

There is also a large body of evidence to support the theory that PD is a result of increased oxidative stress. Evidence supporting this hypothesis includes the facts that there is increased iron,[28] decreased glutathione,[29] decreased superoxide dismutase activity,[30] and increased lipid peroxidation[31] present in the substantia nigra of patients with PD, and there is evidence that antioxidant agents are beneficial to PD patients.[32] The association of complex I deficiency and PD is supportive of this hypothesis also, as a defect in complex I would be likely to give rise to the production of various oxygen radicals by leaking high energy electrons to O_2. Superoxide radicals are easily reduced in aqueous systems to hydrogen peroxide, which can be converted under physiological conditions to form the hydroxyl radical by the conversion of iron from its ferrous to its ferric state via the Fenton reaction. The hydroxyl free radical is highly toxic to cells by causing lipid peroxidation as well as damaging DNA. Dopaminergic neurons are likely to be under an increased oxidative stress because of the oxidative metabolism that catecholamines, in particular dopamine, undergo. MAO catalyzes the oxidation of dopamine, giving rise to hydrogen peroxide, which is normally cleared from the cell by the glutathione system.[33] This MAO-derived hydrogen peroxide is even more likely to give rise to the hydroxyl radical in the presence of a complex I defect and its attendant electron leak. Neuromelanin, which is the pigment deposited over time in the substantia nigra, is believed to be a by-product of the oxidative metabolism of dopamine.[34]

PD has also been found in a number of studies to be more common with increasing age. This has been considered by some to be the inevitable outcome of "normal" aging, as there is a progressive loss of nigral neurons with increasing age.[35] Other explanations include the possibilities that aged neurons are more vulnerable to an insult or that the passage of time rather than aging itself is required, for example as a reaction to a chronic exposure to an exogenous or endogenous toxin. Aging has also been associated on numerous levels with free radical damage. Increased free radical production may therefore be associated with diseases of accelerated aging. Further, aged animals are more vulnerable to MPTP toxicity than young animals.[36] One's susceptibility to extrapyramidal dysfunction as a side effect of neuroleptic medications also increases with advancing age.[37,38]

Whether PD has a genetic basis, and if so how one should categorize the genetic defect, are questions that have been posed by numerous studies in the past, with results that have been variable and at times contradictory. PD has been reported in certain families as autosomal dominantly inherited[39,40] and in some studies as autosomal dominant with variable penetrance;[41] Kondo et al.[42] reported finding a high "heritability," imputing an unknown environmental factor as well. Whether other family members were examined or cases of isolated tremor in family members were included as *forme frustes* of PD are just two of the problems encountered in these studies. Recalculation of the same data with different management of these points can significantly change the conclusions reached.[43] Twin studies done in the 1980s were interpreted as being inconsistent with a significant genetic component.[44] Reconsideration of the data using more rigorous statistical analysis and allowing for a possible prolonged subclinical phase and variability both in defining PD and in accepting atypical cases of PD has changed this conclusion.[45] Proposed potential genetic mechanisms have also expanded to include mitochondrial inheritance, which can be used to generate a model of sporadic disease with low concordance among identical twins.[7] Mitochondrial inheritance either alone or in combination with nuclear inheritance, multiple hereditary traits, or the existence of an inherited vulnerability to an environmental toxin are all possible explanations.

Another genetic mechanism that is a possible cause of PD is the acquisition of mutations, in particular in mitochondrial DNA. Mitochondrial DNA is especially susceptible to oxidative damage, which can give rise to mutations for several reasons.[46] The lack of a protective histone coat and the absence of the extensive repair mechanisms present in nuclear DNA systems, along with the proximity to the ETC, which produces free radicals, place the mitochondrial DNA at a high risk for mutations due to oxidative stress. Mitochondrial DNA likewise evolves 5–10 times faster than nuclear DNA of the same organism. Accumulations of mutations in mitochondrial DNA in senescence and in PD have been reported.[47] The deletion reported is present more so in the striata as compared to the frontal cortices, increases in amount with age, is accelerated in PD, and spans the genes coding for four complex I subunits. Interestingly, the deletion could be considered not only as a cause, but also as a result of complex I deficiency in that free radicals generated by a defective complex I could damage mitochondrial DNA and lead to this deletion. Complex I is situated in the inner mitochondrial membrane and is dependent on the association with the membrane for its integrity; this could lead to a scenario in which a defect in an enzyme can cause a cycle of worsening damage to the same enzyme via several mechanisms. Free radicals generated by a faulty complex I would potentially damage complex I via lipid peroxidation of its associated membrane and also block the ability to regenerate the complex by damaging the DNA required to do so. Ozawa et al.[48] studied the total sequence data of mitochondrial DNA taken from patients with mitochondrial encephalopathies and PD and found distinct clustering of point mutations in both the mitochondrial encephalopathy patients and the PD patients, from which they inferred that PD and mitochondrial encephalopathies are members of the same gene family diverged from a common ancestor. They also found that each patient's unique mutations indicated the existence of the disease-specific type of mutation or combination of mutations, suggesting that not a particular mutation but the type and number of overall mutations is an indispensable factor for the disease. Further, the total number of point mutations seemed to relate closely to the onset of the disease and the life-span of the patients.

An etiology for Parkinson's disease will need to conform with all of the information available to date: the mechanism must fit with the model with a complex genetic pattern, must accept the mitochondrial DNA mutations that have been demonstrated, must explain the evidence for increased oxidative stress and the association with aging, and should at least allow for a toxin to produce a very similar clinical picture. Complex I deficiency could be taken as a "final common pathway" towards parkinsonism. One possible scenario would be that idiopathic PD, being defined as having Lewy bodies, could be the result of a genetically inherited, initially subtle defect in complex I, which over time causes increased free radical generation in the mitochondria, resulting in lipid peroxidation, and mitochondrial DNA mutations, which both lead separately to further deterioration of complex I function. This cycle of degeneration becomes clinically apparent after the loss of approximately 80% of neurons in the substantia nigra. Other toxins affecting complex I in a similar fashion could also give rise to a similar disease state, perhaps making up a subset of "atypical" or non-Lewy body cases. The severity and types of the inherited defects, combined with the exact make up of the acquired mutations could account for the severity of the disease and also explain the overlap with other related degenerative diseases that are frequently seen. Alzheimer's disease has also been reported to have a defect in ETC activity.[49]

In summary, the etiology of Parkinson's disease is still being debated. Complex I deficiency seems to have a role central enough to coincide with the many different theories proposed to date. It may serve as a "final common pathway" to various forms of parkinsonism.

References

1. Langston JW, Ballard P, Tetrud JW, Irwin I. 1983. Chronic parkinsonism in humans due to a product of meperidine-analog synthesis. Science 219:979–980.
2. Chiba K, Trevor A, Castagnoli N Jr. 1984. Metabolism of the neurotoxic tertiary amine, MPTP, by brain monoamine oxidase. Biochem Biophys Res Commun 120:574–578.
3. Langston JW, Irwin I, Langston EB, Forno LS. 1984. 1-Methyl-4-

phenylpyridinium ion (MPP$^+$): Identification of a metabolite of MPTP, a toxin to the substantia nigra. Neurosci Lett 48:87–92.

4. Markey SP, Johannessen JN, Chiueh CC, Burns RS, Herkenham MA. 1984. Intraneural generation of a pyridinium metabolite may cause drug-induced parkinsonism. Nature 311:464–468.

5. Vyas I, Heikkila RE, Nicklas WJ. 1986. Studies on the neurotoxicity of 1-methyl-4-phenyl-1,2,5,6-tetrahydropyridine: Inhibition of NAD-linked substrate oxidation by its metabolite, 1-methyl-4-phenylpyridinium. J Neurochem 46:1501–1507.

6. Javitch JA, D'Amato RJ, Strittmatter SM, Snyder SH. 1985. Parkinsonism-inducing neurotoxin, N-methyl-4-phenyl-1,2,3,6-tetrahydropyridine: Uptake of the metabolite N-methyl-4-phenylpyridine by dopamine neurons explains selective toxicity. Proc Natl Acad Sci USA 82:2173–2177.

7. Ramsay RR, Singer TP. 1986. Energy-dependent uptake of N-methyl-4-phenylpyridinium, the toxic metabolite of 1-methyl-4-phenyl-1,2,3,6-tetra-hydropyridine, by mitochondria. J Biol Chem 261:7585–7587.

8. Poirier J, Barbeau A. 1985. 1-Methyl-4-phenyl-1,2,3,6-tetrahydropyridine-induced inhibition of nicotinamide adenosine dinucleotide cytochrome c reductase. Neurosci Lett 62:7–11.

9. Parker WD, Boyson SJ, Parks JK. 1989. Abnormalities of the electron transport chain in idiopathic Parkinson's disease. Ann Neurol 26:719–723.

10. Mizuno Y, Ohta S, Tanaka M, Takamiya S, Suzuki K, Sato T, Oya H, Ozawa T, Kagawa Y. 1989. Deficiencies in complex I subunits of the respiratory chain in Parkinson's disease. Biochem Biophys Res Commun 163:1450–1455.

11. Mizuno Y, Suzuki K, Ohta S. 1990. Postmortem changes in mitochondrial respiratory enzymes in brain and a preliminary observation in Parkinson's disease. J Neurol Sci 96:49–57.

12. Schapira AHV, Cooper JM, Dexter D, Clark JB, Jenner P, Marsden CD. 1990. Mitochondrial complex I deficiency in Parkinson's disease. J Neurochem 54:823–827.

13. Reichmann H, Riederer P, Seufert S, Jellinger K. 1990. Disturbances of the respiratory chain in brain from patients with Parkinson's disease (abstract). Mov Disord 5(suppl 1):28.

14. Bindhoff LA, Birch-Machin M, Cartlidge NEF, Parker WD, Turnbull DM. 1989. Mitochondrial function in Parkinson's disease. Lancet 2:49.

15. Shoffner JM, Watts RL, Juncos JL, Torroni A, Wallace DC. 1991. Parkinson's disease: A systemic disorder of mitochondrial oxidative phosphorylation (abstract). Neurology 41(suppl 1):152.

16. Dagani F, Ferrari R, Anderson JJ, Baronti F, Bravi D, Davis TL, Mouradian MM, Chase TN. 1991. Altered mitochondrial respiration in Parkinson's disease (abstract). Neurology 41(suppl 1):152.

17. Ferrante C, Bet L, Poaella C, Pifferi S, Amati P, Scarlato G. 1991. Platelet mitochondrial oxygen consumption rate in parkinsonian patients (abstract). Neurology 41(suppl 1):152.

18. Parker WD, Oley CA, Parks JK. 1989. A defect in mitochondrial

electron-transport activity (NADH:coenzyme Q oxidoreductase) in Leber's hereditary optic neuropathy. N Engl J Med 320:1331–1333.

19. Parker WD, Boyson SJ, Luder AS, Parks JK. 1990. Evidence for a defect in NADH:ubiquinone oxidoreductase(complex I) in Huntington's disease. Neurology 40:1231–1233.

20. Kobayashi M, Morishita H, Sugiyama N, Yokochi K, Nakano M, Wada Y, Hotta Y, Terauchi A, Nonaka I. 1987. Two cases of NADH-coenzyme Q reductase deficiency: Relationship to MELAS syndrome. J Pediatr 110:223–227.

21. Tanaka M, Nishikimi M, Suzuki H, Ozawa T, Ichiki T, Kobayashi M, Wada Y. 1987. Variation in the levels of complex I subunits among tissues in a patient with mitochondrial encephalopathy and renal dysfunction. Biochem Int 14:735–739.

22. DiMauro S, Bonilla E, Zeviani M, Nakagawa M, DeVivo DC. 1985. Mitochondrial myopathies. Ann Neurol 17:521–538.

23. Howell N, McCullough D. 1991. Leber hereditary optic neuropathy: Involvement of the mitochondrial ND1 gene and evidence for an intragenic suppressor mutation. Am J Hum Genet 48:935–942.

24. The Parkinson Study Group. 1989. Effect of deprenyl on the progression of disability in early Parkinson's disease. N Engl J Med 321:1364–1371.

25. Tetrud JW, Langston JW. 1989. The effect of deprenyl (selegiline) on the natural history of Parkinson's disease. Science 245:519–522.

26. Elizan TS, Yahr MD, Moros DA, Mendoza MR, Pang S, Bodian CA. 1989. Selegiline use to prevent progression of Parkinson's disease: Experience in 22 de novo patients. Arch Neurol 46:1275–1279.

27. Youngster SK, Sonsalla PK, Sieber BA, Heikkila RE. 1989. Structure–activity study of the mechanism of 1-methyl-4-phenyl-1,2,3,6-tetrahydropyridine (MPTP)-induced neurotoxicity. I. Evaluation of the biological activity of MPTP analogs. J Pharmacol Exp Ther 249:820–828.

28. Sofic E, Reiderer P, Heinsen H, Beckman H, Reynolds GP, Hebenstreit G, Youdim MBH. 1988. Increased iron (III) and total iron content in post mortem substantia nigra of parkinsonian brains. J Neural Transm 74:199–205.

29. Reiderer P, Sofic E, Rausch WD, Schmidt B, Reynolds GP, Jellinger K, Youdim MBH. 1989. Transition metals, glutathione, ferritin, and ascorbic acid in parkinsonian brains. J Neurochem 52:515–520.

30. Saggu H, Cooksey J, Dexter D, Wells FR, Jenner P, Marsden CD. 1989. A selective increase in particulate superoxide dismutase activity in parkinsonian substantia nigra. J Neurochem 53:692–697.

31. Dexter DT, Carter CJ, Wells FR, Javoy-Agid F, Agid Y, Lees A, Jenner P, Marsden CD. 1989. Basal lipid peroxidation in substantia nigra is increased in Parkinson's disease. J Neurochem 52:381–389.

32. Fahn S. 1988. High dose antioxidants in early Parkinson's disease (abstract). Arch Neurol 45:810.

33. Olanow CW. 1990. Oxidation reactions in Parkinson's disease. Neurology 40(suppl 3):32–37.

34. Graham DG. 1979. On the origin and significance of neuromelanin. Arch Pathol Lab Med 103:359–362.

35. McGeer PL, McGeer EG, Suzuki JS. 1977. Aging and extrapyramidal function. Arch Neurol 34:33–35.
36. Jarvis MF, Wagner GC. 1985. Age dependent effects of 1-methyl-4-phenyl-1,2,5,6-tetrahydropyridine (MPTP). Neuropharmacology 24:581–583.
37. Ayd FJ. 1961. A survey of drug-induced extrapyramidal reactions. J Am Med Assoc 175:102–108.
38. Smith JM, Baldessarini RJ. 1980. Changes in prevalence, severity, and recovery in tardive dyskinesia with age. Arch Gen Psychiatry 37:1368–1373.
39. Golbe LI, Di Iorio G, Bonavita V, Miller DC, Duvoisin RC. 1990. A large kindred with autosomal dominant Parkinson's disease. Ann Neurol 27:276–282.
40. Roy M, Boyer L, Barbeau A. 1983. A prospective study of 50 familial cases of Parkinson's disease. Can J Neurol Sci 10:37–42.
41. Mjones H. 1949. Paralysis agitans. A clinical and genetic study. Acta Psychiatr Neurol 24(suppl 54):1–195.
42. Kondo K, Kurland LT, Schull WJ. 1973. Parkinson's disease: Genetic analysis and evidence of a multifactorial etiology. Mayo Clin Proc 48:465–475.
43. Duvoisin RC, Gearing FR, Schweitzer MD, Yahr MD. 1969. A family study of parkinsonism. *In* Progress in Neurogenetics. International Congress Series No. 175, Vol. 1. A Barbeau, JR Brunette (eds). Excerpta Medica, Amsterdam, pp. 492–496.
44. Ward CD, Duvoisin RC, Ince SE, Nutt JD, Eldridge R, Caine DB. 1983. Parkinson's disease in 65 pairs of twins and in a set of quadruplets. Neurology 33:815–824.
45. Golbe LI. 1990. The genetics of Parkinson's disease: A reconsideration. Neurology 40(suppl 3):7–14.
46. Richter C, Park JW, Ames BN. 1988. Normal oxidative damage to mitochondrial and nuclear DNA is extensive. Proc Natl Acad Sci USA 85:6465–6467.
47. Ikeba S, Tanaka M, Ohno K, Sato W, Hattori K, Kondo T, Mizuno Y, Ozawa T. 1990. Increase of deleted mitochondrial DNA in the striatum in Parkinson's disease and senescence. Biochem Biophys Res Commun 170:1044–1048.
48. Ozawa T, Tanaka M, Ino H, Ohno K, Sano T, Wada Y, Yoneda M, Tanno Y, Miyatake T, Tanaka T, Itoyama S, Ikebe S, Hattori N, Mizuno Y. 1991. Distinct clustering of point mutations in mitochondrial DNA among patients with mitochondrial encephalopathies and with Parkinson's disease. Biochem Biophys Res Commun 176:938–946.
49. Parker WD, Filley CM, Parks JK. 1990. Cytochrome oxidase deficiency in Alzheimer's disease. Neurology 40:1302–1303.

Chapter 8

Mosaicism for Levels of Somatic Mutation of Mitochondrial DNA in Different Brain Regions and Its Implications for Neurological Disease

Gino A. Cortopassi, Giulio Pasinetti, and Norman Arnheim

We have developed an assay for a particular class of somatic mutation, deletions of mitochondrial DNA (dmtDNA). The polymerase chain reaction (PCR) has the sensitivity to detect a single mutant DNA molecule.[1–3] Using the PCR we found that a deletion ($\Delta 1$) that occurs at high levels in a rare neuromuscular disease state also occurs at low levels in normal human tissues. The $\Delta 1$ deletion appears to increase with biological age in human tissues such as brain, skeletal muscle, and heart. We recently examined the level of $\Delta 1$ in different brain areas, such as basal ganglia (putamen), mesencephalon, and cerebellum.[4]

Although many biologists believe that deficits of cellular function that increase with age are to some extent the result of an accumulation of deleterious somatic mutations,[5–9] this hypothesis

From Hefti F, and Weiner WJ, (eds.) *Progress in Parkinson's Disease Research—2.* Mount Kisco NY, Futura Publishing Co., Inc., © 1992.

has remained difficult to test. Because the frequencies of somatic mutations are low (between 1/100 and $1/10^9$ genomes), quantitation of their level in human tissues has remained difficult, even with the tools of molecular biology. The few assays of somatic mutation from recently derived, nontransformed human cells that are available are limited to lymphocytic cells,[10–12] and thus may not be representative of other postmitotic cell types such as those found in neuromuscular tissue.

Mutations of the mitochondrial genome have been associated with several types of neuromuscular and neurological disease.[13–16] Symptoms are shared between several mitochondrial diseases, which include myoclonic epilepsy, dementia, lactic acidosis, severe muscle weakness including progressive external ophthalmoplegia, retinopathy, heart block, and stroke. Many of these symptoms can be ascribed directly to a deficit of mitochondrial function. Kearns-Sayre syndrome (KSS) and progressive external ophthalmoplegia (PEO), which are thought to be related syndromes, show sporadic inheritance and are presumably the result of a specific deletion mutation of mtDNA in somatic tissue early in development.[14]

The strong association of mitochondrial mutations with sporadically occurring neurological and neuromuscular disease may be a result of the fact that the mitochondrial genome continues to replicate in postfetal neural tissue,[17] whereas nuclear replication ceases. The high rate of mitochondrial replication may increase the level of mtDNA mutation relative to that of nuclear DNA by four mechanisms: (1) an obligate increase in stochastic errors of replication,[18] (2) increased fixation of unrepaired damage by replication across from the unrepaired lesion,[19] (3) more genetic drift of genomes carrying deleterious mutations,[20] and (4) increased chance for positive selection for a mitochondrial mutation that confers an intracellular selective advantage to the genome carrying it, even though detrimental to the interests of the cell.[21,22]

Recently Ikebe et al.[23] reported an increased level of deleted mitochondrial DNA in basal ganglia (striatum) from patients with Parkinson's disease. The present study examined the level of $\Delta 1$ accumulation in other brain areas. We discuss the possible role of mitochondrial mutations during aging and neurological disease such as Parkinson's.

Methodology and Results

How the Assay Works

The PCR is a technique that allows the amplification of template DNA in vitro, by the use of two oligonucleotide primers, nucleoside triphosphates, and a DNA polymerase (Figure 1). The polymerase catalyzes the template-directed polymerization of triphosphates, beginning at the 3' end of each primer. The PCR can be thought of as two distinct cross feeding reactions, in which the product of one primer extension reaction (primer 1, Figure 1) becomes the template for the other extension reaction (primer 2, Figure 1), and vice versa. When the PCR is 100% efficient, each cycle produces a doubling of the starting template. By repeating this process many times, the PCR can selectively amplify single copy genes from a single sperm molecule, to a copy number of about 100 billion, which is sufficient to be stained and visualized with ethidium bromide.[2]

Our PCR assay for dmtDNA is designed to detect a particular dmtDNA ($\Delta 1$), which accounts for about half of the deleted forms observed in patients with KSS,[16,24,25] and occurs precisely between two 13-bp direct repeats. The strategy for detecting the deleted molecules in a background of normal mtDNA is shown in Figure 2. Using primers 1 and 2, which flank the repeats, and a PCR cycle time lasting 10 minutes, DNA from normal human heart and brain tissue

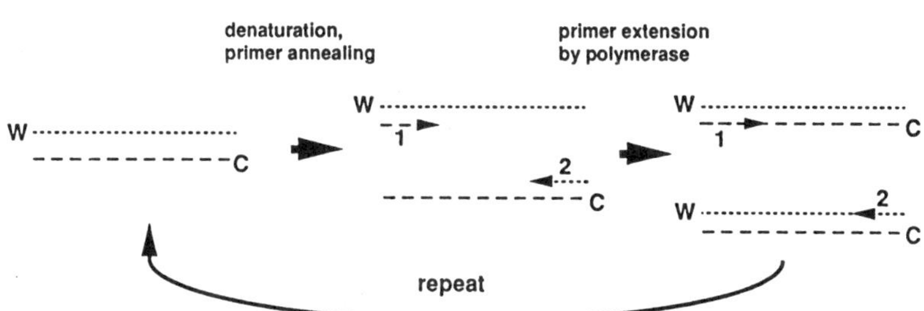

Figure 1.   A schematic of the fundamental cycle of the PCR. W and C refer to the complementary strands of DNA and are positioned at the 3'-OH termini of each chain. Dashed arrows signify primers.

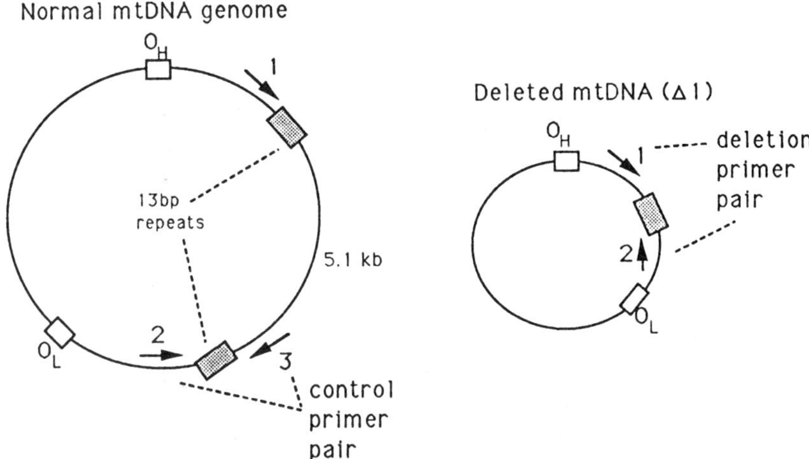

Figure 2. A schematic of a PCR assay for deleted mitochondrial genomes. By limiting cycle time, deleted genomes can be selectively amplified. O_H and O_L refer to origins of heavy and light strand mtDNA synthesis, respectively. Arrows refer to primers, their approximate binding sites, and direction of primer extension. Primers 1 and 2 under short cycle conditions allow the amplification of Δ1 genomes; primers 2 and 3 amplify normal (non-Δ1) mtDNA.

should produce a product of 5.1 kb, which represents the normal undeleted mitochondrial genome (Figure 3). In order to selectively amplify the less frequent Δ1 deletion, which should produce a 520-bp product, the PCR cycle time was shortened 10-fold, to an extent that normal genomes should remain incompletely replicated after each cycle. These short cycle PCRs from adult heart and brain samples make a product that is the size expected for the Δ1 deletion, and restriction mapping and sequencing verified its identity as the Δ1 product.[4]

Increase in Δ1 Mutation with Age

Several human heart and brain DNAs from patients who died from causes unrelated to neuromuscular disease were assayed for Δ1. Δ1 is much more prevalent in adult heart and brain than fetal heart and brain, by a factor of at least 100-fold (Figure 4). The level of dmtDNA in brain is similar or higher than in heart.[4] In order to normalize each sample for the amount of nondeleted dmtDNA, an internal control reaction was run using primers 2 and 3, which

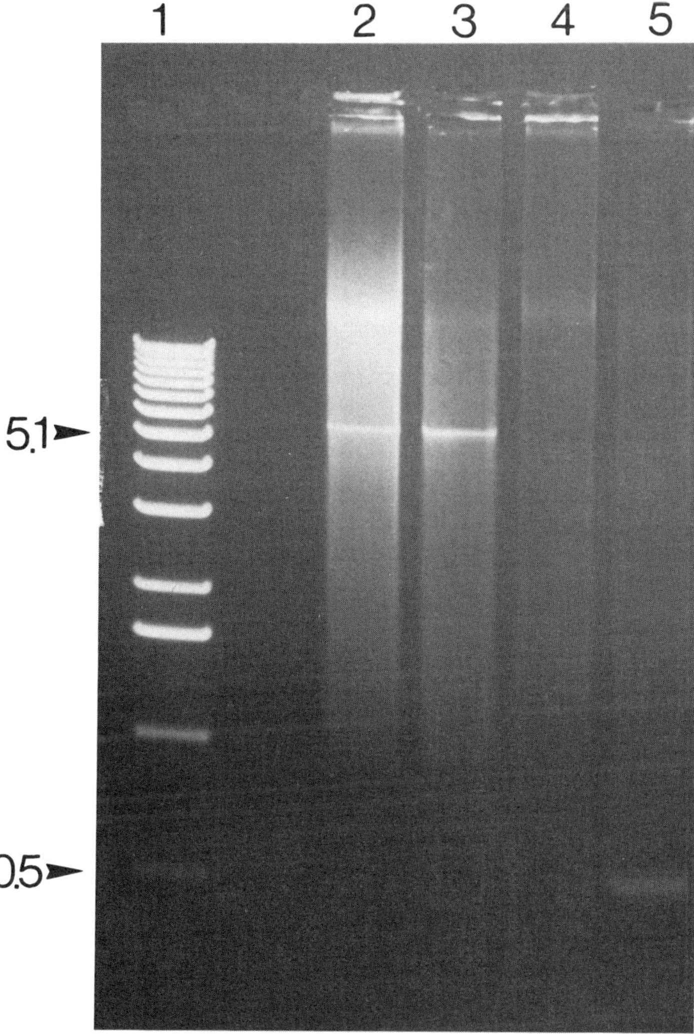

Figure 3. Effect of cycle time on the size of PCR products from normal adult heart using primers 1 and 2. Lane 1, size markers. Lanes 2 and 3, two adult DNAs amplified for 30 long cycles. Lanes 4 and 5, two adult DNAs amplified for 30 short cycles. Approximately 1 μg of total genomic DNA was used in each sample. The arrowheads refer to sizes in kilobases of the products. (Reprinted with permission from Cortopassi and Arnheim.[4])

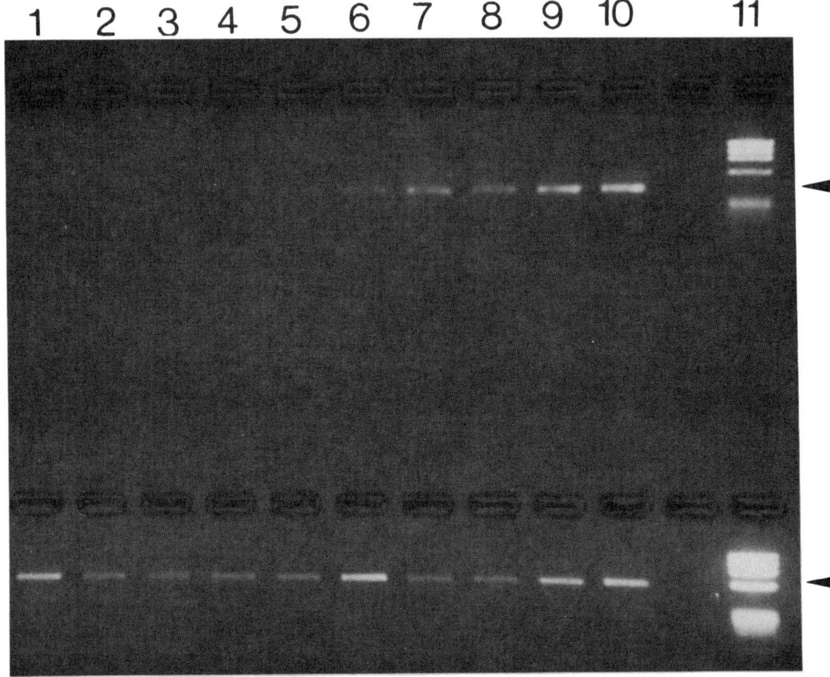

Figure 4.   Assay of heart muscle DNA samples from individuals of different ages. Top row: short cycle amplification of approximately 10-ng of genomic DNA using primers 1 and 2. Lanes 1–10: 22-weeks gestation, 29-weeks gestation, stillborn, and 21, 22, 27, 33, 40, 45, and 53 years, respectively. Lane 11, size markers. Bottom row: parallel samples from the top row were diluted 1000-fold and amplified with primers 2 and 3 as a control for amount of total mtDNA. (Reprinted with permission from Cortopassi and Arnheim.[4])

amplify non-$\Delta 1$ genomes (Figure 2). This is an essential step that allows a fair comparison to be made between the levels of mutant mtDNA in different samples.

Level of dmtDNA in Brain Regions of Parkinsonians and Controls

Levels of $\Delta 1$ were investigated in the basal ganglia (putamen), mesencephalon (including substantia nigra compacta), and cerebellum of parkinsonian patients and controls. Although the level of $\Delta 1$ is consistently higher in putamen and mesencephalon than cerebellum, there is no detectable difference between parkinsonians and controls (Figure 5).

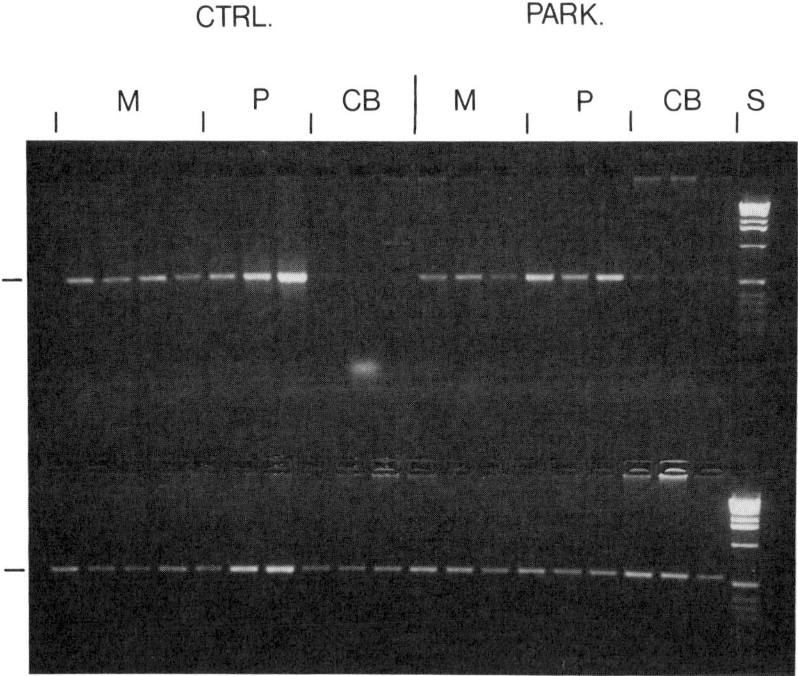

Figure 5. Assay of Δ1 level in different brain regions of Parkinsonians and controls. Top row: control and parkinsonian brain DNAs were amplified with primers 1 and 2 to detect Δ1. M = mesencephalon samples, P = putamen, CB = cerebellum, S = size markers. Bottom row: parallel samples were diluted and amplified with primers 2 and 3, which indicate the amount of normal mtDNA in each sample.

Discussion

Ikebe et al.[23] have presented some data on the presence of Δ1 in brain that agrees, and some that conflicts, with ours. Like us, they find that there is variation in Δ1 level in different brain regions and that brain regions affected in Parkinson's disease tend to have higher levels of Δ1. They report that levels of Δ1 are higher in striatum than cortex of aged individuals. Unlike us, they report that Δ1 is higher in striatum of parkinsonian than nonparkinsonian controls. The reasons for this apparent conflict is unknown. It is possible that cells of the substantia nigra compacta make up too small a fraction of our mesencephalon samples to reflect an actual difference in $\Delta 1$ of nigral cells. On the other hand, it is possible that the higher level of $\Delta 1$ in the striatum claimed by Ikebe et al. may be due to experimental error. Their assay for $\Delta 1$ does not contain an internal control for the level of nondeleted mtDNA, and thus their conclusion that parkinsonians have more dmtDNA could be the result of using different amounts of total mtDNA per sample. Their PCR conditions did not prevent the normal molecules from being amplified. Thus their results might depend strongly on the absolute amount of DNA that was used in each sample. Furthermore, if the level of $\Delta 1$ is continually increasing with age, their results might be explained by the fact that the parkinsonians tested were generally older than the controls. To resolve this issue it is clear that much larger sample sizes should be tested and the level of total mitochondrial DNA and between-age group variance controlled for.

Regardless of the divergence of results between the two groups in the comparisons of parkinsonians and controls, we agree in the observation that the tissues affected in parkinsonism have higher levels of $\Delta 1$ than do regions less affected by Parkinson's, those of cortex[23] and cerebellum (this work). This might mean that the putamen and mesencephalon have an inherently higher susceptibility to accumulate mitochondrial DNA damage, which could be the result of exposure to environmental toxins. It is known that some hydrophobic toxins attack mitochondrial DNA preferentially.[26,27] It is also interesting to note that mitochondrial complex I deficiency occurs in parkinsonism.[28] The $\Delta 1$ deletion encompasses three of the mitochondrially encoded complex I subunits. Further studies are required before one can conclude whether or not $\Delta 1$ or other mtDNA deletions contribute to susceptibility to Parkinson's disease.

References

1. Saiki RK, Gelfand DH, Stoffel S, Scharf SJ, Higuchi R, Horn GT, Mullis KB, Erlich HA. 1988. Primer-directed enzymatic amplification of DNA with a thermostable DNA polymerase. Science 239:487–491.
2. Li H, Gyllensten UB, Cui X-F, Saiki RK, Erlich HA, Arnheim N. 1988. Amplification and analysis of DNA sequences in single human sperm and diploid cells. Nature 335:414–417.
3. Jeffreys AJ, Neumann R, Wilson V. 1990. Repeat unit sequence variation

in minisatellites: A novel source of DNA polymorphism for studying variation and mutation by single molecule analysis. Cell 60:473–485.

4. Cortopassi GA, Arnheim N. 1990. Detection of a specific mitochondrial DNA deletion in tissues of older humans. Nucleic Acids Res 18:6927–6933.

5. Szilard L. 1959. On the nature of the aging process. Proc Natl Acad Sci USA 45:35–40.

5a. Trounce I, Byrne E, Marzuki S. 1989. Decline in skeletal muscle mitochondrial respiratory chain function: Possible factor in ageing. Lancet 1:637–639

6. Orgel LE. 1963. The maintenance of accuracy of proten synthesis, and its relevance to aging. Proc Natl Acad Sci USA 49:517–521.

7. Ames BN. 1989. Endogenous oxidative DNA damage, aging, and cancer. Free Radic Res Commun 7:121–128.

8. Linnane AW, Marzuki S, Ozawa T, Tanaka M. 1989. Hypothesis: Mitochondrial DNA mutation as an important contributor to aging and degenerative diseases. Lancet 1:642–645.

9. Harman D. 1981. The aging process. Proc Natl Acad Sci USA 78:7124–7128.

10. Strauss GH, Albertini RJ. 1979. Enumeration of 6-thioguanine-resistant peripheral blood lymphocytes in man as a potential test for somatic cell mutations arising in vivo. Mutat Res 61:353–379.

11. Langlois RG, Bigbee WL, Jensen RH. 1990. The glycophorin A assay for somatic cell mutations in humans. Prog Clin Biol Res 340C:47–56.

12. Jacobs PA, Brunton M, Court-Brown WM, Doll R, Goldstein H. 1963. Changes of human chromosome count distributions with age: Evidence for a sex difference. Nature 197:1080–1081.

13. Wallace DC. 1989. Mitochondrial DNA mutations and neuromuscular disease. Trends Genet 5:9–13.

14. Holt IJ, Harding AE, Morgan-Hughes JA. 1988. Deletions of muscle mitochondrial DNA in patients with mitochondrial myopathies. Nature 331:717–719.

15. Zeviani M, Moraes CT, DiMauro S, Nakase H, Bonilla E, Schon EA, Rowland CD. 1988. Deletions of mitochondrial DNA in Kearns-Sayre syndrome. Neurology 38:1339–1346.

16. Moraes CT, DiMauro S, Zeviani M, Lombes A, Shanske S, Miranda A, Nakase H, Bonilla E, Werneck LC, Servidio S. 1989. Mitochondrial DNA deletions in progressive external ophthalmoplegia and Kearns-Sayre syndrome. N Engl J Med 320:1293–1299.

17. Gross NJ, Getz GS, Rabinowitz M. 1969. Apparent turnover of mtDNA and mitochondrial phospholipids in the tissues of the rat. J Biol Chem 244:1552–1562.

18. Kunkel TA, Loeb LA. 1981. Fidelity of mammalian DNA polymerases. Science 213:765–767.

19. Loeb LA, Preston BD, Snow ET, Schaaper RM. 1986. Apurinic sites as common intermediates in mutagenesis. Basic Life Sci 38:341–347.

20. Birky CW Jr, Maruyama T, Fuerst P. 1983. An approach to population

and evolutionary genetic theory for genes in mitochondria and chloroplasts, and some results. Genetics 103:513–527.

21. Shoffner JM, Lott MT, Voliavec AS, Soueidan SA, Costigan DA, Wallace
DC. 1989. Spontaneous Kearns-Sayre/chronic external ophthalmoplegia
plus syndrome associated with a mitochondrial deletion: A slip-
replication model and metabolic therapy. Proc Natl Acad Sci USA
86:7952–7956.

22. Shoubridge EA, Karpati G, Hastings KEM. 1990. Deletion mutants are
functionally dominant over wild-type mitochondrial genomes in skeletal muscle fiber segments in mitochondrial disease. Cell 62:43–49.

23. Ikebe S-I, Tanaka M, Ohno K, Sato W, Hattori K, Kondo T, Mizuno Y,
Ozawa T. 1990. Increase of deleted mitochondrial DNA in the striatum
in Parkinson's disease and senescence. Biochem Biophys Res Commun
170:1044–1048.

24. Holt IJ, Harding AE, Morgan-Hughes JA. 1989. Deletions of muscle
mtDNA in mitochondrial myopathies: Sequence analysis and possible
mechanisms. Nucleic Acids Res 17:4465–4469.

25. Mita S, Rizzuto R, Moraes CT, Shanske S, Arnauddo E, Fabrizi GM,
Koga Y, DiMauro S, Schon EA. 1990. Recombination via flanking direct
repeats is a major cause of large-scale deletions of human mitochondrial
DNA. Nucleic Acids Res 18:561–567.

26. Allen JA, Coombs MM. 1980. Covalent binding of polycyclic aromatic
compounds to mitochondrial and nuclear DNA. Nature 287:244–245.

27. Backer JM, Weinstein IB. 1980. Mitochondrial DNA is a major cellular
target for a dihydrodiolepoxide derivative of benzo[a]pyrene. Science
209:297–299.

28. Schapira AH, Cooper JM, Dexter D, Clark JB, Jenner P, Marsden CD.
1990. Mitochondrial complex I deficiency in Parkinson's disease. J
Neurochem 54:823–827.

2

Etiology

Chapter 9

An Overview of the Epidemiology of Parkinsonism

John F. Kurtzke

Epidemiology

Epidemiology may be considered that branch of medical science dealing with the natural history of disease.[1,2] In Figure 1 are denoted the major aspects of the field: its subject matter ("what"); those segments of society for whom this information is required—or at least desirable ("who"); and the ends to which they need employ that knowledge ("uses"). The unit of all epidemiological inquiries of individual diseases is the patient so affected, and therefore primary to all such works is diagnosis. The most basic aspect of epidemiology thereafter is the frequency of the disorder by time and place and by age and sex. Therefore all epidemiology inquiries rest upon case definition and case ascertainment.

Epidemiological measures of frequency are those that enumerate the cases within a defined population, whether that be a nation or any subunit thereof. It is the use of a population denominator that separates epidemiology rates from numerator-only case series collected in clinics or hospitals, and it is the fact of population-based

Supported by the Department of Veterans Affairs (Neuroepidemiology Research Program and Neurology Service). Special thanks to Ms. Robin C. Fisher, Neurology Service, for typing the manuscript.
From Hefti F, and Weiner WJ, (eds.) *Progress in Parkinson's Disease Research—2.* Mount Kisco NY, Futura Publishing Co., Inc., © 1992.

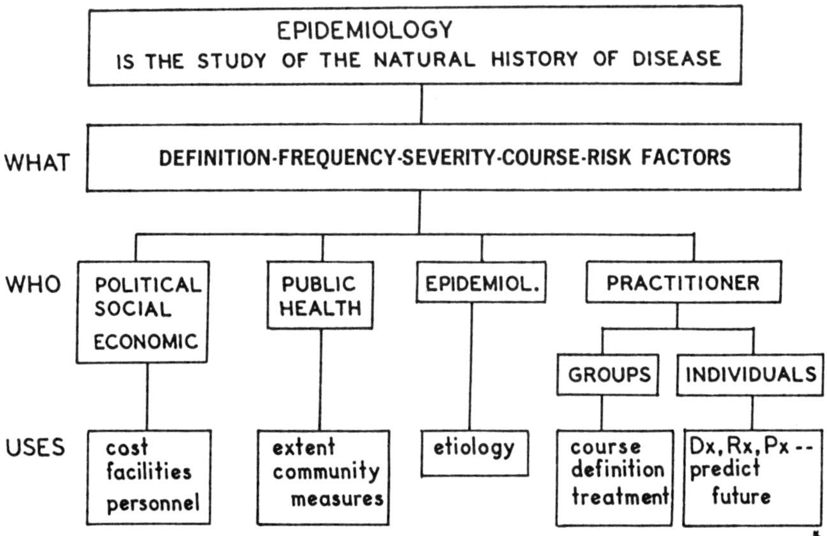

Figure 1. Epidemiology content and uses. Modified from Kurtzke.[3]

data that permits comparisons among different places and times. The epidemiological measurements in common use are the *incidence rate,* the *mortality rate* and the *prevalence "rate."* All are ordinarily expressed as a number per unit of population. Thus ten cases within a community of 20,000 give a rate of 50 per 100,000 population, or 0.5 per 1000 population.

Incidence or Attack Rate. This is defined as the number of new cases of a disease occurring within a unit to time within the specified population. This is most commonly provided as an annual incidence rate per 100,000 population per year. The date of clinical onset of a disease ordinarily defines the time of accession, although on occasion the date of first diagnosis is used. The incidence rate is the preferred measure when seeking etiology by epidemiological means. Note that one considers "onset" as the time when symptoms begin. For a disorder acquired pathologically well before symptom onset, the interval between these two dates is the incubation period. Note also that a patient without symptoms may then not be a "case" even though affected. This can pose problems with autopsy series or seroprevalence studies, as well as with true community surveys. In this last, for an asymptomatic person with pathognomonic physical or laboratory signs, if he is to be included, the date of examination is taken as onset. This is one reason that date of diagnosis is employed throughout in some works.

Mortality or Death Rate. This refers to the number of deaths caused by the disease within a unit time and population, and thus an annual death rate per 100,000 population. The *case fatality ratio* is the proportion of the affected who die from the disease. When this is high, as in ALS or glioblastoma, then death rates are potentially an accurate reflection of the disease. When the case fatality ratio is low, as in epilepsy, then death rate data may be quite biased.

Point Prevalence Rate. This is more properly referred to as a *prevalence ratio* by the purists, since an interval of time is not incorporated unless one does differential calculus. It refers to the number of cases present at one point in time within the community, again expressed per unit of population. Seldom used is another measure, the *period prevalence rate,* which is a count of all cases present over a defined interval of time within the community.

Where there is no migration, and where annual incidence rates are stable, the point prevalence rate equals the average duration of illness in years times the annual incidence rate. Both incidence and prevalence rates arise from specific surveys for the disorder in question within defined populations.

Mortality rates are derived from governmental publications that enumerate causes of death. These lists of deaths by cause and the appropriate death rates are routinely published in most countries, and do provide a resource of great potential value in the study of disease. Their major asset is availability; their major drawback the question of diagnostic accuracy. The causes are coded according to the International Statistical Classification of Diseases, Injuries, and Causes of Death (ICD), a compilation that is revised periodically. The ninth revision of ICD is the one in current use.[4] In this convention a person is allowed only the one underlying cause of death. At certain times and countries, diseases otherwise noted on the death certificate as secondary causes or as associated conditions are retrieved. When this is the situation, the sum of those deaths *with* the disease plus those *due to* the disease (underlying cause) provide the numerator of total deaths attributed to the disorder as recorded on death certificates. In ALS most of the listed deaths are underlying-cause deaths; in epilepsy most are not; parkinsonism falls in between.

Age Adjustment. The sum of all cases within the community

provides a *crude rate, all ages.* When both numerator and denominator are delimited by age or sex, we have *age-specific* or *sex-specific* rates. Rates by age and sex for all age groups from birth onward afford the best description of the frequency of the disease. Differences in crude rates between communities may merely reflect differences in the denominator age structure. This can be taken care of by comparing the age- and sex-specific rates, but that soon becomes unwieldy with multiple surveys. One method to handle this is to calculate a rate for all ages that "adjusts" the observed age-specific rates to those of a common standard age distribution, such as that of the United States in a censal year. The total rate so calculated then provides a *rate, all ages, adjusted to* X *population,* or an *age adjusted (to* X) *rate.*[2] For disorders like stroke or parkinsonism, age adjustment is essential for proper comparisons—although the necessary data to calculate that rate are often not published. Further, adjustment to one standard population does not equate with that to another, and an age adjusted rate, just like the crude rate, is really an average. Like any average it may be misleading when the underlying distribution is badly skewed, a situation clearly present in stroke and parkinsonism. Further, both these states occur in that portion of the age spectrum where denominators are small and therefore can give unstable rates even if the numerators are large.

Diagnostic Classification

In prior years neurologists were comfortable with a grouping of certain disorders into the extrapyramidal or basal ganglion diseases, terms used to encompass those entities characterized by disturbances of movement excluding the pareses and ataxias. The major categories were parkinsonism, chorea, and dystonia; ballismus, athetosis, and miscellaneous completed the list.[15] As a cause of death, no identification was possible before 1949 or 1950, when the sixth revision of the ICD came into effect. For ICD6 and 7, only paralysis agitans was coded (code 350). For ICD8, in use for 1968–1978, the codes were paralysis agitans (342) and hereditary diseases of the striatopallidal system (331), the latter subdivided into hereditary chorea (331.0), dystonia musculorum deformans (331.1), progressive familial myoclonic epilepsy (331.2), and other (331.9).[6]

When Cotzias et al. in 1967 demonstrated the efficacy of

high-dose levodopa in Parkinson's disease,[7] they not only revolutionized treatment for that disorder, they also set in motion a process that has led to the formation and flourishing of movement disorder clinics, associations, journals—and diseases. Among the resulting classifications were those of Fahn[8] and McDowell and Cedarbaum.[9] Even the ICD reacted; the coding in use since 1979 is provided in Table 1.[4] ICD9 was adopted in all countries outside Scandinavia, which retained ICD8. ICD10 has yet to appear. A modest proposal for a classification that epidemiologists could use is cited in Table 2. "Secondary" parkinsonism would be coded to the underlying disease or cause in this schema. The table at least has the advantage of mutually exclusive categories.

Despite the description in 1817 by Sir James Parkinson[10] of "the shaking palsy," it was really Charcot who characterized the full clinical spectrum of paralysis agitans as "rigidité des muscles ... un tremblement existant même au repos ... la perte de la faculté de

Table 1.
Movement Disorders[a]

332	*Parkinson's disease*
332.0	Paralysis agitans
332.1	Secondary parkinsonism
333	*Other extrapyramidal disease and abnormal movement disorder*
333.0	Other degenerative basal ganglion disease (Hallevorden-Spatz; olivopontocerebellar degeneration; parkinsonism with orthostatic hypotension; progressive supranuclear ophthalmoplegia; Shy-Drager; striatonigral degeneration)
333.1	Essential and other specified forms of tremor
333.2	Myoclonus (all varieties)
333.3	Tics of organic origin
333.4	Huntington's chorea
333.5	Other choreas (hemiballismus; paroxysmal choreoathetosis)
333.6	Idiopathic torsion dystonia (dystonia musculorum deformans)
333.7	Symptomatic torsion dystonia (athetoid cerebral palsy, Vogt's disease; double athetosis)
333.8	Fragments of torsion dystonia (blepharospasm; orofacial dyskinesia; writer's cramp; spasmodic torticollis)
333.9	Other and unspecified (restless legs, stiff man syndrome)

[a]Coding according to the International Classification of Diseases, Injuries, and Causes of Death, Ninth Revision (ICD9).[4]

Table 2.
Movement Disorders: Classification of Primary Dyskinesias for Epidemiological Purposes[a]

1. Parkinsonism (Parkinson's disease)
2. Huntington's disease (Huntington's chorea)
3. Wilson's disease (hepatolenticular degeneration)
4. Torsion dystonia (dystonia musculorum deformans)
5. Focal dystonias (torticollis, et al)
6. Gilles de la Tourette syndrome
7. Essential tremor
8. Progressive supranuclear palsy
9. Shy-Drager syndrome ("multiple system atrophy")
10. Striatonigral degeneration
11. Hallevorden-Spatz disease
12. Choreoacanthocytosis
13. Hexosaminidase deficiency
14. Diffuse Lewy body disease
15. Other or undefined dyskinesias

[a]Excluded are infectious or postinfectious conditions (Creutzfeldt-Jakob disease; Sydenham's chorea); the Guamanian ALS-PD complex; olivopontocerebellar degeneration.

garder l'equilibre pendant la progression . . . une tendance à la propulsion ou à la rétropulsion . . .," as well as its age at onset and its differentiation from multiple sclerosis (pp 155–188[11]). We must remember that even today the diagnosis of parkinsonism is entirely a clinical one without pathognomonic laboratory support in vivo.

In the epidemiological studies to be discussed it is often unclear whether secondary parkinsonism is deliberately included or not, and inadvertent inclusion is not unlikely in any case. Thus diagnostic variation may well explain some of the differences observed. Among the reviews of the epidemiology of parkinsonism are those of Hoehn,[12] Kessler,[13,14] Kurland,[15] Kurland et al.,[16,17] Kurtzke,[18] Marttila and Rinne,[19] and Williams et al.[20]

Mortality Data

As noted above, in ICD6 and 7 parkinsonism or paralysis agitans were coded to rubric 350; for ICD8 the code was 342. In ICD9

Parkinson's disease is 332, with 332.0 for paralysis agitans and 332.1 for secondary parkinsonism.

When listed on the death certificate, parkinsonism coded as underlying cause comprised ¼ to ½ of such deaths in the United States, Canada, Norway, and The Netherlands.[15,20] Later information for Norway indicates 38% in 1969–1978 and 46% in 1979–1983 were coded as underlying cause (T.P. Flaten, personal communication October 11, 1990).

For deaths among known parkinsonian patients in Rochester, Minnesota, it was coded as underlying cause in 1/5.[15,21] Among such patients in Baltimore, Maryland, it was listed on the death certificate as underlying cause for 10% and for 28% as a secondary cause.[22] Therefore the death data based on underlying cause will provide about a third of the deaths listed on the certificates, and only 10–20% of known parkinson patients who die.

International Death Rates

Age-adjusted (U.S. 1950) death rates for parkinsonism in the 1950s were available for 24 countries.[23] The rates ranged from 0.5 per 100,000 for Japan, Czechoslovakia, Mexico, and U.S. nonwhites, to 3.8 per 100,000 in Australia (Figure 2). High rates (some 2.5 +) were recorded for the United Kingdom, Ireland, Belgium, The Netherlands, France, and Switzerland, as well as for Israel, Uruguay, and Australia–New Zealand. Scandinavia, Canada, and U.S. whites were intermediate.

Thus parkinson deaths seemed especially common in western Europe, excluding Scandinavia, and in their emigrant nations of Australia, New Zealand, and Israel. The deaths in Israel would have been for immigrants and not the native-born, considering the age at death for parkinsonism. There was a marked white–nonwhite difference in the U.S. We shall see below that morbidity rates for Scandinavia tend to be high. In an abstract of a review of parkinsonism in Europe, de Pedro and Fratiglione stated: "The figures [not cited] for incidence, prevalence and mortality for Parkinsonism in Iceland rank first among those reported in the world."[24]

For every country except Iceland, the age-adjusted death rates were higher for males than for females, the male–female ratio on the rates averaging 1.4–1.[17]

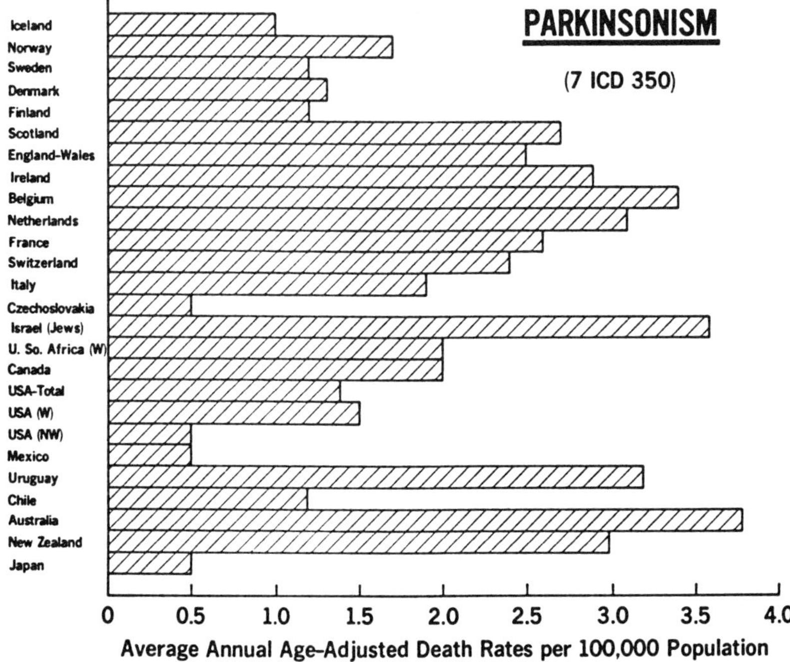

Figure 2. Average annual age-adjusted (U.S. 1950) death rates per 100,000 population, selected countries, 1951–1958. Data of Goldberg and Kurland,[23] from Kurtzke.[18]

Time Trends

Crude death rates for parkinsonism in the United States had remained fairly stable at about 1.4 per 100,000 annually from 1949 to 1961. From 1962 through 1975, the rates fluctuated between 1.4 and 1.6, but there was no consistent pattern indicative of an increase in the death rate.[17] The rates in Great Britain also had varied little for 100 years into the 1960s, once the postencephalitic cases were removed.[25]

Figure 3 shows annual crude death rates for parkinsonism for the United States for 1950–1984, and those for Denmark for 1956–1985.[26] Beginning in 1976 there is a striking increase in the rates in both lands, which has plateaued in Denmark. The recent U.S. deaths were those coded to 332.0 (ICD9). All Danish deaths were listed under 350 (ICD6 and 7) or 342 (ICD8).

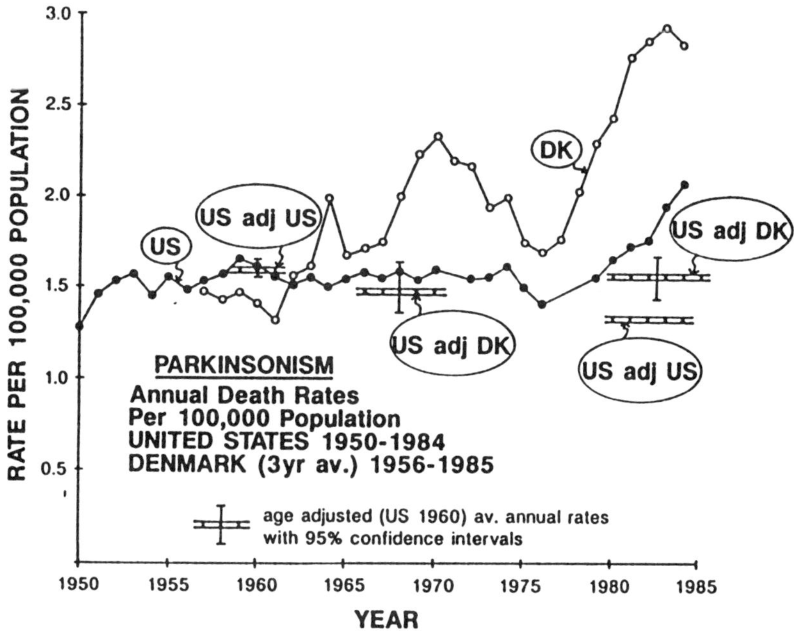

Figure 3. Annual crude death rates per 100,000 population, United States 1950–1984 and Denmark 1956–1985, the latter calculated as 3-year centered moving averages, plus period average annual age-adjusted (U.S. 1960) death rates with 95% confidence intervals: United States 1959–1961 and 1980–1984; Denmark 1966–1970 and 1980–1985. From Kurtzke and Murphy.[26]

The age-adjusted (U.S. 1960) rate, all ages, which had suggested no significant difference between the United States and Denmark in the earlier years, now showed a clear excess in the most recent period for Denmark over the United States. But neither adjusted rate reflected the dramatic rise indicated by the crude rates. Indeed, the recent U.S. adjusted rate was *lower* than that near 1960.

Rates by sex in Denmark demonstrate similar configurations, with the 1976–1984 increase and the notable male excess throughout. However, only the male-adjusted rate had increased significantly over time (Figure 4). The pattern in Denmark for each sex is faithfully duplicated for Norway for 1965–1988, but with the annual crude rates twice as high in the latter country.[27] A peak rate of over 6 per 100,000 population was reached in Norway by 1985, several

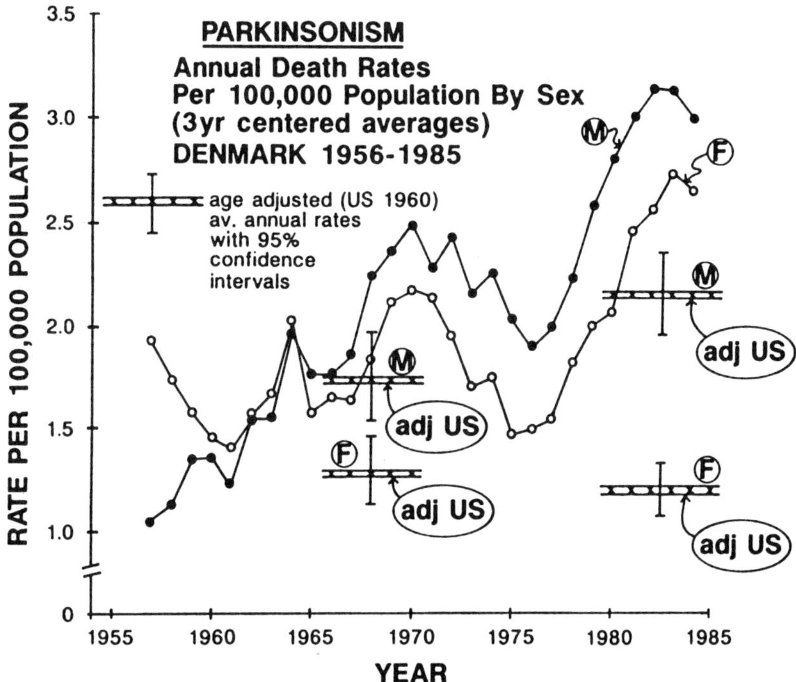

Figure 4.   Annual crude death rates and period average annual age-adjusted rates per 100,000 population by sex, as in Figure 3, Denmark 1956–1985. From Kurtzke and Murphy.[26]

years after the Danish maximum, although with a slight decline thereafter.

In the United States we see clearly a consistent and marked excess of whites over nonwhites, and of males over females (Figure 5). Again though, while the adjusted rates appear significantly higher for males of both races in the recent years than earlier, that for white females is now markedly lower. The increase in the crude rates from 1976 was 54% for white males and 39% for white females. These 1976 to 1984 differences were roughly proportional, blacks and whites, with a similar sex differential.

The paradox of age-adjusted death rates moving in opposite directions requires further attention to the age-specific rates themselves.

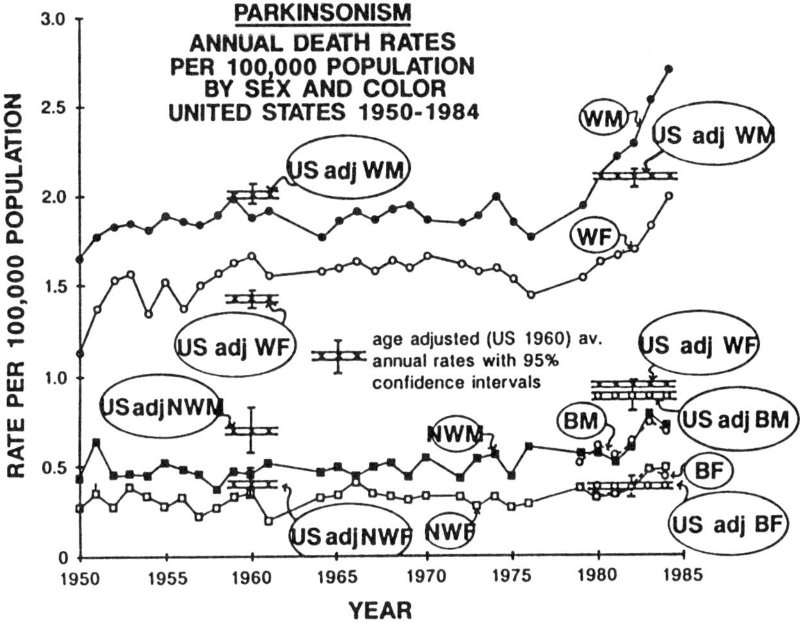

Figure 5.   Annual crude death rates and period average annual age-adjusted rates per 100,000 population by sex, color and race, as in Figure 3, United States 1950–1984. From Kurtzke and Murphy.[26]

Age and Sex

Figure 6 shows average annual age specific death rates by sex and color for 1959–1961 in the United States. Note the maximal rate at age 80 for all groups, and the clear gradation of WM > WF > NWM > NWF. The rate age 75–84 was 27.6 per 100,000 for white males, 20.6 for white females and 23.6 for all whites; similar rates for nonwhites were 8.2 (M), 4.6 (F), and 6.3 (total).[17] For 1965–1971, the configuration was quite similar.[28] The rates at age 75–84 were then 29.0 (WM), 18.6 (WF), and 6.5 (all nonwhites); at age 85 + they were 22.0, 17.3, and 4.3, respectively.

Earlier data for 1955 were also equivalent, but they also afforded an assessment of the marked contribution to Parkinson death rates made by deaths coded as other than underlying cause, material

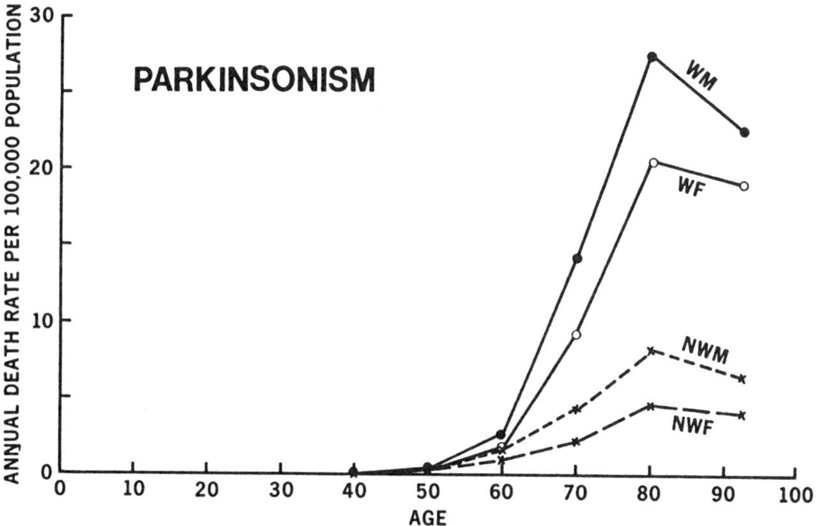

Figure 6.   Average annual age-specific death rates per 100,000 population by sex and color, United States 1959–1961. Data of Kurland et al.;[17] from Kurtzke.[18]

available only for that year.[29] For all deaths recorded on the certificate, the total rate then reached a maximum of some 70 per 100,000 at age 80 for whites, as opposed to the underlying cause rate of about 20 (Figure 7). This configuration was found for each sex and color; in particular, the nonwhite deficit persisted.

The configuration for underlying cause deaths was also not much different for Denmark for 1966–1970 (Figure 8). The maximal rate, both sexes, was at 23.7 per 100,000 age 75–79 with 25.0 male and 22.7 female, quite similar to the rates for U.S. whites. The rate, with small numbers, appeared to remain high for males beyond that age, but that for females fell as in the United States.

Now consider the recent rates. Figure 9 shows a rate, both sexes and colors, of 32.1 per 100,000 age 80–84 (53.5 male, 23.8 female) for the United States 1980–1984. This is the maximal rate age group for blacks (18.2 male, 8.4 female), but for whites the high rates persist or even increase in the 85+ ages. The white male rate is proportionately much higher at this time than was the case for either Denmark or the United States at the earlier intervals. Note too the difference in scale for this and the next figure versus Figures 6 and 8.

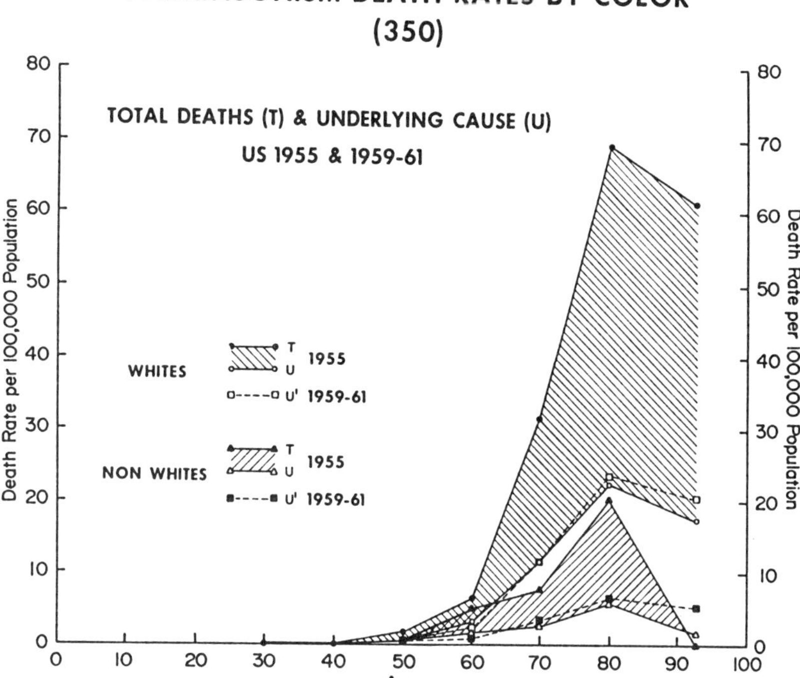

Figure 7.   Annual age-specific death rates per 100,000 population by color and cause: total deaths (T) and underlying cause (U) 1955; underlying cause (U') 1959–1961, United States. Shaded portion indicates the rates as secondary causes of death. From Kurtzke.[18]

This configuration is even more prominent for Denmark 1980–1985 (Figure 10). At age 80–84, the rate, both sexes, is 39.6 per 100,000 with 57.6 male and 29.6 female—quite similar to the recent U.S. rates. The Danish rate 85 +, however, attains 68.2 for males, 28.8 for females, and 41.6 for both sexes.

These are the age-specific rates that provided the discrepant age adjusted rates of Figures 4 and 5, where there had been a marked increase in males only in Denmark and a marked decrease in (white) females only in the United States (the latter male rates had increased moderately), and this despite a higher maximal age specific rate in U.S. women than previously, as well as the similar configuration for both sexes in both lands.

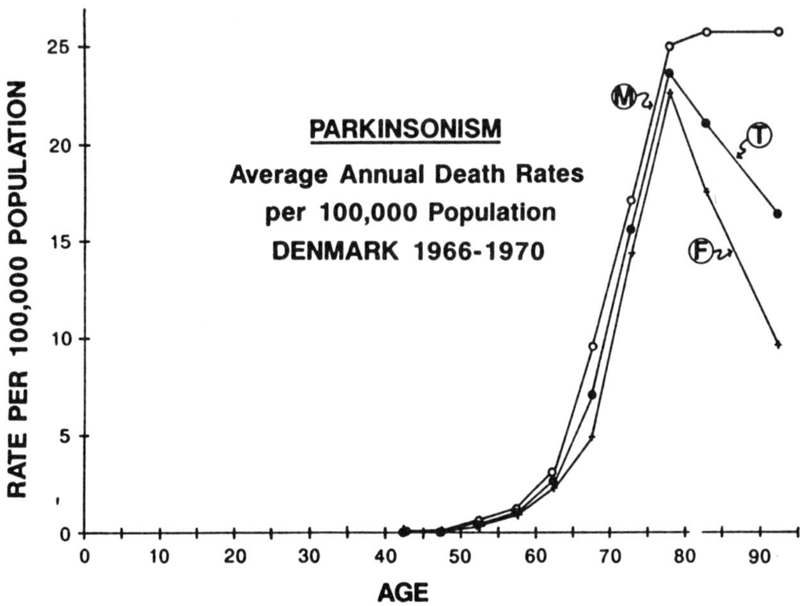

Figure 8. Average annual age-specific death rates per 100,000 population by sex, Denmark 1966–1970.

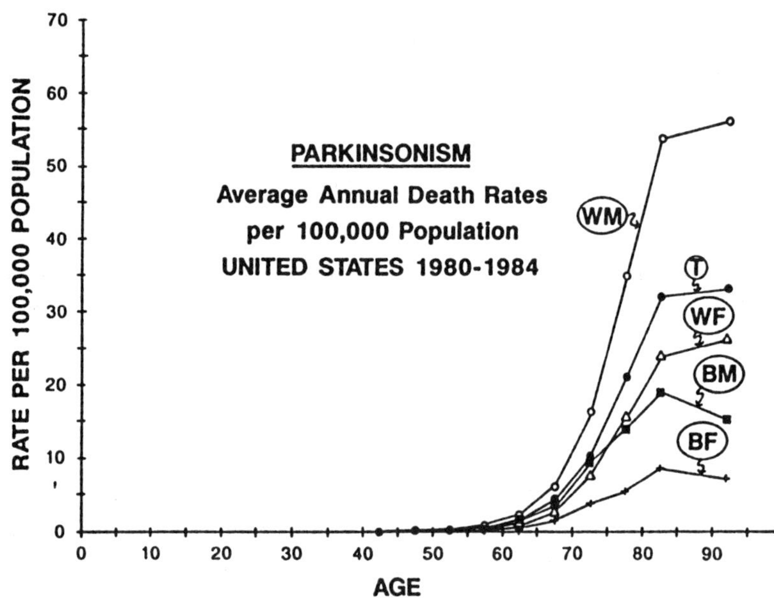

Figure 9. Average annual age-specific death rates per 100,000 population by sex and race, United States 1980–1984.

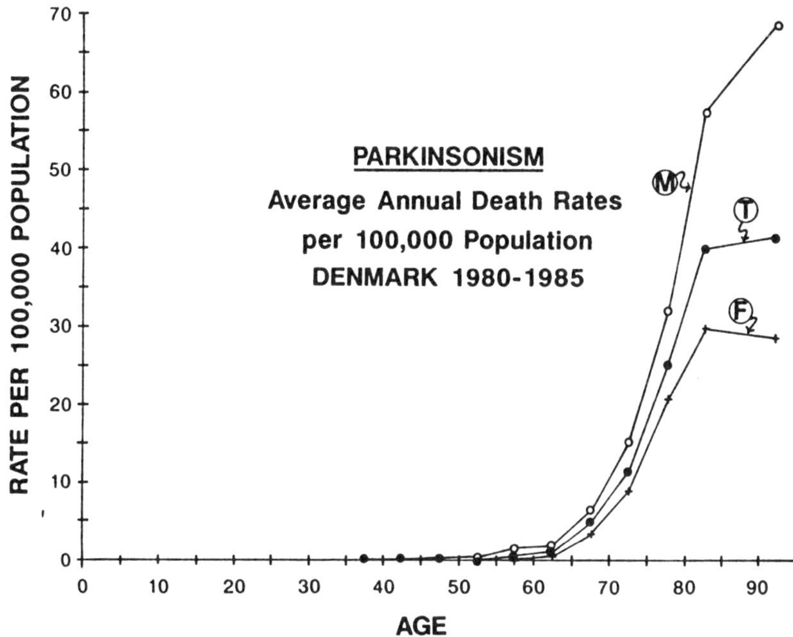

Figure 10. Average annual age-specific death rates per 100,000 population by sex, Denmark 1980–1985.

One explanation for the divergent changes by sex is that the denominator, the population by age, had not changed in parallel fashion for each sex between the intervals in question. There was in fact a progressively increasing female population excess with increasing age over time. Adjusting the recent populations by sex and age so that the increase was proportional to the earlier distributions resulted in much less of a male–female discrepancy in the age-specific and age-adjusted rates. However, the age-specific curves remained largely unchanged: rates still essentially continued to rise with increasing age to the eldest age group, regardless of sex or place (data available).

This change over time could, however, be explained on the basis that parkinsonism patients are living longer with their disease in the 1980s than one or two decades ago. Accordingly, the question was posed: what would the 1980s age-specific death rates look like if all the deaths had occurred 5 years earlier (younger) than actually was the case? When these calculations were made, we did, in fact, return to age-specific death rate configurations that were very similar, by rate, sex, race, and country, to those recorded for the 1960s, as indicated in Figure 11 for Denmark and Figure 12 for the United States.

Even this maneuver, though, did not fully resolve the sex discrepancies over time between the age-adjusted rates. I believe that this is still an artifact caused by differential changes in the denominator populations. The age-specific curves for parkinsonism lie in that part of the age spectrum where population numbers are few and where even minor changes in their composition will affect drastically the age-adjusted rates.

These findings then can be summarized as two: a sharp increase in parkinsonism death rates between 1976 and 1984, and an age-specific death rate curve in the 1980s compatible with deaths then occurring in patients 5 years older than was the case in the

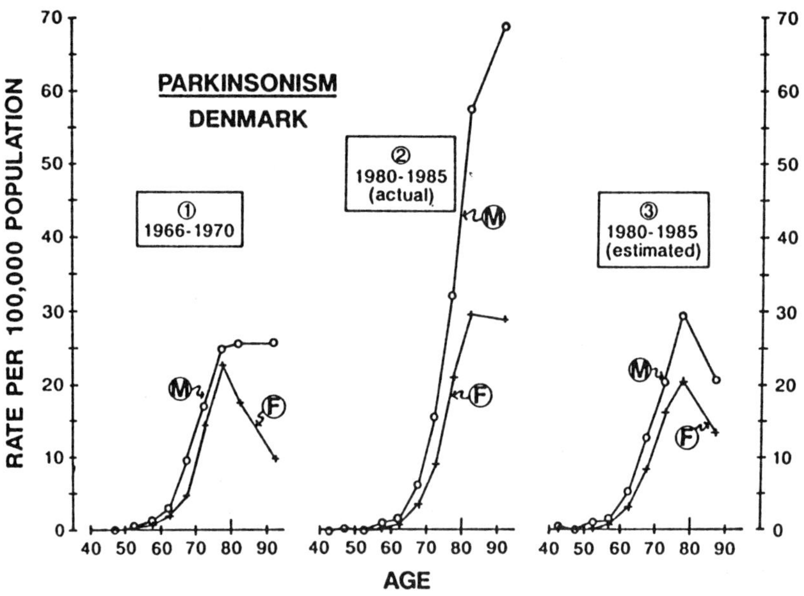

Figure 11. Average annual age-specific death rates per 100,000 population by sex, Denmark: (1) 1966–1970; (2) 1980–1985, actual rates; (3) 1980–1985, estimated rates (adjusted population and all deaths at age 5 years younger). The age 80 indicator is stressed. From Kurtzke and Murphy.[26]

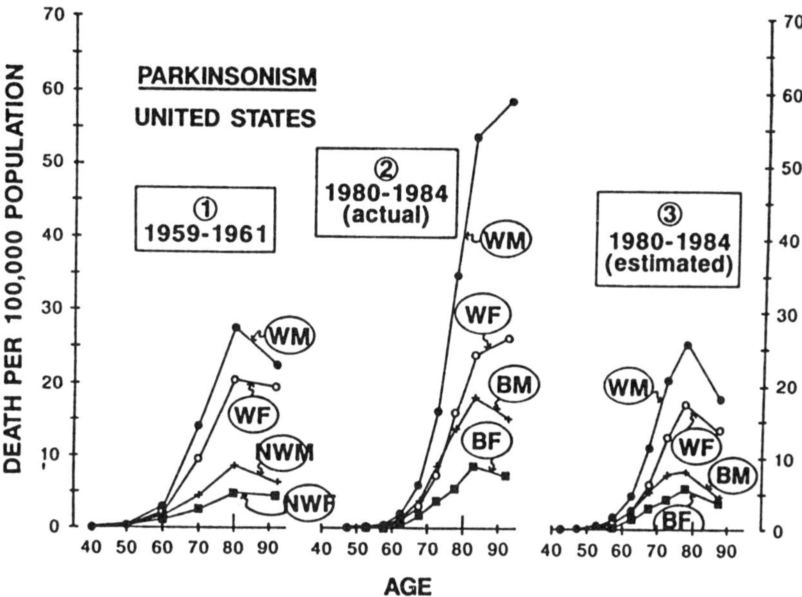

Figure 12. Average annual age-specific death rates per 100,000 population by sex and color/race, United States: (1) 1959–1961; (2) 1980–1984, actual rates; (3) 1980–1984, estimated rates as in Figure 11. The age 80 indicator is stressed. From Kurtzke and Murphy.[26]

1960s. Both are, I believe, attributable to the introduction of levodopa and the other newer antiparkinsonism agents. Diamond et al.[30] concluded there was a progressively favorable reduction of excess mortality due to parkinsonism the earlier that levodopa treatment was initiated. Mortality reduction indicates increased survival. Marttila and Rinne[31] pointed out that this increased survival, which they estimated at 3–6 years overall, would lead to higher prevalence rates as well as, obviously, a higher age at death. In their own Finnish material, the average duration of life after onset of the disease had increased from the 9–10 years of the predopa days to 14 years.[19,32,33]

The material presented here does indeed indicate that there has been an increase by about 5 years in age at death due to parkinsonism, but there is no evidence that this was preferentially for any given age group. The return to the predopa age-specific death rate curve was seen when *all* death ages were reduced by 5 years. This would not have been the case had only the older (late) or the younger (early) deaths been so affected. The increase in the death rates, all ages, is easily attributed to a higher proportion of Parkinson patients under long-term treatment, and thus more likely to have this disorder cited on the certificate as the cause in the event of death. Indeed, Aquilonius et al.[34] have estimated that as early as 1977 virtually all known parkinsonism patients of Sweden and 90% of those of Norway, Denmark, and Finland were under treatment, and with the combination of levodopa and decarboxylase inhibitor.

Race

It is clear from the above that the Parkinson death rate for nonwhites has been consistently lower than that for whites in the United States, and some 90% of nonwhites are blacks.

For 1959–1961, the age adjusted (U.S. 1940) death rates (Table 3) showed a striking and statistically highly significant difference between whites and blacks: the respective rates were 1.3 and 0.4 per 100,000 population, all ages, and 15.0 and 3.7 per 100,000 age 65 +.[35]

The death rates for Oriental Americans (Japanese, Chinese) were equivalent to those for whites; despite small numbers they were also significantly in excess of the rates for blacks. Rates for American Indians did not differ significantly from those for whites— or for blacks, and provide no basis for interpretation.

There was the previously noted uniform and significant male excess in the death rates, regardless of color. This held as well for blacks alone, and was apparently the case for the other races too, although the numbers precluded precision for some of these.

Geography

In the United States 1959–1961, the age-adjusted (U.S. 1940) rates by state of residence at death ranged from 0.5 per 100,000 in Mississippi to 1.9 in Alaska and 1.8 in South Dakota and Vermont. Most of the high rate states were in the northwestern and north central sections of the country.[17]

Because of the age and color differences previously noted, special attention was paid to the distribution by state for whites age 65 +. Their age-adjusted rates are drawn in Figure 13. Again there

Table 3.

Parkinsonism: Deaths and Average Annual Age-Adjusted (U.S. 1940) Death Rates per 100,000 Population, with 95% Confidence Intervals on Rates, by Race and Sex, United States 1959–1961[a]

Age Group and Race	Deaths			Death Rates (95% CI[b])		
	Total	Male	Female	Total	Male	Female
All ages						
Total U.S.	8674	4682	3992	1.2 (1.2–1.2)	1.5 (1.5–1.5)	1.0 (1.0–1.0)
White	8439	4540	3899	1.3 (1.3–1.3)	1.5 (1.5–1.5)	1.1 (1.1–1.1)
Nonwhite	235	142	93	0.4 (0.4–0.5)	0.5 (0.4–0.6)	0.3 (0.2–0.4)
Black	202	116	86	0.4 (0.3–0.5)	0.5 (0.4–0.6)	0.3 (0.2–0.4)
Indian	9	5	4	0.7 (0.3–1.3)	0.8 (0.3–1.9)	0.7 (0.2–1.8)
Japanese	14	12	2	1.1 (0.6–1.8)	1.6 (0.8–2.8)	0.4 (0.0–1.4)
Chinese	6	5	1	1.1 (0.4–2.4)	1.2 (0.4–2.8)	0.7 (0.0–3.9)
Other NW	4	4	0	0.4 (0.1–1.0)	0.6 (0.2–2.2)	— —
Age 65 +						
Total U.S.	7268	3871	3397	14.1 (13.7–14.5)	16.9 (16.4–17.4)	11.9 (11.5–12.3)
White	7114	3776	3338	15.0 (14.5–15.5)	17.9 (17.3–18.5)	12.6 (12.2–13.0)
Nonwhite	154	95	59	4.1 (3.5–4.8)	5.3 (4.3–6.5)	2.9 (2.2–3.7)
Black	131	76	55	3.7 (3.1–4.4)	4.7 (3.7–5.9)	2.9 (2.2–3.8)
Indian	6	4	2	7.8 (2.9–17.0)	9.8 (2.7–25.1)	5.8 (0.7–20.9)
Japanese	11	10	1	11.6 (5.8–20.8)	17.2 (8.3–31.6)	2.5 (0.1–13.9)
Chinese	5	4	1	13.8 (4.5–32.2)	14.8 (4.0–37.9)	9.8 (0.2–54.6)
Other NW	1	1	0	2.3 (0.1–12.8)	3.3 (0.1–18.4)	— —

[a]Data of Kurland et al. [17] From Kurtzke and Goldberg.[35]
[b]95 percent confidence interval, Poisson distribution.

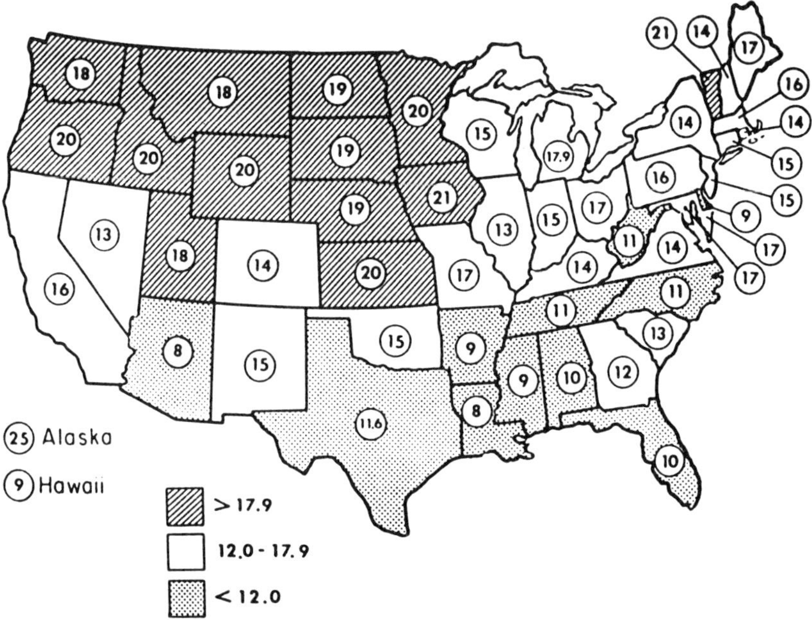

Figure 13. Average annual age-adjusted (U.S. 1940) death rates per 100,000 population for whites age 65 + by state of residence at death, United States, 1959–1961. From Kurland et al.[17]

was an excess in the northwest and a deficit in the south. The distribution was rather reminiscent of that for multiple sclerosis.[18] When death rates by state for both these diseases among whites were directly compared, there was a highly significant correlation between the two; r_s = 0.754, $P < 0.01$ (Figure 14).[36]

Available distributions by sex and color were limited to the nine census regions (CRs) of the United States (Table 4).[35] Since blacks provided 86% of all Parkinson deaths among nonwhites, and 85% of those age 65 +, the nonwhite rates by CR are a close approximation to those for blacks alone. This is even more the situation when we compare the northern United States (defined by the first four CRs with the south (the next three CRs). The two western CRs, Mountain and Pacific, extend from Canada to Mexico. A preponderance of nonblacks among the nonwhites will be found in the Mountain CR (for Indians), and, especially, in the Pacific CR (for all nonblack races), since the latter region comprises not only the westernmost

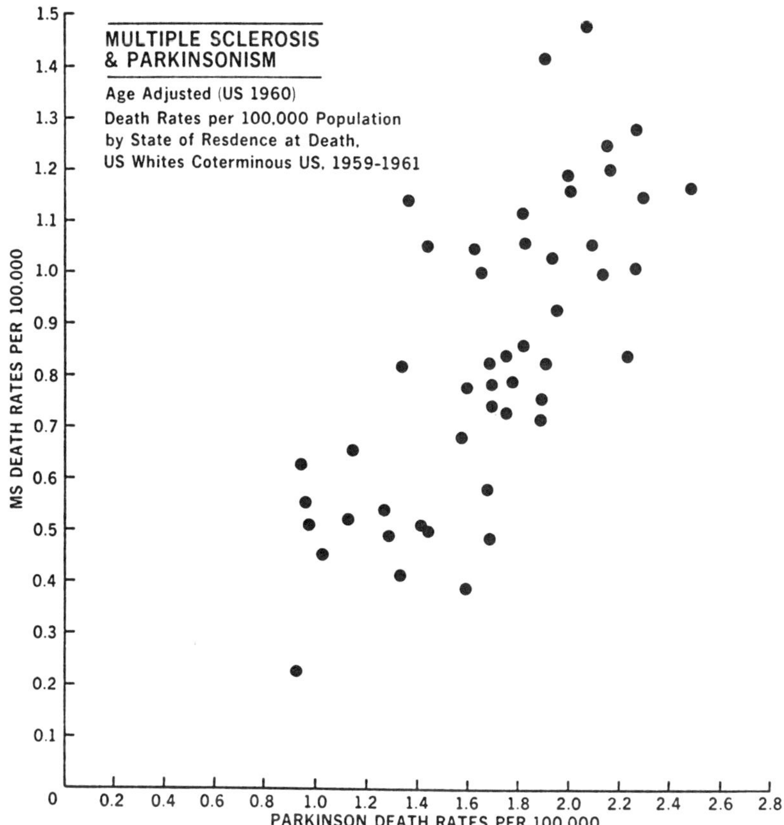

Figure 14.   Average annual age-adjusted (U.S. 1960) death rates per 100,000 population for whites by state or residence at death, compared with analogous death rates from multiple sclerosis, United States 1961–1969. Each point represents both rates for one state of the coterminous US. From Lux and Kurtzke.[36]

states of the coterminous United States, but also includes Alaska and Hawaii. Therefore, when we limit comparisons by color to the seven eastern census regions, we are in fact considering essentially a true white–black relationship within a true north–south division of the country.

It is clear that there was a marked geographic difference in the Parkinson's disease death rates, regardless of age or color. Overall the north–south death rate ratios were 1.4 for whites, all ages and age

Table 4.

Parkinsonism: Average Annual Age-Adjusted (U.S. 1940) Death Rates per 100,000 Population by Age Group (All Ages, Age 65 +), Sex, Color, and Census Region of Residence at Death, United States 1959–1961[a]

Age group and Census Region	White			Nonwhite		
	Total	Male	Female	Total	Male	Female
All ages						
Total U.S.	1.3	1.5	1.1	0.4	0.5	0.3
New England	1.4	1.6	1.2	0.6[b]	1.0[b]	0.3[b]
Middle Atlantic	1.3	1.6	1.1	0.6	0.9	0.4
East North Central	1.3	1.6	1.1	0.6	0.7	0.5
West North Central	1.6	1.9	1.3	0.6	0.5[b]	0.7[b]
South Atlantic	1.1	1.3	0.9	0.3	0.4	0.3
East South Central	1.0	1.2	0.8	0.2	0.2[b]	0.2
West South Central	1.0	1.2	0.8	0.3	0.4	0.2[b]
Mountain	1.2	1.4	1.2	0.6[b]	0.8[b]	0.3[b]
Pacific	1.4	1.6	1.2	0.8	1.1	0.4[b]
Age 65 +						
Total U.S.	15.0	17.9	12.6	4.1	5.3	2.9
New England	15.8	18.1	14.0	6.7[b]	14.5[b]	—[b]
Middle Atlantic	15.0	17.7	12.9	6.5	9.4	4.2
East North Central	15.5	18.7	12.8	5.1	5.6	4.6
West North Central	19.2	23.3	15.7	5.5[b]	5.5[b]	5.5[b]
South Atlantic	12.1	14.6	10.0	3.1	3.8	2.4
East South Central	11.3	13.9	9.0	2.0	1.6[b]	2.4[b]
West South Central	11.3	13.9	9.3	2.3	3.6	1.2[b]
Mountain	14.9	16.4	13.5	8.7[b]	11.5[b]	5.0[b]
Pacific	16.7	19.8	14.4	9.4	13.0	4.8[b]

[a]Data of Kurland et al. [17] From Kurtzke and Goldberg.[35]
[b]Rate based on less than 10 deaths.

65 + ; for nonwhites they were 2.3 and 2.4, respectively. Within each census region, the consistent male excess persisted regardless of color, wherever there were sufficient deaths for reasonably stable rates.

Lilienfeld et al.[37] analyzed U.S. Parkinson deaths by the same measures for 1980–1984, but age adjusted the rates to a different standard. The configuration differs from that in Table 4, but not in any consistent manner by either sex, color, or geography. Compared with the data presented here, the white male rates tended to decrease in the north and increase in the south—but not uniformly, while white female rates almost all decreased and perhaps more so in the north. Taking the age 65 + rates, which seem the more reliable, their north–south death rate ratio is 1.2 for whites; among nonwhites the ratios are 0.9 male and 1.4 female. What does persist is the male and the white preponderance, regardless of geography. The inference remains as to an environmental influence affecting the geographic distribution, but one that would seem to vary more readily than that of multiple sclerosis—assuming all these Parkinson death rates are of equal validity. I suspect the older U.S. death series is, in fact, the more reliable for geographic distributions, the recent series being confounded by the same factors discussed above for the country as a whole.

Morbidity Data

While it is likely that deaths coded to parkinsonism will have been correctly diagnosed, it is clear they reflect only a minority of the affected. Further, it is highly probable that even the cases ascertained in community surveys will represent a notable undercount. Almost all these works rely upon the identification of cases already known to the health care facilities of the area. There are basically two reasons for patients to seek medical help: pain and impaired function. The former is irrelevant in parkinsonism, and the latter almost so in the elderly for even moderate impairment, since they are without occupational or strenuous recreational pressures. Even when dysfunction is bothersome and medical attention sought, the shaking may be dismissed as aging or as senile tremor and the stiffness attributed to "arthritis." Even for neurologists, an early diagnosis of parkinsonism may be difficult, especially if tremor is lacking. It is with these caveats, therefore, that reported morbidity rates should be considered.

Prevalence Rates

Point prevalence rates for parkinsonism in Europe have ranged from 0.7 to 2.5 per 1000 population (Table 5). The highest rates were

Table 5.
Parkinsonism: Point Prevalence Rates per 1000 Population from Community Surveys—Europe

First author (year)	Site	Prev yr.	N	Rate	Notes[a]
Gudmundsson (1967)[38]	Iceland	1963	317	1.7	
Broman (1963)[39]	Göteborg, Sweden	1960	270	0.7	(a)
de Pedro (1984)[40]	Sweden	1980	—	1.7	(b)
de Pedro (1985)[41,42]	Sweden	1984	—	2.5	(c)
Marttila (1976)[43]	Turku CHD, Finland	1971	484	1.2	
Marttila (1990)[33]	Turku CHD, Finland	1985	651	1.5	
Teräväinen (1986)[44]	Helsinki, Finland	1985	196	2.5	
Brewis (1966)[45]	Carlisle, England	1961	80	1.1	(d)
Sutcliffe (1985)[46]	Northampton, England	1982	223	1.1	
Sutcliffe (1985)[46]	Northampton, England	1982	223	0.8	(e)
Mutch (1986)[47]	Aberdeen, Scotland	1984	249	1.6	
Mutch (1986)[47]	Aberdeen, Scotland	1984	249	1.0	(e)
Rosati (1980)[48]	Sardinia, Italy	1972	967	0.7	
Rosati (1980)[48]	Sardinia, Italy	1972	967	0.7	(e)
D'Alessandro (1987)[49]	San Marino	1986	34	1.5	
D'Allesandro (1987)[49]	San Marino	1986	34	1.9	(f)
D'Allesandro (1987)[49]	San Marino	1986	34	1.1	(e)
Chalmanov (1986)[50]	Sofia, Bulgaria	1983	1936	1.7	(g)

[a](a) Hospitalized patients only; (b) estimated from antiparkinson drug sales, "calibrated" for overuse; (c) estimated from antiparkinson drug sales, "refined model"; (d) diagnostic criteria rather strict; (e)age-adjusted U.S. 1960 population; (f)age-adjusted Italy 1980 population; (g) includes secondary parkinsonism.

from Helsinki, Finland,[44] and Sweden,[41,42] although concurrent rates in western Finland were notably lower.[33] Also near 2 per 1000 population was Iceland.[38] That rate is almost 30-years old. Previously, we noted de Pedro's statement that Iceland has the highest rates in the world.[24] Presumably there are later data to support that conclusion, but I have been unable to find them. The rather high rate from Sofia[50] included an appreciable proportion of patients with secondary parkinsonism.

The low rate from Göteborg, Sweden, was based on hospitalized patients only; the author believes the true rate for that community was at least twice the 0.7 observed.[39] Below in Table 10 will be the evidence for incomplete case ascertainment to explain the rate of 0.7 for Sardinia.[48]

Rates in Europe thus lie mostly between 1 and 2.5 per 1000. There is no good evidence for meaningful geographic variation from the few studies available. There is but little support for an increasing prevalence rate that one would expect with the increased survival discussed previously.

Prevalence surveys from outside Europe in general follow the same pattern for whites as just noted (Table 6). There is a curious discrepancy in British Columbia between Vancouver[44] and a nearby rural area.[51] The 95% confidence interval on the rate of 0.7 for the latter is 0.5–0.9, but case ascertainment may well have been incomplete there.

The deficit of blacks with parkinsonism is highly significant in the Baltimore survey[22] and the trend is similar in the smaller survey

Table 6.

Parkinsonism: Point Prevalence Rates per 1000 Population from Community Surveys—Non-European Sites

First author (year)	Site	Prev yr	N	Rate	Notes[a]
Teräväinen (1986)[44]	Vancouver, BC	1985	355	2.3	
Snow (1989)[51]	Rural British Columbia	1988	55	0.7	
Nobrega (1967)[52]	Rochester, Minnesota	1965	75	1.6	
Nobrega (1967)[52]	Rochester, Minnesota	1965	75	1.8	(a)
Kessler (1972)[22]	Baltimore, Maryland, white	1967–9	211	1.3	(b)
Kessler (1972)[22]	Baltimore, Maryland, black	1967–9	17	0.2	(b)
Haerer (1987)[53] +	Copiah County, Mississippi, white	1978	19	1.6	
Anderson (1988)[54]	Copiah County, Mississippi, black	1978	12	1.0	
Pollock (1966)[55]	Wellington, N.Z.	1962	131	1.1	
Jenkins (1966)[56]	Gippsland, Australia	1965	70	0.8	
Harada (1983)[57]	Yonago, Japan	1980	101	0.8	
Harada (1983)[57]	Yonago, Japan	1980	101	0.7	(a)
Li (1985)[58]	Six cities, China	1983	28	0.4	
Li (1985)[58]	Six cities, China	1983	28	0.6	(a)
Schoenberg (1988)[59]	Igbo-Ora, Nigeria	c1978	2	0.1	
Herishanu (1989)[60]	Negev, Israel	1988	156	0.9	(a)
Herishanu (1989)[60]	Negev "focus"	1988	13	5.3	(a)

[a](a) Age adjusted U.S. 1960 population; (b) calculated from community sample.

of Copiah County, Mississippi.[53,54] Rates in Australia–New Zealand from quite old surveys[55,56] do not really support the even older excessively high death rates of Figure 2. Oriental rates may well be lower than in the Occident[57,58]; confidence intervals on the U.S. 1960 age-adjusted rates are 0.57–0.85 for Yonago[57] and 0.40–0.87 for China.[58] For Nigeria[59] the interval is 0.01–0.36, clearly supportive of a low risk for blacks.

Of interest is the rate from three adjoining kibbutzim of the Negev region of Israel.[60] Their rate for parkinsonism, age-adjusted to U.S. 1960 population, was 5.28 per 1000 with a 95% interval of 2.81–9.02 per 1000, clearly the highest frequency reported to date. Conversely, the age-adjusted rate for the entire Negev region was 0.90 (interval 0.77–1.06). These rates were calculated from the data presented and will not be found in the paper.[60] Herishanu et al.[60] noted that the patients of the Negev, whether from the focus or not, were all Ashkenazim (middle European) by birth but had been living in the Negev for 20–40 years or so. Subtracting these 13 cluster patients among their 592 older kibbutz residents from the 156 among the 250,000 Negev population all ages would not alter appreciably the overall adjusted rate of 0.90. Why this cluster should have occurred is not obvious to me—or to the authors.

Among whites, then, a reasonable estimate of prevalence, based upon the better surveys[44,52] is likely to be about 2 per 1000 population. Lower rates may well reflect incomplete case ascertainment. Indeed, Anderson et al.[54] in their door-to-door survey of Copiah County had newly identified 13 (of 31) cases of parkinsonism (42%!) that had previously been undiagnosed. There is little support for the notable geographic variation among whites inferred from the death data, and not much evidence that levodopa has really altered the prevalence of parkinsonism so far. Conversely, the data are so soft and sparse that it is clearly premature to conclude to the contrary on either point. Prevalence rates *are* in general higher in the 1970s and 1980s than in the 1960s, but better case ascertainment could well be the main explanation for this. Racial "protection" for blacks inferred from United States and international death data seems likely to be a valid finding. Whether Oriental rates are truly lower than those for whites is less clear; they seemed not different in the U.S. deaths, but probably are lower in Japan and China. If both are true, this would support environmental influences.

Age, Sex, Race. The death data had indicated a strong relationship of parkinsonism to age, and in prevalence rates this is even more striking. In the Rochester survey, parkinsonism was rarely noted before age 40, whereas 1% of the population over age 60 was affected. Among the oldest age group the prevalence rate exceeded 2%.[52] For other series the curves are similar, even though some absolute rates were notably lower. Table 7 shows age- and sex-specific rates for the Northampton survey.[46] Each rate by age is considerably greater for males than for females, even though the crude rate all ages shows a female excess. Age-adjusted (U.S. 1960) rates do give the more accurate reflection of this difference; the sex ratio on the rates is then 1.30 M–F.

Findings are similar for Aberdeen[47] (Table 8). Again, age adjustment demonstrates the male excess with a 1.54 ratio. Even with the unstable rates for the small series from San Marino[49] the U.S. 1960 age adjustment seems more valid (M–F = 1.26) than the authors' Italian 1980 adjustment (M–F = 0.96) (Table 9). In Sardinia[48] the U.S. adjustment supports the male excess indicated by the crude rates (Table 10). Note in both Italian-area surveys the lower age-specific rates for the eldest groups, in contrast to other series.

Table 7.
Parkinsonism: Age-Specific Prevalence Rates per 1000 Population by Sex, with Age-Adjusted (U.S. 1960) Rates, Northampton District, England, October 1, 1982[a]

Age	Total	Male	Female
< 50	.03	.03	.03
50–59	.64	.92	.36
60–69	2.77	2.84	2.70
70–79	7.02	8.42	6.04
80+	11.36	12.93	10.70
Total	1.08	1.02	1.14
(N)	(226)	(105)	(121)
Age adj[b]	0.76	0.87[c]	0.67[c]

[a]Data of Sutcliffe et al.[46]
[b]U.S. 1960.
[c]M:F ratio = 1.30.

Table 8.
Parkinsonism: Age-Specific Prevalence Rates per 1000 Population by Sex with Age-Adjusted (U.S. 1960) Rates, Aberdeen, Scotland, May 31, 1984[a]

Age	Total	Male	Female
40–44	0.13	0.27	—
45–49	0.76	1.40	0.20
50–54	0.83	1.33	0.39
55–59	0.73	0.67	0.77
60–64	2.40	3.74	1.30
65–69	2.69	3.46	2.11
70–74	7.07	8.56	6.13
75–79	10.20	15.59	7.58
80–84	17.92	10.42	20.77
85 +	22.05	26.58	20.71
Total	1.64	—	—
(N)	(249)	(109)	(140)
Age adj[b]	0.96	1.20[c]	0.78[c]

[a]Data of Mutch et al.[47]
[b]U.S. 1960
[c]M:F ratio = 1.54

This is, I believe, a reflection of incomplete case ascertainment, which in turn provides underestimates for the rates all ages.

Rates in Japan[57] appear to increase with age, as expected from the United States and British data, but at a more modest pace (Table 11). The varying sex differences among the age-specific rates make tenuous the inference of a female preponderance for the (average) total rates. In China[58] the male–female case ratio was 3.67 (22 M, 6 F), a highly significant difference.

Incidence Rates

Average annual incidence rates for parkinsonism have ranged from 5 to 19 per 100,000 population (Table 12). The Swedish rate, as stated above, is less than half that the author thought likely.[39] Other low rates from Italy[48] and Australia[56] are rather old surveys and likely to be incomplete. Noteworthy is the relative stability of the incidence

Table 9.
Parkinsonism: Age-Specific Prevalence Rates per 1000 Population by Sex, with Age-Adjusted (U.S. 1960) Rates, San Marino, April 30, 1986[a]

Age	Total	Male	Female
0–54	0	0	0
55–59	0.80	1.63	0
60–64	3.80	1.78	6.13
65–69	5.73	7.87	4.07
70–74	12.36	13.66	11.28
75–79	19.50	25.64	15.15
80–84	9.49	8.77	9.90
85 +	0	0	0
Total	1.52	1.54	1.50
(N)	(34)	(17)	(17)
Age adj (1980 Italy)	1.85	1.84	1.91
Age adj[b]	1.13	1.30[c]	1.03[c]

[a]Data of D'Alessandro et al.[49]
[b]U.S. 1960.
[c]M:F ratio = 1.26.

Table 10.
Parkinsonism: Age-Specific Prevalence Rates per 1000 Population by Sex, with Age-Adjusted (U.S. 1960) Rates, Sardinia, January 1, 1972[a]

Age	Total	Male	Female
30–39	0.03	0.06	0.01
40–49	0.39	0.35	0.41
50–59	2.05	2.33	1.77
60–69	3.42	3.87	3.00
70–79	3.11	4.06	2.35
80–89	0.83	1.36	0.41
Total	0.66	0.74	0.58
(N)	(967)	(540)	(427)
Age adj[b]	0.66	0.77[c]	0.56[c]

[a]Data of Rosati et al.[48]
[b]U.S. 1960.
[c]M:F ratio = 1.37.

Table 11.
**Parkinsonism: Age-Specific Prevalence Rates per 1000
Population by Sex, with Age-Adjusted (U.S. 1960) Rates,
Yonago, Japan, April 1, 1980[a]**

Age	Total	Male	Female
30–39	.05	0	.09
40–49	.40	.35	.45
50–59	.86	1.03	.72
60–69	2.45	1.45	3.19
70–79	6.98	6.49	7.33
80–89	7.53	9.19	6.63
Total	0.81	0.63	0.97
(N)	(101)	(38)	(63)
Age adj[b]	0.73	0.67[c]	0.79[c]

[a]Data of Harada et al.[57]
[b]U.S. 1960.
[c]M:F ratio = 0.84.

rate in Rochester, Minnesota: the age-adjusted (U.S. 1960) rate of
16.4 for 1967–1979[62] has a 95% confidence interval of 13.6–19.6; the
1935–1966 rate was 18.5[52] with a 16.0–21.3 interval. Even this
apparent difference is entirely due to a lack of three patients age 80 +
in the 13 years of the recent survey.

The Netherlands rate is that from reports of patients seen in 3
years within 60 Sentinel Stations (General) Practices of that country,[61] and here too an underestimate is not unlikely; confidence
interval on that rate is 8.2–14.5.

Thus the more complete Occidental rates would suggest an
annual incidence rate rather close to 20 per 100,000. With a similarly
calculated estimate of 200 for prevalence, an average duration of
some 10 years would be expected. Nine to 10 years is what had been
found in Finland in the predopa era; at present the duration is 14
years.[32] We should then begin to see prevalence rates approaching
300; the highest we have so far is 250 (see above). Median survival in
Rochester too was 10 years for a largely predopa series.[62] The next
update from that community should be of interest. Kurland[15] had
earlier calculated a ''lifetime cumulative incidence'' of 2.5% for
parkinsonism.

Table 12.
Parkinsonism: Average Annual Incidence Rates per 100,000 Population from Community Surveys

First author (year)	Site	Period	N	Rate
Broman (1963)[39]	Göteborg, Sweden	1957–61	—	6(a)[a]
Gudmundsson (1967)[38]	Iceland	1954–63	272	16
Marttila (1976)[43]	Turku CHD, Finland	1969	67	17
Brewis (1966)[45]	Carlisle, England	1955–61	60	12(b)
Hofman (1989)[61]	Netherlands Sentinel Practices	1983–85	51	11
Rosati (1980)[48]	Sardinia, Italy	1961–71	796	5
Jenkins (1966)[56]	Gippsland, Australia	1959–64	35	7
Nobrega (1967)[52]	Rochester, Minnesota	1935–66	191	18
Nobrega (1967)[52]	Rochester, Minnesota	1935–66	191	19(c)
Rajput (1984)[62]	Rochester, Minnesota	1967–79	120	17
Rajput (1984)[62]	Rochester, Minnesota	1967–79	120	16(c)
Rajput (1984)[62]	Rochester, Minnesota	1967–79	120	18(d)
Harada (1983)[57]	Yonago, Japan	1975–79	62	10

[a](a) Author's estimate, hospitalized cases only; (b) diagnostic criteria rather strict; (c) age-adjusted U.S. 1960; (d) age-adjusted U.S. 1970.

The confidence interval on the rate of 10 per 100,000 for Yonago, Japan[57] is 7.8–13.1. If our Occidental rates are indeed close to 20, then this would seem low and in support of the prevalence and mortality rates for Orientals in their home lands.

Age and Sex. Average annual incidence rates for all parkinsonian states in Rochester, Minnesota, are shown in Table 13.[62] The male–female ratio on the age adjusted (U.S. 1960) rates is almost 1.6 for all disorders and for parkinsonism alone. Rates for "idiopathic parkinsonism" from that series were published later[63] and provide then a sex ratio closer to 1.5 (Table 14).

In both tables cases were entered by age at diagnosis, an interval that has averaged near 5 years from onset in that community.[52,62] For parkinsonism this otherwise minor difference makes a marked change in the configuration of the age-specific incidence curve. Figure 15 shows the earlier Rochester series[52] both as published, by date of diagnosis, and then by date of onset.[64] Instead of a dramatically sharp rise to a maximum rate over 170 per 100,000 at age 70–79, there is a more modest peak near 120 per 100,000 at that

Table 13.
Parkinsonian Conditions: Average Annual Age-Specific
Incidence Rates per 100,000 Population by Sex for
All Parkinsonian States[a] Based on Date of Diagnosis,
Rochester, Minnesota, 1967–1979[b]

	Rate per 100,000		
Age at Diagnosis	Total	Male	Female
0–29	0	0	0
30–54	5.3	6.5	4.1
55–64	32.2	41.0	26.0
65–74	113.5	147.1	94.1
75–84	254.4	345.6	209.5
85+	155.4	175.3	148.2
Total	19.7	20.2	19.3
(N)	(138)	(64)	(74)
Age adj U.S. 1960	18.8	24.5[c]	15.5[c]
Age adj U.S. 1970	20.5	—	—
Estimates for parkinson alone:			
Total	17.1	17.6	16.8
(N)	(120)	—	—
Age adj U.S. 1960	16.4	21.3[d]	13.5[d]
Age adj U.S. 1970	17.8	—	—

[a]Parkinson,[118] arteriosclerotic Parkinson,[2] secondary (drug) Parkinson,[10] "parkinsonism plus."[8] [b]Data of Rajput et al.[62] [c]M:F ratio = 1.57. [d]M:F ratio = 1.58.

age, from which the rate age 60–69 differs little. Further, there is then a sharp decline in the eldest age group, not apparent when diagnosis-date rates are considered.

The rates for the recent series[63] (Table 14) are almost identical to the diagnosis-date curve of Figure 15, until the eldest age; five more cases would give the same rate in that age group, and two of these were presumably the excluded "arteriosclerotic parkinson" patients.

Rates from Iceland[38] resemble the onset-date curve for Rochester (Figure 15). Configuration is similar but at lower levels for Carlisle.[45] Incidence rates also peaked at age 70–79 in Finland[19] at about 90 per

Table 14.
Parkinsonism: Average Annual Age-Specific Incidence Rates per 100,000 Population by Sex for Idiopathic Parkinsonism, Presumably Based on Date of Diagnosis, Rochester, Minnesota, 1967–1979[a]

Age	Total	Male	Female
0–39	0	0	0
40–49	4.3	9.0	0
50–59	16.8	22.4	12.2
60–69	56.6	59.5	54.6
70–79	168.3	202.0	151.4
80 +	135.1	236.2	94.6
Total	—	—	—
(N)	(118)	(54)	(64)
Age adj U.S. 1960	15.9	20.2[b]	13.4[b]
Age adj U.S. 1970	17.0	21.3	13.9

[a]Data of Rajput et al.[63] [b]M:F ratio = 1.51.

100,000. In all series the rates for age 60–69 are notably higher than those for age 80 +. Probably the age of maximal risk for parkinsonism is about age 65–75 or so. The sharp rise from about age 50 and, more importantly, the sharp and consistent decline above age 80 strongly indicate that parkinsonism is (an) acquired, exogenous disease(s), and *not* a manifestation of aging or "degeneration."

As to sex, the other surveys support the male preponderance of Rochester with ratios of 1.2–1.4, except for Finland,[19] where age adjusted rates were equivalent between the sexes.

Genetic Factors

Although some recent studies indicated little or no familial tendency to parkinsonism,[65] most investigators had recorded a familial aggregation of cases. In the earliest survey from Rochester, the history of a similar illness in an immediate member of the family

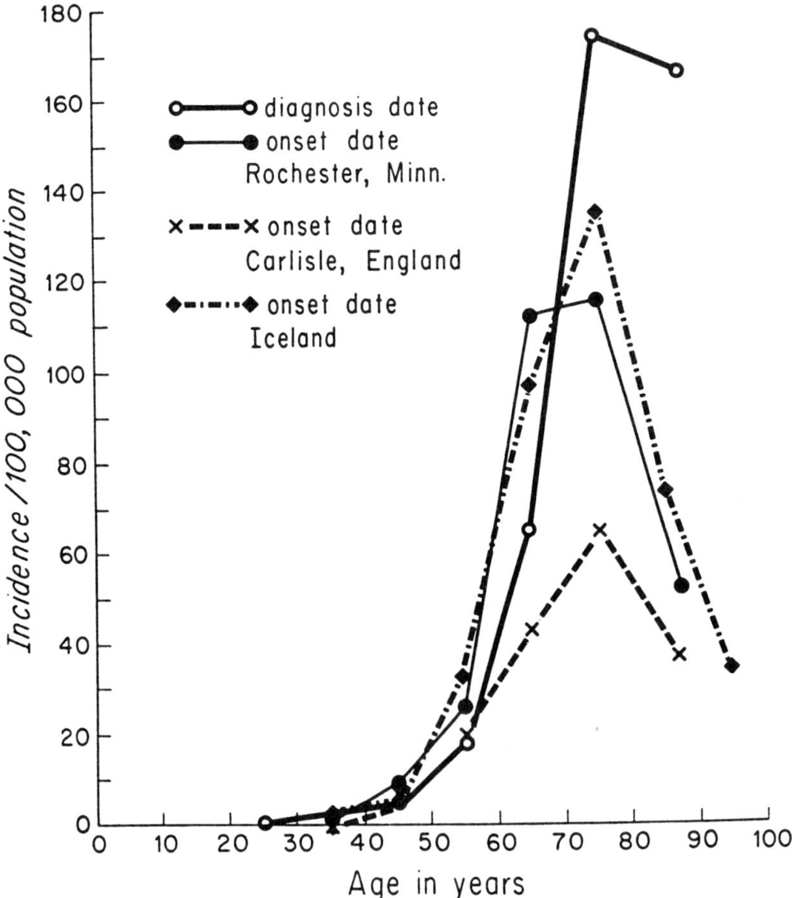

Figure 15.   Average annual age-specific incidence rates per 100,000 population, Rochester Minnesota, 1935–1966;[52] Carlisle, England, 1955–1961;[45] and Iceland, 1954–1963.[38] Rochester rates for age at diagnosis as well as age at onset, others by age at onset. From Kurland and Kurtzke.[64]

was obtained in 16% of the cases of idiopathic parkinsonism.[15] Mjönes[66] in Sweden obtained positive family histories in 41% of the idiopathic and 19% of the arteriosclerotic cases—as well as 42% of the postencephalitic patients. In Iceland, Gudmundsson[38] reported positive family histories for 20% of his idiopathic and arteriosclerotic patients and for 13% of the postencephalitic.

Allan[67] and Mjönes[66] had compiled striking series of pedigrees with parkinsonism in members of several generations, and in a pattern compatible with autosomal dominance with incomplete penetrance. Martin et al.[68] described a frequency of parkinsonism more than twice as great among siblings of index patients as among sibling of controls. The frequency in parents of index cases was three times that of the parents of controls. Similar assertions as to high familial occurrence with a multifactorial genetic basis were made by Young et al.[69] and Kondo et al.[70] Myrianthopoulos et al.[71] recorded an increased familial frequency among phenothiazine-induced parkinsonism patients vs matched patient controls. Actually, Young et al.[69] had concluded that "The distribution of ancestral secondary cases suggests a multifactorial etiology [nongenetic] for most cases of Parkinson's disease."

The reservations as to a genetic etiology raised by Marttila and Rinne[65] and Young et al.[69] received striking support in the work of Ward et al.[72] They followed up 43 monozygotic and 19 dizygotic twin sets in which an index case had Parkinson's disease. Only one monozygotic pair was definitely concordant for parkinsonism, although two or three more monozygotic and one dizygotic pairs were "concordant" when less-than-probable (and indeed unlikely) parkinsonian clinical features were considered in the cotwin. The authors stated that the frequency was no greater in the cotwins than expected in an unrelated matched control group and that environmental agents should be regarded as major factors in the etiology of Parkinson's disease. One might note that data for the prior "positive" family studies were frequently based on assertions of the patient or his family, with documentation of such cases seldom provided in the publications.

Marttila et al. have also approached this question by surveying the nationwide Finnish Twin Cohort for cases of parkinsons.[73] This cohort consists of all same-sexed twins born before 1958 and alive in 1967. They found 42 cases in 41 twin pairs [18 monozygous (MZ), 14 dizygous (DZ), 9 undetermined zygosity]. Only one DZ pair was concordant for Parkinson's disease. Nor was there any excess of Parkinson's disease among the twins: based on Finnish age- and sex-specific prevalence rates, 33 cases were expected among the surviving twins in 1981; 35 were found. They concluded that: "This study . . . suggests that Parkinson's disease is an acquired disease not caused by a hereditary process [p 1217]."[73]

Marsden advertised for twins with parkinsonism in the newsletter of the Parkinson's Disease Society of the United Kingdom.[74] Twenty-two sets of twins with definite Parkinson's disease were ascertained; one MZ and one DZ set were concordant, all others discordant. Marsden agreed that parkinsonism is not a genetic disorder.

While concordant twin cases of Parkinson's disease have recently been recorded,[75,76] Duvoisin[77] has properly observed that this does not negate the previous evidence against a genetic influence. Eldridge and Ince posit a protective factor in utero that protects the unaffected twin; in which case "there may be a genetic predisposition to Parkinson's disease . . . [p 1355]."[78] Robbins, pointing out that hereditary and genetic are not equivalent terms, indicates that the absence of the latter (with which he agrees) does not necessarily negate the former, to which point he hypothesized "a stable genetic defect that arose as a somatic cell mutation, as opposed to a germ cell mutation, very early in embryogenesis [p 412]."[79] This was in support of Duvoisin's suggestion that "impairment of DNA repair mechanisms may be present in Parkinson's disease as well as in other neurodegenerative disorders of adult life [p 410]."[77]

Golbe, in another attempt to retrieve the genetic hypothesis, concludes that (1) parkinsonism is probably not a unitary disease, (2) since some cases are familial their "abnormal gene(s) . . . must be located, sequenced, and transcribed . . . [in order to test] 'sporadic' PD and their relatives . . . [and (3)] intriguing data on mitochondrial and hepatic metabolic defects must be confirmed and extended [p 12]."[80] To me, the evidence to date is overwhelmingly against a genetic etiology for "sporadic" parkinsonism.

Risk Factors

Encephalitis. More than a risk factor, a specific infectious etiology had been claimed for all parkinsonism. It is well known that postencephalitic parkinsonism was an early or late result of von Economo's encephalitis, which followed the influenza pandemic that began in World War I. As this cohort aged, so of course did its mean age at onset for new cases. The proportions such cases contributed to all parkinsonism have dropped precipitously with time; in fact there were none in the recent Rochester survey.[62]

Noting a rising mean age at onset over time for all parkinsonian patients seen at the Massachusetts General Hospital, Schwab et al.[81] and Poskanzer and Schwab[82] propounded that all parkinsonism was a result of subclinical encephalits, and thus the disease would soon disappear. There is strong evidence, discussed elsewhere,[16,83,84] as well as that presented above, that this is not the case: population-based onset ages have been constant over time, incidence rates have been constant through 1979, and increasingly more patients were born well after the 1920s.

Smoking. That cigarette smokers are at lower risk for parkinsonism than nonsmokers was reported from prospective mortality data for U.S. smokers[85,86] as well as in morbidity studies of varied composition.[22,87–89] Even in the twin survey of Ward et al.[72] this difference was found.

A large case–control study in Derby, England, provided a relative risk for smoking up to 20 years earlier of 0.5. "The type of disease, age of onset and rate of progression were associated with a similar reduction in risk . . . [p 577]."[90] Golbe et al., however, were unable to correlate smoking histories with severity, onset age, or progression in a mailed questionnaire survey of Parkinson patients.[91] This study was based on some 3600 questionnaires accepted out of the 6000 returned among the 32,000 mailed to readers of the United Parkinson Foundation newsletter.

In reviewing the material to 1986, Baron concluded that ". . . the totality of evidence does indicate that cigarette smoking has clinically important effects on the dopaminergic systems. . . . This appears to be due to nicotine and could account for the lower risks of Parkinson's disease found in smokers [p 1493]."[92] Baron's judgment as to the inverse relation between smoking and parkinsonism was in accord with all the material noted above, including that of Kessler and Diamond in their earlier review,[88] once the findings of Golbe et al.[91] are discounted.

A major study concluding otherwise was that of Rajput et al., who stated: "The relative risk (RR) for ever smoked and IPD [idiopathic Parkinson's disease] was not significantly different from unity (RR = 0.7, 95% confidence interval = 0.4 to 1.2) [p 226]."[63] They did note a highly significant younger age at diagnosis (68.8 years) for ever-smokers vs never smokers (73.8), "although this needs to be interpreted cautiously [ibid]." The method of analysis used was rather complex. Material consisted of medical records of

Rochester resident IPD patients diagnosed at Mayo Clinic 1967–1979, compared with those of two age- and sex-matched controls per patient. The latter were also Rochester resident patients diagnosed at the same facility and time as the index case. Their data are presented in Table 15. The unmatched odds ratio and confidence intervals calculated therefrom are almost identical with the matched-pair analyses published. Note the upper confidence limit exceeds 1.00 by very little. The body of Table 15, with the ratios of the several subset ratios versus the total, does indicate a progressively increasing deficit of smokers among Parkinson patients: none or past to low to heavy smokers. Further, if we compare current smokers with never plus past-only smokers, statistical significance is attained. Granted, this could be considered a questionable maneuver since the total group does not differ significantly, but I think this is countered by the point

Table 15.
Parkinsonism: Smoking Habits as Recorded in Medical Records of Cases and Matched Controls for Rochester Resident Patients of the Mayo Clinic 1967–1979[a]

Smoking History	Cases	Controls	Ratio Subset C/C Ratio to Total Known C/C Ratio
(a) never smoked	65	126	1.14
(b) ever smoked	39	103	0.83
(c) only in past	25	44	1.25
(d) current	14	59	0.52
(e) ≤20/day	11	34	0.71
(f) >20/day	1	25	0.09
(g) unknown amount	2	0	—
(h) no data	14	7	
Total known	104	229	1.00
Total	118	236	1.09

Unmatched odds ratio (b) vs (a) = 0.73, 95% CI = 0.46–1.18
$$X^2c = 1.34, 0.30 > P > 0.20$$
Unmatched odds ratio (d) vs (a + c) = 0.45, 95% CI = 0.24–0.85
$$X^2c = 5.63, 0.02 > P > 0.01$$

[a]Data of Rayput et al.[63]

that a wide range of deficit is *not* ruled out for the total; the confidence interval is 0.46–1.18.

Presentation of findings of negative correlations or "protective" factors is hampered by the mathematical fact that their odds ratio (OR) or RR can range only from less than 1.0 to 0. By looking at the inverse relationship in Table 15, the risk (OR) of parkinsonism in never smokers is 1.36; that for current nonsmokers is 2.23.

Later series also support a negative relationship between smoking and parkinsonism. In a case–control study of registry subjects from the Sentinel Stations Practices of The Netherlands, an adjusted RR of 0.6, 95% confidence interval (CI) 0.3–1.0, was found comparing ever to never cigarette smokers in 86 cases and 172 controls.[61] No other risk factor tested was statistically significant. An insignificant OR of 0.6 (CI 0.2–1.3) was found for nursing home patients of Hong Kong, with but 34 cases and 105 controls.[93]

Detailed telephone interviews of 31 discordant MZ twins from the series of Ward et al.[72] were conducted by Bharucha et al.[94]: the only statistically significant difference was for cigarette smoking; OR for "smoked more cigarettes than co-twin" was 0.4, $P = 0.03$. Lastly, Reshef et al.[95] in Israel reported a significant negative correlation among 115 chronic hospitalized psychiatric patients with drug-induced parkinsonism between smoking and the severity of the neurological impairments, the heavy smokers being the least impaired and the nonsmokers the worst.

Therefore, cigarette smoking is clearly a protective factor in parkinsonism, and the unpopularity of any such relationship should not deter us from seeking pathophysiological inferences. Yong and Perry[96] found that monoamine oxidase B (MAO-B), the enzyme that converts MPTP into an active neurotoxin, is normal in parkinsonism but is lower in platelets of normal heavy smokers than in nonsmokers. They also observed "that hydrazine, a compound present in tobacco smoke, had a significant effect in mice in protecting dopaminergic nigrostriatal neurons from damage by MPTP [p 265]." MPTP, of course, is the street drug, "synthetic heroin," that was found to be the cause of a permanent parkinsonian state,[97,98] and that has become a leading model of experimental parkinsonism. One might also wonder about nicotine itself in terms of dopamine metabolism—as noted by Baron.[92]

Cancer. Kessler thought the "striking absence of buccal cavity/

pharynx cancer, and a near-absence of lung cancer [he found in case control comparisons of both hospital records and at interview] among male parkinsonians are consistent with the relative infrequency of smoking . . . [p 308]."[99] Rajput et al. recorded no deficit in Rochester: 16% of 118 parkinsons vs 13% of 236 controls (RR = 1.3, NS) had had malignancies diagnosed.[63] In Yonago, Japan, only 10% of the 50 Parkinson deaths were attributed to cancer, versus 19% expected—a difference, however, that is not statistically significant.[57]

Among 406 parkinsonian patients under treatment by Jansson and Jankovic,[100] the number of malignancies recorded in their medical records was 18 for cancers plus 10 for nonmelanoma skin cancer. The authors compared these values with expectations from Third National Cancer Survey data for the former and another NIH publication for the latter (references in ref. 100): respective expectations were 41.9 and 49.9 cases. The problem here is one of cancer case ascertainment in routine neurological records, even though they very carefully adjusted for length of follow-up.

The strongest evidence for cancer protection is still, then, Kessler's hospital series,[99] which he himself noted was subject to considerable bias; and that against is the Mayo series with an insignificant excess (1.3) risk.[63] I believe this relationship warrants the Scottish verdict of "not proved," but it clearly should not to be ignored. The standard epidemiological series are unlikely further to resolve the question because of small size or short duration or both. One approach would be ascertainment of underlying causes of death where parkinsonism is listed as a secondary (contributory, associated condition) cause. These data are probably available for Norway and perhaps Denmark and may well also be retrievable from nonpublished information in the United States.

Rural Residence. Based on histories of 21 early-onset Parkinson patients born and raised in Saskatchewan, Rajput et al. noted a marked excess of rural residence and drinking well water in the first 15 years of life.[101] These findings were supported when extended to all 552 Parkinson patients seen at their clinic.[102] In Hong Kong, Ho et al. had found excess frequencies of prior farming, herbicide/pesticide use, and eating of raw vegetables in their nursing home Parkinson patients.[93] Those factors were not found relevant in Saskatchewan.[101,102]

Tanner et al.[103] studied 100 Parkinson and 200 control patients from three teaching hospitals of China and found a significant *reduced* risk for rural (village) residence, with OR of 0.57, as well as similar significant "protection" for pig or chicken raising and wheat growing; that for well water drinking (0.74) was not significant. Their excess risks were for use of industrial chemicals and quarrying. Zayed et al.[104] also found a significant negative relation with rural living in Quebec, with OR of 0.31; also protective were residence near industry or mining. Their excesses were for occupational exposure to Mn, Fe, and Al.

From the Movement Disorder Clinic of the University of Kansas, Koller et al. reported a significant *excess* of rural residents and well water, with no significant difference in farming or herbicides/ pesticides, with 150 patients and other clinic matched controls.[105] They noted the well water correlation was dependent on the rural. Their work has been extended to 38 sibling pairs, both of whom had Parkinson's disease, contrasted with 38 matched normal sibling sets *and* 38 sib pairs with essential tremor.[106] Rural living and well water drinking (the latter probably dependent on the former) were significantly in excess in PD with OR of 4.3 and 2.8, respectively, but they were equivalently in excess for the essential tremor patients. We may note in closing the lower prevalence in rural British Columbia[51] than in Vancouver[44] (Table 6).

Because of the inconsistency of the findings, I doubt if early rural residence influences the appearance of parkinsonism, either plus or minus. A fortiori, then, the relationships with well water would also appear irrelevant.

Others. Tanner[107] and Tanner and Langston[108] have reviewed the evidence for environmental toxins as the cause of parkinsonism. The conclusions are that no specific chemical or mechanism has yet been defined in this regard.

Golbe et al.[109] found no early dietary factors positively associated with parkinsonism, but they reported significantly reduced OR for ingestion of salad oils, nuts, and plums in a telephone questionnaire of 81 patients vs their sibs. While plums may not have been specifically included, many of the studies considered above have investigated dietary habits, with no consistent results.

Childhood viral infections conferred reduced risk of parkinsonism (but only significant for measles) in the Harvard alumni follow-up of Sasco and Paffenbarger.[110] An incidence series of herpes zoster in Rochester, Minnesota, had a relative risk of parkinsonism of 0.7 (0.2–1.7 CI), while a history of zoster in the Parkinson series[62,63] had an OR of 1.3 (0.2–4.8 CI).[111] Herpes simplex virus type 1 (HSV 1) serum—but not CSF—antibodies were elevated in a sample of 37 Finnish parkinson patients; HSV 2 and cytomegalovirus antibodies were equivalent, case and control, in serum and CSF.[112] This was a follow up of their previous report on antibodies to 15 viruses and *Mycoplasma pneumoniae* in serum of 441 patients, none of which differed from controls except for herpes simplex.[113] I have not found other support for the HSV 1 difference.

Histocompatibility antigens showed no differences in HLA-A or HLA-B loci in Japan;[114] the authors cite equally negative studies from the United States, France, and Finland. No relationships were found in New York for HLA-linked complement markers.[115]

Dementia is a finding in parkinsonism that is increasingly frequent with increasing duration of illness and increasing age.[116,117] One question is how many of these diffuse Lewy body disease[118] rather than parkinsonism.

Comment

Mortality or death rates from parkinsonism based on the underlying cause of death, the usual measure, provide only some ⅓ of all parkinson deaths recorded on the death certificates, and only 10–20% of Parkinson patients who die. Findings based on death data may then be subject to appreciable bias. International death rates in the 1950s were highest in Europe, excluding Scandinavia, and in Israel, Uruguay, and Australia–New Zealand. The Israeli rates were for immigrants to the country. Scandinavian morbidity rates tend to be high and Australian ones low.

Crude death rates had remained quite constant in the United States, Great Britain, and Denmark up to 1976. Beginning in 1976 there was a striking increase in the rates in the United States, Denmark and Norway, which was very steep in the latter two countries and more gradual in the United States. Plateaus were recorded in the mid-1980s in Scandinavia.

Parkinson death rates uniformly show a gradient of white male greater than white female, and, in the United States, greater than black male greater than black female. Age-specific rates were uniform in configuration in the United States and Denmark from the

1950s into the 1970s, with virtually no deaths under age 50, a steep rise to a peak at 77 or 80, and a clear decline beyond. The hierarchy of WM > WF > NWM > NWF persisted at all ages. Death rates in the 1980s were again similar in the United States and Denmark, but were markedly different from previously in configuration: all age-specific rates were higher and the maximum rate was at age 82 or 85+. However, attributing the parkinson deaths to ages 5 years younger provided age-specific curves identical to the earlier ones. This is evidence that age at death, and hence survival, has increased by some 5 years since the introduction and widespread use of levodopa. The increasing crude rates are explained by the same mechanism, with more Parkinson patients now under continued treatment and thus more likely to have this diagnosis on the certificate in the event of death.

Blacks in the United States have death rates about ⅓ those of whites, although for Oriental Americans their death rates are equal to whites. All groups share the male excess. Geographically, in the United States, Parkinson deaths are higher in the north than in the south, again regardless of sex or race.

Prevalence rates for parkinsonism in Europe range from about 1 to 2.5 per 1000 population; the range is similar elsewhere in the Occident. Most of the lower rates are likely to reflect incomplete case ascertainment. A reasonable overall estimate of the prevalence of parkinsonism in whites is some 2 per 1000 population. In Japan and China, prevalence rates are well under 1 per 1000. If the U.S. death rates, equivalent in whites and Orientals, are valid, this suggests a major environmental influence on parkinsonism in Orientals. Both U.S. and African prevalence surveys confirm the death data of marked "protection" against parkinsonism in blacks. Melanin–dopamine neuronal pathways provide a rationale for this finding.

Age-specific prevalence rates rise with age in the better surveys and reach somewhere near 2% of the most elderly as affected with this disease. There is almost uniformly a male excess in all surveys and at all ages at about 1.4 or 1.5 to 1, male to female, in full accord with the death data.

Average annual incidence rates in the surveys more likely to reflect good case ascertainment range from about 15 to almost 20 per 100,000 population in the Occident. Average duration of illness in the predopa days was some 10 years. An incidence rate of 20 times a duration of 10 years would indeed give a prevalence rate of 200 per

100,000—or 2 per 1000. We should perhaps, then, soon be seeing prevalence rates of some 3 per 1000 with the 5-year gain in survival inferred from the death data and confirmed in community-based case material.

Incidence rates also reflect the male excess of the other measures. By age they show in general a very marked rise from virtually 0 about age 40 to either a plateau between age 55 and 80 or a maximum at age 70–79, and thereafter with a very marked decrease in the elder ages. The maximal risk for parkinsonism is probably at about age 65–75, with a very rapid fall-off on either side, younger and older. This configuration is not at all what one would expect from any "degenerative" or "aging" disease, and is most compatible with parkinsonism being (an) acquired, exogenous disease(s).

Despite earlier data—and valiant recent efforts—parkinsonism does not seem to be a hereditary or genetic disease. The lack of concordance in the twin collections of Ward et al.[72] and Marsden[74] and in the Finnish prospective twin cohort[73] seems irrefutable.

As to risk factors in parkinsonism, aside from age, sex, and race, the only one that seems virtually uniform is the "protection" afforded by smoking. I think this is real, and further efforts should be expended to determine whether this is a direct nicotine effect[92] or due to hydrazine[96]—or other mechanisms. It is not unlikely, though, that this is protection against the *manifestation* of parkinsonism and not against its cause(s). In other words, it may delay or minimize either the metabolic defect or the neuronal damage that ultimately leads to symptoms, but may give no clue as to etiology. Similar observations might be made as to the protection among blacks.

I believe parkinsonism has (an) exogenous cause(s), but, if it is a unitary disease, what that cause may be remains unknown.

References

1. Kurtzke JF. 1986. Multiple sclerosis from an epidemiological viewpoint. *In* Multiple Sclerosis. A Critical Conspectus. EJ Field (ed). MTP Press, Lancaster, England, pp 83–142.
2. Kurtzke JF. 1984. Neuroepidemiology. Ann Neurol 16:265–277.
3. Kurtzke JF. 1974. Neurologic needs of the community. Neuroepidemiology. American Academy of Neurology Special Course. *In* JF Kurtzke (ed). Education Marketing Corp, Minneapolis, Minnesota, pp 61–65 + tape cassette.

4. World Health Organization. 1977. Manual of the International Statistical Classification of Diseases, Injuries, and Causes of Death, 9th revision, Vol. I. WHO, Geneva.

5. McDowell FH, Lee JE, Sweet RD. 1978. Extrapyramidal disease. *In* Clinical Neurology, Vol. 3. AB Baker, LH Baker (eds). Harper & Row, Philadelphia, pp 1–67.

6. World Health Organization. 1967, 1969. Manual of the International Statistical Classification of Disease, Injuries and Causes of Death, 1965 revision, Vol. 1, 2. WHO, Geneva.

7. Cotzias GC, VanWoert MH, Schiffer LM. 1967. Aromatic amino acids and modification of parkinsonism. N Engl J Med 276:374–379.

8. Fahn S. 1986. Parkinson's disease and other basal ganglion disorders. *In* Diseases of the Nervous System. Clinical Neurobiology, Vol. II. AK Asbury, GM McKhann, WI McDonald (eds). Heinemann, London, pp 1217–1238.

9. McDowell FH, Cedarbaum JM. 1987. The extrapyramidal system and disorders of movement. *In* Clinical Neurology, Vol. 3. AB Baker, RJ Joynt (eds). Harper & Row, Philadelphia, pp 1–97.

10. Parkinson J. 1986. An Essay on the Shaking Palsy. Sherwood, Neely, and Jones, London. 1817. Special Edition, The Classics of Neurology and Neurosurgery Library. Gryphon Editions, Birmingham, Alabama.

11. Charcot J-M. 1877. Leçons sur les Maladies du Système Nerveux Fautes a la Salpêtrière, Recueillies et Publiées par Bourneville, Tome Premier, Troisieme édition. V. Adrien Delahaye et Cie, Paris.

12. Hoehn MM. 1971. The epidemiology of parkinsonism. *In* Monoamines. Noyaux Gris Centraux et Syndrome de Parkinsonism. J de Ajuriaguerra, G Gautier (eds). George Cie SA, Geneva, pp 281–300.

13. Kessler II. 1973. Parkinson's disease: Perspectives on epidemiology and pathogenesis. Prevent Med 2:88–105.

14. Kessler II. 1978. Parkinson's disease in epidemiologic perspective. Adv Neurol 19:355–384.

15. Kurland LT. 1958. Epidemiology: Incidence, geographic distribution and genetic considerations. *In* Pathogenesis and Treatment of Parkinsonism. WS Fields (ed). Charles C Thomas, Springfield, Illinois, pp 5–43.

16. Kurland LT, Hauser WA, Okazaki H, Nobrega FT. 1969. Epidemiologic studies of parkinsonism with special reference to the cohort hypothesis. *In* Third Symposium on Parkinson's Disease. Livingstone, Edinburgh, pp 12–16.

17. Kurland LT, Kurtzke JF, Goldberg ID, Choi NW, Williams G. 1973. Parkinsonism. *In* Epidemiology of Neurologic and Sense Organ Disorders. LT Kurland, JF Kurtzke, ID Goldberg (eds). Harvard University Press, Cambridge, Massachusetts, pp 41–63.

18. Kurtzke JF. 1985. Neurological system. *In* Oxford Textbook of Public Helath, Vol. 4, Specific Applications. WW Holland, R Detels, G Knox (eds). Oxford University Press, Oxford, England, pp 203–249.

19. Marttila RJ, Rinne UK. 1981. Epidemiology of Parkinson's disease—an overview. J Neural Transm 51:135–148.
20. Williams GR, Kurland LT, Goldberg ID. 1966. Morbidity and mortality with parkinsonism. J Neurosurg 24:138–143.
21. Rajput AH, Offord KP, Beard CM, Kurland LT. 1984. Epidemiology of parkinsonism: Incidence, classification and mortality. Ann Neurol 16:278–282.
22. Kessler II. 1972. Epidemiologic studies of Parkinson's disease: III. A community-based survey. Am J Epidemiol 96:242–254.
23. Goldberg ID, Kurland LT. 1962. Mortality in 33 countries from diseases of the nervous system. World Neurol 3:444–465.
24. de Pedro J, Fratiglione L. 1990. Parkinson's disease (PD) occurrence in Europe (abstract). Acta Neurol Scand H82(suppl 128):33.
25. Duvoisin RC, Schwietzer MD. 1966. Paralysis agitans mortality in England and Wales, 1855–1962. Br J Prev Soc Med 20:27–33.
26. Kurtzke JF, Murphy FM. 1990. The changing patterns of death rates in parkinsonism. Neurology 40:42–49.
27. Flaten TP. 1991. Changing mortality from Parkinson's disease. Neurology 41:329–330.
28. Mason TJ, Fraumeni JF Jr, Hoover R, Blot WJ. 1981. An Atlas of Mortality from Selected Diseases. NIH Publ No 81-2397. USDHHS, PHS, NIH. USGPO, Washington, D.C., May.
29. National Center for Health Statistics. 1965. Vital Statistics of the United States 1955. Supplement: Mortality Data. Multiple cause of death. Estimated number of conditions coded on death certificates. USGPO, Washington, D.C.
30. Diamond SG, Markham CH, Hoehn MM, McDowell FH, Muenter MD. 1987. Multi-center study of Parkinson mortality with early versus later dopa treatment. Ann Neurol 22:8–12.
31. Marttila RJ, Rinne UK. 1979. Changing epidemiology of Parkinson's disease: Predicted effects of levodopa treatment. Acta Neurol Scand 59:80–87.
32. Marttila RJ, Rinne UK. 1988. Natural course of Parkinson's disease: Effect of levodopa on patient survival (abstract). Acta Neurol Scand 77:346.
33. Marttila RJ, Rinne UK. 1990. Temporal changes in the prevalence of Parkinson's disease (abstract). Acta Neurol Scand H82(suppl 128):28.
34. Aquilonius S-M, Granat M, Hartvig P. 1981. Utilization of antiparkinson drugs in Norway, Sweden, Denmark and Finland 1975–1979. Acta Neurol Scand 64:47–53.
35. Kurtzke JF, Goldberg ID. 1988. Parkinsonism death rates by race, sex, and geography. Neurology 38:1558–1561.
36. Lux WE, Kurtzke JF. 1987. Is Parkinson's disease acquired? Evidence from a geographic comparison with multiple sclerosis. Neurology 37:467–471.
37. Lilienfeld DE, Sekkor D, Simpson S, Perl DP, Ehland J, Marsh G, Chan E, Godbold JH, Landrigan PJ. 1991. Parkinsonism death rates by race, sex and geography: A 1980s update. Neuroepidemiology (in press).

38. Gudmundsson KR. 1967. A clinical survey of parkinsonism in Iceland. Acta Neurol Scand 43(suppl 33):1–61.
39. Broman T. 1963. Parkinson's syndrome, prevalence and incidence in Göteborg. Acta Neurol Scand 39(suppl 4):95–101.
40. de Pedro J, Rosenqvist U. 1984. Tracers for paralysis agitans in epidemiological research. II. A model for indirect estimation of the prevalence of the disease. Neuroepidemiology 3:97–107.
41. de Pedro J, Rosenqvist U. 1985. Tracers for paralysis agitans in epidemiological research. III. Refinement of the model for estimation of the prevalence of the disease. Neuroepidemiology 4:161–175.
42. de Pedro J, Rosenqvist U. 1985. Tracers for paralysis agitans in epidemiological research. IV. Trends in national drug policy and measurement of the prevalence of the disease in Sweden. Neuroepidemiology 4:176–185.
43. Marttila RJ, Rinne UK. 1976. Epidemiology of Parkinson's disease in Finland. Acta Neurol Scand 53:81–102.
44. Teräväinen H, Forgash L, Heitanen M, Schilzer M, Schoenberg B, Calne DB. 1986. The age of onset of Parkinson's disease: Etiological implications. Can J Neurol Sci 13:317–319.
45. Brewis M, Poskanzer DC, Rolland C, Miller H. 1966. Neurological disease in an English city. Acta Neurol Scand 42(suppl 24):9–89.
46. Sutcliffe RLG, Prior R, Mawby B, McQuillan WJ. 1985. Parkinson's disease in the district of the Northamptom Health Authority, United Kingdom. A study of prevalence and disability. Acta Neurol Scand 72:363–379.
47. Mutch WJ, Dingwall-Fordyce J, Downie AW, Paterson JG, Roy SK. 1986. Parkinson's disease in a Scottish city. Br Med J 292:534–536.
48. Rosati G, Granieri E, Pinna L, Aiello I, Tola R, DeBastiari P, Pirisi A, Devoto MC. 1980. The risk of Parkinson disease in Mediterranean people. Neurology 30:250–255.
49. D'Alessandro R, Gamberini G, Granieri E, Benassi G, Naccarato S, Manzaroli D. 1987. Prevalence of Parkinson's disease in the Republic of San Marino. Neurology 37:1679–1682.
50. Chalmanov YN. 1986. Epidemiological studies of parkinsonism in Sofia. Neuroepidemiology 5:171–177.
51. Snow B, Wiens M, Hertzman C, Calne D. 1989. A community survey of Parkinson's disease. Can Med Assoc J 141:418–421.
52. Nobrega FT, Glattre E, Kurland LT, Okazaki H. 1967. Comments on the epidemiology of Parkinsonism including prevalence and incidence statistics for Rochester, Minnesota, 1935–1966. Excerpta Med Int Congr Ser 175:474–485.
53. Haerer AF, Anderson DW, Schoenberg BS. 1987. Survey of major neurologic disorders in a biracial United States population: The Copiah County study. South Med J 80:339–343.
54. Anderson DW, Schoenberg BS, Haerer AF. 1988. Prevalence surveys of neurologic disorders: Methodological implications of the Copiah County study. J Clin Epidemiol 41:339–345.

55. Pollock M, Hornabrook RW. 1966. The prevalence, natural history and dementia of Parkinson's disease. Brain 89:429–448.

56. Jenkins AC. 1966. Epidemiology of parkinsonism in Victoria. Med J Aust 2:496–502.

57. Harada H, Nishikawa S, Takahashi K. 1983. Epidemiology of Parkinson's disease in a Japanese city. Arch Neurol 40:151–154.

58. Li S, Schoenberg BS, Wang C, Cheng X-m, Rui D-y, Bolis CL, Schoenberg DG. 1985. A prevalence survey of Parkinson's disease and other movement disorders in the People's Republic of China. Arch Neurol 42:655–657.

59. Schoenberg BS, Osuntokun BO, Adeuja AOG, Bademosi O, Nottidge V, Anderson DW, Haerer AF. 1988. Comparison of the prevalence of Parkinson's disease in black populations in the rural United States and in rural Nigeria: Door-to-door community studies. Neurology 38:645–646.

60. Herishanu YO, Goldsmith JR, Abarbanel JM, Weinbaum Z. 1989. Clustering of Parkinson's disease in southern Israel. Can J Neurol Sci 16:402–405.

61. Hofman A, Collette HJA, Bartells AIM. 1989. Incidence and risk factors of Parkinson's disease in The Netherlands. Neuroepidemiology 8:296–299.

62. Rajput AH, Offord KP, Beard CM, Kurland LT. 1984. Epidemiology of parkinsonism: Incidence, classification, and mortality. Ann Neurol 16:278–282.

63. Rajput AH, Offord KP, Beard CM, Kurland LT. 1987. A case–control study of smoking habits, dementia, and other illnesses in idiopathic Parkinson's disease. Neurology 37:226–232.

64. Kurland LT, Kurtzke JF. 1972. Geographic neuropathology. *In* J Minckler (ed). Pathology of the Nervous System, Vol. 3. McGraw-Hill, New York, pp 2803–2808.

65. Marttila RJ, Rinne UK. 1976. Arteriosclerosis, heredity, and some previous infections in the etiology of Parkinson's disease: A case–control study. Clin Neurol Neurosurg 79:46–56.

66. Mjönes H. 1949. Paralysis agitans: A clinical and genetic study. Acta Psychiatr Neurol Scand 00(suppl 54):1–195.

67. Allan W. 1937. Inheritance of shaking palsy. Arch Intern Med 60:424–436.

68. Martin WE, Young WI, Anderson VE. 1973. Parkinson's disease. A genetic study. Brain 96:495–506.

69. Young WI, Martin WE, Anderson VE. 1977. The distribution of ancestral secondary cases in Parkinson's disease. Clin Genet 11:189–192.

70. Kondo K, Kurland LT, Schull WJ. 1973. Parkinson's disease: Genetic analysis and evidence of a mulitfactorial etiology. Mayo Clin Proc 48:465–475.

71. Myrianthopoulos NC, Kurland AA, Kurland LT. 1962. Hereditary predisposition in drug induced parkinsonism. Arch Neurol 6:5–9.

72. Ward CD, Duvoisin RC, Ince SE, et al. 1983. Parkinson's disease in 65 paris of twins and in a set of quadruplets. Neurology 33:815–824.

73. Marttila RJ, Kaprio J, Koskenvuo M, Rinne UK. 1988. Parkinson's disease in a nationwide twin cohort. Neurology 38:1217–1219.
74. Marsden CD. 1987. Parkinson's disease in twins. J Neurol Neurosurg Psychiatr 50:105–106.
75. Koller W, O'Hara R, Nutt J, Young J, Rubino F. 1986. Monozygotic twins with Parkinson's disease. Ann Neurol 19:402–405.
76. Jankovic J, Reches A. 1986. Parkinson's disease in monozygotic twins. Ann Neurol 19:405–408.
77. Duvoisin RC. 1986. On heredity, twins, and Parkinson's disease. Ann Neurol 19:409–411.
78. Eldridge R, Ince SE. 1984. The low concordance rate for Parkinson's disease in twins: A possible explanation. Neurology 34:1354–1356.
79. Robbins JH. 1987. Parkinson's disease, twins, and the DNA-damage hypothesis (letter). Ann Neurol 21:412.
80. Golbe LI. 1990. The genetics of Parkinson's disease: A reconsideration. Neurology 40(suppl 3):7–14.
81. Schwab RS, Doshay LJ, Garland H, Bradshaw P, Garvey E, Crawford B. 1956. Shift to older age distribution in parkinsonism: A report on 1,000 patients covering the past decade from three centers. Neurology 6:783–790.
82. Poskanzer DC, Schwab RS. 1963. Cohort analysis of Parkinson's syndrome: Evidence for a single etiology related to subclinical infection about 1920. J Chron Dis 16:961–973.
83. Kurtzke JF, Kurland LT. 1973. The epidemiology of neurologic disease. *In* Clinical Neurology, Vol. 3. AB Baker, LH Baker (eds). Harper & Row, Hagerstown, Maryland, pp 1–80.
84. Kurtzke JF, Kurland LT. 1983. The epidemiology of neurologic disease. *In* Clinical Neurology, Vol. 4. AB Baker, LH Baker (eds). Harper & Row, Philadelphia, pp 1–143.
85. Hammond CA. 1966. Smoking in relation to the death rates of one million men and women. *In* Epidemiologic Approaches to the Study of Cancer and Other Chronic Diseases. NCI Monogr No. 19. USGPO, Washington, D.C., pp 127–204.
86. Kahn HA. 1966. The Dorn study of smoking and mortality among U.S. veterans: Report on eight and one-half years of observation. *In* Epidemiologic Approaches to the Study of Cancer and Other Chronic Diseases. NCI Monogr No. 19. USGPO, Washington, D.C., pp 1–125.
87. Baumann RJ, Jameson HD, McKean HE, Haack DG, Weisberg LM. 1980. Cigarette smoking and Parkinson disease: 1. A comparison of cases with matched neighbors. Neurology 30:839–843.
88. Kessler II, Diamond EL. 1971. Epidemiologic studies of Parkinson's disease. I. Smoking and Parkinson's disease: A survey and explanatory hypothesis. Am J Epidemiol 94:16–25.
89. Nefzger MD, Quadfasel FA, Karl VC. 1967. A retrospective study of smoking and Parkinson's disease. Am J Epidemiol 88:149–158.
90. Goodwin-Austen RB, Lee PN, Marmot MG, Stein GM. 1982. Smoking and Parkinson's disease. J Neurol Neurosurg Psychiatr 45:577–581.
91. Golbe LI, Cody RA, Duvoisin RC. 1986. Smoking and Parkinson's

disease. Search for a dose–response relationship. Arch Neurol 43:774–778.

92. Baron JA. 1986. Cigarette smoking and Parkinson's disease. Neurology 36:1490–1496.

93. Ho SC, Woo J, Lee CM. 1989. Epidemiologic study of Parkinson's disease in Hong Kong. Neurology 39:1314–1318.

94. Bharucha NE, Stokes L, Schoenberg BS, Ward C, Ince S, Nutt JG, Eldridge R, Calne DB, Mantel N, Duvoisin R. 1986. A case–control study of twin pairs discordant for Parkinson's disease: A search for environmental risk factors. Neurology 36:284–288.

95. Reshef A, Rabey JM, Bar P, Schlosberg A, Korczyn AD. 1977. Smoking and drug-induced parkinsonism. Neurology 37(suppl 1):121.

96. Yong VW, Perry TL. 1986. Monoamine oxidase B, smoking and Parkinson's disease. J Neurol Sci 72:265–272.

97. Burns RS, LeWitt PA, Ebert MH, Pakkenberg H, Kopin IJ. 1985. The clinical syndrome of striatal dopamine deficiency. Parkinsonism induced by 1-methyl-4-phenyl-1,2,3,6-tetrahydropyridine (MPTP). N Engl J Med 312:1418–1421.

98. Ballard PA, Tetrud JW, Langston JW. 1985. Permanent human parkinsonism due to 1-methyl-4-phenyl-1,2,3,6-tetrahydropyridine (MPTP): Seven cases. Neurology 35:949–956.

99. Kessler II. 1972. Epidemiologic studies of Parkinson's disease. II. A hospital-based survey. Am J Epidemiol 95:308–318.

100. Jansson B, Jankovic J. 1985. Low cancer rates among patients with Parkinson's disease. Ann Neurol 17:505–509.

101. Rajput AH, Uitti RJ, Stern W, Laverty W. 1986. Early onset Parkinson's disease in Saskatchewan—environmental considerations for etiology. Can J Neurol Sci 13:312–316.

102. Bennett V, Rajput AH, Uitti RJ. 1988. An epidemiological survey of agricultural chemicals and incidence of Parkinson's disease (abstract). Neurology 38(suppl 1):349.

103. Tanner CM, Chen B, Wang W, Peng M, Liu Z, Liang X, Kao LC, Gilley DW, Goetz CG, Schoenberg BS. 1989. Environmental factors and Parkinson's disease: A case–control study in China. Neurology 39:660–664.

104. Zayed J, Ducic S, Campanella G, Panisset JC, André P, Masson H, Roy M. 1990. Facteurs environmentaux dans l'étiologie de la maladie de Parkinson. Can J Neurol Sci 17:286–291.

105. Koller W, Vetere-Overfield B, Gray C, Alexander C, Chin T, Dolezal J, Hassanein R, Tanner C. 1990. Environmental risk factors in Parkinson's disease. Neurology 40:1218–1221.

106. Wong GF, Gray CS, Hassanein RS, Koller WC. 1991. Environmental risk factors in siblings with Parkinson's disease. Arch Neurol 48:287–289.

107. Tanner CM. 1989. The role of environmental toxins in the etiology of Parkinson's disease. Trends Neurosci 12:49–54.

108. Tanner CM, Langston JW. 1990. Do environmental toxins cause Parkinson's disease? A critical review. Neurology 40(suppl 3):17–30.

109. Golbe LI, Farrell TM, Davis PH. 1988. Case-control study of early life dietary factors in Parkinson's disease. Arch Neurol 45:1350–1353.
110. Sasco AJ, Paffenbarger RS Jr. 1985. Measles infection and Parkinson's disease. Am J Epidemiol 122:1017–1031.
111. Ragozzino MW, Kurland LT, Rajput AH. 1983. Investigation of the association between herpes zoster and Parkinson's disease. Neuroepidemiology 2:89–92.
112. Marttila RJ, Rinne UK, Halonen P, Madden DL, Sever SL. 1981. Herpes viruses and parkinsonism. Herpes simplex virus types 1 and 2, and cytomegalovirus antibodies in serum and CSF. Arch Neurol 38:19–21.
113. Marttila RJ, Arstila P, Nikoskelainen J, Halonen PE, Rinne UK. 1977. Viral antibodies in the serum of patients with Parkinson's disease. Eur Neurol 15:25–33.
114. Takagi S, Shinohara Y, Tsuji K. 1982. Histocompatibility antigens in Parkinson's disease. Acta Neurol Scand 66:590–593.
115. Nerl C, Mayeux R, O'Neill GJ. 1984. HLA-linked complement markers in Alzheimer's and Parkinson's disease: C4 variant (C4B2) a possible marker for senile dementia of the Alzheimer type. Neurology 34:310–314.
116. Ebmeier KP, Calder SA, Crawford JR, Stewart L, Besson JAO, Mutch WJ. 1990. Clinical features predicting dementia in idiopathic Parkinson's disease: A follow-up study. Neurology 40:1222–1224.
117. Jones R, Godwin-Austen RB, Lowe J. 1988. Age-related variation in Parkinson's disease (abstract). Acta Neurol Scand 77:344.
118. Crystal HA, Dickson DW, Lizardi JE, Davies P, Wolfson LI. 1990. Antemortem diagnosis of diffuse Lewy body disease. Neurology 40:1523–1528.

Chapter 10

Idiopathic Parkinsonism:
More Rapid Progression in Late-Onset Patients

E.Ch. Wolters, J. Tsui, and D.B. Calne

In the prelevodopa era, the rate of spread and of loss of mobility in parkinsonian patients was found to be faster in late-onset disease.[1] Recently Agid et al. have argued, however, that idiopathic parkinsonism (IP) does not progress more rapidly in elderly subjects.[2] Because our clinical impression suggests a positive correlation between the rate of progression in IP and the age of onset, we surveyed our patient population retrospectively. More rapidly advancing disease in the elderly would support the hypothesis of a combination of subclinical insult and age-related decay of the dopaminergic nigrostriatal pathway in the pathogenesis of IP.[3]

We employed dose increments of levodopa/carbidopa and bromocriptine as an index of disease progression because we raise the dosage of these medications as clinical features deteriorate. It is not our practice to alter the intake of other drugs as deficits advance.

Patients and Methods

Age of onset, dosage of medication, and complications of therapy were surveyed in 608 patients with IP. The criteria for diagnosis

This work was supported by a grant from the Medical Research Council of Canada.
From Hefti F, and Weiner WJ, (eds.) *Progress in Parkinson's Disease Research—2*. Mount Kisco NY, Futura Publishing Co., Inc., © 1992.

were those proposed by Schoenberg.[4] The age of onset was determined from discussion with the patient, and where possible, the family. None of the subjects had undergone surgical treatment. The period of observation was limited to 6 years because subsequently the drug intake becomes erratic due to complications of long-term therapy such as fluctuations in response, severe dyskinesia, and psychiatric reactions. Elimination of patients with disease duration over 6 years left 292 subjects suitable for analysis. Only patients living on the last day of the study were included.

The medications at the last out-patient visit were expressed as therapeutic units (1 TU = 1 mg levodopa (in Sinemet) or 1 TU = 0.1 mg of bromocriptine).[5] Another conversion rate of 1 TU = 0.05 mg bromocriptine was also employed for a further check of the dosage equivalence between levodopa/carbidopa and bromocriptine.

Results

An analysis of our patient population revealed a different pattern in sex distribution before and after age 60 years, with a male:female ratio of 2:1 before and 1:1 after this age. The mean age of onset was 57.7 years (range 23–84; males 56, females 60.1). Over all ages, the male–female ratio was 3:2.

We found side effects serious enough to necessitate a change in dosage in 110 of the 292 patients. When dyskinesias or fluctuations in response developed, partial replacement of levodopa/carbidopa by bromocriptine had been undertaken. Psychiatric side effects had resulted in a decrease in bromocriptine dosage in 48 patients (28 males, 20 females) and a decrease in levodopa/carbidopa in 46 patients (28 males, 18 females), with a tendency for these problems to be commoner in older patients. Other complications noted were pulmonary fibrosis ($N = 7$) and erythromelalgia ($N = 4$) due to bromocriptine. Gastrointestinal problems ($N = 5$) occurred with either dopaminomimetic agent. Hypotension, headaches, and impotence did not necessitate dose adjustment.

Figure 1 shows the correlation between the annual dose increment of antiparkinson medication and the age of onset for patients with a history of symptoms for 6 years or less. For the 292 patients as a group, the age of onset correlated positively with the

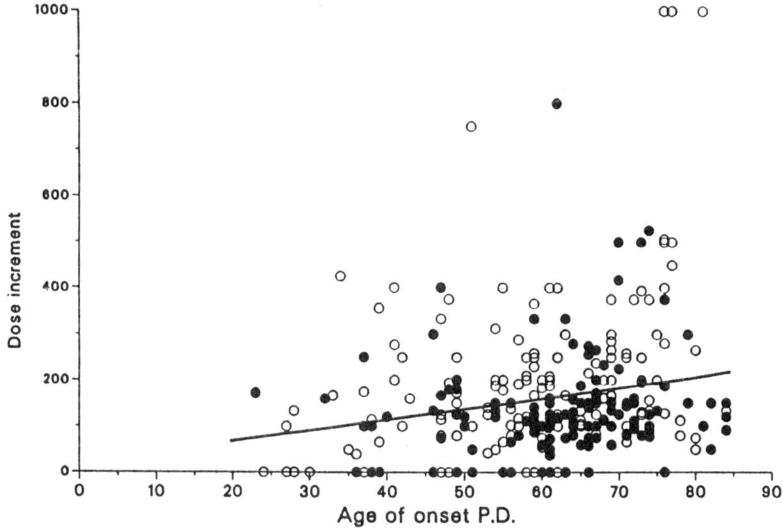

Figure 1.   Relation between the increment of antiparkinson medication over 6 years (expressed in the therapeutic units—see text) and the age on onset in males (○) and females (●). Regression coefficient 2.6, $P < 0.00005$.

dose increment over 6 years (regression coefficient = 2.6, $P < 0.0005$). This correlation held when the results were recalculated with 1 mg levodopa equivalent to 0.05 mg bromocriptine.

Discussion

Previous studies have shown a slightly greater prevalence for the IP in men.[6,7] However, we found a substantially lower frequency of women versus men in younger patients with IP. Over 8% of our patients had onset before 40 years of age; over 50% of the patients had their onset before age 60 years. The adverse reactions to treatment were similar to those reported in the literature.[8] Our patient population conforms to the general profile of subjects with IP. Quinn et al.[9] have reported that dyskinesia and fluctuations in response to levodopa are more prominent in younger patients with IP. This has also been our experience, but it did not distort our analysis because we manage such side effects by reducing levodopa and increasing bromocriptine; the assessment of total therapeutic units takes into account the administration of both levodopa and bromocriptine.

We infer that the rate of increase of dopaminomimetic therapy is an index of the rate of progression of IP because: (1) we adjust dosage according to the severity of symptoms, provided patients do not encounter unacceptable side effects; and (2) dose limiting side effects were more frequent in our older patients. The correlation of increasing dose increments with a higher age of onset was therefore detected in spite of a contrary bias in the data.

The correlation we found between dose increment per year and age of onset supports the notion that IP has a faster course in the elderly. It is consistent with the report by DeJong and Burns[1] on the rate of progress of parkinsonism in the era immediately preceding the advent of dopaminomimetic therapy. They estimated that the rate of advance of symptoms in the average patient aged 65 years was some four times greater than for a patient of 35 years. Our findings are also in accord with the observations of Diamond et al.[8] These workers noted less disability after 4, 5, and 6 years in an early-onset group, compared with a late-onset group. There was also a trend for mortality to be lower in the young-onset group. Taken together these observations all support the hypothesis that age-related loss of neurons plays a part in the pathogenesis of IP.

Agid et al.[2] reported two relevant but conflicting observations. For a similar duration of illness (7.7 years), their late-onset group had more severe deficits than their early-onset group when both were receiving levodopa. This finding is consistent with ours. However, when levodopa was stopped for periods of 18 hours to 7 days, the difference between their early- and late-onset groups disappeared. It may be that variation in the interval between stopping levodopa and recording motor deficits contributed to their findings, particularly since there is a substantial disparity in the rate of clinical deterioration after cessation of levodopa therapy in different individuals.

It is relevant to note that Gibb and Lees[10] have described more marked (24%) loss of nigral cells in young-onset cases at autopsy, but these patients had suffered from IP much longer (12 years) than their elderly group. This disparity in the duration of disease makes it difficult to infer the relative rates of neuronal deaths.

Summary

In a retrospective study of 292 patients with IP, we found a positive correlation between the age of onset and the rate of dose increment per year of antiparkinson drugs for the first 6 years of the disease. Since our practice is to increase treatment according to the severity of symptoms, the dose increment per year expresses the rate of progression of the disease. We conclude that IP advances more rapidly in older patients. This finding is in accord with the hypothesis that aging contributes to the clinical expression of IP.

References

1. DeJong JD, Burns BD. 1967. Parkinson's disease—a random process. Can Med Assoc J 97:49–56.
2. Agid Y, Bonnet AM, Dubois B, Javoy-Agid F, Ruberg M, Sherman D. 1989. Does aging contribute to aggravation of Parkinson's disease? *In* Parkinsonism and Aging. DB Calne, G Comi, D Crippa, R Horowshi, M Trabucchi (eds). Raven Press, New York, pp 115–123.
3. Calne DB, Langston JW. 1983. The aetiology of Parkinson's syndrome. Lancet 2:1457–1459.
4. Schoenberg BS. 1987. Environmental risk factors for Parkinson's disease. The epidemiologic evidence. Can J Neurol Sci 14:407–413.
5. Libman I, Gawel MJ, Riopelle RJ, Bouchard S. 1987. A comparison of bromocriptine (Parlodel) and levodopa-carbidopa (Sinemet) for treatment of "de novo" Parkinson's disease patients. Can J Neurol Sci 14: 576–580.
6. D'Alessandro R, Gamberini G, Granieri E, Benassi G, Naccarato S, Manzaroli D. 1987. Prevalence of Parkinson's disease in the Republic of San Marino. Neurology 37:1679–1682.
7. Mutch WJ, Dingwall-Fordyce I, Downie AW, Paterson JC, Roy SK. 1986. Parkinson's disease in a Scottish city. Br Med J 292:534–536.
8. Diamond SG, Markham CH, Hoehn MM, McDowell FH, Muenter MD. 1989. Effect of age at onset on progression and mortality in Parkinson's disease. Neurology 39:1187–1190.
9. Quinn N, Critchley P, Marsden CD. 1987. Young onset Parkinson's disease. Mov Disord 2:73–91.
10. Gibb WRG, Lees AJ. 1988. A comparison of clinical and pathological features of young- and old-onset Parkinson's disease. Neurology 38:1402–1406.

Chapter 11

The Genetics of Parkinson's Disease—A Review

Roger C. Duvoisin

A significant role for heredity in the etiology of Parkinson's disease (PD) has long seemed attractive, but convincing evidence has been elusive. Many PD patients offer positive family histories, but it has been difficult to establish whether this truly represents familial concentration or merely reflects the population prevalence of the disorder. Occasional familial clusters have been encountered, but it has not been clear whether they truly had PD or some other condition, such as olivopontocerebellar atrophy or essential tremor. The search for evidence of a genetic basis for PD also has been hampered by uncertainties regarding its nosologic independence and until recently by disagreement on its pathological substrate and the significance of the Lewy body.

The first systematic genetic study of paralysis agitans was carried out by Mjones in the late 1930s and early 1940s.[1] His detailed report was the most authoritative statement on the subject for nearly two decades. The problems he encountered still confront those who attempt a clinical genetic analysis of PD. Thus his data and his method of analysis deserve our careful attention. From the perspective of our present knowledge, it is clear that Mjones faced formidable obstacles in his endeavor. PD, paralysis agitans, or "idiopathic parkinsonism" (the terms were used synonymously)

From Hefti F, and Weiner WJ, (eds.) *Progress in Parkinson's Disease Research—2.* Mount Kisco NY, Futura Publishing Co., Inc., © 1992.

was then considered by many authorities to be a syndrome, not a specific entity. Indeed, there was no agreement among pathologists about its morbid anatomy. Postencephalitic parkinsonism still accounted for a large proportion of Parkinson patients seen at the time.[2] Many patients were thought to have vascular or arteriosclerotic parkinsonism as described by Critchley.[3] Neurosyphilis was still a common disorder and a "luetic parkinsonism" complicated differential diagnosis.

Mjones admitted encountering "considerable difficulties" in differentiating these different groups. Present day neurologists who enjoy the advantages of diagnostic and neuroimaging technologies far superior to those available in his day can readily sympathize with that admission. The contribution of olivopontocerebellar atrophy to the clinical spectrum of parkinsonism was not yet appreciated, while striatonigral degeneration and progressive supranuclear palsy had not yet been recognized. Postmortem examination of the brain had been carried out in 11 of Mjones' affected cases, but microscopical examination was done in only four and the substantia nigra was described in only one, a patient who died in 1930. The pathologist found "an almost total loss of cells" and "severe gliosis" in the lateral portion of the nigra but made no mention of Lewy bodies.

Mjones' principle analysis was based on 194 index cases diagnosed as "paralysis agitans" by stated criteria. He had personally examined nearly half the probands; most of his data was collected from medical records at nine separate clinics and hospitals. He found 162 secondary cases among the relatives of 79 of his probands; 46 (11.9%) of the parents and 50 (7.2%) of 694 siblings were affected. Some additional relatives were affected, but the size of the population at risk, i.e., the total number of relatives is not known. Mjones concluded that the disorder was an autosomal dominant with 60% penetrance.

However, Mjones counted monosymptomatic cases or "formes frustes" with tremor alone as secondary cases of PD, accepting their relationship to the index case as a diagnostic feature. He justified this approach on the grounds that "without this factor a number of abortive or incipient secondary cases would undoubtedly have been interpreted as, for example, essential tremor." He also noted in support of his approach that some authorities, e.g., Critchley,[4] considered essential tremor a "forme fruste" of PD.

While there may be some justification for this approach, it is difficult for neurologists today to accept a diagnosis of PD in individuals who only had tremor after hard work (Mjones' cases I,11b and I,43Aa), senile dementia and tremor of the left foot (case II,42Aa), only "tremulous voice" (case II,21Ab), or the members of family I,13 who had tremor of the head and hands for many years, especially since tremor of the head is rare in PD and common in essential tremor. It is also difficult to accept as secondary cases relatives with atypical manifestations such as the sibling (case 14Aa) who had ataxic gait and bilateral Babinski signs.

Fortunately, Mjones provided extensive clinical data in his tables so that it is possible to critically reassess his material. Duvoisin et al.[5] recalculated from these data the prevalence of secondary cases among parents and siblings, excluding the atypical and monosymptomatic cases; the prevalences then fell to 3.4 and 2.8%, respectively. These authors then undertook a smaller study of the prevalence of PD among patient siblings using their spouses and the spouse's siblings over age 25 as a control population. Personally examining 69% of the 424 available family members, they found only four (2.8%) of the index siblings and three (2.1%) of the spouses and spouse siblings to be affected. The difference is not significant and is similar to the recalculated data of Mjones. Five cases of essential tremor were found among the index siblings and five among the control group.

The failure of these authors to confirm a familial concentration of PD argued against a role for heredity. However, they cautiously concluded that "the predicament we face regarding the etiology of Parkinson's disease is reminiscent of the situation that pertained with respect to Down's syndrome prior to the discovery of trisomy, when a genetic explanation was attractive despite inconsistencies with simple mendelism."

A subsequent study of similar design by Martin et al.,[6] based on 130 index cases, yielded nearly identical results: 16 secondary cases of parkinsonism were found among 488 index siblings versus seven among 450 spouses and spouse siblings. Combining the data of these two studies yields a prevalence of 20 (3.2%) secondary cases among 634 index siblings versus 10 (1.7%) among the control group. The difference is not significant.

In a case-control study using age-matched neighbors as controls to assess the significance of positive family histories, Martilla and Rinne[7] elicited reports of 16 (4.4%) secondary cases of PD among the first degree relatives versus 11 (2.5%) among the first degree relatives of the control group. The secondary cases were not examined. Again, the difference fails to reach significance.

Kondo et al.,[8] in a statistical analysis of the Parkinson population studied at the Mayo Clinic, found 9.7% of proband siblings affected. Instead of using a control population, they compared that figure with an expected 0.89% prevalence based on the age-specific prevalence rates for parkinsonism previously reported by Kurland.[9] Applying Falconer's[10] method for estimating the "heritability" of multifactorial disorders, Kondo et al.[8] calculated a heritability of 0.79 and postulated a multifactorial etiology. However, since the methods of ascertainment are different, this type of comparison is of uncertain value. These authors suggested that a study of twins would be the most economical and direct means of assessing the role of genetic factors.

Twin Concordance

Following up on that suggestion, Duvoisin et al. carried out a study of identical twins in the years 1978–1982.[11,12] The first 12 consecutive twin pairs examined were discordant for PD.[11] At the conclusion of the study, 65 pairs of monozygotic (MZ) twins had been examined.[11] They were divided into four groups: 43 pairs of MZ twins in which the proband was considered on clinical grounds to have typical PD (group I); five pairs of MZ twins in which the proband was considered to have atypical parkinsonism but no other etiology could be established (group II), 19 pairs of dizygotic (DZ) twins in which the proband was considered to have typical PD, and 12 additional MZ twin pairs in which the proband was believed to have some disorder other than PD, e.g., Alzheimer's disease, essential tremor, olivopontocerebellar atrophy, or cerebral vascular disease.

One group I cotwin had "definite PD" and one was classified as "possible PD." In comparison, only one DZ twin pair was concordant. The difference, 1/43 vs 1/19 is not significant. A survey of identical twins in the United Kingdom[13] and a large survey of twins by Martilla in Finland using different methods of ascertainment[8] yielded similar findings.[14] These observations led its authors and most other investigators to conclude that genetic factors do not play a significant role in the etiology of PD.[15]

However, recent developments indicate several reasons the twin studies may have underestimated the prevalence of PD among either MZ or DZ cotwins of the probands. First, it has become clear that the contribution of progressive supranuclear palsy (PSP) and multiple system atrophy (MSA) to the clinical spectrum of parkinsonism is greater than was recognized at the time of the twin study.[16,17] It is thus possible that several cases of PSP could have been inadvertently included as probands, an error that would have tended to reduce the observed concordance. Inclusion of MSA cases may also have contaminated the data.

Second, recent experience indicates that cases considered atypical may be found to have typical Lewy body PD at postmortem study.[18,19] A concordant MZ twin pair was rejected from the study as atypical because MSA was suspected, but this pair may in fact have had Lewy body PD. Two MZ twin pairs were rejected because the proband had dementia, but the single concordant DZ twin pair was retained despite the presence of dementia. The proband in this pair had a mild dementia, which was thought not inconsistent with PD, while his cotwin had prominent dementia, which had preceded the onset of parkinsonian motor features by several years and he was thought possibly to have Alzheimer's disease. The validity of so relative a distinction is uncertain, and it may reasonably be argued that accepting this concordant DZ pair was inconsistent with the exclusion of the two MZ pairs with dementia. We now know that the combination of dementia and parkinsonism is consistent with diffuse Lewy body disease, a condition not yet widely recognized at the time.

Third, Johnson et al.[20] have recently recalculated the previous twin study data to assess the effect of assuming that the patients rejected as atypical in fact had PD. They considered the effect of several assumptions. Under the maximum assumption, i.e., that all the atypical cases in fact had PD, the concordance rate among MZ twins for overt clinical disease rises to 6/50, suggesting a significant if still small role for heredity. However, when they employed Smith's equations[21] to compare the prevalence of PD among the cotwins with the population prevalence, they found the confidence intervals so large that these numbers failed to reach significance. Johnson et al.[20] concluded that the available twin study data are inconclusive and do not exclude a genetic component in PD.

Another important limitation of the twin study is that preclinical PD could not be detected. Postmortem studies of "incidental" Lewy body disease show that preclinical PD greatly exceeds clinically overt PD in prevalence. Thus it is possible that many if not most of the cotwins had preclinical PD. The probands were selected for study because they had overt PD, whereas the cotwins were involved only by reason of their twin status. Hence the ratio of clinical to preclinical PD among the cotwins would be expected to be similar to that in the general population. The number of cotwins with preclinical PD would be the product of the number with clinical PD multiplied by the ratio of preclinical to clinical PD in the general population.

Preclinical PD. An estimate of the prevalence of preclinical PD may be derived from studies of "incidental" Lewy bodies in routine autopsies. Forno found Lewy bodies in the pigmented nuclei of the brain stem in 50 (4.7%) of 1069 routine autopsies of nonparkinsonian subjects at a Veterans Administration hospital.[22] In a recent communication, she states that "all but about 2% of the cases studied were over age 40" (personal communication 1989). Thus 98% or 1048 were over age 40 and incidental Lewy bodies were present in 50/1048 or 4.8% of veterans over age 40.

Forno provided morphological evidence that patients with "incidental" Lewy bodies in fact had preclinical PD. The pattern of cell loss and the distribution of Lewy bodies was similar to that observed in PD and was associated with nerve cell loss, neuronal fragmentation, and extraneuronal neuromelanin intermediate in degree between normalcy and the findings in overt PD. On retrospective review of the clinical notes, she found evidence of symptomatology consistent with parkinsonism in one fifth of the cases with Lewy bodies. These cases were probably in the prodromal phase of the disease when there are insufficient manifestations to permit the clinical diagnosis, and this observation is consistent with the common clinical experience of a long prodromal phase in many patients.

Gibb and Lees[23] recently found Lewy bodies in the same distribution associated with evidence of neuronal degeneration in 14 (6.0%) of 234 nonparkinsonians ranging in age from 40 to 99 years and came to the same conclusions. They analyzed their data by 10-year age groups. The prevalence of "incidental" Lewy body disease rose from 3.8% in the 50- to 59-year bracket to 12.8% in the 80- to 89-year bracket. These authors also reviewed previous reports of incidental Lewy bodies. Comparing the combined data to the epidemiological survey of PD in Glasgow, Scotland, by Mutch et al.,[24] they concluded that the prevalence of preclinical PD was 10–15 times greater than that of clinically overt disease.

More recently, Forno and Langston have examined an additional 1199 postmortem brain specimens and found incidental Lewy bodies in 76 (6.3%), a prevalence similar to what she found in her earlier study.[25] The prevalence increased sharply with age from 1.8% in the sixth decade to 11.9% in the ninth decade of life. Adding Fornos' new data with that of Woodard,[26] Gibb and Lees and Tomonaga's[27] similar survey of Lewy bodies in the locus ceruleus yields combined data (Table 1) showing a rising prevalence of preclinical PD with age reaching 12.2% in the ninth decade. There seems to be a further increase in the prevalence of Lewy bodies in the tenth and eleventh decades, but the numbers are too small to permit the conclusion that the prevalence is still rising beyond age 80. Age-adjusted to the 1980 U.S. population aged 40 and above, these data project a prevalence for preclinical PD of 4020/10,[5] approximately 12 times larger than the prevalence of PD in the general population over age 40 of 345/100,000 determined in the most recent U.S. epidemiological study, that of Schoenberg et al.[28]

The remarkably high prevalence of preclinical PD, especially in the oldest age groups, has profound implications for the analysis of family and twin study data. It is consistent with a very low penetrance of the presumed PD gene. Multiplying by 12, the two affected MZ cotwins found in the American twin study yields 24

Table 1.
Prevalence of Incidental Lewy Bodies at Different Ages
(Combined Data of Woodard,[26] Forno et al.,[25] Tomonaga,[27] and Gibb and Lees[23])[a]

Age Group (years)	Autopsies (N)	With LBD (N)	%
40–49	70	0	0
50–59	340	7	2.1
60–69	647	32	4.9
70–79	483	50	10.4
80–89	395	48	12.2
90–99	63	11	17.5
100+	4	1	25.0

[a]The differences between the successive age groups 70 and above are not significant.

additional MZ cotwins with preclinical PD and a total concordance of 26/43 (0.60), consistent with a very large genetic contribution.

The Twin Follow-Up Study. These considerations have led my colleagues and me to resurvey the participants of the old twin study to determine whether some of the apparently unaffected cotwins may have progressed in the past decade to a clinical phase of the disease and to use [18F]fluorodopa positron emission tomography (PET) to detect preclinical PD in those cotwins who still appear to be unaffected.[29] The use of PET scanning for this purpose was suggested by the work of Calne and colleagues, who demonstrated impaired striatal dopamine uptake with fluorodopa PET in persons exposed to the dopaminergic neurotoxin MPTP but who were asymptomatic[30] and in patients with Guamanian ALS presenting no overt features of parkinsonism.[31]

The follow-up survey is still underway, but some preliminary data may be mentioned here. Thus far, we have concentrated our efforts on the group I (typical PD) and group II (atypical PD) twin pairs. As of December 31, 1990, follow-up information had been obtained on 32 of the original 43 pairs of identical (MZ) twins and on all five pairs of the atypical MZ twins. The data are summarized in Table 2.

One group I cotwin, normal in 1980, developed symptoms of PD in 1986, 6 years after the pair had been examined by the twin study team and 26 years after the proband had first become affected! The cotwin of the pair considered "possibly"concordant died 2 years after being examined. No evidence of PD developed in that time and hence it appears appropriate to consider that pair discordant.

The probands experienced a higher mortality than their cotwins,

Table 2.
Follow-Up Data on Subjects of Original American Twin Study

	Group I		*Group II*	
	Probands	*Cotwins*	*Probands*	*Cotwins*
Living	17	23	1	1
Deceased	14	5	2	1
Lost	12	15	2	2
Total	43	43	5	4

presumably reflecting the adverse effect of PD on life expectancy. Postmortem examinations, including neuropathological studies of the brain, have been carried out in one of the deceased probands from each of these groups. Both autopsied probands were from discordant twin pairs. The pathological diagnosis in the group I proband was pallidoluysian atrophy. There were no Lewy bodies or neurofibrillary tangles. The postmortem diagnosis in the proband from group II was striatonigral degeneration.

Correcting for the single misdiagnosis in group I and adding the additional concordant pair alters the clinical concordance rate slightly from 1/43 (4.7%) to 2/42 (7.1%). It is possible that an additional clinically affected cotwin may be found among the 15 group I cotwins still "lost" to follow-up, but it seems doubtful at this point that the concordance for clinically overt PD will be increased to more than 3/42 or 4/42 (9.5%).

In the 1983 report,[12] four of 70 siblings over age 60 were reported also to have PD. Two additional siblings have become affected since the original study, bringing the known total to 6/70 (8.6%). One nontwin sibling who was clinically normal in 1980 later developed PD at age 81, 31 years older than the age at which the proband had first developed symptoms, while the cotwin remains clinically unaffected at age 78!

Fluorodopa PET scanning was performed at the University of British Columbia PET Centre in Vancouver, BC, Canada under the direction of Dr. Donald Calne. To date, seven of the clinically normal group I cotwins have undergone fluorodopa PET scanning—one has an abnormal scan consistent with PD. Thus the combined concordance now becomes 3/42 (7.1%). We have not found a high prevalence of subclinical PD; however, it must be admitted that we do not know what proportion of persons with preclinical PD can be detected by PET scanning. It would be prudent to defer drawing any conclusions before the completion of the follow-up study. It is possible that further PET scanning might reveal additional cases with subclinical nigrostriatal impairment.

In summary, these data essentially reaffirm the findings of the original twin studies. Ward et al.[12] had recognized that further observation of the twins might reveal an increase in concordance for PD but predicted that the increase "would be small." We have now found a small increase, but we are still left with the conclusion to which Johnson et al.[20] arrived, namely that the twin study data were insufficient to assess the possible role of genetic factors in the etiology of PD. It would appear that a twin study of sufficient size to yield definitive data may not be practical.

Perhaps the most important finding of the twin follow-up study is the remarkably late age of onset of PD in the eighth and ninth decades in the recently affected nontwin siblings and the unexpectedly long period of discordance of 26 years in the one MZ twin pair to become concordant in the years since the original twin study was carried out. Allowance must be made for the markedly age-related expression of PD and a large intrafamilial variation in age of onset in analyzing clinical data for evidence of a presumed underlying gene defect.

Familial Parkinsonism

Family Clusters of Parkinsonism

It is clear that PD can, at least in some families, occur in a hereditary pattern. Such family clusters present at this time the major opportunity available to clarify the possible genetic etiology of PD. Adequately studied clinically and pathologically, they also provide unique opportunities to assess the range of variation in the clinical expression of Lewy body disease. Whether the underlying gene defect(s) responsible for the disorder in these families also accounts for sporadic PD, which may be only *apparently* sporadic, remains to be determined.

Numerous reports of patients with two or more secondary cases among their first-degree relatives have been published over the past century. Examples include the report of Allan,[32] an early clinical geneticist, of a collection of familial cases and the brief report of Bell and Clark,[33] who also provided an annotated bibliography of previous similar reports. Unfortunately, the authors of these early reports provided little clinical description and no pathological confirmation, so that one cannot determine whether their subjects had PD or some other disorder. Indeed, unusually early onset, atypical features, and the description of ataxia in some individuals suggest that some represent kindreds of multiple system atrophy. Consequently these reports, although provocative, are only of historical interest.

Mjones[1] described in his genetic study of PD, nine families in which the disease occurred in three generations and two families with affected members in four generations. He presented pedigree charts for seven of these families. These show a pattern of direct transmission in most cases, which supports his conclusion of autosomal dominant inheritance. He explains the preponderance of males in his material to a lower penetrance of the genotype in women, an interpretation that merits our attention today. Mjones emphasized a very large intrafamilial variation in clinical features including age of onset, some affected members exhibiting mild disease or "formes frustes" for many years while others pursued a course of rapid deterioration.

From the data in his extensive tables, one can reconstruct his pedigree charts to conform to current practice. A typical example (Figure 1) illustrates the pedigree of his family I,9. These pedigrees and the data provided fail to convincingly document examples of familial PD. Most appear to have essential tremor and some may have other disorders. Unfortunately, there is no postmortem confirmation of PD in any of these families. Yet, despite its limitations, Mjones' study remains of interest today. He recognized many of the problems we still face in studying familial PD, e.g., the significance of atypical and oligosymptomatic cases, the intrafamilial as well as interfamilial variation in clinical features and age of onset, and the meaning of associated neurological disorders, notably senile psychosis or dementia. He also tried to deal with the problem of the late age of onset of PD and to calculate cumulative morbidity risks.

Roy et al.[34] and Barbeau and Roy[35] drew attention to 50 familial cases of parkinsonism they identified on screening a clinic population of 684 patients. They believed these represented subsets of familial parkinsonism distinct from "classic idiopathic parkinsonism." These included several familial clusters of an akinetic–rigid Parkinson syndrome they thought was recessively inherited. In pedigree 023 of Roy et al.,[34] illustrated in their Figure 5 as "probably pseudo-dominant," a mother and four of her seven daughters were affected, while her two sons were spared. They also identified an "essential tremor-related" parkinsonism in 28 cases illustrated by their pedigree DCD-2, in which three of ten offspring of a man said to have essential tremor had "mixed parkinsonism" and two of three children of one of these also had essential tremor. They felt that about 15% of parkinsonism is due to various hereditary disorders produc-

Mjone's Pedigree

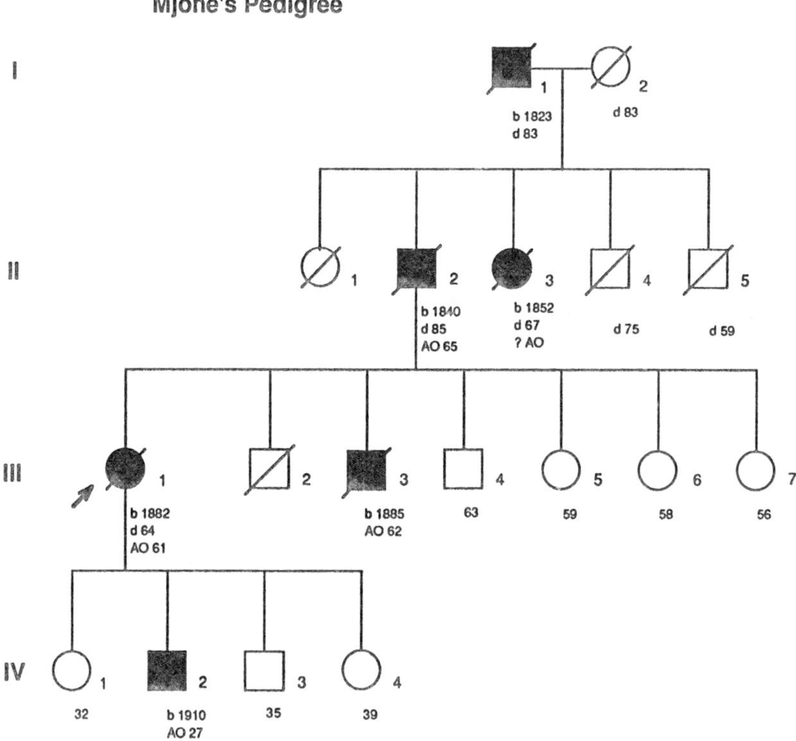

Figure 1.   Pedigree chart of Mjones' family 1,9 redrawn to conform to modern usage showing birthdates and age at death or at the time of the study. [1] AO = age at onset. The proband, indicated by the arrow had the onset of the disease at age 61. Examined in 1943 (see Mjones, p.154) she had tremor, rigidity, cogwheeling, and a "parkinsonian mask." Mentally, she was "sluggish with prolonged reaction time." Her brother had the onset at age 62 of tremor and a "parkinsonian mask." Her son (see Mjones, p.44) developed progressive "mental insufficiency" at age 20 with "lack of concentration and paranoid ideas." He was hospitalized repeatedly during the years 1937–1940 for symptoms interpreted as "postencephalitic disturbances." Sialorrhea and "some lack of facial expression and slowness of movement" were found. A physician examining this patient in 1940 noted "parkinsonian mask, no tremor or rigidity. . .slowing of thought processes." Historical information only was available on the reportedly affected members of generations I and II. The proband's grandfather, born in 1804, was said to have had "definite tremor in whole body, most pronounced in arms, walked bent forward, became lame, same symptoms as proband." He died at age 83. Her father had only tremor of the hands with "no effect on working capacity," and her affected aunt had "increased tremor in hands, walked bent forward. . ."

ing phenocopies of PD, while the remainder represent sporadic idiopathic parkinsonism.[34]

These families resemble Mjones' pedigrees, which also contained both individuals without tremor and many secondary cases with tremor alone. It seems quite possible that postural tremor similar to that of essential tremor could be the sole manifestation of PD for many years in some patients with the "benign tremulous form of PD" and that this may occur in such familial clusters. However, without pathological confirmation, it remains unclear what conditions these families had.

Degl'Innocenti et al.[36] recently reported a family in which seven members in five sibships of the same generation were affected with clinically typical PD. The pattern of familial concentration was consistent with autosomal dominant inheritance. Although postmortem confirmation was not available, the clinical descriptions are typical of PD and, in the era of CT and MRI scanning, the probability that the diagnosis is correct seems high.

Large Parkinson Disease Kindreds

Two larger pedigrees of dominantly inherited Lewy body parkinsonism with postmortem confirmation recently have been described and a third is presently under study. The first of these was initially reported by Spellman[37] in 1962. He identified an Iowa family with nine affected individuals in four generations in a pattern consistent with autosomal dominant inheritance (Figure 2). In subsequent reviews, this family was considered atypical for PD because of the early age of onset, rapid progression, and the description of limb ataxia in one case and of extensor plantar responses in another. This family was subsequently studied by Muenter et al.[38] and reported in 1986 in a program abstract. By that time, three additional members had been affected and a postmortem study had become available. The illness presented initially a typical Parkinson syndrome in the second or third decade of life with bradykinesia, rigidity, mild tremor, stooped posture, and impaired postural reflexes. The clinical course was rapidly progressive with the subsequent appearance of dementia. Severe involvement of the pigmented nuclei of the brain stem and the limbic cortex with nerve cell loss, gliosis, and Lewy bodies were found on postmortem study.

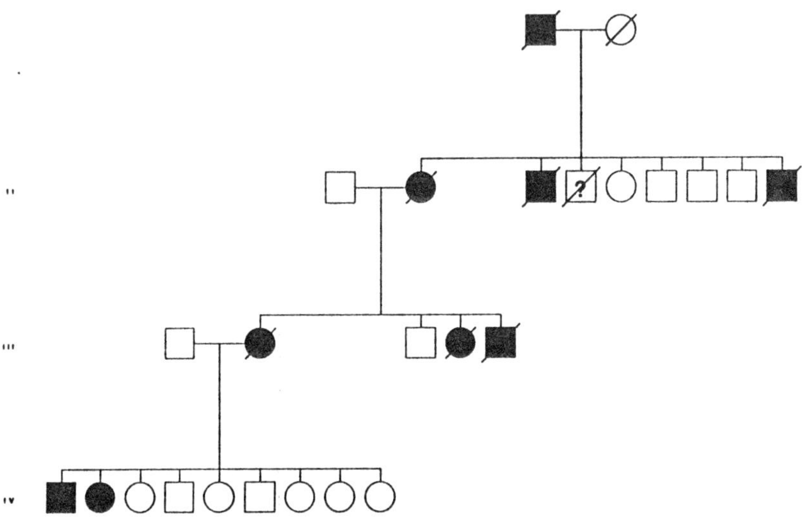

Figure 2. Pedigree of the family reported by Spellman[37] and later by Muenter et al.[38] redrawn after Spellman.

This family therefore represents diffuse Lewy body disease of young adult onset.

The largest PD pedigree studied to date is that recently reported by Golbe et al.[39] These authors found that four patients seen at the Parkinson Research Group at Robert Wood Johnson Medical School (RWJMS) over a period of 8 years were members of a large kindred. A fifth case had first been seen in consultation by the present author in 1965. These patients had not previously been aware of their relationships. They were descendants of several individuals who had emigrated to the United States from the village of Contursi in the Campania region of southern Italy between 1890 and 1920. The coincidence of their common origin from the same village aroused suspicion that they were related. After diligently pursuing their genealogies, relationships were identified that showed that they were in fact members of two possibly related families. Our colleagues at the University of Naples, Italy, Prof. V. Bonavita, and Dr. G. Di Iorio, found that these two families were linked by a common ancestor who lived in Contursi during the late 18th century. They also found collateral descendants presently living in Italy. Thus a single large pedigree had been identified distributed between two continents with an autosomal dominant PD. The pedigree is illustrated in Figure 3. It is the largest kindred with autopsy-proven Lewy body PD presently known.

A total of eight living and 33 deceased members of the "Contursi" pedigree had been affected with a Parkinson syndrome somewhat atypical for PD due to a relatively early adult onset, minimal tremor, and an aggressive course with death occurring a mean of 9.7 years after symptom onset. There were 23 men and 18 women. The age of onset varied from 28 to 68 years (mean 46.5 ± 10.8 SD). However, in other respects, including responsiveness to levodopa therapy, the condition appears clinically typical of PD. Histological confirmation of typical Lewy body disease is available thus far in two affected members.

The high clinical penetrance in this pedigree indicates that a single gene defect may be responsible. Only the finding that the duration of the disease in deceased members was somewhat longer in those who had lived out their lives in Italy than those who had lived in the United States suggests the possible effect of an environmental factor, but this difference could represent an artifact due to the lack of a standard manner of observation. Most importantly, the pedigree is sufficiently large to allow DNA linkage studies in search of an underlying gene defect.

A third kindred (Figure 4) more typical in age of onset, is presently under observation (M.H. Mark and R.C. Duvoisin, unpublished data). The proband has been previously described as a clinically atypical case with pathologically typical Lewy body PD by Sage et al. (see case 1, JP, in that report).[19] I learned after following this patient for several years that his maternal aunt living in Nova Scotia was thought to have PD. A year after the proband's death, his brother in Nova Scotia was diagnosed with PD. Examination confirmed the diagnosis in the brother and uncovered two other family members with minimal manifestations consistent with PD, such as facial hypomimia and/or stooped posture, insufficient in themselves to justify the clinical diagnosis.

The pattern observed in this Nova Scotia family, counting the oligosymptomatic family members, appears consistent with autosomal dominant inheritance and incomplete penetrance. Fluorodopa PET scanning is planned in the oligosymptomatic and clinically unaffected members. An interesting point is the clinical atypicality of the proband, indicating an appreciable degree of intrafamilial

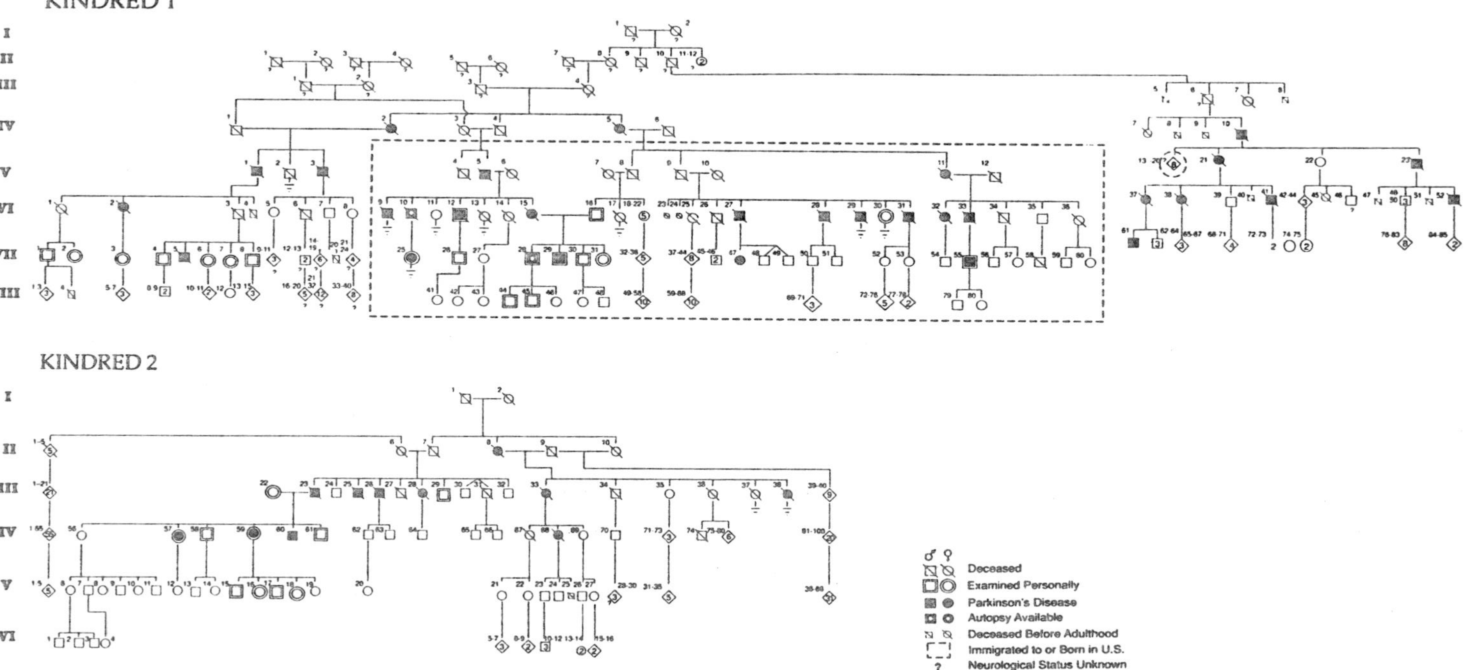

Figure 3. The Contursi pedigree. (Reproduced with permission from Golbe et al.[39]

Nova Scotia Pedigree

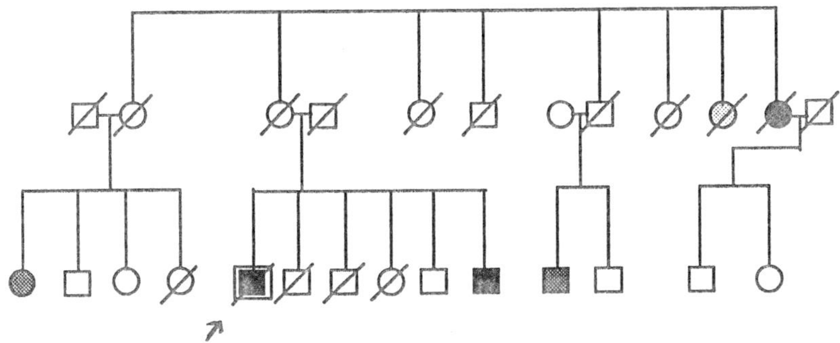

Figure 4. The Nova Scotia pedigree presently under study by Mark and Duvoisin (unpublished data). The proband, JP, is indicated by the arrow.

variability of clinical manifestations. Without a postmortem examination, it would not have been recognized that the proband, his sibling, and his aunt had the same disorder.

Comparison of the Three Kindreds. The question naturally arises whether these three kindreds of documented Lewy body parkinsonism represent different disorders or variations of the same disorder. The question cannot be definitively answered from presently available clinical and pathological data. It will only be definitively resolved by molecular analysis of DNA from members of these families. However, several considerations favor the interpretation that they represent a single disorder.

All three share a similar Lewy body pathology. Several recent postmortem series of patients with diffuse Lewy body disease have established this disorder as part of the spectrum of Lewy body disease.[40,41] Kosaka argues that it represents an extended form of PD.[42]

The three kindreds may be seen as steps in a continuum with some degree of overlap between them. The Iowa kindred represents the most severe disease of the three and has the earliest age of onset. The Contursi kindred is intermediate in age of onset and severity, while the third with a later age of onset is the mildest and most typical. Dementia was severe in the Iowa kindred in the later stages of the disease, as is often the case in juvenile onset PD,[42] minimal in the Contursi kindred, and was not noted in the third kindred. These considerations suggest the possibility that the same gene defect could account for all three kindreds, diffuse Lewy body disease perhaps representing a more severe mutation of the same gene.

Additional Multiplex Families. Are these large kindreds a special small group accounting only for a small percentage of the patients with PD encountered in the population at large or are they representative of PD generally? This question will probably be fully resolved only when a gene marker becomes available. However, a preliminary review of small multiplex families with three or more affected persons in two generations collected from patients under our care and in which postmortem confirmation of Lewy body disease has been obtained suggests that the latter possibility is the more likely.

In view of the negative results of previous family studies, we have been somewhat surprised that we have been able to identify a considerable number of such families. The reason appears to be that we have made persistent and repeated efforts to obtain data on all first- and second-degree relatives of patients followed over periods of years. We have found that detailed informative family histories in PD patients are usually positive. However, relatively few individuals in the age range affected are able to provide a detailed account of even their first-degree relatives at their first consultation. Consequently, most family histories recorded in clinical practice and documented in medical charts are not negative but uninformative.

Good patient rapport established over time and the help of interested family members willing to research their family genealogies are necessary to gathering an informative family history. The existence of secondary cases has often become evident only after periods of years. Part of the reason is, undoubtedly, the relatively advanced age at PD onset in many cases. It is thus understandable that epidemiological surveys in which patients and their families were interviewed and examined by an investigating team on only one or two occasions have failed to uncover many secondary cases.

These multiplex families can usefully supplement the opportunity provided by the larger kindreds described above to carry out DNA linkage studies with the view of ultimately mapping a gene defect. Pending the discovery of a gene marker in the larger kindreds, they also make it possible to address such questions as whether diffuse Lewy body disease (Lewy body dementia), juvenile PD, the benign tremulous form of PD, and other variants are within the range of intrafamilial variation and therefore varying expressions of the same disease. These families will also help define intrafamilial as well as interfamilial variations in age of onset, predominant clinical manifestations, rate of progression, etc. The data already available suggest the hypothesis that Lewy body PD is part of the clinical range of expression of an autosomal dominant disorder with partial age-related penetrance, long premorbid and prodromal phases, and marked variability of clinical manifestations extending beyond the motor syndrome of parkinsonism upon which our traditional concept PD is based.

References

1. Mjones H. 1949. Paralysis agitans. A clinical genetic study. Acta Psychiatr Neurol Scand 25(suppl 54):1–195.
2. Dimsdale H. 1946. Changes in parkinson syndrome in 20th century. QJ Med 15:155–170.
3. Critchley M. 1929. Arteriosclerotic parkinsonism. Brain 52:23–83.
4. Critchley M. 1949. Observations on essential (heredofamilial) tremor. Brain 72:113–139.
5. Duvoisin RC, Gearing F, Schweitzer M, Yahr MD. 1969. A family study of parkinsonism. *In* Progress in Neurogenetics. A Barbeau, JR Brunette (eds). Excerpta Medica, Amsterdam, pp 492–496.
6. Martin WE, Young WI, Anderson VE. 1976. Parkinson's disease. A genetic study. Brain 96:495–506.
7. Martilla RJ, Rinne UK. 1976. Arteriosclerosis, heredity and some previous infections in the etiology of Parkinson's disease. Clin Neurol Neurosurg 79:46–56.
8. Kondo K, Kurland LT, Schull WJ. 1973. Parkinson's disease, genetic

analysis and evidence of a multifactorial etiology. Mayo Clin Proc 48:465–475.

9. Kurland LT. 1958. Epidemiology: Incidence, geographic distribution and genetic considerations. *In* Pathogenesis and Treatment of Parkinsonism. W Fields (ed). Charles C. Thomas, Springfield, IL, pp 5–49.

10. Falconer DS. 1965. The inheritance of liability to certain disease estimated from the incidence among relatives. Ann Hum Genet 29:51–76.

11. Duvoisin RC, Eldridge R, Williams A, Nutt J, Calne DB. 1981. Twin study of Parkinson's disease. Neurology 31:77–80.

12. Ward CD, Duvoisin RC, Ince SE, Nutt J, Eldridge R, Calne DB. 1983. Parkinson's disease in 65 pairs of twins and in a set of quadruplets. Neurology 33:815–824.

13. Marsden CD. 1987. Parkinson's disease in twins. J Neurol Neurosurg Psychiatr 50:105–106.

14. Martilla RJ, Kaprio J, Kostenvuo MD, Rinne UK. 1988. Parkinson's disease in a nationwide twin cohort. Neurology 38:1217–1219.

15. Duvoisin RC. 1986. Genetics of Parkinson's disease. Adv Neurol 45:307–312.

16. Duvoisin RC, Golbe LI, Lepore FE. 1987. Progressive supranuclear palsy. Can J Neurol Sci 14:547–554.

17. Quinn NP. 1989. Multiple system atrophy—the nature of the beast. J Neurol Neurosurg Psychiatr Special suppl:78–89.

18. Quinn NP, Luthert P, Honavar M, Marsden CD. 1989. Pure akinesia due to Lewy Body Parkinson's disease: A case with pathology. Mov Disord 4:85–89.

19. Sage JI, Miller DC, Golbe LI, Walters A, Duvoisin RC. 1990. Clinically atypical expression of pathologically typical Lewy-body parkinsonism. Clin Neuropharmacol 13:36–47.

20. Johnson WG, Hodge SE, Duvoisin RC. 1990. Twin studies and the genetics of Parkinson's disease—a re-appraisal. Mov Disord 5:187–194.

21. Smith C. 1974. Concordance in twins: Methods and interpretation. Am J Hum Genet 26:454–466.

22. Forno LS. 1969. Concentric hyaline intraneuronal inclusions of Lewy type in the brains of elderly persons (50 incidental cases): relationship to parkinsonism. J Am Geriatr Soc 17:557–575.

23. Gibb WRG, Lees AJ. 1988. The relevance of the Lewy body to the pathogenesis of idiopathic Parkinson's disease. J Neurol Neurosurg Psychiatr 51:745–752.

24. Mutch WJ, Dingwall-Fordyce I, Downie AW, Paterson JG, Roy SK. 1986. Parkinson's disease in a Scottish city. Br Med J 1:534–536.

25. Forno LS, Langston JW. 1990. Lewy bodies and aging (abstract 52). J Neuropathol Exp Pathol 40:278.

26. Woodard JS. 1962. Concentric hyaline inclusion body formation in mental disease. Analysis of 27 cases. J Neuropathol Exp Neurol 21:442–449.

27. Tomonaga M. 1983. Neuropathology of the locus ceruleus: A semiquantitative study. J Neurol 230:231–240.

28. Schoenberg BS, Anderson DW, Haerer AF. 1985. Prevalence of Parkinson's disease in the biracial population of Copiah County, Mississippi. Neurology 35:841–845.
29. Zimmerman TR, Bhatt M, Calne DB, Duvoisin RC. 1991. Parkinson's disease in monozygotic twins: A follow up (abstract 508S). Neurology 41(suppl 1):255.
30. Peppard RF, Guttman M, Martin WRW, Clark C, Eisen A, Calne DB. 1989. Dopaminergic deficits demonstrated in caucasian amyotrophic lateral sclerosis using positron emission tomography (abstract). Neurology 39 (suppl 1):400.
31. Calne DB, Langston JW, Martin WR, et al. 1985. Positron emission tomography after MPTP: Observations relating to the cause of Parkinson's disease. Nature 317:246–248.
32. Allan W. 1927. Inheritance of the shaking palsy. Arch Intern Med 60:424–436.
33. Bell J, Clark AJ. 1927. A pedigree of paralysis agitans. Ann Eugen 1:445–462.
34. Roy M, Boyer L, Barbeau A. 1983. A prospective study of 50 cases of familial Parkinson's disease. Can J Neurol Sci 10:37–42.
35. Barbeau A, Roy M. 1984. Familial subsets of idiopathic Parkinson's disease. Can J Neurol Sci 11:144–150.
36. Degl'Innocenti F, Maurello MT, Marini P. 1989. A parkinsonian kindred. Ital J Neurol Sci 10:307–310.
37. Spellman GG. 1962. Report of familial cases of parkinsonism. JAMA 179:160–162.
38. Muenter MD, Howard FM, Okazaki H, et al. 1986. A familial Parkinson–dementia syndrome (abstract). Neurology 36(suppl 1):115.
39. Golbe LI, Di Iorio G, Bonavita V, Miller DC, Duvoisin RC. 1990. Autosomal dominant Parkinson's disease. Ann Neurol 27:276–282.
40. Byrne E, Lennox G, Lowe J, Godwin-Austen RB. 1989. Diffuse Lewy body disease: Clinical features in 15 cases. J Neurol Neurosurg Psychiatr 52:709–717.
41. Burkhardt CR, Filley C, Kleinschmidt-DeMasters BK, de la Monte SM, Norenberg MD, Schneck SA. 1988. Diffuse Lewy body disease and progressive dementia. Neurology 38:1520–1528.
42. Kosaka K. 1990. Diffuse Lewy body disease in Japan. J Neurol 237:192–204.

3

Dopaminergic Neurotransmission

Chapter 12

Molecular Cloning of D_1 and D_2 Dopamine Receptors

David R. Sibley, Frederick J. Monsma, Jr,
Charles R. Gerfen, and Lawrence C. Mahan

Dopamine receptors belong to a large superfamily of neurotransmitter receptors that are coupled to their specific effector functions via guanine nucleotide binding regulatory (G) proteins. Multiple criteria have been used to define two major subfamilies of dopamine receptors, which are referred to as D_1 and D_2.[1] D_1 receptors have been described as being coupled to the stimulation of adenylyl cyclase activity[2] through the G_s regulatory protein, although recent evidence has suggested that some D_1 receptors may activate phospholipase C.[3–5] In contrast, D_2 receptors have been suggested to be linked to various cellular responses[6] including inhibition of adenylyl cyclase activity, inhibition of phosphatidylinositol turnover, increase in K^+ channel activity, and inhibition of Ca^{2+} mobilization. The G protein(s) linking the D_2 receptors to these responses have not been identified, although D_2 receptors have been shown to both copurify and functionally reconstitute with both "G_i" and "G_0" related proteins. Both dopamine receptor subtypes are predominantly found in the central nervous system (CNS) where they are critical for the regulation of cognitive function and motor control. In order to better understand the function and regulation of the D_1 and D_2 receptors at

From Hefti F, and Weiner WJ, (eds.) *Progress in Parkinson's Disease Research—2.* Mount Kisco NY, Futura Publishing Co., Inc., © 1992.

the biochemical and molecular level, we have initiated experimentation to clone cDNAs and/or genes for these receptor subtypes.

D_1 Dopamine Receptor Cloning

As alluded to above, evidence has accumulated suggesting heterogeneity in the D_1 category of dopamine receptors. D_1 receptors have recently been described in both renal[3] and brain[4] tissue, which stimulate phospholipase C activity independently from that of adenylyl cyclase. We have also shown, using *Xenopus* oocyte expression experiments, that rat striatal mRNA encodes D_1 receptors that are coupled to phospholipase C and Ca^{2+} mobilization in a cAMP-independent fashion.[5] These data suggest that there may be multiple D_1 receptors linked to different signal transduction pathways or that a single, multifunctional D_1 receptor exists. In order to investigate these possibilities and to characterize the D_1 receptor(s) on a molecular level, we have cloned the D_1 receptor subtype expressed in mouse NS20Y neuroblastoma cells.[7] We have previously shown that these cells express functional D_1 receptors coupled to the stimulation of cAMP generation.[8,9]

NS20Y cell poly(A)$^+$ RNA was used to first synthesize cDNA by reverse transcription followed by polymerase chain reaction (PCR) amplification with a pair of highly degenerate primers derived from the third and sixth transmembrane regions of the previously cloned adrenergic, D_2 dopaminergic, and serotonin receptors. This process resulted in the amplification of several cDNA fragments that were preliminarily characterized by DNA sequence analysis. One of these fragments was found to exhibit considerable sequence homology to previously cloned G protein-coupled receptors and was used to screen a rat striatal cDNA library in order to isolate a full-length clone. One clone (pB73D1) with an insert of 3.6 kb was isolated and found to hybridize strongly with the ^{32}P-labeled PCR fragment on dot-blot analysis. The nucleotide sequence of this cDNA was found to exhibit >90% homology in the region of the PCR fragment, the divergence of which is probably attributable to species differences (mouse vs rat).

The longest open reading frame in this cDNA codes for a putative 487-residue protein with a theoretical molecular weight of 54,264 Da. Although the neighboring sequence of the first ATG in this reading frame is similar to Kozak's consensus initiation sequence, this is also true for the second and third methionine codons at positions 39 and 46, respectively. Since the human D$_1$ receptor lacks the initial methionine codon seen in the rat sequence (see below), it is assumed that translation begins at the second methionine codon resulting in a 446-residue protein. Hydrophobicity analysis of the translated protein reveals seven clusters of 24 hydrophobic residues, predicted to represent transmembrane-spanning domains, connected by three extracellular and three intracellular loops. Figure 1 thus depicts this putative rat D$_1$ receptor protein as it is believed to be organized in the plasma membrane. This pattern is similar to that observed for other cloned G protein-coupled receptors where the NH$_2$ terminus is proposed to be extracellular and the COOH terminus projects into the cytoplasm. The NH$_2$ terminus and second extracellular loop contain consensus sites for *N*-linked glycosylation while the predicted third cytoplasmic loop exhibits one consensus recognition site for phosphorylation by the cAMP-dependent protein kinase (Figure 1). In addition, the long COOH terminus contains several serine and threonine residues, possibly representing additional sites for regulatory phosphorylation.

Comparison of the deduced amino acid sequence for the pB73D1 cDNA clone with the sequences of various catecholamine receptors indicated that the regions of highest identity appear to occur within the predicted transmembrane spanning domains. Within these regions, the pB73D1 protein exhibits sequence homologies of 44% with the rat D$_2$ dopaminergic receptor; 44%, 43%, and 40% with the human beta$_1$-, beta$_2$-, beta$_3$-adrenergic receptors, respectively; and 43% and 42% with the hamster alpha$_{1B}$- and human alpha$_{2A}$-adrenergic receptors, respectively. When compared with various serotonin receptors, the transmembrane regions of the pB73D1 protein exhibited homologies of 40% for 5-HT$_{1A}$ and 37% for both 5-HT$_{1C}$ and 5-HT$_2$ receptors. The NH$_2$ and COOH termini and the extracellular and intracellular loops are significantly more divergent among these receptors. It is interesting to note that within the third putative transmembrane-spanning domain of pB73D1, there is a conserved aspartate residue that is common to all biogenic amine receptors that have been sequenced thus far.[10] Moreover, the fifth transmembrane-spanning domain of pB73D1 also contains two serine residues that are conserved among catecholamine receptors and are critical for the recognition of agonist ligands possessing a

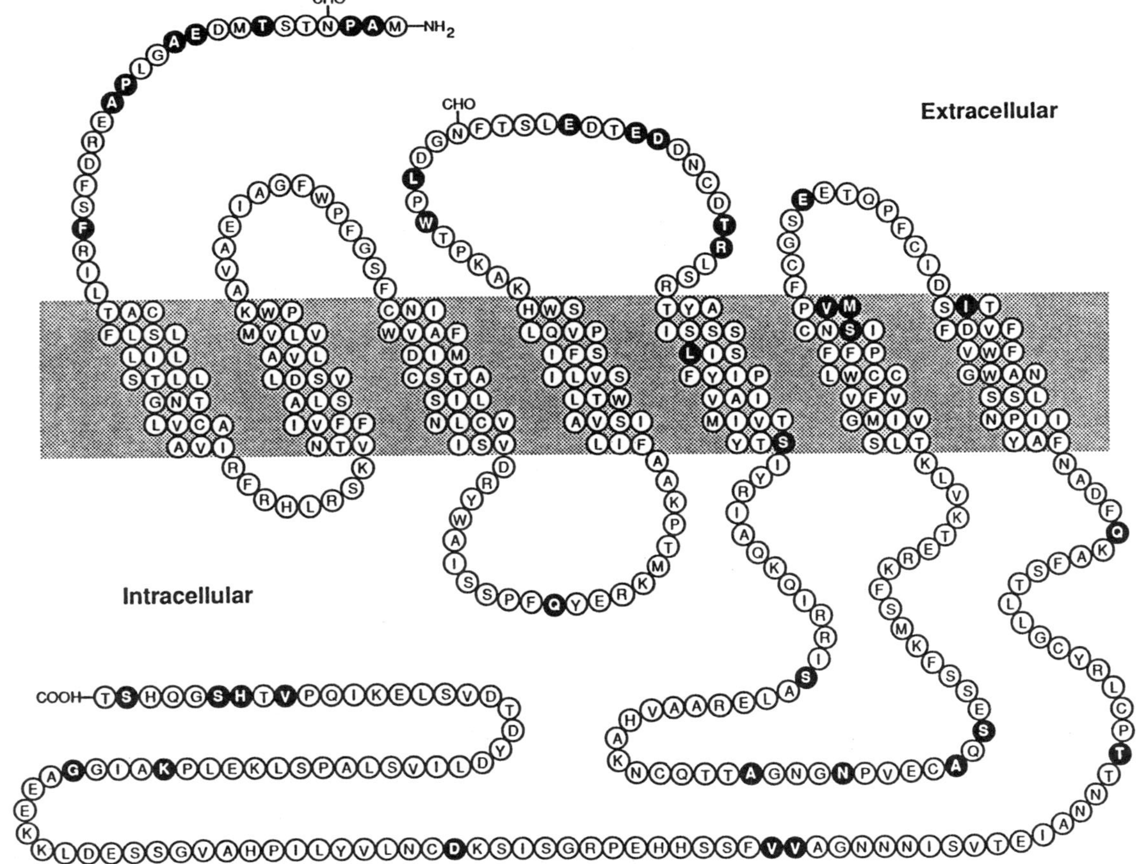

Figure 1. The rat D$_1$ dopamine receptor linked to adenylyl cyclase activation. Transmembrane spanning domains are defined on the basis of hydropathy analysis. Solid circles indicate amino acids that differ between the rat and human proteins. Potential N-linked glycosylation sites are indicated with CHO.

catechol group.[10] These observations would tend to suggest the pB73D1 clone encodes a receptor for an endogenous catecholamine ligand.

In an initial attempt to establish the identity of pB73D1, we analyzed the tissue distribution of its corresponding mRNA by Northern blot and in situ hybridization analyses.[7] Northern blot analysis in various neural tissues reveals a transcript size of 4.1 kb, which is predominantly located in the striatum with lesser amounts in the cortex and retina. In contrast, little to no mRNA is observed in the cerebellum, hippocampus, olfactory bulb, mesencephalon, or pituitary. In situ hybridization analysis also indicates a high abundance of mRNA in the striatum as well as in the olfactory tubercle. Approximately half of the medium-sized neurons in the striatum are identified using this technique. The tissue distribution of pB73D1 mRNA is remarkably similar to that of the D_1 dopamine receptor, as demonstrated by receptor binding and autoradiography studies.[1]

To definitively establish the identify of the receptor encoded by the pB73D1 clone, the cDNA insert was subcloned into the pCD-SRα vector for expression in eukaryotic cells. The resulting plasmid, pSRα-D_1, was used to transiently transfect COS-7 cells. [³H]SCH-23390, a D_1 selective radiolabeled antagonist, binds to transfected COS-7 membranes in a saturable fashion with high specific activity (400 fmol/mg protein) and an affinity (0.3 ± 0.03 nM) in good agreement with that found in the rat striatum.[7] No specific binding was detected in COS-7 cells that had not been transfected with pSRα-D_1 or transfected with the pCD-SRα vector alone. The ability of a variety of dopaminergic ligands to compete for specific [³H]SCH-23390 binding to transfected COS-7 cell membranes was examined. (+)-SCH-23390 is the most potent agent (0.2 ± 0.01 nM) and is approximately 200-fold more potent than its enantiomer, (−)-SCH-23388 (41 ± 1.2 nM). The nonselective dopaminergic antagonist (+)-butaclamol also exhibits high affinity (2.8 ± 0.2 nM) and is more than four orders of magnitude more potent than its inactive isomer, (−)-butaclamol (31 ± 0.8 μM). The D_2-selective antagonist spiperone exhibits relatively low affinity (290 ± 7 nM) as do the serotonin antagonists, ketanserin (0.42 ± 0.031 μM) and mianserin (0.18 ± 0.042 μM). The endogenous agonist, dopamine, is also able to completely inhibit [³H]SCH-23390 binding (0.64 ± 0.092 μM). This rank order of potency as well as the absolute affinities (K_i) of these compounds agree well with those previously demonstrated for striatal D_1 receptors.[1,7]

It was also demonstrated that pSRα-D_1-transfected COS-7 cells exhibit D_1 receptor-mediated stimulation of cAMP production.[7] Dopamine stimulates cAMP production by approximately twofold in these transfected cells. In contrast, no response to dopamine is observed in nontransfected cells. The D_1 selective agonists (+)SKF-38393 and (±)SKF-82958 also stimulate cAMP accumulation to a similar extent as dopamine. Although SKF-38393 has been reported to be a partial agonist at D_1 receptors, its fuller efficacy observed here is probably due to presence of spare receptors resulting from overexpression of receptor protein. In addition, the stimulation by SKF-38393 exhibits appropriate stereoselectivity with the (−) isomer exhibiting a lower potency. Finally, the beta-adrenergic agonist, epinephrine, also exhibits a low potency relative to dopamine as expected for a D_1 receptor. In these experiments, the beta-adrenergic antagonist propranolol was included in the assays to preclude stimulation of the endogenous COS-7 cell beta-adrenergic receptor. These expression data thus confirm that the cDNA that we have cloned encodes a functional D_1 dopamine receptor protein.[7] Recently, the gene for the human D_1 receptor has also been cloned and expressed, shown to be intronless, and to reside on human chromosome 5.[11–13] The homology between the human and rat D_1 receptors is quite high, being approximately 91% at the amino acid level (Figure 1).

It is important to emphasize that the D_1 receptor that has been cloned[7,11–13] is one that is functionally coupled to the stimulation of adenylyl cyclase. Recently, unique D_1 receptors have been described in kidney[3] and brain,[4] which stimulate phospholipase C activity independently from the activation of adenylyl cyclase. We have also shown, using *Xenopus* oocyte expression experiments, that rat striatum contains mRNA encoding D_1 receptors that can couple to phospholipase C, inositol phosphate production, and Ca^{2+} mobilization in a cAMP-independent fashion.[5] It is interesting that the mRNA that codes for this D_1 receptor-stimulated phospholipase C response is 2.5 kb in size[5] in comparison with the 4.1-kb D_1 receptor mRNA observed here. Moreover, in preliminary experiments, we have found that when mRNA is transcribed from the pB73D1 D_1 receptor cDNA clone and injected into *Xenopus* oocytes, dopamine will stimulate cAMP accumulation twofold but is incapable of producing a Ca^{2+} mobilization response.[7] These findings suggest that the striatum contains two separate D_1 receptor proteins that are coupled to different signal transduction pathways. Further experimentation involving the cloning and expression of the other D_1 receptor subtype(s) will be required to confirm this hypothesis.

D_2 Dopamine Receptor Cloning

As indicated above, D_2 receptors have also been demonstrated to be linked to multiple cellular responses.[6] One means of achieving the diversity of second messenger pathways associated with D_2 receptor activation would be the existence of multiple D_2 receptor subtypes, each being coupled with a different G protein-linked response. Efforts towards elucidating D_2 receptor diveristy were recently advanced by the cloning of a cDNA encoding a rat D_2 receptor.[14] This receptor exhibits considerable amino acid homology with other members of the G protein-coupled receptor superfamily for which cDNAs and/or genes have been cloned. When expressed in mammalian cells, the cloned D_2 receptor exhibits pharmacologically specific radioligand binding activity and is functionally coupled to the inhibition of adenylyl cyclase activity.[14–17] Subsequent to the initial report on the cloning of the D_2 receptor,[14] we described the identification and cloning of a cDNA encoding an RNA splice variant of this rat D_2 receptor gene.[18] The cDNA isolated by our laboratory codes for a D_2 receptor isoform that is predominantly expressed in the brain and contains an additional 29 amino acids in the third cytoplasmic loop, a region believed to be involved with G protein coupling. This is the first example of a novel G protein-coupled receptor isoform generated by alternative RNA splicing.

As part of an effort to isolate cDNAs encoding dopamine receptor subtypes, we initially constructed a lambda ZAP II cDNA library using mRNA purified from rat striatum, the region of the brain known to contain the highest levels of both D_1 and D_2 dopamine receptors. This library was screened with a mix of two 36 mer synthetic oligonucleotides, the sequence of which was derived from amino acids 352–363 of the rat D_2 receptor cDNA.[14] This region corresponds to the sixth transmembrane-spanning domain and is known to exhibit very high homology among previously cloned G protein-coupled receptors. Out of 1×10^6 recombinants screened, a total of 15 positive clones were isolated. Restriction analysis and partial sequence information indicated that five of these clones were related to the rat D_2 receptor cDNA previously reported. One of the clones containing an insert of 2.5 kb was completely sequenced. The longest open reading frame in this cDNA codes for a 444-amino acid protein with a molecular weight of 50,887 Da. Figure 2 depicts this D_2 receptor protein as it is believed to be organized in the plasma membrane. The nucleotide and amino acid sequence within the coding region is identical to the rat D_2 receptor cDNA previously reported,[14] with the notable exception of an additional 87-bp sequence coding for a 29-amino acid insertion between residues 241 and 242. This is located within the predicted third cytoplasmic loop approximately 30 amino acids away from the carboxy terminus of the fifth transmembrane-spanning domain. In addition to this insertion sequence, and a slightly extended 5' untranslated sequence, we also noted five base differences within the 3' untranslated region in comparison with the previously published sequence.[14,18] Subsequent sequence analysis indicated that all five of the D_2 receptor-related cDNAs isolated from this library contained the identical 87-bp insertion sequence. The nucleotide sequences delineating the boundaries of this insertion sequence correspond with consensus exon sequences for RNA splice junctions, suggesting that the cDNA resulted from alternative RNA splicing.

In order to confirm the D_2 subtype identity of this cDNA clone and to determine if the 29-amino acid insertion sequence results in a major alteration in the ligand binding properties of the D_2 receptor, the cDNA was inserted into the SV40 promoter-driven vector, pEUK-C1, for expression in eukaryotic cells. The resulting plasmid (pEUK-D2L) was used to transiently transfect COS-7 cells. Three days after transfection, membranes were prepared, and the binding of the D_2 dopaminergic antagonist [³H]methylspiperone was examined. [³H]Methylspiperone bound to the membranes in a saturable fashion with high specific activity (1 pmol/mg protein) and an affinity (62.1 ± 2.1 pM) in good agreement with that found in the rat striatum.[1,18] No specific binding activity was detected in COS-7 cells that had not been transfected with pEUK-D2L or transfected with the pEUK-C1 vector alone. A variety of dopaminergic ligands were examined for their ability to compete for specific [³H]methylspiperone binding to transfected COS-7 cell membranes. The high-affinity D_2-selective antagonist, spiperone (36 ± 3.8 pM) is the most potent

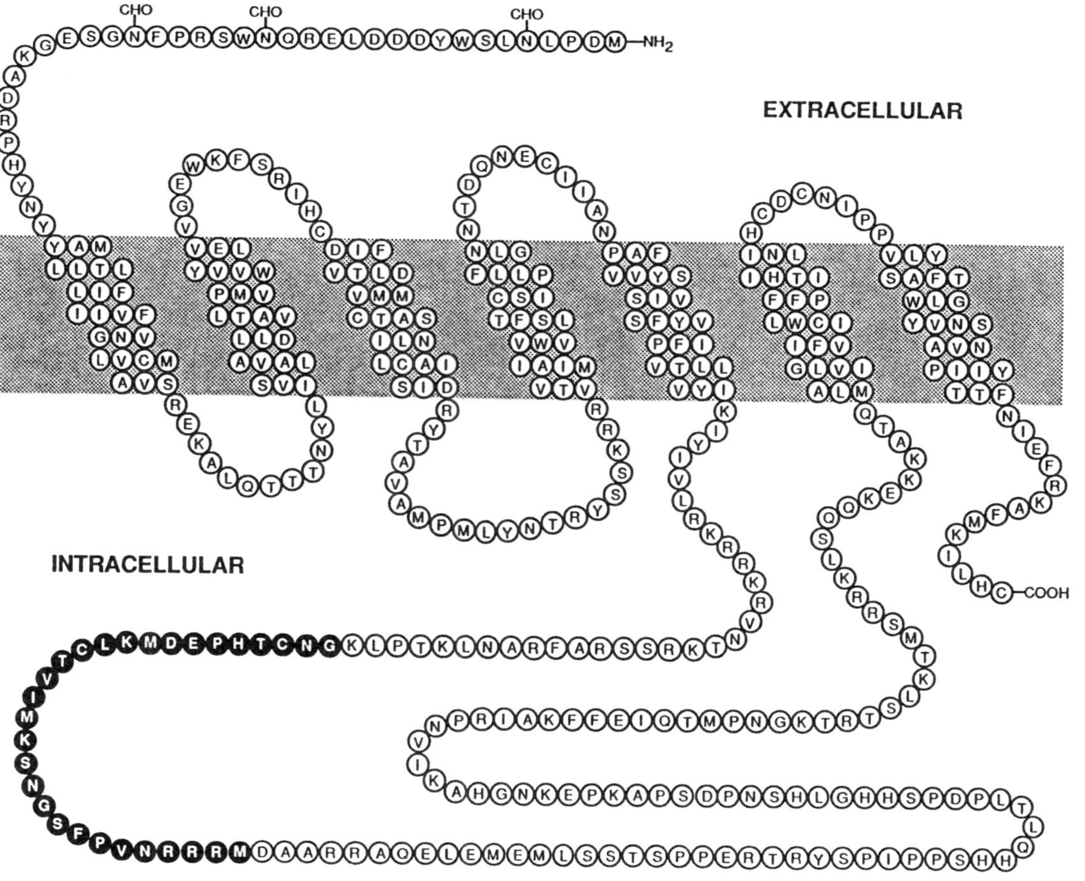

Figure 2. The rat D_2 dopamine receptor. The shaded amino acids indicate the splice variation insertion sequence.

agent followed by the non-selective dopaminergic antagonist (+)-butaclamol (0.52 ± 0.01 nM), which is more than four orders of magnitude more potent than its inactive isomer, (−)-butaclamol (> 10 μM). The D_2-selective antagonist (−)-sulpiride (7.9 ± 0.42 nM) also exhibits high affinity whereas the D_1-selective antagonist SCH-23390 (0.41 ± 0.047 μM) does not. This rank order of potency as well as the absolute affinities (K_i) of the antagonists agree well with those previously demonstrated for D_2 receptors.[1] Dopamine is also able to completely inhibit [³H]methylspiperone binding (K_i = 0.71 ± 0.012 μM) although the competition curve is homogeneous (Hill coefficient = 1) and not significantly affected by guanine nucleotides indicating the absence of appropriate G protein coupling in the COS-7 cells. These experiments indicate that the insertion sequence does not appear to affect the basic properties of ligand recognition for the D_2 receptor.[1,18]

In order to verify the expression of the D_2 receptor variant containing the insertion sequence and to determine the relative proportions of the two receptor isoforms, we subjected various rat tissues to Northern blot analysis using an oligonucleotide probe to a consensus region as well as an insert sequence-specific probe.[18] The tissues expressing the highest levels of the 2.9-kb D_2 receptor mRNA are the striatum and pituitary. The retina showed a moderate abundance of mRNA, with low levels being observed in the mesencephalon and cortex and trace quantities detected in the olfactory bulb and hippocampus. Little to no mRNA was found in the cerebellum and kidney. This tissue distribution corresponds closely to that previously determined for D_2 receptor expression. Of greatest interest, however, is the fact that in all of the tissues examined, the amount of mRNA detected with the two probes is very similar and in no instance did the consensus probe detect greater quantities of mRNA.

To further investigate the relative distributions of the two mRNAs encoding the D_2 receptor isoforms, we performed in situ hybridization analysis in the rat forebrain with the two oligonucleotide probes used for the Northern analysis.[18] Identical patterns of labeling were obtained in a coronal section of rat brain, which includes the striatum using both the consensus region probe and the insert sequence probe. The highest labeling occurred in the striatal neurons, where about 50% of the medium-sized neurons were labeled. Larger-sized (putatively cholinergic interneurons) cells in the striatum also exhibited labeling.

It is interesting that in the Northern blot and in situ hybridization analyses, there did not appear to be any difference in the levels of mRNA detected using the two oligonucleotide probes.[18] If any tissue or brain area expressed mRNA containing the insertion sequence at a level equal to or less than the one lacking the insertion, then the consensus probe should detect mRNA levels that are at least twofold greater than those seen with the insert probe. These experiments thus indicate that not only is the longer D_2 receptor variant (which we propose designating D_{2L}) expressed in brain and other tissues, but in those areas that have been examined (especially the striatum), it appears to be the major if not exclusive isoform. Further experiments directed at determining the actual levels of the receptor proteins will be required to confirm this point. Recent experiments using antipeptide antibodies to the D_2 receptor have demonstrated that, at least in the striatum, the longer D_2 receptor protein is, in fact, more prevalent.[19] Presently, the location of predominant expression of the shorter D_2 receptor lacking the insertion sequence (no designated D_{2S}) is unclear.

In most instances, the genes for the G protein-coupled receptor family have demonstrated a lack of introns within their coding sequences, thus precluding the generation of receptor diversity through alternative RNA splicing. Our current data,[18] however, on the rat D_2 receptor now provides the first example of G protein-coupled receptor isoforms that are generated through alternative RNA splicing. These isoforms are defined by the presence or absence of an internal 29-amino acid sequence within the receptor protein. This observation has been confirmed recently by several other groups for rat,[20–24] human,[25–28] bovine,[29] and mouse[30] D_2 receptors. This RNA splice variation could have arisen either through the existence of a "cassette exon" or through alternative internal acceptor or donor sites within the precursor mRNA. The isolation and sequencing of the rat[24] and human[26–28] D_2 receptor gene have recently been achieved and the gene shown to contain an 87-bp "cassette" exon encoding the splice variation sequence. The location of this optional amino acid sequence is particularly intriguing as it occurs within the predicted third cytoplasmic loop of the receptor. Recent mutagenesis studies using the beta₂-adrenergic catecholamine receptor have indicated that this region is highly involved in G protein-receptor coupling.[10] It is thus tempting to speculate that the two D_2 receptor isoforms are coupled to different G proteins, thus resulting in the diversity of responses associated with D_2 receptor activation. Recent data have suggested, however, that both receptor isoforms will inhibit adenylyl cyclase activity[27,31] as well as activate K^+ channels.[32] Further work involving the stable expression of the two D_2 receptor isoforms in cells exhibiting a variety of G protein-linked effector systems will thus be required to test this hypothesis.

References

1. Creese I, Fraser CM (eds). 1987. Receptor Biochemistry and Methodology: Dopamine Receptors, Vol. 8. Liss, New York, pp 1–245.
2. Kebabian JW, Agui T, van Oene JC, Shigematsu K, Saavedra JM. 1986. The D_1 dopamine receptor: New perspectives. Trends Pharmacol 7:96–99.
3. Felder RA, Felder CC, Eisner GM, Jose PA. 1989. The dopamine receptor in adult and maturing kidney. Am J Physiol 257:F315–F327.
4. Undie AS, Friedman E. 1990. Stimulation of a dopamine D_1 receptor enhances inositol phosphates formation in rat brain. J Pharmacol Exp Ther 253:987–992.
5. Mahan LC, Burch RM, Monsma FJ Jr, Sibley DR. 1990. Expression of striatal D_1 dopamine receptors coupled to inositolphosphate production and Ca^{2+} mobilization in *Xenopus* oocytes. Proc Natl Acad Sci USA 87:2196–2200.
6. Vallar L, Meldolesi J. 1989. Mechanisms of signal transduction at the dopamine D_2 receptor. Trends Pharmacol Sci 10:74–77.
7. Monsma FJ Jr, Mahan LC, McVittie LD, Gerfen CR, Sibley DR. 1990. Molecular cloning and expression of a D_1 dopamine receptor linked to adenylyl cyclase activation. Proc Natl Acad Sci USA 87:6723–6727.
8. Monsma FJ Jr, Brassard DL, Sibley DR. 1989. Identification and characterization of D_1 and D_2 dopamine receptors in cultured neuroblastoma and retinoblastoma clonal cell lines. Brain Res 492:314–324.
9. Barton AC, Sibley DR. 1990. Agonist-induced desensitization of D_1 dopamine receptors linked to adenylyl cyclase activity in cultured NS20Y neuroblastoma cells. Mol Pharmacol 38:531–541.
10. Strader CD, Sigal IS, Dixon RAF. 1989. Structural basis of beta-adrenergic receptor function. FASEB J 3:1825–1832.
11. Dearry A, Gingrich JA, Falardeau P, Fremeau RT Jr, Bates MD, Caron MG. 1990. Molecular cloning and expression of the gene for a human D_1 dopamine receptor. Nature 347:72–76.
12. Zhou QY, Grandy DR, Thambi L, Kushner JA, Van Tol HHM, Cone R, Pribnow D, Salon J, Bunzow JR, Civelli O. 1990. Cloning and

expression of human and rat D$_1$ dopamine receptors. Nature 347:76–80.

13. Sunahara RK, Niznik HB, Weiner DM, Stormann TM, Brann MR, Kennedy JL, Gelernter JE, Rozmahel R, Yang Y, Israel Y, Seeman P, O'Dowd BF. 1990. Human dopamine D$_1$ receptor encoded by an intronless gene on chromosome 5. Nature 347:80–83.

14. Bunzow JR, Van Tol HHM, Grandy DK, Albert P, Salon J, Christie M, Machida CA, Neve KA, Civelli O. 1988. Cloning and expression of a rat D$_2$ dopamine receptor cDNA. Nature 336:783–787.

15. Neve KA, Henningsen RA, Bunzow JR, Civelli O. 1989. Functional characterization of a rat dopamine D$_2$ receptor cDNA expressed in a mammalian cell line. Mol Pharmacol 36:446–451.

16. Albert PR, Neve KA, Bunzow JR, Civelli O. 1990. Coupling of a cloned rat dopamine-D$_2$ receptor to inhibition of adenylyl cyclase and prolactin secretion. J Biol Chem 265:2098–2104.

17. Vallar L, Muca C, Magni M, Albert P, Bunzow J, Meldolesi J, Civelli O. 1990. Differential coupling of dopaminergic D$_2$ receptors expressed in different cell types. J Biol Chem 265:10320–10326.

18. Monsma FJ Jr, McVittie LD, Gerfen CR, Mahan LC, Sibley DR. 1989. Multiple D$_2$ dopamine receptors produced by alternative RNA splicing. Nature 342:926–929.

19. McVittie LD, Ariano MA, Sibley DR. 1991. Characterization of anti-peptide antibodies for the localization of D$_2$ dopamine receptor in rat striatum. Proc Natl Acad Sci USA 88:1441–1445.

20. Giros B, Sokoloff P, Martres MP, Riou JF, Emorine LJ, Schwartz JC. 1989. Alternative splicing directs the expression of two D$_2$ dopamine receptor isoforms. Nature 342:923–926.

21. Miller JC, Wang Y, Filer D. 1990. Identification by sequence analysis of a second rat brain cDNA encoding the dopamine (D$_2$) receptor. Biochem Biophys Res Commun 166:109–112.

22. O'Dowd BF, Nguyen T, Tirpak A, Jarvie KR, Israel Y, Seeman P, Niznick HB. 1990. Cloning of two additional catecholamine receptors from rat brain. FEBS Lett 262:8–12.

23. Rao DD, McKelvy J, Kebabian J, MacKenzie RG. 1990. Two forms of the rat D$_2$ dopamine receptor as revealed by the polymerase chain reaction. FEBS Lett 263:18–22.

24. O'Malley KL, Mack KJ, Gandelman KY, Todd RD. 1990. Organization and expression of the rat D$_{2A}$ receptor gene: Identification of alternative transcripts and a variant donor splice site. Biochemistry 29:1367–1371.

25. Selbie LA, Hayes G, Shine J. 1989. The major dopamine D$_2$ receptor: Molecular analysis of the human D$_{2A}$ subtype. DNA 8:683–689.

26. Grandy DK, Marchionni MA, Makam H, Stofko RE, Alfano M, Frothingham L, Fischer JB, Burke-Howie KJ, Bunzow JR, Server AC, Civelli O. 1989. Cloning of the cDNA and gene for a human D$_2$ dopamine receptor. Proc Natl Acad Sci USA 86:9762–9766.

27. Dal Toso R, Sommer B, Ewert M, Herb A, Pritchett DB, Bach A, Shivers BD, Seeburg PH. 1989. The dopamine D$_2$ receptor: Two molecular forms generated by alternative splicing. EMBO J 8:4025–4034.

28. Gandelman KY, Harmon S, Todd RD, O'Malley KL. 1991. Analysis of the structure and expression of the human dopamine D_{2A} receptor gene. J Neurochem 56:1024–1029.

29. Chio CL, Hess GF, Graham RS, Huff RM. 1990. A second molecular form of D_2 dopamine receptor in rat and bovine caudate nucleus. Nature 343:266–269.

30. Montmayeur JP, Bausero P, Amlaiky N, Maroteaux L, Hen R, Borelli E. 1991. Differential expression of the mouse D_2 dopamine receptor isoforms. FEBS Lett 278:239–243.

31. Rinaudo MS, Monsma FJ Jr, Black LE, Mahan LC, Sibley DR. 1990. Expression and characterization of D_2 dopamine receptor isoforms in transfected mammalian cell lines. Soc Neurosci Abstr 16:209.

32. Einhorn LC, Falardeau P, Caron MG, Oxford GS. 1990. Both isoforms of the D_2 dopamine receptor couple to a G protein-activated K^+ channel when expressed in GH_4 cells. Soc Neurosci Abstr 16:382.

Chapter 13

Cloning of the Dopamine Receptors

Olivier Civelli, James R. Bunzow, Hubert H.M. Van Tol, Qun-Yong Zhou, and David K. Grandy

Dopamine is the predominant catecholamine neurotransmitter in the mammalian brain and is involved in the regulation of a number of physiological activities, predominantly, movement, emotional stability, and prolactin secretion.[1-8] These activities are associated with three principal dopaminergic pathways: (1) The nigrostriatal pathway controls movements; partial degeneration of this system contributes to the pathogenesis of Parkinson's disease. (2) The mesocorticolimbic pathway is involved in emotional stability; imbalance in this pathway is thought to contribute to the etiology of schizophrenia. (3) The tuberoinfundibular pathway regulates prolactin secretion from the pituitary and influences lactation and fertility.

Classically, dopamine was thought to exert its effects by binding to two G protein-coupled receptors, known as the D_1 and D_2 receptors.[9] These receptors can be differentiated pharmacologically, biologically, physiologically, and by their anatomical distribution (for review see ref. 10). Because of their importance in pathophysiology, the dopamine receptors have been the subjects of intense pharmacologic and physiological research. Their structures have remained mostly unknown until recently with the application of molecular biological approaches.

This work was supported by a grant from NIMH, R 01 MH45614.
From Hefti F, and Weiner WJ, (eds.) *Progress in Parkinson's Disease Research—2.* Mount Kisco NY, Futura Publishing Co., Inc., © 1992.

Cloning of the D$_2$ Dopamine Receptor

The cloning of the D$_2$ dopamine receptor resulted from the use of a strategy based on the sequence homology expected to exist among G protein-coupled receptors. The β_2-adrenoreceptor coding sequence was used as a hybridization probe to screen a rat genomic library under low-stringent hybridization conditions. By screening the equivalent of three genomes, 90 positive clones were identified, from which 20 were characterized and partially sequenced. This allowed the characterization of the clones encoding the rat β_1-adreno,[11] the serotonin 1a,[12] the muscarinic 4 (Bunzow et al., unpublished) and another clone, RGB-2, which as described below, encodes the dopamine D$_2$ receptor.[13]

The RGB-2 clone contained a DNA fragment that could be translated into a protein that shared 48% amino acid identity with the sixth and the seventh transmembrane domains of the β_2-adrenoreceptor. The RGB-2 genomic fragment hybridized to a 2.8-kb rat brain mRNA and was subsequently used to screen a rat brain cDNA library. One positive clone, containing a 2.5-kb insert, was sequenced, and its corresponding peptide sequence was determined. This clone encodes a 415-amino acid protein with all the expected characteristics of a G protein-coupled receptor. Therefore it appeared that RGB-2 could be a G protein-coupled receptor.

To determine the ligand specificity of RGB-2, the tissue distribution of its mRNA was analyzed in order to relate RGB-2 expression to the distribution of a known receptor. Northern blot analysis showed that RGB-2 mRNA sequences are expressed throughout the rat brain with the highest levels found in the striatum. Importantly, the RGB-2 mRNA is present in high levels in the intermediate and anterior lobe of the pituitary. These data suggested that RGB-2 could encode a dopamine D$_2$ receptor. To investigate this possibility the RGB-2 cDNA was expressed in a heterologous cell system, and the binding characteristics of the resulting protein were determined.

The full-length RGB-2 cDNA was cloned into a plasmid containing the metallothionein promoter, and this construct was cotransfected with pRSVneo (a selectable marker conferring resistance to the antibiotic neomycin) into mouse Ltk$^-$ cells. This fibroblast cell line does not express endogenous mouse RGB-2 mRNA sequences. Stable transfectants (expressing RGB-2) were isolated, and membranes from one of these clones, L-RGB2Zem-1 were prepared and analyzed for their ability to bind dopamine ligands.[13]

L-RGB2Zem-1 membranes bound D_2 dopamine agonists and antagonists with the same pharmacological profile as do rat striatal membranes. These studies used the antagonist [^{3}H]spiperone whose binding was shown to be saturable (950 fmol/mg protein) and of high affinity (48 pM). [^{3}H]Spiperone binding to L-RGB2Zem-1 membranes was displaced by several antagonists with the stereo-specificity expected of a D_2 receptor and with the same K_is as determined in rat striatal membranes. Finally, as determined using compounds that detect more than one receptor type, the transformed Ltk − cells expressed only one type of receptor. Therefore, RGB-2 encodes a protein that possesses the D_2 receptor binding characteristics. The next step was to show that this D_2 receptor was functional, i.e., couples to a second-messenger system.

D_2 receptors are present on lactotroph cells of the anterior pituitary, where they regulate prolactin secretion. The somatomam-motroph cell line GH_4C1 is derived from a rat pituitary tumor and is known to secrete prolactin. This cell line, however, does not bind dopamine and represents an excellent cell system in which to study exogenously expressed D_2 receptor activity. GH_4C1 cells were transfected with the RGB-2 cDNA metallothionein construction and several stably transformed cells were cloned and raised. One, GH_4ZR7, was found to express high levels of RGB-2 mRNA.[14]

We then analyzed the effects of dopamine binding on the levels of intra- and extracellular cAMP. Since the D_2 receptor is expected to inhibit cAMP levels, VIP (vasointestinal peptide) was used to first stimulate endogenous cAMP production. Dopamine inhibited both basal and VIP-stimulated cAMP levels in media from GH_4ZR7 cells. Furthermore, intracellular cAMP levels were inhibited, albeit at a less pronounced level, probably due to the lower recovery of intracellular cAMP. The stereospecificity of these inhibitions was demonstrated using isomers of sulpiride: the active enantiomer (−)-sulpiride blocked the inhibition while (+)-sulpiride had no effect.

To demonstrate that the changes in cAMP levels were the result of an inhibition of adenylate cyclase, dopamine was added to membranes of VIP- or forskolin-stimulated GH_4ZR7 cells and adenylate cyclase activity was measured. Dopamine inhibited adenylate cyclase activity by 45%. This inhibition was stereoselective since the agonist quinpirole was active, while its enantiomer LY181990 did not have any significant effect.

Finally, the inhibition of prolactin (PRL) secretion by dopamine, was assayed in GH_4ZR7 cells. VIP and thyrotropin-releasing hormone (TRH) are known to enhance PRL release by a cAMP-dependent and a cAMP-independent mechanism, respectively. Dopamine was able to inhibit PRL secretion stimulated by both hormones. These inhibitions were reversed by the active antagonist (−)-sulpiride but not (+)-sulpiride. Therefore, we had demonstrated that the RGB-2 cDNA encodes a D_2 dopamine receptor that is functional, since it can couple to inhibitory G protein and since this coupling results in an inhibition of adenylate cyclase activity as measured by the drop in cAMP levels and in an inhibition of PRL secretion.

Cloning of the Dopamine D_1 Receptor

The success of the homology approach in the cloning of the D_2 receptor opened the door for the cloning of other dopamine receptors, in particular the D_1 receptor.

We took advantage of the polymerase chain reaction (PCR) -based approach, which had been developed to clone several thyroid G protein-coupled receptors.[15] This approach consists of synthesizing two sets of synthetic oligonucleotides, corresponding to two highly conserved regions among all the G protein-coupled receptor (in general found in transmembrane domains III and VI). These oligonucleotides are used as primers in a PCR reaction for specific amplification of cDNAs containing complementary sequences. The cDNAs used for the D_1 receptor cloning were synthesized from rat striatum. To direct the PCR approach toward the specific cloning of the D_1 receptor, our group has used the fact that G_s coupled catecholamine receptors have a putative third cytoplasmic loop of 52–78 amino acids.[16] Therefore our total population of PCR products were size-fractionated and products in the expected range were sequenced. Of 24 PCR products, seven encoded potential G protein-coupled receptors, one of which was later shown to be the D_1 receptor.

The demonstration that the cloned receptor was the D_1 receptor was accomplished by applying techniques similar to those used in the D_2 receptor studies. First the putative D_1 receptor human gene or rat cDNA were expressed by transient expression in COS-7 cells. Membrane proteins from the transfected cells were tested for their ability to bind D_1 receptor ligands. The specific antagonist SCH-23390 was found to have the highest affinity for the cloned receptor, the overall pharmacologic profile was: SCH-23390 > (+)-butaclamol >> SCH-23388 >> spiperone or haloperidol. This pharmacological profile is that of a D_1 receptor binding site. The biological activity of the cloned receptor was studied upon stable or transient transfection of different cells and analysis of dopamine simulation of adenylyl cyclase activity. The cloned receptor was shown to stimulate adenylyl cyclase activity according to a pharmacologic profile expected for the D_1 receptor. Therefore the D_1 dopamine receptors had been cloned.

The Two Forms of the D_2 Receptor

By analyzing human pituitary cDNAs, we found out that there exist not one but two dopamine D_2 receptor forms.[17] These two forms exist in human, rat, and bovine and differ in 29 amino acid residues located in the putative third cytoplasmic loop of the receptor.

Several data were obtained about the 29-amino acid addition. First, the additional residues do not modify the affinity or the profile of the D_2 receptor for antagonists.[17] Second, they do not affect significantly the ability of the receptor to inhibit cAMP production,[18] as could have been expected from their location in the third cytoplasmic loop. Third it was found that the 29-amino acid addition contains two potential glycosylation sites but thus far nothing is known about their importance if any.[17] Fourth, it was also found that the two forms of the D_2 receptor coexist in all tissues analyzed but that their ratio varies. The short form is the least abundant. Its concentration is very low in the pituitary but represents about half of the D_2 receptor mRNA in the pons or medulla.[19,20] Fifth, the generation of the two forms of D_2 receptor was shown to be the result of an alternative splicing event occurring during the maturation of the D_2 receptor pre-mRNA.[17,18,20] This was demonstrated by the discovery of an 87-bp exon encoding the additional amino acid residues. These studies also led to the description of the organization of the D_2 receptor gene, with the coding part of the D_2 receptor encoded by seven exons, one of which (exon 5 in ref. 17) is alternatively spliced.

In summary, the two D_2 receptor forms have not been shown to differ in their pharmacological or biological activities. They are generated by alternative splicing and coexist in a tissue specific ratio. The differences in their biological significance, if any, has still to be demonstrated.

Acknowledgments: We would like to thank Julie Tasnady for preparation of the manuscript.

References

1. Hornykiewicz O. 1966. Dopamine and brain function. Pharmacol Res 18:925.
2. Lee T, Seeman P, Rajput A, Farley IJ, Hornykiewicz O. 1978. Receptor basis for dopaminergic supersensitivity in Parkinson's disease. Nature 273:59.
3. Arnt J. 1987. Behavioral studies of dopamine receptors: Evidence for regional selectivity and receptor multiplicity. *In* Dopamine Receptors: Receptor Biochemistry and Methodology, Vol. 8. I Creese, CM Fraser (eds). Alan R. Liss, New York, p 199.
4. Seeman P. 1987. Dopamine receptors and the dopamine hypothesis of schizophrenia. Synapse 1:133.
5. Seeman P. 1987. Dopamine receptors in human brain diseases. *In* Dopamine Receptors: Receptor Biochemistry and Methodology, Vol. 8. I Creese, CM Fraser (eds). Alan R. Liss, New York, p 233.
6. Carlsson A. 1988. The current status of the dopamine hypothesis of schizophrenia. Neuropsychopharmacology 1:179.
7. MacLeod RM. 1976. Regulation of prolactin secretion. *In* Frontiers in Neuroendocrinology, Vol. 4. L Martin, WF Ganong (eds). Raven Press, New York, p 169.
8. Caron MG, Beaulieu M, Raymond V, Gagne B, Drouin J, Lefkowitz J, Labrie F. 1978. Dopaminergic receptors in the anterior pituitary gland. J Biol Chem 253:2244.
9. Kebabian JW, Calne DB. 1979. Multiple receptors for dopamine. Nature 277:93.
10. Creese I, Fraser CM (eds). 1987. *In* Dopamine Receptors: Receptor Biochemistry and Methodology, Vol. 8. Alan R. Liss, New York, p 1.
11. Machida CA, Bunzow JR, Searles RP, Van Tol H, Tester B, Neve KA, Teal P, Nipper V, Civelli O. 1990. Molecular cloning and expression of the rat β_1-adrenergic receptor gene. J Biol Chem 265:12960.
12. Albert PR, Neve KA, Bunzow JR, Civelli O. 1989. Coupling of a cloned rat dopamine D_2 receptor to inhibition of adenylyl cyclase and prolactin secretion. J Biol Chem 265:2098.
13. Bunzow JR, Van Tol HHM, Grandy DK, Albert P, Salon J, Christie M,

Machida CA, Neve KA, Civelli O. 1988. Cloning and expression of a rat D$_2$ dopamine receptor cDNA. Nature 336:783.

14. Albert PR, Zhou QY, Van Tol HHM, Bunzow JR, Civelli O. 1990. Cloning, functional expression, and mRNA tissue distribution of the rat 5-hydroxytryptamine 1A receptor gene. J Biol Chem 265:5825.

15. Libert F, Parmentier M, Lefort A, Dinsart C, Van Sande J, Maenhaut C, Simon MJ, Dumont JE, Vassart G. 1989. Selective amplification and cloning of four new members of the G protein-coupled receptor family. Science 244:569.

16. Zhou QY, Grandy DK, Thambi L, Kushner JA, Van Tol HHM, Cone R, Pribnow D, Salon J, Bunzow JR, Civelli O. 1990. Cloning and expression of human and rat D$_1$ dopamine receptors. Nature 347:76.

17. Grandy DK, Marchionni MA, Makam H, Stofko RE, Alfano M, Frothingham L, Fischer JB, Burke-Howie KJ, Bunzow JR, Server AC, Civelli O. 1989. Cloning of the cDNA and gene for a human D$_2$ dopamine receptor. Proc Natl Acad Sci USA 86:9762.

18. Dal Toso R, Sommer B, Ewert M, Herb A, Pritchett DB, Bach A, Shivers BD, Seeburg PH. 1989. The dopamine D$_2$ receptor: Two molecular forms generated by alternative splicing. EMBO J 8:4025.

19. Giros B, Sokoloff P, Martres MP, Riou JF, Emorine LJ, Schwartz JC. 1989. Alternative splicing directs the expression of two D$_2$ dopamine receptor isoforms. Nature 342:923.

20. O'Malley KL, Mack KJ, Gandelman KY, Todd RD. 1990. Organization and expression of the rat D$_2$A receptor gene: Identification of alternative transcripts and a variant donor splice site. Biochemistry 29:1367.

Chapter 14

Selective Regulation of Striatal Neurons by the Action of Dopamine at D_1 and D_2 Dopamine Receptors

Alexia E. Pollack and G. Frederick Wooten

The pharmacologic action of both endogenous dopamine and exogenously administered levodopa or dopamine agonists is mediated by dopamine receptors. At least five dopamine receptor subtypes have now been cloned and their amino acid sequences inferred.[1-5] The D_1 and D_2 dopamine receptor subtypes appear to be expressed in highest concentrations in the striatum and are much better characterized pharmacologically than the more recently described D_3 to D_5 receptor subtypes.[6]

The D_1 dopamine receptor appears to be positively linked to adenylate cyclase, while the D_2 subtype appears to be linked negatively.[6] Both agonist and antagonist drugs that are highly selective for the D_1 and D_2 dopamine receptors have been developed. These compounds have greatly facilitated research on the behavioral and pharmacologic effects of the selective activation of D_1 and D_2 receptors. For example, D_1 but not D_2 dopamine agonists increase, and D_1, but not D_2, antagonists decrease metabolic activity in the substantia nigra pars reticulata and medial segment of globus pallidus.[7] This effect of D_1

This work was supported by NIH grant DA 03787 and the Harrison Endowment of the University of Virginia.
From Hefti F, and Weiner WJ, (eds.) *Progress in Parkinson's Disease Research—2.* Mount Kisco NY, Futura Publishing Co., Inc., © 1992.

agonists is dramatically amplified in states of dopamine supersensitivity.[8] In contrast, D_2 agonists appear to be much more efficacious as anti-Parkinson agents than are D_1 agonists.[9,10]

These observations, as well as several other lines of evidence, have raised the question of whether D_1 and D_2 dopamine receptor subtypes are selectively expressed by subpopulations of neurons in the striatum. Harrison et al., using the retrogradely transported neurotoxin volkensin, presented evidence strongly suggesting that striatal D_1 receptors are selectively expressed by neurons that comprise the striatonigral pathway.[11] Gerfen et al. have shown that striatal neurons retrogradely labeled by intranigral injections of tracer substances express D_1 dopamine receptor mRNA.[12] The intrastriatal microinjection of a selective cholinergic neuronal toxin resulted in a selective reduction of D_2, but not D_1 dopamine, receptor binding sites.[13] More recently, Le Moine et al. have shown a high incidence of colocalization of D_2 receptor mRNA with both preproenkephalin (PPE)[14] and choline acetyltransferase mRNA[15] in the striatum. Together these data strongly suggest that D_1 and D_2 dopamine receptors are selectively expressed by different subpopulations of striatal neurons.

One prediction emerging from these mostly anatomical data is that the action of dopamine at D_2 receptors in the striatum would be a powerful site for the regulation of enkephalin. Enkephalins and their precursor molecule PPE appear to be expressed selectively by the subpopulation of striatal neurons projecting to the external segment of the globus pallidus.[16] The evidence reviewed above would suggest that these neurons may selectively express the D_2 dopamine receptor. We have designed experiments to determine if dopaminergic regulation of striatal PPE mRNA was regulated through the selective action of dopamine at either D_1 or D_2 dopamine receptors.

Methods

Rats received a unilateral stereotaxic injection of the neurotoxin 6-hydroxydopamine (6-OHDA) into the left substantia nigra pars reticulata followed by the administration of D_1 or D_2 dopamine receptor agonists for 7 days. Striatal levels of PPE mRNA were determined by dot-blot analysis.[17] Because dopamine agonists are known to inhibit the release of striatal acetylcholine, additional experiments were designed to determine if dopaminergic regulation of striatal PPE mRNA was mediated at least in part by a dopaminergic effect on striatal cholinergic neurons. Rats received a unilateral stereotaxic injection of 6-OHDA into the left substantia nigra pars compacta followed by the administration of the muscarinic cholinergic antagonist scopolamine for 7 days. Unlesioned rats were treated chronically with the D_2 dopamine antagonist eticlopride with or without coadministration of scopolamine. Striatal levels of PPE mRNA were determined by dot-blot analysis.

Two synthetic oligonucleotide probes complementary to PPE mRNA were used in all hybridizations.[18,19] In addition, a synthetic oligo(dT) 30mer was used to "normalize" the dot blots following hybridization with PPE probes to adjust for RNA sample loading errors.

Results and Discussion

Differential Regulation of Striatal Preproenkephalin mRNA by D_1 and D_2 Dopamine Receptors

Eight days after 6-OHDA lesion there was a twofold increase in PPE mRNA in the striatum ipsilateral to the lesion, which was apparent by both Northern and dot-blot analysis. Four days following lesion there was a 50% increase in PPE mRNA in the ipsilateral striatum and the 100% increase seen at 8 days was sustained at 14 and 30 days after lesion.

Treating 6-OHDA-lesioned animals with the D_2 agonist quinpirole for 7 days dose-dependently attenuated the increase in striatal PPE mRNA ipsilateral to a 6-OHDA lesion. A 7-day course of quinpirole (0.1 or 1.0 mg/kg/2X day) brought PPE mRNA levels in the striatum ipsilateral to a 6-OHDA lesion to sham lesion levels. The effect of quinpirole in attenuating the increase in PPE mRNA resulting from a 6-OHDA lesion was blocked by coadministration of the D_2 dopamine antagonist eticlopride. When quinpirole administration was delayed for 7 days following a 6-OHDA lesion, quinpirole attenuated, but did not entirely reverse, the lesion-induced increase in striatal PPE mRNA.

In contrast, treatment of 6-OHDA-lesioned rats with the D_1 dopamine agonist SKF 38393 for 7 days dose-dependently augmented the increase in striatal PPE mRNA ipsilateral to a 6-OHDA lesion.

The coadministration of quinpirole and SKF 38393 in several dose combinations to 6-OHDA-lesioned rats attenuated the lesion-induced increase in striatal PPE mRNA.

Taken together these results suggest that the action of dopamine at D_1 and D_2 dopamine receptors differentially regulates PPE mRNA levels in the striatum and that the primary and proximate effect of dopamine at D_2 dopamine receptors in striatum inhibits enkephalin synthesis.

Evidence that Dopaminergic Regulation of Striatal Preproenkephalin mRNA Levels is Mediated in Part through Cholinergic Interneurons

Administration of scopolamine for 7 days dose-dependently attenuated, but did not entirely reverse, the 6-OHDA lesion-induced increase in striatal PPE mRNA. Treatment with the D_2 antagonist eticlopride for 14 days dose-dependently increased striatal PPE mRNA. Chronic treatment with 1 mg/kg/day of eticlopride increased striatal PPE mRNA 24% compared to vehicle-treated control animals, while 5 mg/kg/day increased PPE mRNA 61% compared to controls. In contrast, there was no effect on striatal PPE mRNA levels following a 14-day course of treatment with 0.1 mg/kg/day of eticlopride.

Coadministration of scopolamine blocked, but did not entirely reverse, the eticlopride-induced increase in striatal PPE mRNA. These results suggest that the D_2 dopamine receptor-mediated regulation of striatal enkephalin can be modulated by cholinergic influence.

Conclusions

These results taken together suggest that the regulation of PPE mRNA expression in the striatopallidal projection is mediated directly by the action of endogenous dopamine on D_2 dopamine receptors expressed on striatopallidal neurons and indirectly via the action of endogenous dopamine on D_2 dopamine receptors expressed by striatal cholinergic interneurons (Figure 1). This interpretation is supported by the recent observation of Le Moine et al. that D_2 dopamine receptor mRNA is expressed by two specific populations of striatal neurons—large aspiny interneurons that express ChAT, and medium spiny neurons that express PPE mRNA and comprise a portion of the striatopallidal pathway. Thus, these results provide an addition to the substantial body of evidence that dopamine receptor subtypes are selectively expressed by different populations of striatal neurons. Specifically, striatopallidal neurons that synthesize PPE appear to selectively express D_2 dopamine receptors, and the action

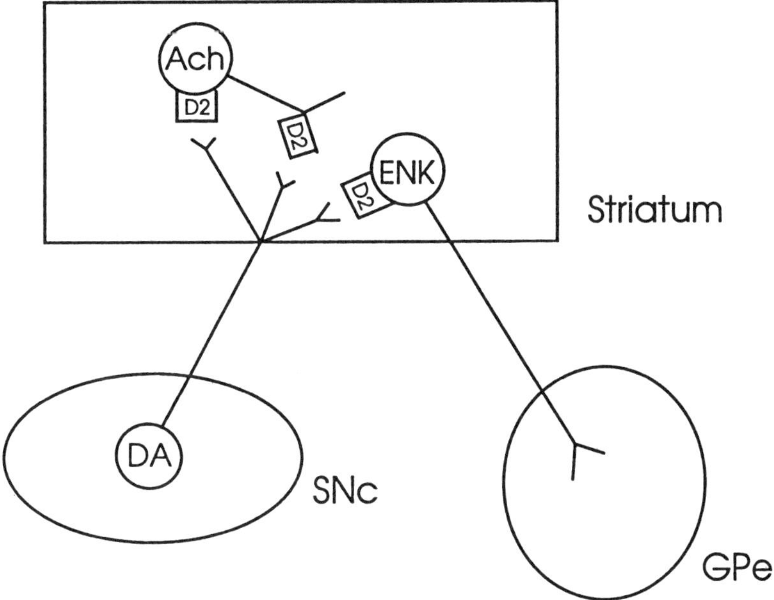

Figure 1. Model of dopaminergic interaction with cholinergic and enkephalinergic neurons in the striatum. Abbreviations: Ach: acetylcholine; DA: dopamine; D_2: D_2 dopamine receptor; ENK: enkephalin; GPe: external segment of globus pallidus; SNc: substantia nigra pars compacta.

of dopamine at those receptors appears to attenuate the levels of PPE mRNA in these neurons.

Acknowledgments: The authors thank Rose Powell for her assistance in the preparation of the manuscript.

References

1. Bunzow JR, Van Tol HHM, Grandy DK, Albert P, Salon J, Christie M, Machida CA, Neve KA, Civelli O. 1988. Cloning and expression of a rat D_2 dopamine receptor cDNA. Nature 336:783–787.
2. Dearry A, Gingrich JA, Falardeau P, Fremeau RT Jr, Bates MD, Caron MG. 1990. Molecular cloning and expression of the gene for a human D_1 dopamine receptor. Nature 347:72–76.
3. Sokoloff P, Giros B, Martres M-P, Bouthenet M-L, Schwartz J-C. 1990. Molecular cloning and characterization of a novel dopamine receptor (D_3) as a target for neuroleptics. Nature 347:146–151.
4. Van Tol HHM, Bunzow JR, Guan H-C, Sunahara RK, Seeman P, Niznik HB, Civelli O. 1991. Cloning of the gene for a human dopamine D_4 receptor with high affinity for the antipsychotic clozapine. Nature 350:610–614.

5. Sunahara RK, Guan H-C, O'Dowd BF, Seeman P, Laurier LG, Ng G, George SR, Torchia J, Van Tol HHM, Niznik HB. 1991. Cloning of the gene for a human D_5 receptor with higher affinity for dopamine than D_1. Nature 350:614–619.

6. Stoof JC, Kebabian JW. 1984. Two dopamine receptors: Biochemistry, physiology, and pharmacology. Life Sci 35:2281–2296.

7. Trugman JM, James CL, Wooten GF. 1990. Regulation of basal ganglia glucose utilization by the D_1 dopamine receptor. Soc Neurosci Abstr 16:81.

8. Trugman JM, Wooten GF. 1987. Selective D_1 and D_2 dopamine agonists differentially alter regional cerebral glucose utilization in rats with unilateral 6-hydroxydopamine substantia nigra lesions. J Neurosci 7:2927–2935.

9. Nomoto M, Janner P, Marsden CD. 1985. The dopamine D_2 agonist LY 141865, but not the D_1 agonist SKF 38393, reverses parkinsonism induced by MPTP in the common marmoset. Neurosci Lett 57:37–41.

10. LeWitt P, Schlick P, Hussain M, Kesaree N, Kareti D, Berchou R. 1988. Selective D_1 agonist (SK&F 38393) in parkinsonism. Neurology 38(suppl 1):258.

11. Harrison MB, Wiley RG, Wooten GF. 1990. Selective localization of striatal D_1 receptors to striatonigral neurons. Brain Res 528:317–322.

12. Gerfen CR, Engber TM, Mahan LC, Susel Z, Chase TN, Monsma FJ Jr, Sibley DR. 1990. D_1 and D_2 dopamine receptor regulated gene expression of striatonigral and striatopallidal neurons. Science 250:1429–1432.

13. Dawson VL, Dawson TM, Filloux FM, Wamsley JK. 1986. Evidence for dopamine D_2 receptors on cholinergic interneurons in the rat caudate-putamen. Life Sci 42:1933–1939.

14. Le Moine C, Normand E, Guitteny AF, Fouque B, Teoule R, Bloch B. 1990. Dopamine receptor gene expression by enkephalin neurons in rat forebrain. Proc Natl Acad Sci USA 87:230–234.

15. Le Moine C, Tison F, Bloch B. 1990. D_2 dopamine receptor gene expression by cholinergic neurons in the rat striatum. Neurosci Lett 117:248–252.

16. Cuello AC, Paxinos G. 1978. Evidence for a long leu-enkephalin striatopallidal pathway in rat brain. Nature 271:178–180.

17. Romano GJ, Shivers BD, Harlan RE, Howells RD, Pfaff DW. 1987. Haloperidol increases proenkephalin mRNA levels in the caudate-putamen of the rat: A quantitative study at the cellular level using in situ hybridization. Mol Brain Res 2:33–41.

18. Angulo JA, Cadet JL, Woolley CS, Suber F, McEwen BS. 1990. Effect of chronic typical and atypical neuroleptic treatment on proenkephalin mRNA levels in the striatum and nucleus accumbens of the rat. J Neurochem 54:1889–1894.

19. Young WS, Bonner TI, Brann MR. 1986. Mesencephalic dopamine neurons regulate the expression of neuropeptide mRNAs in the rat forebrain. Proc Natl Acad Sci USA 83:9827–9831.

Chapter 15

Effects of Dopamine Agonists on Neuronal Activity in the Basal Ganglia of Normal and Dopamine-Denervated Rats

Judith R. Walters, Mark D. Kelland, Kai-Xing Huang, and Debra A. Bergstrom

The striatum, according to current anatomical perspective, is organized into multiple parallel tracks or minicircuits through which information flows from the cortex to the globus pallidus and substantia nigra (for review see refs. 1 and 2). In the matrix compartment of the striatum, afferents originating in a cortical column or set of columns appear to connect with cells within a small cluster.[3] Recent evidence suggests that cells from individual interdigitating striatal clusters project, in turn, to either the substantia nigra or globus pallidus.[4] It is unclear how information is processed by these minicircuits as it passes from cortical efferent to striatal efferent. However, the dilemma of individuals with Parkinson's disease calls attention to the importance of one aspect of this processing—that which is mediated by the dopamine input to the striatum.

The dopaminergic projection from the substantia nigra to the striatum terminates mainly on the stalks of the spines of the striatal efferent neurons.[5] These same spines also receive excitatory input from the cortex and/or thalamus.[6] Thus, dopamine terminals are well positioned to exert a modulatory effect on information passing through the striatum. It has been hypothesized that stimulation of striatal output cells is associated with activation of motor commands and the specification of movement parameters.[2,7,8] Recent studies, however, argue against basal ganglia control of movement initiation and parameter specification and provide support for a role in control of postural holding mechanisms and the switching on or off or blending of various motor programs initiated elsewhere.[9–11] How dopamine affects neuronal transmission directing these processes is an interesting and unresolved problem, currently being explored by a variety of techniques. At issue are fundamental questions regarding the roles of the different dopamine receptor subtypes in modulating basal ganglia output, the net effect of dopamine receptor stimulation on specific striatal efferents, and the compensatory mechanisms induced by reductions in dopamine input to the striatum.

This chapter will review results from a series of studies in which a neurophysiological approach was taken to evaluate the effects of dopamine and dopamine agonists on basal ganglia output in normal rats and rats with unilateral nigrostriatal dopamine cell lesions. The following section presents background information from a variety of neurophysiological, biochemical, and anatomical studies, which has led to some general predictions about how the neuronal activity of cells in the basal ganglia output nuclei is altered by changes in dopamine receptor stimulation in normal and disease states. Subsequent sections will describe results from *in vivo* neurophysiological experiments aimed at exploring these predictions. In these investigations, extracellular single unit recording techniques were used to determine the changes in firing rates of cells in the rat globus pallidus (analogous to the external segment of the globus pallidus in higher species) and the substantia nigra pars reticulata induced by systemic administration of dopamine agonists.

Background: Anatomical, Biochemical, and Neurophysiological Considerations

Most *in vivo* electrophysiological studies have indicated that dopamine exerts an inhibitory influence on the activity of striatal neurons.[12–21] On the other hand, a few studies have reported evidence supporting an excitatory effect of dopamine in the striatum.[19,22–25] Moreover, in studies in which drugs are administered systemically, effects on silent cells are not typically assessed, leaving open the possibility that the ability of dopamine or dopamine agonists to activate silent striatal cells could be underestimated. Thus, expectation that dopamine and dopamine agonists act by reducing striatal output needs to be laced with a few caveats regarding the need for activity to be present in output cells in order for any inhibition to be significant, the limited reports of excitatory effects of dopamine, and the unexplored possibility of effects on silent striatal cells.

To the extent that dopamine agonists do inhibit striatal output, however, current evidence suggests this would mean a reduction in inhibitory input to cells of the globus pallidus and substantia nigra, targets of the striatal efferents (for review, see ref. 26 and Figure 1). The striatopallidal pathway has been shown to utilize GABA and enkephalin as cotransmitters and should, therefore, be inhibitory. The striatonigral pathway also utilizes GABA but contains different cotransmitters: substance P, substance K, and dynorphin. While GABA and dynorphin are clearly inhibitory, substance P and substance K are more commonly found to be excitatory. However, iontophoretic studies indicate that the latter peptides affect the firing rates of only a subpopulation of cells in the substantia nigra[27] (a fact consistent with the scarcity of receptors for these substances in this area[28]), and the effect of stimulating the striatonigral pathway has been shown to be inhibitory on substantia nigra pars reticulata neurons.[29,30] In summary, therefore, data from neurophysiological investigations of the effects of dopamine on striatal efferents and the effects of striatal efferents on their target cells lead to the prediction that systemically administered dopamine agonists should bring about an increase in the activity of pallidal and nigral neurons.

Another strategy for generating hypotheses about how drug or lesion treatment affects neuronal activity in a given region is the use of data from techniques that assess change in transmitter synthesis or transmitter levels. The assumption is that these changes will reflect changes in transmitter release. Measurements of striatal peptide levels and levels of peptide mRNA transcripts provide, in some cases, different predictions about the effects of dopamine agonists and antagonists on activity of striatal efferents (see ref. 26 for review).

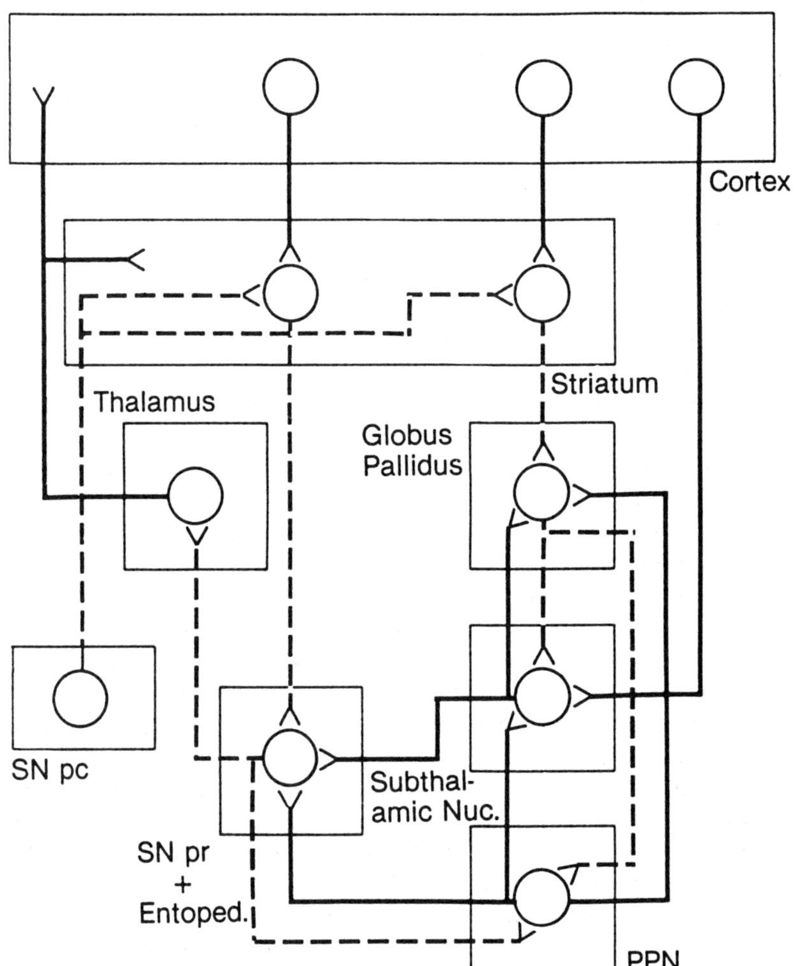

Figure 1. Schematic diagram of the main connections of the basal ganglia output nuclei discussed in the chapter. Pathways believed to be inhibitory are indicated by broken lines, those believed to be excitatory by solid lines. Abbreviations: SN pc: substantia nigra pars compacta; SN pr: substantia nigra pars reticulata; Entoped.: entopeduncular nucleus; PPN: pedunculopontine tegmental nucleus.

Data from these studies are consistent with predictions from neurophysiological studies with respect to the striatopallidal projection but inconsistent with respect to the striatonigral and striatoentopeduncular projections. Dopamine receptor blockade increases the levels of enkephalin and enkephalin mRNA, implying that the activity of striatopallidal enkephalinergic neurons is decreased by dopamine and increased by dopamine blockade. On the other hand, dopamine receptor blockade tends to cause a decrease in substance P and substance K and their peptide precursors' mRNA, while dopamine agonists induce increases in the levels of these indicators. Changes in peptide precursor mRNA levels and receptor binding studies in 6-hydroxydopamine (6-OHDA)-lesioned rats[31,32] also suggest that dopamine induces a net decrease in striatopallidal neuronal activity and a net increase in striatonigral activity. Thus, these studies, like the neurophysiological studies discussed above, would predict that dopamine agonists should cause disinhibition of pallidal cells by reducing activity in the inhibitory striatopallidal pathway, but they would disagree with predictions from the neurophysiological data with respect to effects on cells in the substantia nigra pars reticulata.

Finally, it should be pointed out that in addition to a site of action in the striatum, there are at least a couple of other sites at which dopamine agonists could act to affect neuronal activity in nuclei downstream from the striatum. First, these drugs could exert direct effects in the downstream areas: D_2 receptors are described as being sparse but widespread in the globus pallidus, and striatonigral neurons are known to have D_1 receptors on their terminals.[33–35] Early studies determined that iontophoresed dopamine has the ability to attenuate the effects of iontophoresed GABA on neurons in the globus pallidus and substantia nigra.[36,37] More recent studies, however, attempting to determine which dopamine receptor subtype was mediating this effect, found that both the active and inactive enantiomers of quinpirole mimicked this effect of dopamine and both the active and inactive enantiomers of SKF 38393 affected substantia nigra pars reticulata activity (ref. 38 and H.S. Pan and J.R. Walters, unpublished observations). Thus, the effect of iontophoresed dopamine on GABA-mediated inhibition does not appear to involve D_1 or D_2 dopamine receptors (but also see ref. 39); the possibility of other dopamine receptor subtypes could be considered.[40–42] More relevant to the present discussion, however, is the observation that dopamine, when applied alone via iontophoresis, did have some modest effects on the tonic activity of pallidal and nigral neurons. In the substantia nigra pars reticulata firing rates of approximately 50% of the cells were stimulated by iontophoresed dopamine; the average increase was 28% of baseline.[36] Thus, in this brain region, some dopamine agonist-induced increases in rate could be mediated by direct actions in the substantia nigra itself, but agonist-induced decreases in rate would appear to be mediated by indirect mechanisms. In the globus pallidus, fewer cells (30%) were directly affected by iontophoresed dopamine, and the net change was an increase of less than 10%.[37] This suggests that any significant effects of systemically administered dopamine agonists on neuronal activity in globus pallidus are likely to be indirectly mediated.[37]

Second, direct or indirect effects of dopamine agonists on the activity of neurons in the subthalamic nucleus might contribute to the net effects of dopamine agonists on globus pallidus and substantia nigra pars reticulata neuronal activity. In the rat, the globus pallidus and the cortex both project to the subthalamic nucleus which, in turn, projects back to the globus pallidus (Figure 1), to the entopeduncular nucleus (analogous to the internal globus pallidus in higher species) and to the substantia nigra. The question that arises in assessing the potential for the subthalamic nucleus to affect neuronal activity (especially tonic activity) in the globus pallidus and substantia nigra pars reticulata is whether the tonically firing cells in the latter nuclei are intrinsically active and/or whether they are "driven" by excitatory input from the subthalamic nucleus. The subthalamic nucleus is the major target of the inhibitory output from the globus pallidus. If the subthalamic nucleus does act as a significant driving force for the globus pallidus, as has been suggested,[43] then either this excitatory input is subject to feedback regulation by the pallidal cells themselves, or the subthalamic input to the globus pallidus originates from a separate subpopulation of cells in the subthalamic nucleus that are not innervated by the globus pallidus. Anatomical evidence would appear to support the former possibility.[44] A similar set of reciprocal connections exists between the basal ganglia output nuclei and the pedunculopontine tegmental nucleus.[45,46] These considerations suggest that if dopamine agonists attenuate activity in inhibitory striatal efferents, the resulting increase in neuronal firing rates in the globus pallidus and substantia nigra pars reticulata would tend to be dampened by reduced excitatory input from the subthalamic nucleus (and perhaps the pedunculopontine tegmental nucleus).

Effects of Systemically Administered Dopamine Agonists on Neuronal Activity in the Globus Pallidus

Nonselective D_1/D_2 Agonists Stimulate Activity of a Major Pallidal Cell Type

Initial studies, designed to explore the predictions discussed above, examined the effects of systemic administration of nonselective (mixed D_1/D_2) dopamine agonists and indirect acting agonists (e.g., apomorphine and *d*-amphetamine, respectively) on the single unit activity of cells in the globus pallidus. It was found that these drugs do induce marked increases (typically 80–100% above baseline) in the firing rates of the predominant cell type in the globus pallidus of locally anesthetized gallamine-immobilized rats[47–49] (Table 1, Figure 2). This cell type (which will be referred to as the type II pallidal cell) is spontaneously active, typically firing 10–80 spikes/sec and is identified by its biphasic positive/negative extracellularly recorded action potential. The excitatory effect of amphetamine and apomorphine-like drugs on these cells appears to be related to the ability of these drugs to directly or indirectly increase dopamine receptor stimulation, since the effects were reversed by dopamine antagonists. Moreover, drugs such as *d*-lysergic acid diethylamide (LSD), fluoxetine, *l*-amphetamine, and clonidine, interacting primarily with serotonin or norepinephrine receptors, do not significantly affect the activity of these pallidal cells.[47,50,51] It can also be said that these actions of dopamine agonists on neuronal activity in the globus pallidus are not due to changes in nigral dopamine cell activity, because dopamine cell firing can be inhibited by doses of agonists that are significantly less than those required to stimulate the activity of pallidal neurons.[48]

Thus, the finding that dopamine agonists induce very substantial increases in firing rates of the predominant cell type in the globus pallidus is consistent with the idea that tonically active inhibitory striatopallidal neurons innervating these pallidal cells are inhibited by dopamine. To the extent that an increase in neuronal activity in the globus pallidus should induce increased release of GABA in the

Table 1.
Effects of Dopamine Agonists on Single Unit Activity of Substantia Nigra Pars Reticulata and Globus Pallidus Cells in Normal Rats and in Rats with Unilateral 6-OHDA-Induced Lesions of Nigrostriatal Pathway[a]

	Substantia nigra pars reticulata					Globus pallidus				
	% cells no change	% cells with rate up	% cells with rate down	% of baseline	N	% cells no change	% cells showing increase	% cells showing decrease	% of baseline	N
Control										
SKF-38393										
10.0 mg/kg	46	46	8	112±6	13	68	21	10	103±4	19
20.0 mg/kg	30	50	20	137±18	10	47	40	14	117±6	43
Quinpirole										
0.3 mg/kg	67	33	0	114±4	15	38	62	0	127±9	13
1.0 mg/kg	67	33	0	112±6	12	25	75	0	153±11	12
Apomorphine										
0.3 mg/kg	34	36	30	116±10	44	10	90	0	195±12	21
6-OHDA										
SKF 38393										
10.0 mg/kg	22	11	66	58±14	9	31	41	28	125±14	29
Quinpirole										
0.3 mg/kg	27	36	36	94±12	11	27	73	0	160±12	15
1.0 mg/kg	29	0	71	78±5	7	—	—	—	—	—
Apomorphine										
0.3 mg/kg	0	13	87	34±14	8	16	56	28	197±35	18

[a]Data taken from refs. 51, 54, 65, 69, and 70.

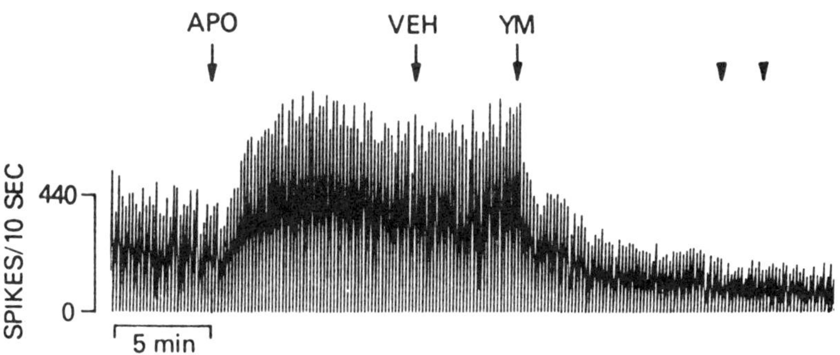

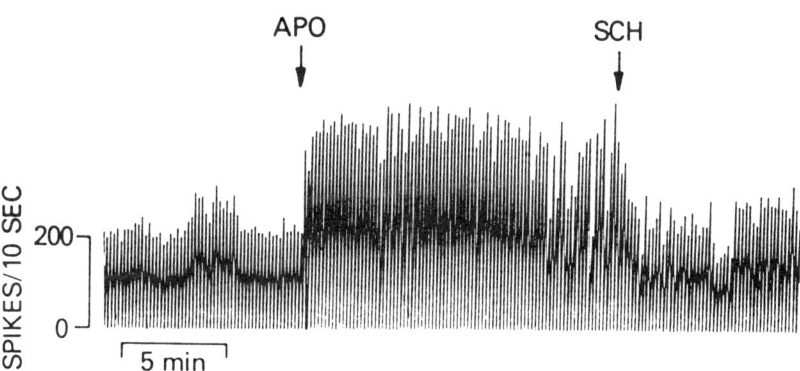

Figure 2.   The effects of the nonselective D_1/D_2 dopamine agonist apomorphine on the single unit activity of globus pallidus neurons in control immobilized, locally anesthetized rats. Apomorphine (APO; 0.32 mg/kg, IV) significantly increased the firing rates of these pallidal type II neurons, as was typically seen. Vehicle (VEH, 0.4 ml) for the YM-09151-2 (YM) exerted no effect on firing, but the selective D_2 antagonist, YM-091551-2 itself (0.2, 0.2, 0.4 mg/kg IV, given at the times indicated by the arrows) effectively reversed the agonist-induced rate increases. Similarly, the D_1 antagonist SCH-23390 (SCH, 0.2 mg/kg IV) also reversed the rate increase induced by apomorphine. Data taken from refs. 47, 48, and 61.

subthalamic nucleus, one would expect that the activity of excitatory subthalamic cells projecting back to the globus pallidus would be reduced, thus attenuating the effect of the reduction in striatal inhibition (Figure 1). If such an effect occurs, the gain in the system is evidently such that a substantial increase in pallidal activity still takes place. Perhaps the net effect of the globus pallidus type II neurons on the subthalamic neurons projecting back to the globus pallidus is small. Understanding how the globus pallidus sustains the increase in activity induced by dopamine agonists in terms of the net effects of striatal and subthalamic input is an interesting issue, especially in view of the fact that the other basal ganglia output nuclei, the entopeduncular nucleus and the substantia nigra pars reticulata (discussed below), also have inhibitory input from the striatum and excitatory input from the subthalamic nucleus, yet current models addressing basal ganglia mechanisms predict that neuronal activity in these latter two basal ganglia nuclei is significantly dampened by dopamine agonist treatment or striatopallidal lesion, resulting in diminished inhibitory control of thalamic neurons.[52]

Role of Striatum in Pallidal Stimulation by Apomorphine

The idea that the striatopallidal neurons play a major role in mediating the effect of D_1/D_2 agonists such as apomorphine on pallidal cell firing rates was examined in a study in which the striatum was lesioned with quinolinic acid.[53] In normal animals, this study found that apomorphine induced significant increases in the firing rate of 90% of the pallidal type II neurons (Figure 2). The increase in rate averaged over 90%.[53] In rats that had relatively effective striatal lesions, as determined by behavioral and biochemical measures, the same dose of apomorphine induced increases in pallidal cell activity in only 45% of cells and the increase averaged only 18% above baseline. Three cells showed decreases in rate. Thus, removal of the striatopallidal pathway markedly reduced the excitatory effect of apomorphine on the activity of the pallidal neurons.[53]

These results are consistent with the idea that striatal efferents play an important role in mediating the effect of apomorphine in the globus pallidus. However, less supportive of the idea that apomorphine acts by reducing activity in tonically active, inhibitory striatopallidal neurons is the finding that the firing rates of the pallidal cells recorded 1 week after the striatal lesions were not at all elevated. There was no significant difference between the average rates of the cells sampled in normal and lesioned animals.[53] This observation either suggests that compensatory mechanisms are activated fairly rapidly after the lesion to bring pallidal rates back to normal or raises questions about the extent to which pallidal cells are tonically inhibited by striatopallidal neurons.

Role of Dopamine Receptor Subtypes in Pallidal Stimulation by Apomorphine

Further studies have shown that the kinds of changes in firing rates in the globus pallidus induced by systemic administration of drugs such as amphetamine and apomorphine require stimulation of both D_1 and D_2 receptors and appear to involve a synergistic interaction between the two receptors (Table 1, Figure 3). These changes can be reversed by either a D_1 or a D_2 antagonist[51,54] (Figure 2). Similar observations have been made in studies investigating the roles of D_1 and D_2 receptors in mediating behavioral effects of dopamine agonists (see ref. 55 for review). Processes mediated by stimulation of D_1 and D_2 receptors also interact to induce *c-fos* expression in the striatum.[56]

The mechanism underlying the synergistic interaction between the two receptor subtypes as well as the exact location of the receptors involved in mediating these effects remain unclear. Debate exists as to whether the two receptors are on the same striatal cell or on different cells, i.e., whether the synergistic interaction between the two receptors goes on intracellularly, perhaps at the level of a second-messenger system, or intercellularly, involving an additional transmitter–receptor system. Bertorello et al.[57] have presented evidence for D_1 and D_2 interactions at the single cell level in a study showing synergistic effects of D_1 and D_2 agonists on Na^+,K^+-ATPase activity in a dispersed striatal cell preparation. They argue that it would be unlikely for the two receptors to be inducing a synergistic effect in a dispersed cell preparation if the different receptor subtypes were on different neurons. In addition, *in vivo* iontophoretic studies on effects of D_1 and D_2 agonists on the activity of neurons in the striatum[58] and the accumbens[59] support the idea that the two receptors are located on the same neuron, although other researchers[22,60] have failed to find evidence for interaction between the two receptors at the single cell level in the striatum. Evidence supporting

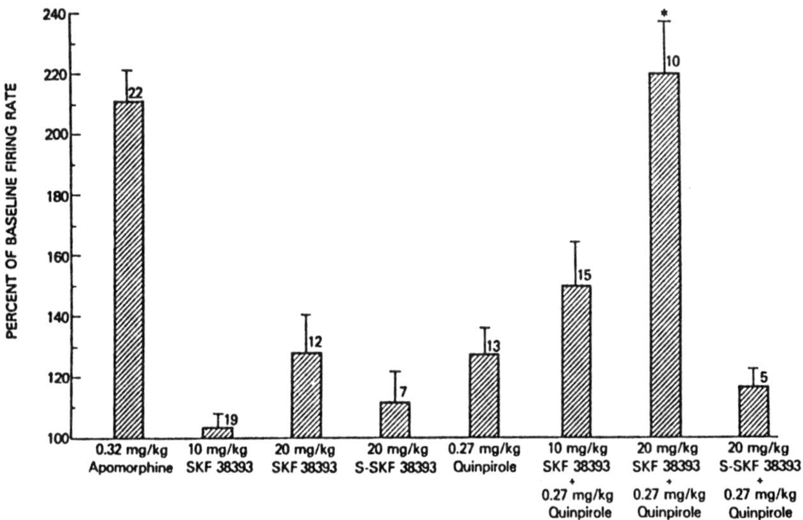

Figure 3.   Effects of various dopamine agonists on the single unit activity of globus pallidus neurons. Drugs were administered intravenously as a single bolus injection while pallidal unit activity was monitored. When more than one drug was given, as in the experiments investigating the combined effects of quinpirole and SKF 38393, SKF 38393 was either administered concurrently with quinpirole or given 3–15 minutes prior to quinpirole. Bars represent the standard error of the mean. Only one dose or dose combination was studied per rat. The number above each bar indicates the number of cells studied. *Denotes a statistically significant difference ($P < 0.05$) relative to quinpirole (0.27 mg/kg) and SKF 38393 (10 and 20 mg/kg). Data taken in part from ref. 51.

the concept that the dopamine receptor subtypes are largely segregated in the striatum[32] has also been presented.

Apomorphine Exerts a Different Effect on a Second Pallidal Cell Type

It should be pointed out that the excitatory effect of apomorphine and D_1/D_2 receptor stimulation on neuronal activity in the globus pallidus, discussed above, describes the response of the predominant cell type in the globus pallidus, the type II pallidal cells, which was initially the exclusive focus of these studies. These are spontaneously active cells identified by their biphasic positive/negative extracellularly recorded action potentials firing in the range of 10–80 spikes/sec with an extracellular action potential duration of approximately 0.8 msec. However, a second population of cells with distinctive neurophysiological properties has been identified recently, also characterized by spontaneous activity but exhibiting a biphasic negative/positive action potential when recorded extracellularly (ref. 21 and M.D. Kelland and J.R. Walters, unpublished observations). These cells, termed pallidal type I cells, fire in the range of 5–75 spikes/sec and have extracellular action potentials of 1–2 msec duration. In contrast to the dramatic increase in activity seen with the positive/negative type II pallidal cells when apomorphine is administered, the negative/positive type I pallidal cells show mainly a decrease in firing rate with systemically administered apomorphine. These type I pallidal cells have not yet been tested for their response to D_1 and D_2 agonists administered separately. The effect of apomorphine on this cell type raises interesting questions about globus pallidus circuitry. Possible explanations for the opposite responses of the two cell types to systemic apomorphine include different striatal innervations, different intrapallidal connections, and selective inputs from the subthalamic nucleus. Another interesting issue raised by these findings is whether the outputs of these two cell types differentially innervate the areas targeted by the globus pallidus, i.e., the subthalamic nucleus, the substantia nigra, and the pedunculopontine tegmental nucleus.

Effect of Dopamine Depletion or Receptor Blockade on Activity of Type II Globus Pallidus Neurons

Blockade of dopamine receptors does not induce the kind of dramatic changes in pallidal cell firing rates that are observed with increases in dopamine receptor stimulation. When the effect of systemic administration of either haloperidol or the D_1 antagonist SCH-23390 on pallidal cell activity was examined, it was found that doses of these dopamine receptor antagonists that effectively block the effects of dopamine agonists on pallidal activity had themselves no significant effect on firing rate.[48,61] Determination of the effects of SCH-23390 (1 mg/kg) on the firing pattern of pallidal cells by analysis of interspike interval histograms over a 10-minute period after IV administration also revealed no significant change (J.H. Carlson and J.R. Walters, unpublished observations). Thus, acute increases in dopamine receptor stimulation are more effective in producing marked changes in pallidal activity than are acute decreases.

To further explore the role of dopamine in regulating the activity of the globus pallidus and the compensatory changes occurring when dopamine cells drop out as they do in Parkinson's disease, we examined the firing rate and pattern of the type II globus pallidus neurons in intact rats and in rats that had survived unilateral lesions of the nigrostriatal pathway for 3 days, 1 week, or 6–11 weeks.[62] In locally anesthetized animals, there was no change in the overall average firing rate of pallidal type II cells 3 days after the lesion, although a more irregular firing pattern with a frequent increase in bursting was observed. One week after the lesion, a decrease in firing rate of approximately 20% was observed and the firing pattern remained significantly more irregular. There is some evidence to suggest that cells firing in a bursting mode release more transmitter than cells firing at the same rate in a nonbursting mode;[63] thus, the increased bursting may partially offset the decrease in rate. At 6–9 weeks after lesion, firing rate was still decreased by 20% and the firing pattern remained irregular although less so than at 3 days and 1 week.[62] These observations are consistent with the idea that loss of dopamine leads to increased activity in inhibitory striatopallidal neurons; in addition, they indicate that the net effect of this lesion also involves alterations in the pattern of pallidal cell firing. Whether the increased bursting is due to changes in striatal firing patterns initiated by loss of dopamine receptor stimulation or is a consequence of other, perhaps subthalamically mediated, mechanisms is unclear.

Compensatory Changes in Receptor Sensitivity in Response to Dopamine Cell Lesion

Compensatory changes in neurotransmitter receptor sensitivity associated with neurons downstream from a lesion can provide indirect evidence for lesion-induced alterations in neuronal input to these neurons.[31] Evidence suggests that dopamine cell lesion brings about compensatory changes in downstream neuronal systems, which may at least partially compensate for the effect of the lesion. Thus, dopamine receptor up-regulation in the striatum, as well as GABA, benzodiazepine, and opiate receptor down-regulation in the striatum and globus pallidus has been documented following dopamine cell lesion.[31]

We have investigated the functional correlates of these compensatory receptor changes in neurophysiological studies in which GABA and enkephalin agonist effects on pallidal activity were determined with the use of iontophoretic techniques (ref. 64 and H.S. Pan and J.R. Walters, unpublished observations). It was found that lesions of the striatonigral pathway reduce the sensitivity of pallidal cells to enkephalin agonists. In normal animals, when applied by microiontophoresis, the nonselective opioid receptor agonist D-Ala2,D-Leu5-enkephalin (DADLE) reduced the activity of about 45% of globus pallidus neurons tested by more than 80% of baseline firing rate, partially inhibited about 30% of the cells, and had no effect on the remaining 25%. The mu opioid receptor-selective agonist D-Ala2,MePhe4,Gly-o15-enkephalin (DAGO) exerted a similar effect, while the delta opioid receptor-selective agonist D-Pen2,5-enkephalin (DPDPE) was less effective. In animals with unilateral 6-OHDA lesion of the nigrostriatal pathway, cells in the globus pallidus ipsilateral to the lesion became significantly less sensitive to all three opioid compounds. The sensitivity of pallidal neurons to iontophoretically applied GABA was also significantly attenuated in the lesioned rats. These results indicate that the functional states of the opioid and GABA receptors are altered by the changes in endogenous transmitter exposure induced by dopamine cell lesion. The development of subsensitivity to enkephalin and GABA in the globus pallidus after striatal dopamine denervation further supports the idea that nigrostriatal dopamine neurons tonically inhibit the activity of striatopallidal neurons utilizing GABA and enkephalins as transmitters. Interestingly, this compensatory functional receptor change apparently cannot fully reverse the overactivity of the striatopallidal neurons since, as described above, pallidal neurons continue to fire at a slower rate in lesioned animals as compared to controls.[62]

Effects of Dopamine Agonists on Pallidal Activity in 6-OHDA-Lesioned Rats

In the dopamine-depleted rats, the combined effect of compensatory changes in dopamine receptor function and downstream changes in neurotransmitter synthesis and receptor sensitivity would seem likely to result in an altered response in downstream nuclei when dopamine agonists are administered a few weeks after 6-OHDA dopamine cell lesion. In fact, in nigrostriatal lesioned rats, the nonselective D_1/D_2 agonist apomorphine produces exaggerated increases, relative to those observed in control rats, in the discharge rates of many type II pallidal neurons[65] (Table 1, Figure 4). Interestingly, however, about 28% of the type II pallidal cells recorded in the lesioned animals actually showed a decrease in rate after apomorphine, a response which, with respect to apomorphine, was very rare to nonexistent in this population of cells in normal animals (Figure 2). This response does not appear to be a simple "supersensitive" response, but rather a qualitative change in the effect of apomorphine on pallidal cell activity, a change that would seem to be linked to the D_1 component of apomorphine's effect since only the D_1 agonist induced any decreases in the activity of pallidal positive/negative type II cells when administered alone[65] (Table 1). D_2 agonist effects are consistently excitatory in both the normal and lesioned rats, although significantly more so in the latter animals. These data suggest that after chronic reduction of the dopamine innervation to the striatum there is a nonuniform change in the influence dopamine agonists exert on input to the globus pallidus so that a subpopulation of type II pallidal cells now receive a net increase in inhibition, perhaps associated with a more dominant D_1 mediated effect. This raises the possibility that the net effect of D_1 receptor stimulation is sometimes excitatory rather than inhibitory in the striatum, especially in the 6-OHDA-lesioned rats. A possible excitatory effect of dopamine on striatal output is also suggested by the response of type I pallidal cells to apomorphine in control rats, as described above.[21] Consideration of the effects of D_1 drugs on firing rates of cells in the substantia nigra pars reticulata of 6-OHDA lesioned rats, described below, provides further support for this idea.

Effects of Dopamine Agonists on Neuronal Activity in the Substantia Nigra Pars Reticulata

Dopamine Agonists Variably Affect Activity of Substantia Nigra Pars Reticulata Cells

The substantia nigra pars reticulata, like the pallidal complex, is a major basal ganglia output nucleus. Both receive inhibitory input

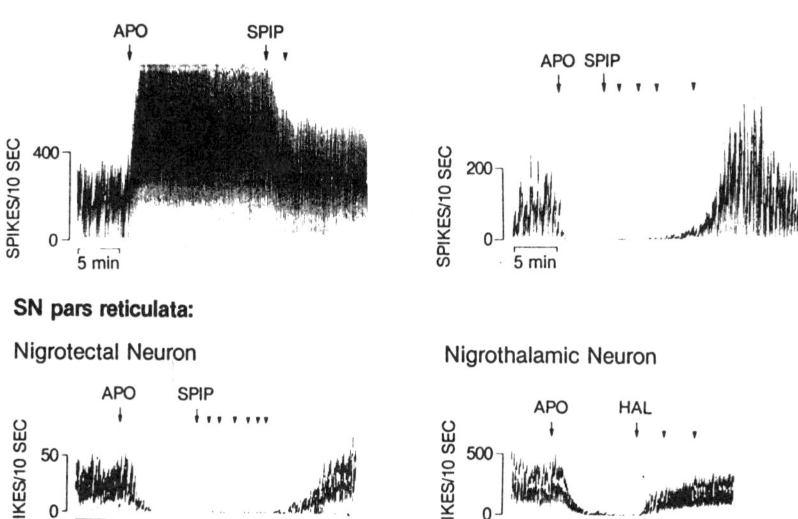

Figure 4. The effects of apomorphine on the single unit activity of globus pallidus neurons and substantia nigra pars reticulata neurons in rats with unilateral 6-OHDA-induced lesions of the nigrostriatal pathway 6–10 weeks prior to the recording experiments. Apomorphine (APO; 0.32 mg/kg, IV) induced significant increases and decreases in the firing rates of pallidal neurons type II in these lesioned animals. Of 18 neurons recorded in lesioned animals, 10 had firing rates that increased by an average of 296 ± 36% of baseline, rates of five cells decreased by 55 ± 19%, and the rates of three cells were not significantly changed (<20%). The dopamine antagonist spiperidol (SPIP; 0.2 mg/kg, IV, given at the times indicated by the arrows) partially to fully reversed the rate changes. Data taken from ref. 65. In the substantia nigra of 6-OHDA-treated animals, apomorphine (0.32 mg/kg) significantly and consistently inhibited the firing rates of reticulata cells that were identified as either nigrotectal or nigrothalamic neurons by antidromic activation from the superior colliculus or the ventromedial thalamic nucleus. The firing rates of 87% of the neurons recorded ($N = 8$) were significantly inhibited with an average inhibition of 79 ± 5%; the firing rate of one of eight cells increased 25% following apomorphine administration. Spiperidol (cumulative dose, 1 mg/kg) and haloperidol (HAL; cumulative dose, 0.6 mg/kg) effectively reversed the decreases in firing rates induced by apomorphine. Data taken from refs. 68 and 69.

from the striatal nucleus and excitatory inputs from the subthalamic and pedunculopontine tegmental nuclei. The substantia nigra pars reticulata is generally considered most similar to the entopeduncular nucleus, the analog of the internal segment of the globus pallidus in higher species, since these two areas have similar inputs and, unlike the globus pallidus proper (which corresponds to the external segment in higher species), both project to the thalamus. A potentially important difference between the substantia nigra pars reticulata and the globus pallidus is the fact that substance P and dynorphin are peptide cotransmitters with GABA in striatonigral neurons whereas, as discussed above, the striatal innervation of the globus pallidus contains enkephalin and GABA. Thus, it is clear that different striatal neurons project to the globus pallidus and to the substantia nigra pars reticulata.

Neurophysiological investigations of the effects of dopamine agonists on the activity of substantia nigra pars reticulata neurons, especially in 6-OHDA-lesioned rats, have raised interesting questions about the nature of dopaminergic modulation of striatonigral activity. When the effects of dopamine agonists on the activity of cells in the substantia nigra pars reticulata were first examined, it was expected that these cells would respond in a manner similar to those in the globus pallidus: apomorphine would inhibit the inhibitory striatonigral neurons and induce an increase in firing rates of the reticulata cells. In fact, when effects of D_1 and D_2 agonists, administered separately, are compared in the two nuclei, responses are not dramatically different[65,70] (Table 1). However, when both D_1 and D_2 receptor subtypes are stimulated together, as with apomorphine administration, differences become more obvious, at least when reticulata neurons are compared with the type II pallidal cells. Apomorphine induced more variable changes in the activity of cells in the substantia nigra pars reticulata[67–69] than are observed with the pallidal type II cells (Figures 2 and 5). The rates of about 36% of the substantia nigra pars reticulata cells are excited by more than 20%, 30% are inhibited by more than 20%, and the rest show no significant rate change[67] (Table 1). The overall average change in rate is slightly positive. As in the globus pallidus, lesion of the striatum with kainic acid attenuates the change in substantia nigra pars reticulata neuronal activity induced by apomorphine.[67]

In contrast to the variable response in firing rate observed in the

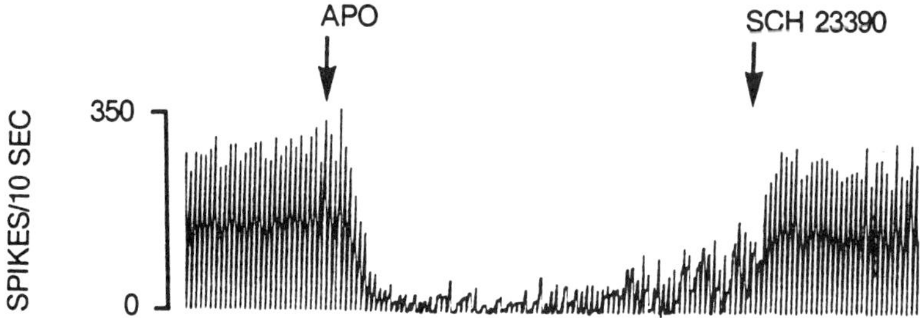

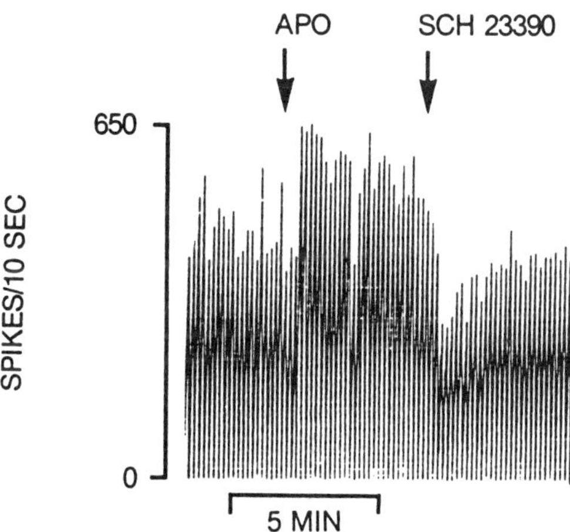

Figure 5. The effects of apomorphine on the single unit activity of substantia nigra pars reticulata neurons in control immobilized, locally anesthetized rats. In response to 0.32 mg/kg apomorphine (APO; IV) administration, the firing rates of approximately one third of the reticulata cells recorded decreased (upper trace), rates of approximately one third of the cells increased (lower trace), and the rates of the remaining one third of cells did not significantly change. Changes in firing rates were effectively reversed by the D_1 antagonist SCH-23390 (SCH; 1.0 mg/kg) as illustrated above or by the D_2 antagonist YM-09151-2 (0.2–1.0 mg/kg; data not shown). Data taken from refs. 61, 67, and 70.

substantia nigra pars reticulata after apomorphine, the type II cells in the globus pallidus, as discussed above, are almost exclusively stimulated by apomorphine.[48] On the other hand, if the responses of the recently described type I pallidal cell (ref. 21 and M.D. Kelland and J.R. Walters, unpublished observations) are considered together with the type II, it could be argued that in control animals there is little difference in the overall responses of the cells in the two nuclei to systemically administered apomorphine. The most common response in both nuclei in the locally anesthetized preparation is an increase in rate, but both nuclei also have a population of cells that fire more slowly after apomorphine administration. In the substantia nigra pars reticulata, however, unlike the globus pallidus, there is no obvious difference in the extracellular waveform between the cells that respond to systemic apomorphine with increases in rate and those responding with decreases; antidromic identification has shown that the two major targets of the substantia nigra pars reticulata neurons, the thalamus and the superior colliculus, both receive input from each type of cell.[67]

Role of Dopamine Receptor Subtypes in Substantia Nigra Effects of Apomorphine

Because the substantia nigra pars reticulata cells show variable changes in firing rate in response to dopamine receptor stimulation in control animals, less has been done to explore synergistic interactions between D_1 and D_2 receptor subtypes in this region. This phenomenon has been easier to demonstrate in this brain area in 6-OHDA-lesioned animals, as described below. Nevertheless, two observations suggest that a synergistic interaction between processes mediated by D_1 and D_2 receptors does play a critical role in regulating the activity of cells in the substantia nigra in unlesioned animals. First, the effects induced by systemically administered apomorphine on reticulata neuronal activity can be reversed by administration of a D_1 antagonist[61] (Figure 5) as well as a D_2 antagonist, regardless of whether apomorphine stimulates or inhibits the activity of the cell. Second, D_1 and D_2 agonists induce a more varied distribution of responses in pars reticulata cell activity when administered together than when administered individually.[70] These results suggest that processes mediated by the D_1 and D_2 dopamine receptor subtypes interact to elicit potentiated dopamine agonist-induced changes in the activity of cells in the substantia nigra pars reticulata, as they do to induce changes in cellular activity in the globus pallidus. The fact that synergistic D_1/D_2 interactions have an effect on neuronal activity in both of these basal ganglia output nuclei supports the idea that the site of the interaction is in the striatum and fundamental to dopamine's regulation of striatal output.

Effects of Dopamine Agonists on Substantia Nigra Pars Reticulata Activity in 6-OHDA-Lesioned Rats

In animals with unilateral 6-OHDA-induced lesion of the nigrostriatal dopamine cells, the responses of substantia nigra pars reticulata neurons to apomorphine administration are qualitatively different from those observed in the normal rat.[68,69] In these lesioned animals, apomorphine consistently inhibits substantia nigra pars reticulata neuronal activity (Figure 4, Table 1). In addition, in these animals, quinpirole and especially SKF 38393, administered separately, can both induce significant inhibitions of single unit activity.[69] Moreover, smaller doses of the two selective agonists, which induce no significant effect when given alone, cause a marked inhibition of substantia nigra pars reticulata cell activity when given together.[69–71] Thus, D_1 and D_2 receptor subtypes clearly interact in this preparation, as well as in control animals, to induce decreases in the activity of substantia nigra pars reticulata cells.

These results suggest that the trend observed in the globus pallidus, toward seeing more decreases in neuronal activity after D_1/D_2 receptor stimulation in 6-OHDA-lesioned rats as compared to control, is even more evident in the substantia nigra pars reticulata, where the net effect of D_1 agonists switches from being modestly excitatory in normal rats to being consistently inhibitory in the lesioned rats. One explanation for these results is that in the 6-OHDA-treated animals, D_1 agonists, and agents such as apomorphine, which stimulate both D_1 and D_2 receptors, produce an increase in the activity of striatonigral neurons, thereby increasing inhibitory input to the substantia nigra. Although contrary to the general view that dopamine is inhibitory in the striatum,[58] this idea is supported by changes in striatal levels of mRNA transcripts of striatonigral peptide neurotransmitters and by the increased 2-

deoxyglucose accumulation observed in the substantia nigra of lesioned rats after D_1 agonists, effects which suggest that D_1 agonists induce increases in the firing rates of the striatonigral cells.[72] *In vivo* iontophoretic studies of D_1 agonist effects in the striatum of 6-OHDA-lesioned rats further support this possibility.[24]

These results raise the following question: if dopamine receptor stimulation is exerting a more profound excitatory effect in the striatum of animals with 6-OHDA lesions, as compared to controls, is this a "supersensitive" response, i.e., an exaggeration of the normal, or a more qualitative change in the way dopamine agonists affect striatal cells? The "supersensitive" response view would imply that dopamine stimulates striatonigral neurons in both the normal and lesioned animals, although more potently in the lesioned animals, and that dopamine cell loss induces a tonic decrease in the activity of the striatonigral cells. This perspective is supported by the fact that there is a marked up-regulation of GABA receptor sensitivity in the substantia nigra pars reticulata after 6-OHDA cell lesion.[31,73] On the other hand, dopamine agonists are more likely to excite rather than inhibit substantia nigra pars reticulata cell activity in the normal animal, at least under the conditions of local anesthesia and immobilization applied during the neurophysiological recording experiment.

The second view, i.e., that dopamine denervation induces a qualitative change in the way dopamine affects striatal cell activity, implies that the net effect of dopamine receptor stimulation is generally excitatory with respect to striatonigral output in the lesioned rats but generally inhibitory in the normal animals. This possibility is supported by *in vivo* iontophoretic studies of D_1 agonist effects in the striatum of 6-OHDA-lesioned rats.[24] In addition, recent intracellular recording studies carried out in vitro in striatal slices from control and 6-OHDA-lesioned rats indicate that the effect of the D_1 agonist SKF 38393 on striatal cell excitability is predominantly inhibitory in striatal tissue from control rats but more frequently excitatory in striatal tissue from dopamine denervated animals.[66] Finally, the effects of D_1 agonists on reserpine-treated animals, described below, indicate that the system is capable of mediating a number of different responses to dopamine receptor stimulation and support the idea that more is involved in these phenomena than straightforward changes in receptor number or affinity.

Effects of D_1 Agonists on Substantia Nigra Pars Reticulata Activity in Reserpine-Treated Rats

A second strategy for studying the consequences of depleting dopamine, in addition to 6-OHDA-induced dopamine cell lesions, is the use of animals treated subchronically with reserpine. We have recently compared the responses of substantia nigra pars reticulata neurons to D_1 agonist administration in these two animals models. The effects observed in the reserpine-treated rats were surprisingly different from those observed in 6-OHDA-lesioned rats. In rats treated with 1 mg/kg/day of reserpine for 6 days,[74,75] systemic administration of SKF 38393 brought about an increase in the firing rates of substantia nigra pars reticulata neurons, which was substantially greater than that seen in controls. After reserpine treatment, 10 mg/kg of SKF 38393 induced an average increase in firing rates of approximately 90% over baseline compared with 18% in controls.[75] This effect was persistent: SKF 38393 induced a similar change in rats treated with reserpine for 6 days and then allowed a 5-day washout period. In comparison, as described above, the same dose of SKF 38393 inhibited substantia nigra pars reticulata firing rates by an average of 75% below baseline in 6-OHDA-lesioned rats previously tested with apomorphine for effective turning.[75] Time course differences do not account for these opposite effects: 7 days after 6-OHDA lesion, SKF 38393 did not induce effects similar to those seen after reserpine. These results demonstrate that monoamine depletion and dopamine cell degeneration both affect D_1 neuronal transmission, but in opposite ways. In addition, they raise questions about which model is more relevant to Parkinson's disease and also point to considerable plasticity in D_1 mechanisms regulating striatal output.

Conclusion

Extracellular single unit recording studies have shown that neuronal activity in basal ganglia output nuclei is affected by dopamine receptor stimulation. While stimulation of either D_1 or D_2 receptors alone produces relatively modest changes in firing rates in the globus pallidus and the substantia nigra pars reticulata in normal rats, stimulation of both D_1 and D_2 receptors results in substantial alterations in neuronal transmission in these areas. Some of these responses to dopamine agonist administration are consistent with the hypothesis that dopamine receptor stimulation exerts an inhibitory effect on the activity of inhibitory striatal output cells; however, other responses cannot be explained by such a mechanism, and additional mechanisms are clearly involved. A further interesting finding, potentially relevant to Parkinson's disease, is the fact that a dramatic change in substantia nigra and globus pallidus single unit response to dopamine receptor stimulation occurs in animals with 6-OHDA-induced lesions of the nigrostriatal dopamine pathway, while a very different change occurs in animals depleted of dopamine via reserpine treatment. These divergent responses to dopamine receptor stimulation in rats depleted of dopamine by two different strategies indicates that the mechanisms triggered by dopamine receptor stimulation are quite plastic and are capable of mediating a range of responses. Hopefully, attempts to delineate the mechanisms underlying these neurophysiological phenomena will provide insight into how dopamine modulates information processing in the basal ganglia and lead to improved strategies for compensating for dopamine cell loss in Parkinson's disease.

References

1. Goldman-Rakic PS, Selemon LD. 1990. New frontiers in basal ganglia research. TINS 13:241–244.
2. Alexander GE, Crutcher MD. 1990. Functional architecture of basal ganglia circuits: Neural substrates of parallel processing. TINS 13:266–271.
3. Selemon LD, Goldman-Rakic PS. 1985. Longitudinal topography and interdigitation of corticostriatal projections in the rhesus monkey. J Neurosci 5:776–794.
4. Selemon LD, Goldman-Rakic PS. 1990. Topographic intermingling of striatonigral and striatopallidal neurons in the rhesus monkey. J Comp Neurol 297:359–376.
5. Smith AD, Bolam JP. 1990. The neural network of the basal ganglia as revealed by the study of synaptic connections of identified neurones. TINS 13:259–265.
6. Dube L, Smith AD, Bolam JP. 1988. Identification of synaptic terminals of thalamic or cortical origin in contact with distinct medium-size spiny neurons in the rat neostriatum. J Comp Neurol 267:455–471.
7. Alexander GE, Crutcher MD, DeLong MR. 1990. Basal ganglia-thalamocortical circuits: Parallel substrates for motor, oculomotor,

"prefrontal" and "limbic" functions. *In* Progress in Brain Research, Vol. 85. HBM Uylings, GG Van Eden, et al., eds. Elsevier Science Publishers, pp. 119–146.

8. Chevalier G, Deniau JM. 1990. Disinhibition as a basic process in the expression of striatal functions. TINS 13:277–280.

9. Mink JW, Thach WT. 1991. Basal ganglia motor control. I. Nonexclusive relation of pallidal discharge to five movement modes. J Neurophysiol 65:273–300.

10. Mink JW, Thach WT. 1991. Basal ganglia motor control. II. Late pallidal timing relative to movement onset and inconsistent pallidal coding of movement parameters. J Neurophysiol 65:301–329.

11. Mink JW, Thach WT. 1991. Basal ganglia motor control. III. Pallidal ablation: Normal reaction time, muscle cocontraction, and slow movement. J Neurophysiol 65:330–351.

12. Bloom FE, Costa E, Salmoiraghi GC. 1965. Anesthesia and the responsiveness of individual neurons of the caudate nucleus of the cat to acetylcholine, norepinephrine and dopamine administered by microelectrophoresis. J Pharmacol Exp Ther 150:244–252.

13. Connor JD. 1970. Caudate nucleus neurones: Correlation of the effects of substantia nigra stimulation with iontophoretic dopamine. J Physiol 208:691–703.

14. Bunney BS, Aghajanian GK. 1973. Electrophysiological effects of amphetamine on dopaminergic neurons. *In* Frontiers in Catecholamine Research. E. Usdin, S. Snyder, (eds). Pergamon Press, New York, pp. 957–962.

15. Ben-Ari Y, Kelly JS. 1974. Iontophoretic and intravenous effects of the neuroleptic, alpha-flupenthixol, on dopamine evoked inhibition. J Physiol 242:66P.

16. Siggins GR. 1978. Electrophysiological role of dopamine in striatum: Excitatory or inhibitory? *In* Psychopharmacology: A Generation of Progress. MA Lipton, A DiMascio, KF Killam (eds). Raven Press, New York, pp 143–157.

17. Skirboll LR, Grace AA, Bunney BS. 1979. Dopamine auto- and postsynaptic receptors: Electrophysiological evidence for differential sensitivity to dopamine agonists. Science 206:80–82.

18. Hu XT, Wang RY. 1988. Comparison of effects of D_1 and D_2 dopamine receptor agonists on neurons in the rat caudate putamen: An electrophysiological study. J Neurosci 8:4340–4348.

19. Akaoka H, Saunier F, Chouvet G. 1987. Neuronal responses to dopamine in rat striatum: Comparison between dopamine iontophoretic application and nigro-striatal pathway stimulation. Biogen Amines 4:407–412.

20. Alloway KD, Rebec GV. 1984. Apomorphine-induced inhibition of neostriatal activity is enhanced by lesions induced by 6-hydroxydopamine but not by long-term administration of amphetamine. Neuropharmacology 23:1033–1039.

21. Kelland MD, Boldry RC, Huang K-X, Chase TN, Walters JR. 1991. Dizocilpine (MK-801), but not NBQX, alters dopamine (DA)-mediated

changes in striatopallidal neuronal activity and behavior. Soc Neurosci Abstr 17:1349.

22. Kitai ST, Sugimori M, Kocsis JD. 1976. Excitatory nature of dopamine in the nigro-caudate pathway. Exp Brain Res 24:351–363.

23. Kitai ST. 1981. Electrophysiology of the corpus striatum and brain stem integrating system. *In:* VB Brooks, (ed). Handbook of Physiology, Vol. 2, The Nervous System.) Bethesda, American Physiological Society, pp 997–1015.

24. Weick BG, Walters JR. 1988. The D_1 selective agonist SKF 38393 can activate striatal neurons in 6-hydroxydopamine lesioned rats. Soc Neurosci Abstr 14:1077.

25. Akaike A, Ohno Y, Sasa M, Takaori S. 1987. Excitatory and inhibitory effects of dopamine on neuronal activity of the caudate nucleus neurons in vitro. Brain Res 418:262–272.

26. Graybiel AM. 1990. Neurotransmitters and neuromodulators in the basal ganglia. TINS 13:244–254.

27, Lanthorn TH, O'Donohue TL, Shults CW, Chase TN, Walters JR. 1984. The effects of ionophoretically applied substance K (SK) on single unit activity in the rat substantia nigra (SN). Soc Neurosci Abstr 10:1121.

28. Danks JA, Rothman RB, Cascieri MA, Chicchi GG, Liang T, Herkenham M. 1986. A comparative autoradiographic study of the distributions of substance P and eledoisin binding sites in rat brain. Brain Res 385:273–281.

29. Collingridge GL, Davies J. 1981. The influence of striatal stimulation and putative neurotransmitters on identified neurons in the rat substantia nigra. Brain Res 212:345–359.

30. Waszczak BL, Walters JR. 1986. Endogeneous dopamine can modulate inhibition of substantia nigra pars reticulata neurons elicited by GABA iontophoresis or striatal stimulation. J Neurosci 6:120–126.

31. Pan HS, Penney JB, Young AB. 1985. γ-Aminobutyric acid and benzodiazepine receptor changes induced by unilateral 6-hydroxydopamine lesions of the medial forebrain bundle. J Neurochem 45:1396–1404.

32. Gerfen CR, Engber TM, Mahan LC, Susel Z, Chase TN, Monsma FJ. Jr, Sibley DR. 1990. D_1 and D_2 dopamine receptor-regulated gene expression of striatonigral and striatopallidal neurons. Science 250:1429–1432.

33. Boyson SJ, McGonigle P, Molinoff PB. 1986. Quantitative autoradiographic localization of the D_1 and D_2 subtypes of dopamine receptors in rat brain. J Neurosci 6:3177–3188.

34. Martres M-P, Bouthenet M-L, Sales N, Sokoloff P, Schwartz J-C. 1985. Widespread distribution of brain dopamine receptors evidenced with [^{125}I]iodosulpride, a highly selective ligand. Science 228:752–755.

35. Richfield EK, Debowey DL, Penney JB, Young AB. 1986. Basal ganglia and cerebral cortical distribution of dopamine D_1 and D_2 receptors in neonatal and adult cat brain. Neurosci Lett 73:203–208.

36. Waszczak BL, Walters JR. 1983. Dopamine modulation of the effects of

the γ-amino butyric acid on substantia nigra pars reticulata neurons. Science 220:218–221.

37. Bergstrom DA, Walters JR. 1984. Dopamine attenuates the effects of GABA on single unit activity in the globus pallidus. Brain Res 310:23–33.

38. Weick BG, Walters JR. 1987. Do D_1/D_2 receptor interactions occur directly in the substantia nigra pars reticulata? Soc Neurosci Abstr 13:489.

39. Waszczak BL. 1990. Differential effects of D_1 and D_2 dopamine receptor agonists on substantia nigra pars reticulata neurons. Brain Res 513:125–135.

40. Sokoloff P, Giros B, Martres M-P, Bouthenet M-L, Schwartz J-C. 1990. Molecular cloning and characterization of a novel dopamine receptor (D_3) as a target for neuroleptics. Nature 347:146–151.

41. Van Tol HHM, Bunzow JR, Guan H-C, Sunahara RK, Seeman P, Niznik HB, Civelli O. 1991. Cloning of the gene for a human dopamine D_4 receptor with high affinity for the antipsychotic clozapine. Nature 350:610–614.

42. Sunahara RK, Guan H-C, O'Dowd BF, Seeman P, Lauier LG, Ng G, George SR, Torchia J, Van Tol HHM, Niznik HB. 1991. Cloning of the gene for a human dopamine D_5 receptor with higher affinity for dopamine than D_1. Nature 350:614–619.

43. Kitai ST, Kita H. 1987. Anatomy and physiology of the subthalamic nucleus: A driving force of the basal ganglia. *In* The Basal Ganglia-2. Structure and Function—Current Concepts. MB Carpenter, A Jayaraman, (eds). Plenum, New York, pp 357–373.

44. Canteras NS, Shammah-Lagnado SJ, Silva BA, Ricardo JA. 1990. Afferent connections of the subthalamic nucleus: A combined retrograde and anterograde horseradish peroxidase study in the rat. Brain Res 513:43–59.

45. Saper CB, Loewy AD. 1982. Projections of the pedunculopontine tegmental nucleus in the rat: Evidence for additional extrapyramidal circuitry. Brain Res 252:367–372.

46. Moriizumi T, Nakamura Y, Tokuno H, Kitao Y, Kudo M. 1988. Topographic projections from the basal ganglia to the nucleus tegmenti pedunculopontinus pars compacta of the cat with special reference to pallidal projections. Exp Brain Res 71:298–306.

47. Bergstrom DA, Walters JR. 1981. Neuronal responses of the globus pallidus to systemic administration of *d*-amphetamine: Investigation of the involvement of dopamine, norepinephrine and serotonin. J Neurosci 1:292–299.

48. Bergstrom DA, Bromley SD, Walters JR. 1982. Apomorphine increases the activity of rat globus pallidus neurons. Brain Res 238:266–271.

49. Bergstrom DA, Bromley SD, Walters JR. 1982. Time schedule of apomorphine administration determines the degree of globus pallidus excitation. Eur J Pharmacol 78:245–248.

50. Bergstrom DA, Bromley SD, Walters JR. 1984. Dopamine agonists

increase pallidal unit activity: Attenuation by agonist pretreatment and anesthesia. Eur J Pharmacol 100:3–12.

51. Carlson JH, Bergstrom DA, Walters JR. 1987. Stimulation of both D_1 and D_2 dopamine receptors appears necessary for full expression of postsynaptic effects of dopamine agonists: A neurophysiological study. Brain Res 400:205–218.

52. DeLong MR. 1990. Primate models of movement disorders of basal ganglia origin. TINS 13:281–285.

53. Pan HS, Engber TM, Chase TN, Walters JR. 1990. The effects of striatal lesion on turning behavior and globus pallidus single unit response to dopamine administration. Life Sci 46:73–80.

54. Walters JR, Bergstrom DA, Carlson JH, Chase TN, Braun AR. 1987. D_1 dopamine receptor activation required for postsynaptic expression of D_2 agonist effects. Science 236:719–722.

55. Clark D, White FJ. 1987. Review: D_1 dopamine receptor—the search for a function: A critical evaluation of the D_1/D_2 dopamine receptor classification and its functional implications. Synapse 1:347–388.

56. Paul ML, Graybiel AM, Robertson HA. 1990. Synergistic activation of the immediate-early gene *c-fos* in striosomes by D_1 and D_2-selective dopamine agonists. Soc Neurosci Abstr 16:954.

57. Bertorello AM, Hopfield JF, Aperia A, Greengard P. 1990. Inhibition by dopamine of (Na^+, K^+)ATPase activity in neurostriatal neurons through D_1 and D_2 dopamine receptor synergism. Nature 347:386.

58. Hu X-T, Wachtel SR, Galloway MP, White FJ. 1990. Lesions of the nigrostriatal dopamine projection increase the inhibitory effects of D_1 and D_2 dopamine agonists on caudate-putamen neurons and relieve D_2 receptors from the necessity of D_1 receptor stimulation. J Neurosci 10:2318–2329.

59. White FJ. 1987. D_1 dopamine receptor stimulation enables the inhibition of nucleus accumbens neurons by a D_2 receptor agonist. Eur J Pharmacol 135:101–105.

60. Shen R, Freeman AS, Asdourian D, Chiodo LA. 1989. The role of D_1 and D_2 dopamine receptors in regulating the electrophysiological activity of caudate neurons in the rat. Soc Neurosci Abstr 15:1000.

61. Carlson JH, Bergstrom DA, Walters JR. 1986. Neurophysiological evidence that D_1 dopamine receptor blockade attenuates postsynaptic but not autoreceptor-mediated effects of dopamine agonists. Eur J Pharmacol 23:237–251.

62. Pan HS, Walters JR. 1988. Unilateral lesion of the nigrostriatal pathway decreases the firing rate and alters the firing pattern of globus pallidus neurons in the rat. Synapse 2:650–656.

63. Gonon FG. 1988. Nonlinear relationship between impulse flow and dopamine released by rat midbrain dopaminergic neurons as studied by in vivo electrochemistry. Neuroscience 24:19–28.

64. Pan HS, Walters JR. 1988. Lesion of the nigrostriatal dopamine pathway induces functional down regulation of delta-opiate and GABA receptors in the globus pallidus. Soc Neurosci Abstr 14:1157.

65. Carlson JH, Bergstrom DA, Demo SD, Walters JR. 1990. Nigrostriatal

lesion alters neurophysiological responses to selective and nonselective D_1 and D_2 dopamine agonists in globus pallidus. Synapse 5:83–93.

66. Thompson LA, Walters JR, Twery MJ. 1991. SKF-38393 increases the excitability of striatal neurons in vitro following chronic dopaminergic denervation. Soc Neurosci Abstr 17:850.

67. Waszczak BL, Lee EK, Ferraro T, Hare TA, Walters JR. 1984. Single unit responses of substantia nigra pars reticulata neurons to apomorphine: Effects of anesthesia and striatal lesions. Brain Res 306:307–318.

68. Waszczak BL, Lee EK, Tamminga CA, Walters JR. 1984. Effect of dopamine system activation on substantia nigra pars reticulata output neurons: Variable single-unit responses in normal rats and inhibition in 6-hydroxydopamine-lesioned rats. J Neurosci 4:2369–2375.

69. Weick BG, Walters JR. 1987. Effects of D_1 and D_2 dopamine receptor stimulation on the activity of substantia nigra pars reticulata neurons in 6-hydroxydopamine lesioned rats: D_1/D_2 coactivation induces potentiated responses. Brain Res 405:234–246.

70. Walters JR, Bergstrom DA, Carlson JH, Weick BG, Pan HS. 1987. Stimulation of D_1 and D_2 dopamine receptors: Synergistic effects on single unit activity in basal ganglia output nuclei. *In* Neurophysiology of Dopaminergic Systems: Current Status and Clinical Perspectives. LA Chiodo, AS Freeman (eds). Lakeshore Publ. Co., Detroit, MI, pp 285–316.

71. Weick BG, Walters JR. 1987. D_1 dopamine receptor stimulation potentiates neurophysiological effects of bromocriptine in rats with lesions of the nigrostriatal dopamine pathway. Neuropharmacology 26:641–644.

72. Trugman JM, Wooten GF. 1987. The effects of L-Dopa on regional cerebral glucose utilization in rats with unilateral lesions of the substantia nigra. Brain Res 379:264–274.

73. Weick BG, Engber TM, Susel Z, Chase TN, Walters JR. 1990. Responses of substantia nigra pars reticulata neurons to GABA and SKF 38393 in 6-hydroxydopamine lesioned rats are differentially affected by continuous and intermittent levodopa administration. Brain Res 523:16–22.

74. Huang K-X, Walters JR. 1992. D_1 stimulation inhibits dopamine cell activity following reserpine pretreatment but not chronic SCH-23390: An effect blocked by NMDA antagonists. J Pharmacol Exp Ther 260:409–416.

75. Huang K-X, Walters JR. 1991. D_1 agonist has opposite effects on neuronal transmission in the basal ganglia of two animal models of Parkinson's disease: Effects blocked by NMDA antagonist. Soc Neurosci Abstr 17:1349.

Chapter 16

Investigations of Adaptive Changes Associated with Lesioning Dopaminergic Neurons with 6-Hydroxydopamine

*George R. Breese, Hugh E. Criswell,
Gary E. Duncan, Kevin B. Johnson,
Peter E. Simson, Robert A. Mueller,
Karl F. Jensen, and James O'Callaghan*

In the early 1960s, it was established that lesioning of the dopaminergic neurons in the substantia nigra contributed to Parkinson's disease.[1,2] The discovery that MPTP, a recreational drug toxic to dopaminergic neurons, can produce parkinsonism symptoms, has fortified this conclusion.[3–5] The observation that a phenylethylamine analog, 6-hydroxydopamine (6-OHDA), destroys catecholamine-containing neurons in the periphery,[6] led to studies to determine whether this drug would have a similar destructive action on central catecholaminergic neurons. From these latter studies, two ap-

Unpublished data and recent literature were supported by U.S. Public Health Service grants HD-03110, HD-23042, NS-21345, and MH-33127.
From Hefti F, and Weiner WJ, (eds.) *Progress in Parkinson's Disease Research—2.* Mount Kisco NY, Futura Publishing Co., Inc., © 1992.

proaches emerged destroying central dopaminergic neurons in brain with this neurotoxin. One approach involved microinjection of 6-OHDA into the region containing dopaminergic cell bodies,[7] while the other involved the administration of 6-OHDA into the ventricular system.[8,9] In order to provide a predictable animal model of parkinsonism, studies also were undertaken to lesion dopaminergic neurons with 6-OHDA in rhesus monkeys.[10] After determining that intraventricular administration of 6-OHDA in this primate was unacceptable because of generalized neurotoxicity, Kraemer et al.[10] devised a means to microinject 6-OHDA into the substantia nigra to destroy dopaminergic neurons. Careful application of this treatment led to symptoms in monkeys resembling those in Parkinson's patients,[10] with minor nonspecific neurological impairment.

Since the development of these procedures to reduce dopamine-containing neurons in brain with 6-OHDA, there has been considerable effort to understand the adaptive changes that accompany destruction of dopaminergic neurons. Progress made in this area of dopaminergic mechanisms will be reviewed.

Behavioral Recovery from 6-OHDA Lesions

Treatment of rats with 6-OHDA to destroy catecholaminergic neurons in brain was demonstrated to disrupt food and water intake,[11] as well as cause deficits in performance of tasks such as self-stimulation and avoidance.[12,13] However, some deficits induced by 6-OHDA treatment were found to recover over time.[10–13] Two possible explanations were proposed to account for this adaptation and recovery of function: (1) adaptive change within the remaining parts of the dopaminergic system or (2) an adaptation of other neural systems that could compensate for the loss of dopamine-containing neurons. To explore the potential involvement of adaptation within dopaminergic neurons, 6-OHDA-lesioned rats were pretreated with a dose of α-methyltyrosine that did not affect behavioral responses in control animals, but was sufficient to interfere with the synthesis of catecholamines. This treatment was found to reinstate many deficits that were observed after acute administration of the 6-OHDA neurotoxin but which became less visible with time.[10–13] These results clearly indicated that a change in the function of remaining dopaminergic neurons or their modulating or effector output systems was responsible for the neurological adaptation that followed acute lesions to dopaminergic neurons.

Changes in Receptor Function after Dopaminergic Lesions

There is considerable literature that indicates that peripheral denervation leads to postsynaptic supersensitivity.[14] Since our laboratory demonstrated that destruction of central noradrenergic neurons increased the central response to a noradrenergic agonist,[15] we next evaluated whether behavioral supersensitivity would be observed after dopaminergic agonist administration to lesioned rats. This was accomplished by administering L-dopa to 6-OHDA-lesioned rats.[16] This treatment resulted in a marked increase in locomotor activity or an increase in turning after unilateral lesions of the nigrostriatal dopaminergic pathway in rats.[16,17] This evidence of a remarkable increase in central catecholamine receptor sensitivity following 6-OHDA treatment led to further attempts to understand the basis of this adaptive change in behavioral responsiveness.

One immediate question raised about the supersensitive L-dopa response in dopaminergic-lesioned rats concerned the mechanism by which decarboxylation of L-dopa to dopamine occurs once dopamine-containing neurons are destroyed. Data from this investigation indicated that although L-dopa was decarboxylated in lesioned rats, it was decarboxylated less efficiently than in unlesioned controls.[18] Additionally, destruction of serotoninergic neurons was found to diminish the decarboxylation of L-dopa further in lesioned rats, indicating that serontonin-containing neurons were an additional site, but not the only site, at which the aromatic amino acid decarboxylase transforms dopa to dopamine in the 6-OHDA-lesioned rat.[18] Since serotonin-containing neurons are reported to be reduced in Parkinson's disease,[19] one potential reason for the subsequent loss of the effectiveness of L-dopa in the treatment of parkinsonism could be the loss of monamine-containing neurons other than those containing dopamine.[18]

Responses to Dopamine Agonists in 6-OHDA-Lesioned Rats

Subsequent studies in the 6-OHDA-lesioned rats demonstrated that the action of a number of drugs purported to act on dopaminergic receptors are enhanced following the lesion. These drugs included apomorphine, piribedil, and bromocriptine.[20] In contrast to this result, pretreatment with reserpine and α-methyltyrosine was found to antagonize the action of piribedil, suggesting that its action was dependent upon endogenous catecholamines.[20] Paradoxically, the action of apomorphine was only slightly affected by the reserpine/α-methyltyrosine treatment (unpublished data). These paradoxical findings were not understood until the later discovery that more than one dopamine receptor type is present in brain.[21]

Kebabian et al.[21] proposed the existence of two major receptor systems for dopamine in brain. In this scheme, the D_1 dopamine receptor was associated with activation of adenylate cyclase and the D_2-dopamine receptor was associated with inhibition of adenylate cyclase.[21] The development of an antagonist that selectively inhibited the action of dopamine to stimulate adenylate cyclase provided an important new tool for investigating the function of the receptor subtypes.[21] This compound is SCH-23390. Subsequently, an agonist acting specifically on D_2-dopamine receptors, quinpirole,[24] and an agonist acting on D_1-dopamine receptors, SKF-38393,[29] were discovered. Moreover, the classical neuroleptic drugs were found to act primarily on D_2-dopamine receptors,[25] but with only moderate selectivity.

One difficulty with the purported D_1-dopamine antagonist, SCH-23390, was that it also antagonized the behavioral effects of dopamine agonists thought to act on D_2-dopamine receptors in normal rats.[21] Breese and Mueller[26] confirmed this observation, but demonstrated that this effect of SCH-23390 on a D_2-dopamine-induced response was not observed in rats lesioned with 6-OHDA. This basic observation was also reported by Arnt.[27] As a result of these findings, it was proposed that D_1-dopamine receptors control the function of D_2-dopamine receptors.[26] This "coupling" of D_1- and D_2-dopamine receptors provided an explanation for the action of SCH-23390 to antagonize D_2-dopamine agonists in unlesioned animals and for the reserpine/α-methyltyrosine combination to block the action of agonists for this receptor subtype.[26] Subsequently, Walters et al.[28] demonstrated a facilitatory interaction between D_1-and D_2-dopamine agonists. Further, Jackson et al.[29] demonstrated that inclusion of a D_1-dopamine agonist with a D_2-dopamine agonist in rats given the reserpine and α-methyltyrosine treatment restored the response of the D_2-dopamine agonist. All these data suggested coupling of the function of postsynaptic D_1- and D_2-dopamine receptors.[26]

In unlesioned rats, administration of the D_1-dopamine agonist, SKF 38393 did not produce a major behavioral response,[23] although sniffing was reported to be increased.[30] In contrast, when SKF 38393 was administered to neonatally 6-OHDA-lesioned rats after prior exposure of the lesioned rats to D_1-dopamine receptor activation, several behaviors linked to dopaminergic action were observed.[31] This result provided clear evidence that D_1-dopamine receptors had a potent function in the CNS.[31]

Demonstration of D_1-Dopamine Receptor Priming in Rats Lesioned as Neonates

In contrast to the potent action of SKF 38393 in the neonatally lesioned rats that had been treated previously with other dopamine agonists, the D_1-dopamine agonist SKF 38393 gave little response when administered for the first time to naive neonatally 6-OHDA-lesioned animals.[32] In fact, there was little behavioral difference from that observed after saline injection. Since marked locomotor responses were observed after a D_1-dopamine agonist in rats that had received other dopamine agonists before the first SKF 38393 injection, a basis of the lack of response in the drug-naive lesioned rats were sought.[32] It was observed that administering SKF 38393 repetitively at 1-week intervals progressively increased activity with a maximal response observed with dose 4.[32] This phenomenon resulting from the repeated D_1-dopamine agonist exposure to neonatally 6-OHDA-lesioned rats is referred to as "priming" of D_1-dopamine receptor sensitivity.[32]

Criswell et al.[33,34] have recently extended work on this phenomenon in rats lesioned as neonates with 6-OHDA. Importantly, this work demonstrated that priming of D_1-dopamine sensitivity could not be elicited in rats lesioned with 6-OHDA as adults or in unlesioned controls. In the neonatally lesioned rats, priming was relatively permanent, lasting at least 6 months, even if injections were halted. Further, it was found that priming could not be related to conditioning to the environment where the injection of the agonist occurred.[33] Repeated administration of the D_2-dopamine agonist did not cause an increase in locomotor activity, but did increase the effectiveness of the D_1-dopamine agonist.[32,33] However, in contrast to this latter finding, simultaneous administration of D_2-dopamine antagonist with each dose of the D_1-dopamine agonist had no influence on the action of SKF 38393 to prime the D_1-dopamine receptor, indicating that a permissive effect of the D_2-dopamine receptor is not a prerequisite for priming of D_1-dopamine receptors.[33] Further, it was observed that microinjection of the D_1-agonist into the nucleus accumbens caused a progressive increase in locomotor activity with each microinjection,[33] suggesting that priming is due to a local action of the D_1-agonist in at least one terminal field. These data provide evidence that priming of D_1-dopamine receptors is a form of permanent neural adaptation.[34] The role this phenomenon may play in the normal physiology or in the consequence of neuropathology of dopaminergic function has yet to be determined.

Several investigations have demonstrated that prior treatment with an NMDA antagonist prevents long-term potentiation (LTP), a model system of neuronal learning.[35,36] Since priming might be considered a form of neuronal adaptation or learning, it was reasoned that pretreatment with an NMDA antagonist prior to the administration of the D_1-dopamine agonist might prevent priming of D_1-dopamine receptor sensitivity. In accord with this supposition, Criswell et al.[34] found that treatment with MK 801, an NMDA antagonist, prevented priming. This finding gives credence to the view that priming of D_1-dopamine receptor sensitivity is a form of neuronal learning. Another implication of this finding is that priming requires activation of a neural circuit that includes glutamate transmission. Additional work will be necessary to resolve whether this latter observation is at odds with our earlier microinjection studies in the nucleus accumbens.[33] Conceivably, the glutamatergic synapses involved are in the accumbens or activated elsewhere as a result of D_1-receptor activation in that structure.

D_1-Dopamine Receptor Desensitization

Whereas repeated administration of the D_1-dopamine receptor agonist SKF 38393 resulted in sensitization of behavioral responses, a new D_1-dopamine agonist from Abbott laboratories (A-68930) appears to differ from SKF 38393 on this measure. This latter compound inhibits the activity response to SKF 38393 when administered 1 day before SKF 38393 treatment.[37] As a consequence of this report, we have examined the action of this agonist on responses to SKF 38393 in neonatally lesioned rats. These preliminary data in a group of rats used for general screening have confirmed this early report, showing that the response to SKF 38393 is reduced at 1 and 3 days and does not recover fully until 14 days after a single exposure to the Abbott D_1-agonist (unpublished data). This compound could provide yet another new tool by which D_1-dopamine receptor function can be evaluated.

D_1- and D_2-Dopamine Receptor Responses in Adult and Neonatally Lesioned Rats

As already described, administration of SKF 38393, a D_1-dopamine receptor agonist, produces a marked behavioral response in rats lesioned as neonates. In contrast, it was determined that rats lesioned as adults with 6-OHDA do not usually exhibit such a marked supersensitivity to the D_1-dopamine receptor agonist.[32] Responses in this latter group can vary from little response to activity equivalent to that in neonatally lesioned rats. Conversely, on average, neonatally lesioned rats show less sensitivity to the D_2-dopamine receptor agonist quinpirole, when compared to responses of adult-lesioned rats.[32] We continue to search for the biological basis of the differences between rats lesioned as neonates and those lesioned as adults.

When L-dopa is administered to rats lesioned as neonates, a significant portion of these rats will exhibit self-injurious behavior.[38] This behavioral response to L-dopa is rarely observed in rats lesioned as adults.[38] While this behavioral response has been attributed to effects on D_1-dopamine receptors in the neonatally lesioned rat, it has been demonstrated that activation of D_2-dopamine receptors can play a facilitatory role is self-injurious behavior.[38] D_2-dopamine receptor activation alone, however, does not produce self-injurious behavior in neonates or adult-lesioned rats.[38]

The behavioral differences between neonatal and adult lesioned rats led to our hypothesis that neonatally lesioned rats provide an animal model of the neurological deficit in Lesch-Nyhan disease, while the adult-lesioned rat is a model of parkinsonism.[38] The results thus far obtained in these animal models could be important in determining strategies for the treatment of these disease states. For example, data in the adult-lesioned rats suggest that SKF 38393 would not be effective in parkinsonism, whereas a D_2-dopamine receptor agonist should be efficacious. Clinical reports seem to support such a prediction.[39] However, given the reported coupling between D_1- and D_2-dopamine receptors,[26,28,31,32] it will be of considerable interest to know whether combining the two agonist treatments could have therapeutic benefits not seen with either agonist alone. It is also conceivable that combining L-dopa with drugs affecting D_1-dopamine function may influence the therapeutic effectiveness and unwanted side effects that can accompany L-dopa therapy. Data obtained in the neonatally lesioned rats suggest that D_1-dopamine antagonists may provide a therapeutic advantage in the treatment of aggressive behavior in the mentally retarded.[38,40,41]

Relationship of Receptor Binding to Behavioral Supersensitivity in Lesioned Rats

Given the marked behavioral supersensitivity to dopamine agonists in the 6-OHDA-lesioned rats, we explored whether binding of ligands to the dopamine receptors would reflect this behavioral change. Using binding to caudate and nucleus accumbens membranes from control and lesioned rats, it was apparent that binding of ligands for D_1 and D_2-dopamine receptors was not altered.[42] This was subsequently confirmed in a separate study.[43] Because we have observed electrophysiological differences in the sensitivity to D_1- and D_2-dopamine agonists in the dorsal–lateral versus the medial portions of the striatum,[44] an autoradiographic evaluation of receptor binding and measurement of D_1-dopamine mRNA in dopamine-rich brain sites has been undertaken. Like the homogenate binding studies, it appears that there is no increase in the number of D_1-dopamine receptors compared to control in any subregion of the caudate in lesioned rats.[45]

We have evaluated the action of a D_1-dopamine agonist on adenylate cyclase activity in striatal homogenates from control and neonatally lesioned rats. A small significant increase in adenylate cyclase activity with SKF 38393 was observed in the lesioned rats, but this response has been variable (unpublished data). Several years ago, Breese et al.[46] found no increase in striatal cAMP in vivo after L-dopa administration in rats lesioned as adults with 6-OHDA.

However, there was a marked increase in cGMP in the cerebellum after L-dopa administration that was attributable to the elevated locomotor activity.[46] However, it was observed that apomorphine administered to adult-lesioned rats often increased cGMP in striatum.[46] Because it has been reported that a D_1-dopamine agonist increased cGMP in striatum in control rats,[47] our earlier result concerning the change in cGMP in lesioned rats after apomorphine should be explored in more detail with specific D_1 and D_2-dopamine agonists.

Changes in Other Neurotransmitter Systems after 6-OHDA-Induced Lesions

Several investigations have been undertaken to explore the involvement of other neurotransmitter systems following lesions to dopaminergic neurons. The first of these studies examined the sensitivity of GABA receptors in the substantia nigra, because this is one of the major output areas for the striatum.[48] It was found that turning behavior in adult and neonatal lesioned rats was equally affected when muscimol was unilaterally microinjected into this site.[48] However, only the neonatally lesioned rats exhibited self-mutilatory behavior after bilateral administration of this GABA agonist in the substantia nigra reticulata.[48] This observation raised the possibility that integration of the behavioral responses occurred at this site or at a site central to this brain region.

Subsequent investigations evaluated the action of neonatal 6-OHDA lesions on peptides associated with dopaminergic function. It was demonstrated that enkephalin content was increased in striatum after this lesion.[49] The increase in this peptide was accompanied by an increase in messenger RNA.[49] In contrast to this change, tackykinin content (i.e., substance P and substance K), as well as message for these peptides, was decreased.[49] These changes were found to occur during ontogeny after neonatal 6-OHDA treatment.[50] It has not yet been evaluated how these changes influence responses to dopamine agonists.

Effect of Dopaminergic Neurons on Brain Proteins

Because dopamine receptor levels were not altered after lesioning of dopaminergic neurons, it was believed that other second or third components in the receptor messenger system linked to dopaminergic receptor function might be affected. Because the protein DARPP-32 was found in brain regions associated with dopaminergic innervation,[51] this was one of the proteins examined in lesioned rats. It was found that neither the content of this protein nor its mRNA were altered in rats lesioned as neonates.[52] Furthermore, using an antibody to the phosphorylated form of the protein, it was also found that the relative degree of phosphorylation of DARPP-32 was also unaltered or was below the detection limits of the assay[52] (unpublished data). Thus, we have not been able to link this protein directly with changes in dopaminergic function. However, there was an unexpected, fortuitous finding in our evaluation of phospho-DARPP-32 in brain. It was discovered that another protein was present in the lesioned rats that was not present in control rats[52] (unpublished data). While this protein has a lower molecular weight than phospho-DARPP-32, it can be surmised that this is a phosphorylated protein with some structural characteristics similar to DARPP-32, because it was visualized with an antibody to phospho-DARPP-32. Identification of this protein will obviously be a priority of our future research.

c-Fos is an immediate early gene-derived protein that was found to be induced after seizure activity.[53] Robertson et al.[54] demonstrated that L-dopa would increase *c-fos* on the lesioned side of a unilateral 6-OHDA-lesioned rat. Based upon this finding, it seemed possible that examining CNS tissue for *c-fos* immunoreactivity after D_1-agonist administration to neonatally lesioned rats might identify the specific neurons involved in the supersensitive response. Therefore, Mueller et al.[55] examined the effect of the D_1-dopamine agonist on *c-fos* expression in neonatally 6-OHDA lesioned rats and found that 3 mg/kg of SKF 38393 increased *fos*-like immunoreactivity in the lesioned rats but not in unlesioned rats. The D_2-dopamine agonist quinpirole produced no increase in striatum of lesioned or control rats, indicating that this change in *c-fos* is specific to D_1-dopamine receptors.[55] This conclusion has been reported by Robertson et al.[56] based upon investigations of D_1- and D_2-dopamine agonists in adult rats with unilateral 6-OHDA lesioning of dopaminergic neurons. Recently, Johnson et al.[57] have demonstrated that a new D_1- agonist (A-68930) increased *fos*-like immunoreactivity in brain of lesioned rats and noted the close association between *c-fos* expression and the location of D_1-dopamine receptor message in brain. Presently, this change in *c-fos* in the lesioned rats is the only biochemical measure that we have encountered that proportionately reflects the degree of behavioral supersensitivity of D_1-dopamine agonists in lesioned rats. However, it remains unclear if *c-fos* expression is a requisite step in the production of "priming" of D_1-dopamine receptors in neonatally lesioned rats.

Conclusion

The present review has presented the pathway taken from establishing an approach for destroying dopaminergic neurons in brain with 6-OHDA to data currently being collected to evaluate the consequences of this lesion.[7–18] With the use of a tyrosine hydroxylase inhibitor, we were able to demonstrate that mechanisms within the dopaminergic system were responsible for the recovery of functions observed after the lesion.[10–13] While an increased presynaptic release of dopamine from surviving neurons is an important component of the adaptation,[58,59] our efforts focused upon the post-synaptic supersensitivity to dopamine agonists.[31–34,42–46] The fact that both D_1-and D_2-dopamine receptor subtypes contribute to the super sensitive response of L-dopa provided additional avenues for research.[31,32,42] From this work came concepts of D_1/D_2 receptor coupling and priming of D_1-dopamine receptors.[26,31,33,34] The fact that the D_1-dopamine receptor priming has many characteristics of neuronal learning no doubt will have implications for dopaminergic function, but presently this relationship is not yet understood. The fact that *c-fos* expression reflects behavioral supersensitivity[55] and that a protein is found in greater abundance in lesioned rats compared to unlesioned rats[52] suggests that secondary and tertiary mechanisms may be involved in receptor supersensitivity. Perhaps we will eventually unravel the biochemical responses that are linked to *c-fos* protein expression and the formation of the unknown protein after the 6-OHDA lesion. Once this is accomplished, our understanding of the biochemical steps involved in orchestrating the supersensitive behavioral responses to D_1-dopamine receptor activation in neonatally lesioned rats may be realized. Such information could provide new approaches by which disease associated with a loss of dopaminergic neurons can be treated.

Acknowledgments   The excellent typing of the manuscript was performed by Ms. Doris Lee.

References

1. Ehringer H, Hornykiewicz O. 1960. Verteilung von Noradrenalin und Dopamin (3-Hydroxytyramin) im Gehirn des Menschen und ihr Verhalten bei Erkrankungen des extrapyramidalen System. Klin Wochenschr 38:1238–1239.
2. Bernheimer H, Birkmayer W, Hornykiewicz O. 1963. Zur Biochemie des Parkinsonsyndroms des Menschen, Klin Wochenschr 41:564–569.
3. Davis GC, Williams AC, Markey SP, Ebert MH, Caine ED, Reichert CM, Kopin IJ. 1979. Chronic parkinsonism secondary to intravenous injection of meperidine analogues. Psychiatry Res 1:249–254.
4. Langston JW, Ballard P, Tetrud JW, Irwin I. 1983. Chronic parkinsonism in humans due to a product of meperidine-analog synthesis. Science 219:979–980.
5. Ballard PA, Langston JW, Tetrud J, Burns RS. 1983. Chemically induced chronic parkinsonism in young adults: Clinical and neuropharmacology aspects. Neurology 33(suppl 2):90.
6. Tranzer JP, Thoenen H. 1968. An election microscopic study of selective, acute degeneration of sympathetic nerve terminals after administration of 6-hydroxydopamine. Experientia 24:155–156.
7. Ungerstedt U. 1968. 6-Hydroxydopamine induced degeneration of central monamine neurons. Eur J Pharmacol 5:107–110.
8. Breese GR, Traylor TD. 1970. Effects of 6-hydroxydopamine on brain norepinephrine and dopamine: Evidence for selective degeneration of catecholamine neurons. J Pharmacol Exp Ther 174:413–420.
9. Uretsky NJ, Iversen LL. 1970. Effects of 6-hydroxydopamine on catecholamine neurons in brain. J Neurochem 17:269–278.
10. Kraemer GW, McKinney WT, Prange AJ Jr, Breese GR, McMurray TM, Kemnitz J. 1976. Isoniazid: Behavioral and biochemical effects in rhesus monkeys. Life Sci 19:49–60.
11. Breese GR, Smith RD, Cooper BR, Grant LD. 1973. Alterations in consummatory behavior following intracisternal injection of 6-hydroxydopamine. Pharmacol Biochem Behav 1:319–328.
12. Cooper BR, Breese GR, Grant LD, Howard JL. 1973. Effects of 6-hydroxydopamine treatments on active avoidance responding: Evidence for involvement of brain dopamine. J Pharmacol Exp Ther 185:358–370.
13. Cooper BR, Konkol RJ, Breese GR. 1978. Effects of catecholamine depleting drugs and *d*-amphetamine on self-stimulation of the substantia nigra and locus coeruleus. J Pharmacol Exp Ther 204:59q2–605.
14. Breese GR. 1975. Chemical and immunochemical lesions by specific neurotoxic substances and antisera. *In* Handbook of Psychopharmacol-

ogy, Vol. 1. LL Iversen, SD Iversen, SH Snyder (eds). Plenum Press, New York, pp 137–189.

15. Breese GR, Moore RA, Howard JL. 1972. Central actions of 6-hydroxydopamine and other phenylethylamine derivatives on body temperature in the rat. J Pharmacol Exp Ther 180:591–602.

16. Hollister AS, Breese GR, Cooper BR. 1974. Comparison of tyrosine hydroxylase and dopamine-beta-hydroxylase inhibition with the effects of various 6-hydroxydopamine treatments on *d*-amphetamine induced motor activity. Psychopharmacologia 36:1–16.

17. Ungerstedt U. 1971. Post-synaptic supersensitivity after 6-hydroxydopamine induced degeneration of the nigra-striatal dopamine system. Acta Physiol Scand Suppl 367:69–93.

18. Hollister AS, Breese GR, Mueller RA. 1979. Role of monoamine neural systems in L-dihydroxyphenylalanine stimulated activity. J Pharmacol Exp Ther 208:37–43.

19. Scatton B, Javoy-Agid F, Montfort JC, Agid Y. 1984. Neurochemistry of monoaminergic neurons in Parkinson's disease. *In* Catecholamines: Neuropharmacology and Central Nervous System-Therapeutic Aspects. E Usdin, A Carlsson, A Dahlstrom, V Engel (eds). Alan R. Liss, New York. pp 43–52.

20. Breese GR, Mueller RA, Napier TC, Duncan GE. 1986. Neurobiology of D_1 dopamine receptors after neonatal-6-OHDA treatment: Relevance to Lesch-Nyhan disease. *In:* Neurobiology of Central D_1 Dopamine Receptors. (eds). GR Breese and I Creese. New York, Plenum Press 204: pp 197–215.

21. Kebabian JW, Briggs C, Britton DR, Asin K, DeNinno M, MacKenzie RG, McKelvy JF, Schoenleber R. 1990. A68930: A potent and specific agonist for the D_1 dopamine receptor. Am J Hypotension 3:40S–42S.

22. Iorio LC, Barnett A, Billard W, Gold EH. 1986. Benzazepines: Structure–activity relationships between D_1 receptor blockade and selected pharmacological effects. Adv Exp Med Biol 204:1–14.

23. Setler PE, Sarau HM, Zirkle CL, Saunders HL. 1978. The central effects of a novel dopamine agonist. Eur J Pharmacol 50:419–430.

24. Tsuruta K, Frye EA, Grewe CW, Cote TE, Eskay RL, Kebabian TW. 1981. Evidence that LY-141865 specifically stimulates the D_2 dopamine receptor. Nature 292:463–465.

25. Seeman P. 1980. Brain dopamine receptors. Pharmacol Rev 32:229–313.

26. Breese GR, Mueller RA. 1985. SCH-23390 antagonism of a D_2 dopamine agonist depends upon catecholaminergic neurons. Eur J Pharmacol 113:109–114.

27. Arnt J. 1985. Hyperactivity induced by stimulation of separate D_1 and D_2 receptors in rats with bilateral 6-OHDA lesions. Life Sci 37:717–723.

28. Walters JR, Bergstrom DA, Carlson JH, Chase TN, Braun AR. 1987. D_1-dopamine receptor activation required for postsynaptic expression of D_2 agonist effects. Science 236:719–722.

29. Jackson DM, Ross SB, Edwards SR. 1989. Dopamine D_2-agonist induced behavior depression is reversed by dopamine D_1-agonists. J Neural Transm 75:213–220.

30. Molloy AG, Waddington JL. 1987. Assessment of grooming and other behavioral responses to the D_1 dopamine receptor agonist SK & F 38393 and its *R*- and *S*-enantiomers in the intact adult rat. Psychopharmacology 92:164–168.

31. Breese GR, Baumeister A, Napier TC, Frye GD, Mueller RA. 1985. Evidence that D_1 dopamine receptors contribute to the supersensitive behavioral responses induced by L-dihydroxyphenylalanine in rats treated neonatally with 6-hydroxydopamine. J Pharmacol Exp Ther 235:287–295.

32. Breese GR, Napier TC, Mueller RA. 1985. Dopamine agonist-induced locomotor activity in rats treated with 6-hydroxydopamine at differing ages: Functional supersensitivity of D_1 dopamine receptors in neonatally lesioned rats. J Pharmacol Exp Ther 234:447–455.

33. Criswell HE, Breese GR, Mueller RA. 1989. Priming of D_1 dopamine receptor responses: Long lasting supersensitivity to D_1 dopamine agonist following repeated administration to neonatal 6-hydroxydopamine lesioned rats. J Neurosci 9:125–133.

34. Criswell HE, Mueller RA, Breese GR. 1990. Long-term D_1-dopamine receptor sensitization in neonatal-6-OHDA-lesioned rats is blocked by an NMDA antagonist. Brain Res 512:284–290.

35. Collinridge GL, Bliss TVP. 1987. NMDA receptors—their role in long-term potentiation. Trends Neurosci 10:288–293.

36. Goddard GV, McIntyre DC, Leech CK. 1969. A permanent change in brain function resulting from daily electrical stimulation. Exp Neurol 25:295–330.

37. DeNinno MP, Schoenleber R, MacKenzie R, Britton DR, Asin KE, Briggs C, Trugman JM, Ackerman M, Artman L, Bednarz L, Bhatt R, Curzon P, Gomaz E, Kang CH, Stittsworth J, Kebabian JW. 1992. A68930: A potent agonist selective for the dopamine D_1 receptor. Eur J Pharmacol 199:209–219.

38. Breese GR, Baumeister AA, McCown TJ, Emerick SG, Frye GD, Mueller RA. 1984. Behavioral differences between neonatal and adult 6-hydroxydopamine-treated rats: Relevance to neurological symptoms in clinical syndromes with reduced dopamine. J Pharmacol Exp Ther 231:343–354.

39. Braun AR, Fabbrini G, Mouradian MM, Serrati C, Barone P, Chase TN. 1987. Selective D_1 dopamine receptor agonist treatment of Parkinson's disease. J Neural Trans 68:41–50.

40. Breese GR, Criswell HE, McQuade RD, Iorio LC, Mueller RA. 1989. Pharmacological evaluation of SCH-12679: Evidence for an in vivo antagonism of D_1 dopamine receptors. J Pharmacol Exp Ther 252:558–567.

41. Criswell HE, Mueller RA, Breese GR. 1989. Clozapine antagonism of D_1 and D_2 dopamine receptor-mediated behaviors. Eur J Pharmacol 159:141–147.

42. Breese GR, Duncan G, Napier TC, Bondy SC, Emerick S, Iorio LC, Mueller RA. 1987. 6-Hydroxydopamine treatments enhance behavioral responses to intracerebral microinjection of D_1 and D_2 dopamine

agonists into nucleus accumbens and striatum without changing dopamine antagonist binding. J Pharmacol Exp Ther 240:167–176.

43. Duncan G, Criswell H, McCown TJ, Paul I, Mueller RA, Breese GR. 1987. Behavioral and neurochemical response to haloperidol and SCH-23390 in rats treated neonatally or as adults with 6-hydroxydopamine. J Pharmacol Exp Ther 243:1027–1034.

44. Simson PE, Johnson KB, Jurevics HA, Criswell HE, Napier TC, Duncan GE, Mueller RA, and Breese BR. Augmented sensitivity of D_1-dopamine receptors in lateral but not medial striatum following 6-hydroxydopamine-induced lesions in the neonatal rat. J Pharmacol Exp Ther (submitted).

45. Criswell HE, Simson PE, Breese GR. 1991. Augmented dopamine receptor sensitivity in lateral, but not medial, caudate following neonatal-6-hydroxydopamine lesions. Soc Neurosci 17:821.

46. Breese GR, Mueller RA, Mailman RB. 1979. Effect of dopaminergic agonists and antagonists on in vivo cyclic nucleotide content: Relation of guanosine 3':5'-monophosphate (cGMP) changes in cerebellum to behavior. J Pharmacol Exp Ther 209:262–270.

47. Altar CA, Boyar WC, Kim HS. 1990. Discriminatory roles for D_1 and D_2-dopamine receptor subtypes in the in vivo control of neostriatal cyclic GMP. Eur J Pharmacol 181:17–21.

48. Breese GR, Hulebak KL, Napier TC, Baumeister AA, Frye GD, Mueller RA. 1987. Enhanced muscimol-induced behavioral responses after 6-OHDA lesions: Relevance to susceptibility for self-mutilation behavior in neonatally lesioned rats. Psychopharmacology 91:356–362.

49. Sivam SP, Breese GR, Napier TC, Mueller RA, Hong JS. 1987. Neonatal and adult 6-hydroxydopamine-induced lesions differentially alter tachykinin and enkephalin gene expression. J Neurochem 49:1623–1633.

50. Sivam SP, Krause JE, Breese GR, Hong H-S. 1991. Dopamine-dependent postnatal development of enkephalin and tachykinin neurons of rat basal ganglia. J Neurochem 56:1499–1508.

51. Foster GA, Schultzber M, Hokfelt T, Goldstein M, Hemmings HC Jr, Quimet CC, Walaas SI, Greengard P. 1987. Development of a dopamine- and cyclic adenosine 3':5'-monophosphate-regulated phosphoprotein (DARPP-32) in the prenatal rat central nervous system, and its relationship to the arrival of presumptive dopaminergic innervation. J Neurosci 7:1994–2018.

52. Breese GR, O'Callaghan J, Ehrlich M, Criswell HE, Mueller RA, Greengard P. 1990. Absence of a change in DARPP-32 protein or mRNA in eonatal-6-OHDA-lesioned rats. Soc Neurosci 16:1179.

53. Morgan JI, Cohen DR, Hempstead JL, Curran T. 1987. Mapping patterns of *c-fos* expression in the central nervous system after seizure. Science 237:192–197.

54. Robertson HA, Peterson MR, Murphy K, Robertson GS. 1989. D_1-dopamine receptor agonists selectively activate striatal *c-fos* independent of rotational behavior. Brain Res 503:346–349.

55. Mueller RA, Grimes LM, Criswell HE, Carter LS, McGimsey WC, Stumpf W, Breese GR. 1989. D_1 dopamine agonist induces *c-fos* protein in the striatum of 6-OHDA-lesioned rats. Soc Neurosci 15:430.

56. Robertson HA, Peterson MR, Murphy K, Robertson GS. 1989. D_1 dopamine receptor agonists, selectively activate *c-fos* independent of rotational behavior. Brain Res 503:346–349.

57. Johnson KB, Jensen KF, Coates NH, Mueller RA, Criswell HE, Duncan GE, Breese GR, Caron MG, Fremeau RT Jr. 1991. Induction of *c-fos*-like immunoreactivity by the selective D_1-dopamine agonist A-68930 in neonatally-6-OHDA-lesioned rats: Comparison with D_1 receptor mRNA localization. FASEB 5:A413.

58. Zigmond MJ, Acheson AL, Stachowiak MK, Stricker EM. 1984. Neurochemical compensation after nigrostriatal bundle injury in an animal model of preclinical parkinsonism. Arch Neurol 41:856–861.

59. Zigmond MJ, Berger TW, Grace AA, Stricker EM. 1989. Compensatory responses to nigrostriatal bundle injury: Studies with 6-hydroxydopamine in an animal model of parkinsonism. Mol Chem Neuropathol 10:185–200.

Chapter 17

DARPP-32, A Protein Phosphatase Inhibitor Enriched in Dopamine-Innervated Brain Regions and Regulated by Multiple Extracellular Signals

Jean-Antoine Girault

Dopamine acts on target cells through at least two classes of receptors, referred to as D_1 and D_2 receptors.[1] Recent cloning of members of these two classes has shown the likely existence of some heterogeneity within each of them (see Chapters 12 and 13 in this book). Nevertheless, the presently best characterized coupling mechanisms for dopamine receptors are stimulation of the adenylyl cyclase by D_1 receptors and inhibition of the cyclase and opening of potassium channels by D_2 receptors.[1,2] Since the only known target for cAMP in mammalian cells (olfactory neurons excepted) is cAMP-dependent protein kinase (PKA), understanding the actions of dopamine through D_1 receptors at a molecular level requires the identification of proteins phosphorylated by PKA in neurons bearing the D_1 receptor. Several years ago it was shown that some protein substrates for PKA in brain are found only in restricted brain areas.[3,4]

From Hefti F, and Weiner WJ, (eds.) *Progress in Parkinson's Disease Research—2*. Mount Kisco NY, Futura Publishing Co., Inc., © 1992.

Some of these phosphoproteins were of special interest since they were detected only in regions known to receive an abundant dopaminergic innervation.[3,4] Three such proteins have now been purified and sequenced and their physiological role is being examined.[5-7] The best characterized among these proteins is DARPP-32 (*d*opamine- and c*A*MP-*r*egulated *p*hospho*p*rotein with an apparent M_r of 32,000 on SDS-polyacrylamide gel electrophoresis) (see ref. 8 for a review). DARPP-32 has been purified to homogeneity,[6] its primary structure has been determined by direct protein sequencing,[9] and its cDNA has been cloned.[10,11] In rat striatal slices, dopamine was found to stimulate the phosphorylation of DARPP-32.[12] DARPP-32 bears sequence homologies with protein phosphatase inhibitor 1 and, when phosphorylated by PKA, DARPP-32 was shown to inhibit protein phosphatase 1 (ref. 13 and see below). Hence, it was proposed that D_1-mediated regulation of phosphatase 1 activity was an important action of dopamine on postsynaptic cells.[8]

The regional, cellular, and subcellular distribution of DARPP-32 has been studied using a variety of methods including microdissection after focal brain lesions, immunocytochemistry, and in situ hybridization.[14-16] DARPP-32 is a cytosolic protein, highly enriched in the striatal medium-sized spiny neurons that project into the substantia nigra and the globus pallidus. DARPP-32 is highly concentrated in the caudate-putamen, where it is located in the cell bodies and dendrites of medium-sized spiny neurons, and in the substantia nigra and globus pallidus, where it is located in the terminals of these neurons.[17] DARPP-32 is also abundant in neurons of the nucleus accumbens, the anterior olfactory nucleus, the olfactory tubercle, the bed nucleus of the stria terminalis, and portions of the amygdaloid complex.[15] Intermediate levels are found in some cortical and hippocampal neurons, and in cerebellar Purkinje cells.[15] DARPP-32 is also found in some nonneuronal cells, in brain (choroid plexus epithelial cells, pituicytes, tanycytes, and some astrocytes),[14,15,18,19] and in the periphery (kidney, eye ciliary processes, adipose tissue, parathyroid gland, etc.).[14,15,19-22] At a gross level, there appears to be a close overlap between the expression of DARPP-32 and that of dopamine D_1 receptors, as measured by binding studies. There are nevertheless some mismatches (e.g., choroid plexus, which contains high levels of DARPP-32 and no D_1

receptor), and the exact degree of coexpression of the two proteins remains to be determined using double in situ hybridization or immunocytochemistry. In the case of the caudate-putamen, recent evidence suggests some degree of segregation of D_1 and D_2 receptors, the former being preferentially expressed in striatonigral neurons and the latter in striatopallidal neurons.[23] It will therefore be of great interest to determine whether or not the expression of DARPP-32 is restricted to the D_1-containing medium-sized spiny neurons. Interestingly, there appears to be some overlap between the expression of DARPP-32 and that of inhibitor 1, although inhibitor 1 is more widely expressed than DARPP-32.[24] In particular, medium-sized striatonigral neurons contain both phosphoproteins.[24,25]

In its amino-terminal region, DARPP-32 displays a high degree of homology with protein phosphatase inhibitor 1, a protein initially isolated from rabbit skeletal muscle.[26] Like inhibitor 1, DARPP-32 is phosphorylated by PKA on a threonine, a rather unusual phosphorylation site for this kinase.[27] Both proteins are dephosphorylated by protein phosphatases 2A and 2B (calcineurin),[13,28] a calcium/calmodulin-activated phosphatase that is abundant in brain.[29] Like inhibitor 1, DARPP-32 becomes a potent inhibitor of phosphatase 1 ($K_i \sim 1$ nM) when it is phosphorylated by PKA on threonine-34.[13] Phosphatase 1 is a widespread, broad-spectrum phosphoprotein phosphatase that is involved in many regulatory processes (see ref. 30 for a review). Although the role of phosphatase 1 and its cAMP-induced inhibition via inhibitor 1 has been well characterized in skeletal muscle,[30] very little is known on phosphatase 1 in central neurons. Three points therefore appear to be especially important for the understanding of the role of DARPP-32 in the action of dopamine: (1) the identification of the isoform(s) of phosphatase 1 present in neurons which contain DARPP-32 and the characterization of their substrates; (2) the determination of the regulation of the phosphorylation and dephosphorylation of DARPP-32; and (3) the elucidation of the biochemical differences between inhibitor 1 and DARPP-32 with a special emphasis on the specific properties of DARPP-32 that may explain its preferential expression in dopamine-innervated cells. In the present chapter we will discuss recent advances that have been made concerning the second and third of these points. We will also examine some of the possible implications of this work in relation with Parkinson's disease.

Phosphorylation State-Specific Antibodies: A Tool for Studying Regulation of DARPP-32 Phosphorylation in Intact Cells

Determination of the phosphorylation state of a protein in intact cells and of its regulation is usually carried out by [32P]phosphate prelabeling or by "back-phosphorylation."[31] In the case of DARPP-32, the first method is limited by the existence of several sites of phosphorylation for several kinases on the molecule (see below) and the second method is limited by its lack of sensitivity. We have therefore developed a different approach based on the use of phosphorylation state-specific antibodies, in collaboration with John Kebabian's group at Abbott Laboratories.[32,33] A synthetic peptide of ten residues, encompassing the cAMP-dependent phosphorylation site, was phosphorylated in vitro with purified PKA. The phosphopeptide was separated from remaining dephosphopeptide and from nucleotide di- and triphosphate by HPLC, coupled to a carrier (*Limulus polyphemus* hemocyanin), and used to immunize rabbits and mice. The serum of several immunized animals reacted only with phospho-DARPP-32, but not with dephospho-DARPP-32. Some of the positive mice were selected for the production of monoclonal antibodies, one of which (Mab-23) was used in subsequent studies. Mab-23 reacted with phospho-DARPP-32 but not with dephospho-DARPP-32 using dot blot, western blot and radioimmunoassays. On the other hand, Mab-23 reacted equally well with phospho-inhibitor 1, a predictable finding given the very high sequence homology (9/10 identical residues) between DARPP-32 and inhibitor 1 in the region surrounding the phosphorylation site, which was used for designing the synthetic peptide. On western blots, Mab-23 revealed the presence of phospho-DARPP-32 in striatal homogenates that had been incubated with PKA and ATP, and in striatal neurons in culture that had been treated with 100 μM forskolin. No phospho-DARPP-32 was detectable in the corresponding (untreated) controls. In addition to phospho-DARPP-32, Mab-23 reacted with unidentified proteins of higher molecular weight that were not affected by forskolin treatment. The presence of these cross-reacting antigens made it necessary in all experiments to separate the proteins by electrophoresis and to use western blotting in order to study the phosphorylation of DARPP-32. Using this approach, it was shown by Gretchen Snyder that incubation of slices from rat substantia nigra in the presence of dopamine or ʟ-dopa induced the phosphorylation of DARPP-32 (Snyder and Greengard, personal communication). This effect was mediated by stimulation of the D_1 receptor since it was mimicked by SKF 38393 and blocked by SCH-23390 but not by sulpiride (Snyder and Greengard, unpublished observations). These observations demonstrate that rationally designed phosphorylation state-specific antibodies are a valuable tool for studying DARPP-32 phosphorylation state in intact cells. They also provide evidence that the state of phosphorylation of DARPP-32 is regulated by dopamine acting on D_1 receptors, not only in the cell bodies and dendrites of medium-sized striatonigral neurons, but also in the terminals of these neurons in the substantia nigra.

Stimulation of Glutamate NMDA Receptors Induces Dephosphorylation of DARPP-32

The threonine phosphorylated by PKA on DARPP-32 is dephosphorylated in vitro by phosphatases 2A and 2B.[13,34] Phosphatase 2B is a protein phosphatase that is activated by Ca^{2+} and by Ca^{2+}/calmodulin and is identical to calcineurin.[29] Phosphatase 2B is abundant in brain and is highly enriched in striatonigral neurons.[35] Since stimulation of the NMDA type of glutamate receptor induces a Ca^{2+} influx into striatal neurons, we examined the effects of stimulation of NMDA receptors on the state of phosphorylation of DARPP-32.[36] Rat striatal slices, incubated in physiological conditions, were prelabeled with [^{32}P]phosphate for 90 minutes and exposed to various drugs for 5 minutes. Slices were homogenized in denaturing conditions, DARPP-32 was immunoprecipitated with specific antibodies, and the amount of [^{32}P]phosphate incorporated into seryl and threonyl residues was determined (PKA phosphorylates a threonine). Treatment of the slices with 50 μM forskolin increased phosphorylation of threonine by 300%. This increase was completely prevented by simultaneous application of 100 μM NMDA. The effect of NMDA was mediated through NMDA receptors since it was blocked by a noncompetitive antagonist (MK 801, 10 μM) and by a competitive antagonist (AP5, 100 μM). None of these treatments had any effect on DARPP-32 serine phosphorylation. The total level of DARPP-32, measured by immunoblotting, was unchanged by NMDA treatment, showing that the effects of NMDA were not due to proteolysis of DARPP-32. It was also verified that NMDA did not block the stimulation of PKA by forskolin-induced cAMP production, using direct measurement of the activated form of the kinase and quantification of the phosphorylation state of other PKA substrates. Therefore, the most likely explanation of the inhibition by NMDA of the forskolin-stimulated threonine phosphorylation of DARPP-32 is that NMDA stimulated dephosphorylation of DARPP-32, presumably by stimulation of phosphatase 2B. This observation demonstrates that a neurotransmitter can act on a target neuron by stimulating a protein phosphatase. It has now been shown that stimulation of NMDA receptors in several brain regions, including hippocampus and striatum, induces dephosphorylation of another phosphoprotein substrate for calcineurin, MAP 2.[37] The observation that stimulation of dopamine D_1 receptors and glutamate NMDA receptors have opposing effects on the state of phosphorylation of DARPP-32 may provide a molecular basis for some of the opposing physiological effects that have been described for these neurotransmitters in the striatum.

DARPP-32, But Not Inhibitor 1, is Phosphorylated by Casein Kinase II

While the amino-terminal parts of inhibitor 1 and DARPP-32 are highly homologous, their carboxy-terminal moieties are completely different. Among the features specific to DARPP-32, are a long stretch of acidic residues, of presently unknown function, and a putative phosphorylation site for casein kinase II. Using purified proteins and purified enzymes, it was found that casein kinase II phosphorylates DARPP-32 but not inhibitor 1.[38] In vitro, casein kinase II incorporates more than 2 moles of phosphate per mole of DARPP-32. Phosphopeptide sequencing has shown that the two main phosphorylation sites are serines 102 and 45. Studies carried out with [^{32}P]phosphate-prelabeled rat striatal slices have shown that serine 102 is labeled in intact cells.[38] In vitro phosphorylation of DARPP-32 by casein kinase II makes it a better substrate for PKA, by increasing the V_{max} of phosphorylation by 2.2.[38] It is therefore interesting to speculate that phosphorylation of DARPP-32 by casein kinase II in intact cells might modulate its responsiveness to PKA and, consequently, to dopamine. Casein kinase II is a widespread enzyme that seems generally to have a modulatory function.[39] It is enriched in brain neurons, including striatonigral neurons.[40] In nonneuronal cell lines, casein kinase II activity is increased by growth factors including epidermal growth factor, insulin, and insulin-like growth factor I.[39,41,42] In rat striatal slices, among a variety of neurotransmitters and growth factors tested, only insulin modestly enhanced casein kinase II activity (~50%) and DARPP-32 serine phosphorylation (~25%).[43] It is an exciting possibility that insulin, or some more potent, as yet unidentified, growth factor regulates DARPP-32 serine phosphorylation and may affect its responsiveness to dopamine in striatal neurons.

Possible Functional Implications and Consequences for Parkinson's Disease

DARPP-32 is a phosphorylation state-dependent inhibitor of phosphatase 1, which is highly enriched in neurons that receive a dopaminergic innervation, including the striatonigral neurons. DARPP-32 is the target of several identified phosphorylation and dephosphorylation pathways (Figure 1). Although much remains to be learned concerning the physiological role of DARPP-32 in these neurons, it is likely that dopamine, acting on D_1 receptors, will inhibit phosphatase 1 activity by inducing DARPP-32 phosphorylation. This could have several consequences, the simplest being a reinforcement of other D_1 effects, by preventing dephosphorylation of other substrates for PKA. In addition, by preventing dephosphorylation of substrates for protein kinases different from PKA, phospho-DARPP-32 could potentiate other second messenger pathways. Conversely, phospho-DARPP-32 could reinforce desensitization mechanisms of some receptors (i.e., by preventing dephosphorylation of a receptor whose desensitization is phosphorylation-dependent). These propositions are only working hypotheses at present, but they suggest that DARPP-32 may have an important regulatory role in striatal neurons. In this regard, it is striking that phosphorylation of DARPP-32 is regulated directly by the two most important pathways impinging on striatal neurons, the

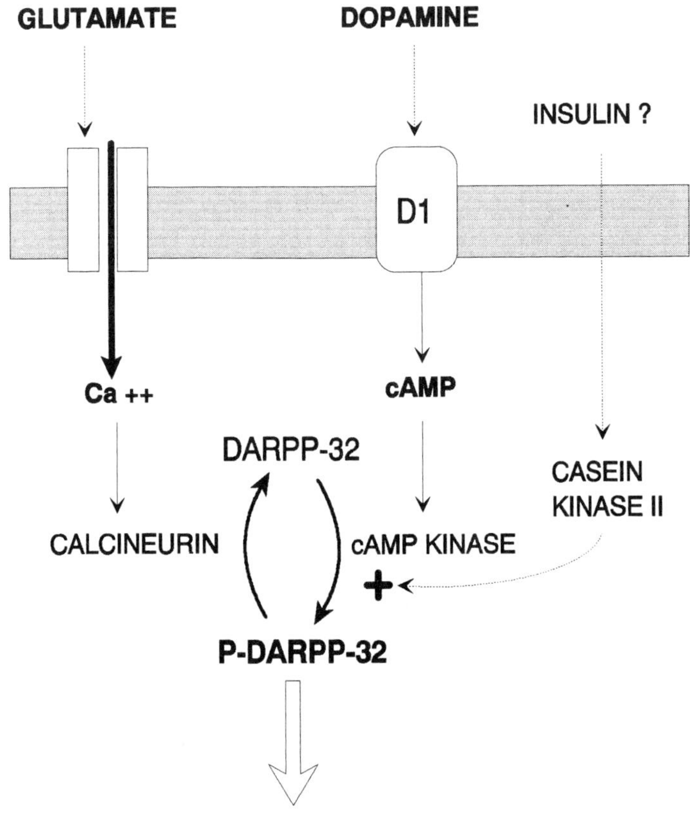

Figure 1.   Schematic representation of the phosphorylation–dephosphorylation pathways converging on DARPP-32. DARPP-32 is phosphorylated on a threonine (T) by cAMP-dependent protein kinase (PKA). This phosphorylation pathway is stimulated by dopamine acting on D_1 receptors. DARPP-32 is a potent inhibitor of phosphatase 1 when phosphorylated on threonine. Glutamate stimulates NMDA receptors, thereby producing a Ca^{2+} influx, directly through the receptor channel or indirectly through voltage-sensitive Ca^{2+} channels. Ca^{2+} activates the Ca^{2+}/calmodulin-stimulated protein phosphatase 2B, also called calcineurin. Calcineurin dephosphorylates the threonine residue phosphorylated by PKA. Therefore stimulation of calcineurin antagonizes the effects of PKA on DARPP-32, as indicated by a minus sign on the scheme. DARPP-32 is also phosphorylated on serine (S) by casein kinase II. Casein kinase II activity and DARPP-32 phosphorylation are stimulated by insulin in striatal slices. Phosphorylation of DARPP-32 by casein kinase II facilitates the action of PKA in vitro, as indicated by a plus sign on the scheme.

corticostriatal glutamatergic neurons, and the nigrostriatal dopaminergic neurons.

What happens when dopaminergic neurons are destroyed? Experimentally, destruction of dopaminergic neurons in rats or monkeys,[44,45] as well as chronic blockade of dopaminergic receptors[46] did not alter the expression of DARPP-32. Furthermore, in postmortem samples from caudate nucleus and putamen of human patients affected by Parkinson's disease, or supranuclear palsy, a related disease, the levels of DARPP-32, and several other phosphoproteins, were normal.[47] These observations suggest that the components of the postsynaptic machinery underlying the effects of dopamine on striatal neurons are not affected, despite the prolonged disappearance of dopaminergic neurons. Therefore, the decreased efficiency of current dopaminergic therapeutics after several years of disease cannot be attributed to transynaptic degeneration or postsynaptic lesions. This type of evidence supports the view that improved dopaminergic treatment (e.g., drugs with better pharmacokinetic properties) should be efficient even after many years of disease. Another consequence of these observations, and of our present knowledge of the regulation of DARPP-32, is that it may be possible to reinforce dopamine action by facilitating DARPP-32 threonine phosphorylation. At least two theoretical ways of attaining this aim are suggested by our results. One would be to prevent DARPP-32 dephosphorylation by blocking NMDA receptors. Another would be to enhance casein kinase II activity, and DARPP-32 serine phosphorylation, thereby facilitating its phosphorylation by PKA in response to dopamine. Interestingly, blockade of NMDA receptors has been reported to compensate for some of the behavioral effects secondary to destruction of dopaminergic neurons or blockade of dopamine receptors.[48–51] Obviously NMDA antagonists may exert their effects at several biochemical and anatomical levels. For instance, a direct effect of these compounds on the output structures of the basal ganglia is likely[52] and may be especially relevant in the complete absence of dopamine. We have also suggested,[53] in agreement with some behavioral observations,[54] that NMDA antagonists (and perhaps anticholinergic agents) may potentiate dopamine effects on striatonigral neurons by preventing DARPP-32 dephosphorylation in the striatum. These two mechanisms are not mutually exclusive. The first could correspond to a compensatory mechanism for the complete absence of dopamine, while the second could be critical for reinforcing an impaired, but still existing, dopaminergic transmission. At present, these novel approaches are speculative, but they provide potential targets for clinical pharmacologists in the future.

References

1. Kebabian JW, Calne DB. 1979. Multiple receptors for dopamine. Nature 277:93–96.
2. Freedman JE, Weight FF. 1988. Single K^+ channels activated by D_2 dopamine receptors in acutely dissociated neurons from rat corputs striatum. Proc Natl Acad Sci USA 85:3618–3622.
3. Walaas SI, Nairn AC, Greengard P. 1983. Regional distribution of calcium- and cyclic adenosine 3':5'-monophosphate-regulated protein phosphorylation systems in mammalian brain. II. Soluble systems. J Neurosci 3:302–311.
4. Walaas SI, Nairn AC, Greengard P. 1983. Regional distribution of calcium- and cyclic adenosine 3':5'-monophosphate-regulated protein phosphorylation systems in mammalian brain. I. Particulate systems. J Neurosci 3:291–301.
5. Hemmings HC Jr, Greengard P. 1989. ARPP-21, a cAMP-regulated phosphoprotein M_r = 21,000 enriched in dopamine-innervated brain regions. I. Purification and characterization of the protein from bovine caudate nucleus. J Neurosci 9:851–864.
6. Hemmings HC Jr, Nairn AC, Aswad DW, Greengard P. 1984. DARPP-32, a dopamine- and adenosine 3':5'-monophosphate- regulated phosphoprotein enriched in dopamine-innervated brain regions. II Purification and characterization of the phosphoprotein from bovine caudate nucleus. J Neurosci 4:99–110.
7. Horiuchi A, Williams KR, Kurihara T, Nairn AC, Greengard P. 1990. Purification and cDNA cloning of ARPP-16, a cAMP-regulated phosphoprotein enriched in basal ganglia, and of a related phosphoprotein, ARPP-19. J Biol Chem 265:9476–9484.
8. Hemmings HC Jr, Walaas SI, Ouimet CC, Greengard P. 1987. Dopaminergic regulation of protein phosphorylation in the striatum: DARPP-32. Trends Neurosci 10:377–383.
9. Williams KR, Hemmings HC Jr, LoPresti MB, Konigsberg WH, Greengard P. 1986. DARPP-32, a dopamine- and cyclic AMP-regulated neuronal phosphoprotein. Primary structure and homology with protein phosphatase inhibitor-1. J Biol Chem 261:1890–1903.
10. Ehrlich ME, Kurihara T, Greengard P. 1990. Rat DARPP-32: Cloning, sequencing and characterization of the cDNA. J Mol Neurosci 2:1–10.
11. Kurihara T, Lewis RM, Eisler J, Greengard P. 1988. Cloning of cDNA for DARPP-32, a dopamine- and cyclic AMP-regulated neuronal phosphoprotein. J Neurosci 8:508–517.
12. Walaas SI, Aswad DW, Greengard P. 1983. A dopamine- and cyclic

AMP-regulated phosphoprotein enriched in dopamine-innervated brain regions. Nature 301:69–71.

13. Hemmings HC Jr, Greengard P, Tung HYL, Cohen P. 1984. DARPP-32, a dopamine-regulated neuronal phosphoprotein, is a potent inhipitor of protein phosphatase-1. Nature 310:503–505.

14. Hemmings HC Jr, Greengard P. 1986. DARPP-32, a dopamine- and adenosine 3′:5′-monophosphate-regulated phosphoprotein: Regional, tissue, and phylogenetic distribution. J Neurosci 6:1469–1481.

15. Ouimet CC, Miller PE, Hemmings HC Jr, Walaas SI, Greengard P. 1984. DARPP-32, a dopamine- and adenosine 3′:5′-monophosphate-regulated phosphoprotein enriched in dopamine-innervated brain regions. III. Immunocytochemical localization. J Neurosci 4:111–124.

16. Schalling M, Djurfeldt M, Hokfelt T, Ehrlich M, Kurihara T, Greengard P. 1990. Distribution and cellular localization of DARPP-32 mRNA in rat brain. Mol Brain Res 7:139–149.

17. Ouimet CC, Greengard P. 1990. Distribution of DARPP-32 in the basal ganglia: An electron microscopic study. J Neurocytol 19:39–52.

18. Meister B, Hokfelt T, Tsuruo Y, Hemmings HC Jr, Ouimet CC, Greengard P, Goldstein M. 1988. DARPP-32, a dopamine- and cyclic AMP-regulated phosphoprotein in tanycytes of the mediobasal hypothalamus: Distribution and relation to dopamine and luteinizing hormone-releasing hormone neurons and other glial elements. Neuroscience 27:607–622.

19. Meister B, Villar MJ, Schalling M, Ehrilich M, Greengard P, Hokfelt T. 1989. Demonstration of DARPP-32 in pituicytes of the neurohypophysis—decreased expression after administration of hypersmotic stimuli. Acta Physiol Scand 137:461–462.

20. Meister B, Fried G, Hokfelt T, Hemmings HC Jr, Greengard P. 1988. Immunohistochemical evidence for the existence of a dopamine- and cyclic AMP-regulated phosphoprotein (DARPP-32) in brown adipose tissue of pigs. Proc Natl Acad Sci USA 85:8713–8716.

21. Meister B, Fryckstedt J, Schalling M, Cortes R, Hokfelt T, Aperia A, Hemmings HC Jr, Nairn AC, Ehrlich M, Greengard P. 1989. Dopamine- and cAMP-regulated phosphoprotein (DARPP-32) and dopamine DA1 agonist-sensitive Na^+,K^+-ATPase in normal tubule cells. Proc Natl Acad Sci USA 86:8068–8072.

22. Stone RA, Laties AM, Hemmings HC Jr, Ouimet CC, Greengard P. 1986. DARPP-32 in the ciliary epithelium of the eye: A neurotransmitter-regulated phosphoprotein of brain localizes to secretory cells. J Histochem Cytochem 34:1465–1468.

23. Gerfen CR, Engber TM, Mahan LC, Susel Z, Chase TN, Monsma FJ Jr, Sibley DR. 1990. D_1 and D_2 dopamine receptor-regulated gene expression of striatonigral and striatopallidal neurons. Science 250:1429–1432.

24. Gustafson EL, Girault J-A, Hemmings HC Jr, Nairn AC, Greengard P. 1991. Immunocytochemical localization of phosphatase inhibitor 1 in rat brain. J Comp Neurol 277:170–188.

25. Nairn AC, Hemmings HC Jr, Walaas SI, Greengard P. 1988. DARPP-32 and phosphatase inhibitor-1, two structurally related inhibitors of protein phosphatase-1, are both present in striatonigral neurons. J Neurochem 50:257–262.

26. Aitken A, Bilham T, Cohen P. 1982. Complete primary struture of protein phosphatase inhibitor-1 from rabbit skeletal muscle. Eur J Biochem 126:235–246.

27. Hemmings HC Jr, Williams KR, Konigsberg WH, Greengard P. 1984. DARPP-32, a dopamine- and adenosine 3':5'-monophosphate-regulated neuronal phosphoprotein. I. Amino acid sequence around the phosphorylated threonine. J Biol Chem 259:14486–14490.

28. King MM, Huang CY, Chock PB, Nairn AC, Hemmings HC Jr, Chan KF, Greengard P. 1984. Mammalian brain phosphoproteins as substrates for calcineurin. J Biol Chem 259:8080–8083.

29. Klee CB, Cohen P. 1988. The calmodulin-regulated protein phosphatase. *In* Molecular Aspects of Cellular Regulation. P Cohen, CB Klee (eds). Elsevier Biomedical Press, Amsterdam. pp 225–248.

30. Cohen P. 1989. The structure and regulation of protein phosphatases. Annu Rev Biochem 54:453–508.

31. Forn J, Greengard P. 1978. Depolarizing agents and cyclic nucleotides regulate the phosphorylation of specific neuronal proteins in rat cerebral cortex slices. Proc Natl Acad Sci USA 75:5195–5199.

32. Chen J, Zei-Jing Huang, Kebabian J, Girault J-A, Czernik AJ, Greengard P. 1989. Production of serum antibodies specific for the phosphorylated form of DARPP-32 (abstract). FASEB J 2:A550.

33. Czernik AJ, Girault J-A, Nairn AC, Chen J, Snyder GL, Kebabiab J, Greengard P. 1991. Production of phosphorylation-state specific antibodies. Methods Enzymol 201:264–283.

34. Hemmings HC Jr, Nairn AC, Elliott JI, Greengard P. 1990. Synthetic peptide analogs of DARPP-32 (M, 32,000 dopamine- and cAMP-regulated phosphoprotein), an inhibitor of protein phospatase-1. Phosphorylation, dephosphorylation, and inhibitory activity. J Biol Chem 265:20369–20376.

35. Goto S, Matsukado Y, Mihara Y, Inoue N, Miyamoto E. 1986. The distribution of calcineurin in rat brain by light and electron microscopic immunohistochemistry and enzyme-immunoassay. Brain Res 397:161–172.

36. Halpain S, Girault J-A, Greengard P. 1990. Activation of NMDA receptors induces dephosphorylation of DARPP-32 in rat striatal slices. Nature 343:369–372.

37. Halpain S, Greengard P. 1990. Activation of NMDA receptors induces rapid dephosphorylation of the cytoskeletal protein MAP2. Neuron 5:237–246.

38. Girault J-A, Hemmings HC Jr, Williams KR, Nairn AC, Greengard P. 1989. Phosphorylation of DARPP-32, a dopamine- and cAMP-regulated phosphoprotein, by casein kinase II. J Biol Chem 264:21748–21759.

39. Krebs EG, Eisenman RN, Kuenzel EA, Litchfield DW, Lozeman FJ, Luscher B, Sommercorn J. 1988. Casein kinase II as a potentially

important enzyme concerned with signal transduction. Cold Spring Harbor Symp Quant Biol 53:77–84.

40. Girault JA, Hemmings HC Jr, Zorn SH, Gustafson EL, Greengard P. 1990. Characterization in mammalian brain of a DARPP-32 serine kinase identical to casein kinase II. J Neurochem 55:1772–1783.

41. Ackerman P, Osheroff N. 1989. Regulation of casein kinase II activity by epidermal growth factor in human A-431 carcinoma cells. J Biol Chem 264:11958–11965.

42. Klarlund JK, Czech MP. 1988. Insulin-like growth factor I and insulin rapidly increase casein kinase II activity in BALB/c 3T3 fibroblasts. J Biol Chem 263:15872–15875.

43. Zorn SH, Girault J-A, Greengard P. 1989. Regulation of the phosphorylation of DARPP-32 by casein kinase II. Soc Neurosci Abstr 15:835.

44. Raisman R, Girault J-A, Moussaoui S, Feuerstein C, Jenner P, Marsden CD, Agid Y. 1990. Lack of change in striatal DARPP-32 levels following nigrostriatal dopaminergic lesions in animals and in parkinsonian syndromes in man. Brain Res 507:45–50.

45. Walaas SI, Greengard P. 1984. DARPP-32, a dopamine- and adenosine 3':5'-monophosphate-regulated phosphoprotein enriched in dopamine-innervated brain regions. I Regional and cellular distribution in the rat brain. J Neurosci 4:84–98.

46. Grebb JA, Girault J-A, Ehrlich M, Greengard P. 1990. Chronic treatment of rats with SCH-23390 or raclopride does not affect the concentrations of DARPP-32 or its mRNA in dopamine-innervated brain regions. J Neurochem 55:204–207.

47. Girault J-A, Raisman-Vozari R, Agid Y, Greengard P. 1989. Striatal phosphoproteins in Parkinson disease and progressive supranuclear palsy. Proc Natl Acad Sci USA 86:2493–2497.

48. Bormann J. 1989. Memantine is a potent blocker of N-methyl-D-aspartate (NMDA) receptor channels. Eur J Pharmacol 166:591–592.

49. Carlsson M, Carlsson A. 1989. The NMDA antagonist MK-801 causes marked locomotor stimulation in monoamine-depleted mice. J Neural Transm 75:221–226.

50. Olney JW, Price MT, Labruyere J, Salles KS, Friedrich G, Mueller M, Silverman E. 1987. Anti-parkinsonian agents are phencyclidine agonists and N-methyl-aspartate antagonists. Eur J Pharmacol 142:319–320.

51. Schmidt WJ, Bubser M. 1989. Anticataleptic effects of the N-methyl-D-aspartate antagonist MK-801 in rats. Pharmacol Biochem Behav 32:621–623.

52. Klockgether T, Turski L. 1989. Excitatory amino acids and the basal ganglia: Implications for the therapy of Parkinson's disease. Trends Neurosci 12:285–286.

53. Girault J-A, Halpain S, Greengard P. 1990. Excitatory amino acid antagonists and Parkinson's disease. Trends Neurosci 13:325–326.

54. Schmidt WJ, Bubser M, Hauber W. 1990. Excitatory amino acids and Parkinson's disease. Trends Neurosci 13:46.

Chapter 18

Heterogeneity of Dopamine Receptors and Their Possible Role in Mediating Antiparkinsonian Responses

Menek Goldstein

The therapeutic response of parkinsonian patients to L-dopa treatment provided a rationale for clinical trials with various dopamine (DA) agonists. Clinical studies indicate that DA agonists are effective in ameliorating parkinsonian symptomatology, but treatment with these drugs is not as effective as with L-dopa and the occurrence of untoward side effects limits their usefulness. The question of whether the therapeutic effectiveness of DA formed from administered L-dopa is due to the stimulation of only DA D_2 (D_2), or also of other DA receptor subtypes, is of importance for designing new antiparkinsonian agents. The recent discoveries of the existence of multiple DA receptors in the central nervous system suggest that specific DA receptor subtypes may mediate distinct antiparkinsonian responses elicited by selective DA agonists. Pharmacologic and biochemical studies have characterized the two major DA receptor subtypes, D_1 and D_2 receptors (D_1 and D_2R), as being linked to activation and inhibition, respectively, of the adenylate cyclase

These studies were supported by a grant from the National Institutes of Health (NH 06801).
From Hefti F, and Weiner WJ, (eds.) *Progress in Parkinson's Disease Research—2.* Mount Kisco NY, Futura Publishing Co., Inc., © 1992.

system. Although the antiparkinsonian effects of DA agonists seem to be associated with stimulation of D_2R, nevertheless the involvement of D_1R and of other DA receptor subtypes in mediating the antiparkinsonian effects of DA agonists cannot be excluded.

The antiparkinsonian response of selective DA receptor subtype agonists can be evaluated in nonhuman primate models that mimic the symptomatology of Parkinson's disease. In this chapter I will review some of our studies with DA agonists on amelioration of parkinsonian symptoms in two such models. The effects of selective DA agonists on tremor and occurrence of abnormal involuntary movements (AIMs) in monkeys with surgical unilateral ventromedial tegmental (VMT) lesions of the brain stem, and on the relief of parkinsonian-like symptoms (PLS) and on the occurrence of AIMs in monkeys with 1-methyl-4-phenyl-1,2,3,6-tetrahydropyridine (MPTP)-induced hemiparkinsonism will be described. In addition, the possible role of the multiple DA receptor subtypes in mediating antiparkinsonian activity will be discussed.

D_1R Subtypes and DA Agonist-Elicited Antiparkinsonian Activity

The gene encoding the human and rat D_1R was cloned and characterized.[1,2] The pharmacological and functional profiles of the D_1R expressed in transfected cells are characteristic of a D_1R coupled to the stimulatory adenylate cyclase system. More recently, a gene was cloned with great homology to the D_1R and designated as D_5R.[3] The D_5R has a similar pharmacologic profile to the D_1, with the exception that it has a tenfold higher affinity for DA. The D_5R subtype, like the D_1R, is positively linked to the adenylate cyclase system. The finding that both receptor subtypes mediate stimulation of adenylate cyclase raises the question of whether redundancy of these subtypes reflects some still unknown differences such as different abilities to undergo desensitization. The behavioral functions that are assumed to be mediated by D_1 are probably mediated by D_5 and/or by both D_1 and D_5R. Since the D_5 subtype has a higher affinity for the transmitter DA than the D_1 subtype, it is likely that the former is of greater physiological significance than the latter. Thus, the antiparkinsonian effects elicited by administration of low doses of L-dopa might be due to stimulation of D_5 rather than D_1R. The functional responses elicited by D_1 and D_5R subtypes cannot be differentiated until selective D_1 and D_5 agonists and/or antagonists become available.

The antiparkinsonian effects of DA agonists in animal models that mimic Parkinson's disease were evaluated with mixed D_1 agonists prior to the characterization of the D_5 receptors. The selective D_1 agonists such as SKF 38393 or CY 208-24, by themselves, do not exert antiparkinsonian responses in monkeys with unilateral surgical VMT lesions or in those with MPTP-induced hemiparkinsonism,[4,5] but these agonists potentiate the antiparkinsonian effects of the selective D_2 agonists in both primate models.[4,5] The combination of D_1 with D_2 agonists potentiate the relief of tremor and PLS, as well as the occurrence of AIMs elicited by selective D_2 agonists in both primate models that mimic parkinsonian symptomatology. Since the selective D_1 agonists probably also stimulate D_5 receptors, it remains to be elucidated whether the interaction between D_2 and D_1R and/or D_5R produces synergistic functional responses.

The findings that D_1 (and probably D_5) coexist with D_2R in distinct neuronal populations of the striatum suggest that this phenomenon occurs at the cellular level.[6] At the biochemical level the stimulation of D_1 (or D_5R) increases the formation of cyclic AMP (cAMP), while stimulation of D_2R decreases the formation of cAMP. It seems paradoxical that an interaction between two receptor subtypes produces opposing effects biochemically and synergistic effects behaviorally. However, these receptor subtypes might not only be linked to adenylate cyclase but rather to multiple transduction pathways. Multiple D_1R subtypes that stimulate adenylate cyclase and phospholipase C activities were described in peripheral tissues.[7] Furthermore, a synergism between D_1 and D_2R in mediating Na^+, K^+-ATPase inhibition was reported.[8] It is noteworthy that the inhibition of Na^+, K^+-ATPase occurs at low concentrations of DA (at a concentration of 10^{-9} M, half maximal inhibition was obtained), suggesting that this inhibitory response is mediated by a DA receptor subtype with pharmacologic characteristics similar to those of a D_5R subtype.

D_2R Subtypes and DA Agonist-Elicited Antiparkinsonian Activity

The classification of multiple D_2R is based on the findings that multiple mRNAs encoding for D_2R arise from alternative splicing of a D_2 gene sequence.[9–11] The mRNAs differ by 87 bases, which encode for an additional 29 amino acids in the third cytoplasmic loop of the receptor. The AA insert is located in a domain of the receptor that probably interacts with GTP binding proteins of various signal transduction pathways.[12] The binding profile to DA agonists and antagonists of the two isoforms (D_2 short and D_2 long) expressed in transfected cells shows no significant differences, but differences in the transduction mechanisms or posttranslational changes (glycosylation) resulting in different molecular weights could not be ruled out. Since the level of the expression of the D_2 long form in the striatum is seven times higher than the D_2 short form, it could be assumed that the antiparkinsonian activity of DA agonists is mainly associated with stimulation of the former form.

The effects of selective and nonselective D_2 agonists on PLS were investigated in the nonhuman primate models. The results of our studies have shown that selective D_2 agonists such as quinpirole or (+)-PHNO ameliorate parkinsonian symptoms and induce AIMs in monkeys with surgical unilateral VMT lesions and in those with MPTP-elicited hemiparkinsonism. The amelioration of different PLS symptoms (e.g., tremor, rigidity) by D_2 agonists is dose-dependent, and the dose-response curves for amelioration of each of these symptoms (e.g., tremor, rigidity) are similar. This indicates that the tested D_2 agonists nonselectively stimulate D_2R subtypes that mediate distinct behavioral responses. A subtype-selective DA agonist that ameliorates specifically distinct motor dysfunctions without inducing severe untoward side effects will be therapeutically advantageous over the available nonselective ones.

Although at present only the D_2R forms that arose from alternative splicing of the D_2 gene sequence were described, it seems likely that other D_2 genes may be discovered in the future. Thus, studies on the interactions of DA agonists with specific D_2R subtypes might lead to the discovery of more selective antiparkinsonian agents.

D_3R Subtype and Its Role in Mediating DA Agonist-Elicited Antiparkinsonian Activity

The findings that a receptor subtype, D_3, is expressed in the brain and differs in its pharmacology and signaling systems from D_1

and D_2R subtypes[13] raises the obvious question of whether some motor functions are mediated by this receptor subtype. The high binding affinity of the D_3R for DA and for the D_2 agonists quinpirole and pergolide suggest that the antiparkinsonian effects exerted by these agonists might, in part, be mediated by the D_3R subtype. Since the binding of DA agonists to the D_3R subtype is apparently not regulated by GTP, and since the D_3 subtype is localized in different brain regions than the D_2R,[13] it might be possible to utilize these criteria for differentiation of these two DA receptor subtypes. It is noteworthy that DA receptors on corticostriatal terminals are also not regulated by GTP,[14] suggesting that a population of these receptors might represent the D_3 subtype. This idea is supported by our previous studies that have shown that GTP-elicited inhibition of pergolide binding to striatal DA receptors is enhanced on the decorticated side of the striatum.[15] Thus, removal of D_3R by decortication may shift the striatal D_2/D_3 ratio in favor of the D_2 which could account for the increased modulation of pergolide binding by GTP.

If indeed decortication removes a D_3R population in the striatum, then the binding profile of DA agonists with high affinity for D_3 and D_2R (high), such as quinpirole or pergolide, may differ on the decorticated side from that of the intact side of the striatum. To test this idea we have hypothetically projected binding profiles, which are illustrated in Figures 1–4. If we assume that 50% of the [³H]spiroperidol ([³H]Spi) binding in the intact striatum is associated with high agonist affinity sites,[16,17] and that of the 50%, approximately 30% is due to the D_2 (high) and approximately 20% to the D_3, then the displacement profile of [³H]Spi binding by quinpirole could be illustrated on the intact and lesioned sides of the striatum as depicted in Figures 1 and 3. Treatment with GTP/NaCl converts all D_2 (high) sites to D_2 (low) without affecting D_3 (Figure 2), resulting in approximately 20% of D_3 and 80% D_2 (low). On the other hand, decortication eliminates the D_3 sites, leaving 30% D_2 (high) and 50% D_2 (low) sites (Figure 3). Treatment of striatal membranes from the decorticated side with GTP/NaCl converts all the D_2 (high) to D_2 (low) sites, resulting in a monophasic displacement curve (Figure 4). An experimental confirmation of these hypothetical displacement curves will corroborate the idea that D_3R are associated with corticostriatal DA receptors and that a population of D_2 (high) is identical to D_3R.

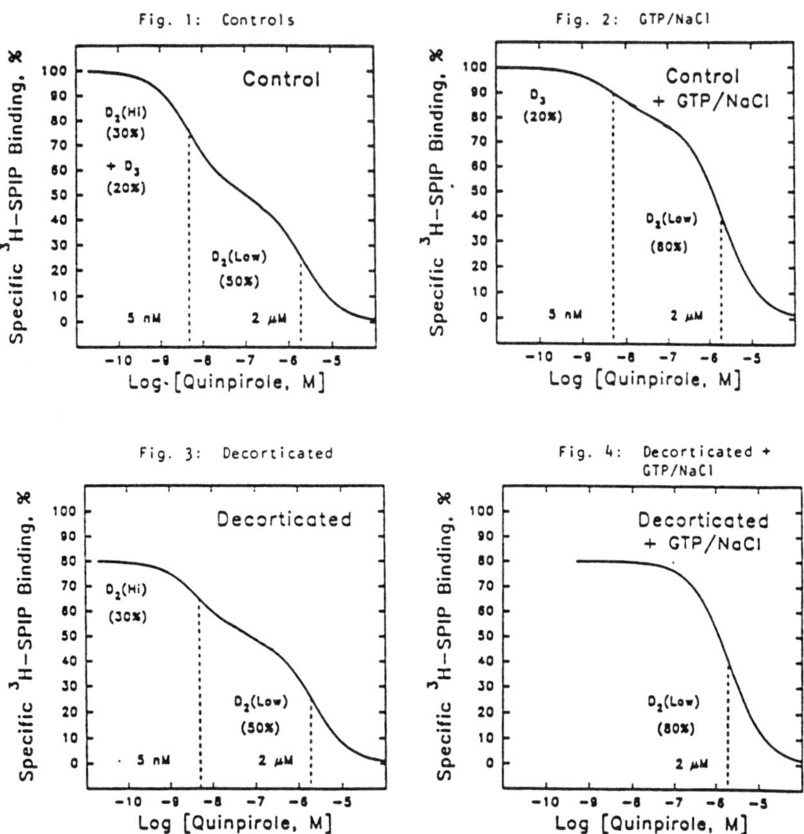

Figures 1–4. Hypothetical displacement curves of striatal [³H]spiperone ([³H]SPIP) binding by quinpirole under various experimental conditions.

To determine the functional response of stimulation of D_3R, the rotational behavior elicited by DA agonists could be compared in rats with unilateral 6-OHDA lesions of the nigrostriatal neurons with those with dual lesions (unilateral 6-OHDA and unilateral cortical ablation). If cortical ablation results in a decrease of striatal D_3R, then the rotational response elicited by low doses of DA agonists with high affinities for D_3R (e.g., pergolide or quinpirole) might be diminished. The dual lesion model might be useful in evaluating the functional responses elicited by stimulation of the D_3R subtype.

References

1. Dearry A, Gingrich JA, Falardeau P, Fremeau RT Jr, Bates MD, Caron MG. 1990. Molecular cloning and expression of the gene for a human D_1 dopamine receptor. Nature 347:72–76.
2. Zhou Q-Y, Grandy DK, Thambi L, Kushner JA, Van Tol HHM, Cone R, Pribnow D, Salon J, Bunzow JR, Civelli O. 1990. Cloning and expression of human and rat D_1 dopamine receptors. Nature 347:76–80.
3. Sunahara RK, Guan H-G, O'Dowd BF, Seeman P, Laurier LG, Ng G, George SR, Torchia J, Van Tol HHM, Niznik HB. 1991. Cloning of the gene for a human dopamine D_5 receptor with higher affinity for dopamine D_1. Nature 350:614–619.
4. Goldstein M, Deutch AY. 1988. The therapeutic potential of D_1 and D_2 dopamine agonists in Parkinson's disease. *In* Progress in Parkinson Research. F Hefti, WJ Weiner (eds). Plenum Press, New York, pp 61–66.
5. Goldstein M. 1986. Selective dopamine agonists as putative antiparkinsonian agents. *In* Recent Developments in Parkinson's Disease. S Fahn, CD Marsden, P Jenner, P Teychenne (eds). Raven Press, New York, pp. 183–189.
6. Seeman P, Niznik HB, Guan H-C, Booth G, Ulpian C. 1989. Link between D_1 and D_2 dopamine receptors is reduced in schizophrenia and Huntington's diseased brain. Proc Natl Acad Sci USA 80:10156–10160.
7. Felder CC, Jose PA, Axelrod J. 1989. The dopamine agonist SKF 82526 stimulates phospholipase activity independent of adenylate cyclase. J Pharmacol Exp Ther 248:171–175.
8. Bertorello AM, Hopfield JF, Aperia A, Greengard P. 1990. Inhibition by dopamine of $(Na^+ + K^+)$ATPase activity in neostriatal neurons through D_1 and D_2 dopamine receptor synergism. Nature 347:386–388.
9. Giros B, Sokoloff P, Martres M-P, Riou J-F, Emorine LJ, Schwartz J-C. 1989. Alternative splicing directs the expression of two D_2 dopamine receptor isoforms. Nature 342:923–926.
10. Monsma FJ Jr, McVittie LD, Gerfen CR, Mahan LC, Sibley DR. 1989. Multiple D_2 dopamine receptors produced by alternative RNA splicing. Nature 342:926–929.
11. Dal Toso R, Sommer B, Ewert M, Herb A, Pritchett DB, Bach A, Shivers BD, Seeburg PH. 1989. The dopamine D_2 receptor: Two molecular forms generated by alternative splicing. EMBO J 8:4025–4034.
12. Chio CL, Hess GF, Graham RS, Huff RM. 1990. A second molecular form of D_2 dopamine receptor in rat and bovine caudate nucleus. Nature 343:266–269.
13. Sokoloff P, Giros B, Martres M-P, Bouthenet M-L, Schwartz J-C. 1990. Molecular cloning and characterization of a novel dopamine receptor (D_3) as a target for neuroleptics. Nature 347:146–151.
14. Schwarcz R, Creese I, Coyle J, Snyder SH. 1978. Dopamine receptors localised on cerebral cortical afferents to rat corpus striatum. Nature 271:766–768.
15. Goldstein M, Lew JY, Sauter A, Lieberman A. 1980. The affinities of ergot compounds for dopamine agonist and dopamine antagonist

receptor sites: Ergot compounds and brain function: Neuroendocrine and neuropsychiatric aspects. Adv Biochem Psychopharmacol 23:75–83.
16. Seeman P, Watanabe M, Grigoriadis D, Tedesco JL, George SR, Svensson U, Nilsson JLG, Neumeyer JL. 1985. Dopamine D_2 receptor binding sites for agonists: A tetrahedral model. Mol Pharmacol 28:391–399.
17. Wreggett KA, Seeman P. 1984. Agonist high- and low-affinity states of the D_2 dopamine receptor in calf brain: Partial conversion by guanine nucleotide. Mol Pharmacol 25:10–17.

4

Cell Biology

Chapter 19

Neuroplasticity and Parkinson's Disease

Thomas H. McNeill, Heng-Wei Cheng, Jose A. Rafols, and Nozomu Mori

The ability of neurons to adapt or modify their structure in response to changes in intrinsic and/or extrinsic environmental cues, i.e., neuroplasticity, is a fundamental prerequisite for the formation of the neuroanatomical networks that are achieved in the developing brain.[1–3] In addition, it has been reported that a "plastic" nervous system is critical for the day-to-day maintenance of normal brain function [1,4–6] and that the ability of target neurons to remodel their neuronal circuitry in response to naturally occurring phenomena such as cell loss and/or partial neuronal deafferentation plays an important role in maintaining the functional integrity of the central nervous system (CNS) in normal aging.[7–10] Conversely, it has been proposed that there is a diminished capacity in the plastic response of aged neurons to response to the loss of their afferent input [11–13] and that alteration of a neuron's normal compensatory response to the loss of a neighboring neuron may serve as a common pathophysiological mechanism in the progression of neurodegenerative disorders such as Alzheimer's disease.[8,10]

Recently, we reported that there is a significant reduction in the

Funding for these research studies was supported by USPPS grants AG 05445, AG 09793, NS 14705, AG 00300, and the National Parkinson Foundation.
From Hefti F, and Weiner WJ, (eds.) *Progress in Parkinson's Disease Research—2.* Mount Kisco NY, Futura Publishing Co., Inc., © 1992.

size of the dendritic arbor of medium spiny I (MSI) neurons of the putamen in advanced Parkinson's disease (PD),[14] the principle target population for both dopaminergic nigrostriatal and glutamatergic corticostriatal afferent fibers.[15,16] Data from our postmortem brain study suggest that there is a significant decline in both the length and number of individual dendritic segments per MSI neuron as well as an increase in the number of atrophic MSI neurons characterized by truncated dendrites with few dendritic spines and irregular swellings. Whether these pathological changes reflect a deficit in the plastic response of striatal target cells to respond to: (1) the loss of dopaminergic afferent fibers from the substantia nigra;[17–19] (2) the combination of the dopaminergic deficit characteristic of PD and age-associated pathological changes in other afferent projection pathways such as those from the cortex or thalamus;[18–21] or (3) the direct pathological involvement of putamenal neurons in advanced PD is currently unknown. However, we hypothesize that the reduction in the size of the dendritic arbor of MSI neurons severely reduces the volume of dendritic neuropil that is available to receive and process information from remaining dopaminergic axons, thus, limiting the efficacy of L-dopa replacement therapy. Evidence from the clinical literature is consistent with this hypothesis and suggests that there is a progressive lack of striatal responsiveness to L-dopa treatment in advanced PD and may reflect a shift in the pathogenesis of PD from purely a presynaptic (i.e., nigrostriatal) to both a pre- and postsynaptic (i.e., striatum) disease state. However, while data from our previous studies have suggested a possible link between the declining efficacy of L-dopa treatment in chronic PD and altered neuronal plasticity of striatal target neurons, the cellular events that lead to the atrophy of striatal dendrites in advanced PD is currently unknown.

In order to address this issue, studies conducted in our laboratory over the last several years have examined the plastic response of MSI target neurons to the loss of different afferent projection pathways and the influence of aging on these processes. Specifically, we have studied the time-dependent morphological and molecular changes that characterize the differential response of surviving afferent fibers and target neurons following partial deafferentation of the ST based on either a homotypic or heterotypic pattern of reinnervation. Our studies have concentrated on the structural changes that occur in striatal target neurons (dendritic morphology and spine density) following lesions of either the dopaminergic nigrostriatal or glutamatergic corticostriatal systems. In addition, we have recently initiated studies to correlate our morphological findings with changes in mRNA levels for two growth-associated proteins (SCG-10 and GAP-43) as markers of plasticity and neurite outgrowth.

The following review summarizes data from our previous animal studies and has provided the basis for us to formulate several working hypotheses regarding the cellular events that may lead to the regression of the dendritic arbor of MSI striatal neurons in advanced PD. These include: (1) striatal target neurons are differentially affected by deafferentation lesions of the corticostriatal or nigrostriatal pathways; (2) the influence of age on reactive synaptogenesis in the ST is lesion specific; (3) the cellular events that govern neurite outgrowth following neuronal deafferentation are similar to those that regulate the spatial and temporal growth of neural processes during early development; and (4) neurite outgrowth during reactive synaptogenesis is differentially regulated in the brain based on the type of axonal remodeling required to form new synaptic circuits at the lesion site, i.e., paraterminal (SCG-10) or collateral (GAP-43) axonal sprouting.

Neurocircuitry of the Striatum

Based on previous experimental and clinical findings,[22–25] the ST (i.e., caudate nucleus and putamen) has been shown to be critically involved in the integration and coordination of normal motor function and is characterized by a relatively uncomplicated cytological organization that facilitates the study of reactive synaptogenesis following lesions of different afferent projection pathways. Anatomically, the chief cell type found in the ST is the MSI neuron, which comprises approximately 95% of all neurons found in the ST.[26,27] MSI neurons form synaptic specializations with afferent axons from distinct sets of topographically and neurochemically defined neurons in the cortex, thalamus, and midbrain (Figure 1). These include: (1) dopaminergic perikarya from the pars compacta of the SN,[28,29] which project topographically to the ST and form predominantly axospinous synapses on MSI neurons;[15,30,31] (2) glutamatergic neurons from layers II–V of the cerebral cortex, which project differentially to the patch and matrix compartments of the

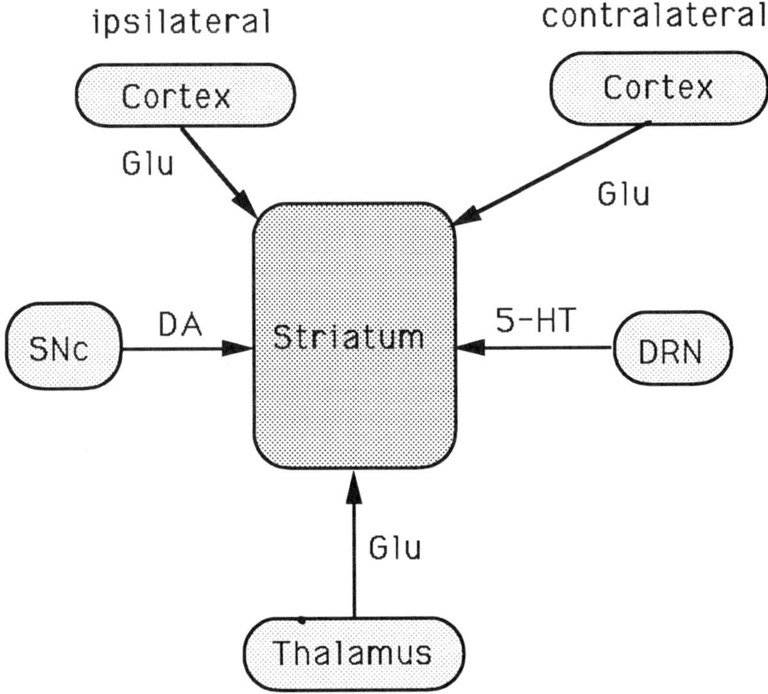

Figure 1. Schematic diagram of the principal afferent projection pathways to the striatum. These include: glutamatergic (Glu) fibers from the cortex and thalamus; dopaminergic (DA) fibers from the pars compacta of the substantia nigra (SNc); and serotonergic (5-HT) axons from the dorsal raphe nucleus of the midbrain (DRN).

ST[25,32] and synapse on MSI neurons to form the bilateral corticostriate pathway;[33–36] (3) putative glutamatergic cells from the intralaminar nuclei of the thalamus that also synapse on MSI neurons of the ST and form the thalamostriatal pathway;[33,37] and (4) serotonergic neurons of the dorsal raphe, which synapse on both spiny and aspiny striatal cells.[38–40] In turn, the ST sends topographically organized efferent fibers to both the pars reticulata of the SN and the internal segment of the globus pallidus.[41] These fibers originate from separate populations of medium-sized neurons of the ST[25,42,43] that contain the neurotransmitters GABA,[44–46] some of which colocalize the neuropeptide, enkephalin[47,48] or substance-P.[49,50] In addition, numerous other synaptically active molecules such as somatostatin, NPY, neurotensin, and Ach form a complex network of intraneurons within the ST and are thought to play an important role in the integration and regulation of striatal motor function.[25,51]

Effect of Nigrostriatal Deafferentation on Dendritic Morphology of Striatal Target Neurons

Since partial dopaminergic deafferentation is the neuropathological hallmark of PD, our initial studies examined the effect of dopaminergic deafferentation on the morphology of MSI neurons of the ST, the principal target population for afferent nigrostriatal fibers, using the dopaminergic neurotoxin 6-hydroxy/dopamine (6-OHDA). For our study adult (6 month) and aged (20 month) C57BL/6N mice were pretreated with imipramine (25 mg/kg) and given unilateral injections of 4.5 μg of 6-OHDA in 4.5 μl of 0.1% ascorbic acid stereotaxically. Mice were killed at 2 weeks postinjection and the ST was processed for Golgi staining while the SN was fixed in 4% paraformaldehyde and processed for tyrosine hydroxylase (TH) immunocytochemistry and cell counts. Quantitative analysis of the dendritic arbor of MSI neurons were analyzed as described previously,[52] and data were collected from the caudal level of the ST, an area that receives a dense topographic projection from the dopaminergic neurons of the pars compacta of the SN[25,29] and contains a high density of D-2 DA receptors.[53]

As expected, mice treated with the unilateral injection of 6-OHDA had a significant loss of immunoreactive TH-containing neurons from the pars compacta (A9) and pars lateralis (A8) of the SN on the side of the injection at 14 days postinjection.[54,55] Cell loss ranged between 84% and 95% for both the adult and aged mice and was distributed throughout the rostral–caudal extent of the SN. In contrast, TH-containing neurons of the ventral tegmental area (A10) did not show a significant decline in cell number following the 6-OHDA lesion.

A summary of the data from our quantitative dendritic analysis is presented in Tables 1–3. We found that while there was no significant difference in dendritic variables related to changes in the total dendritic arbor (i.e., total dendritic length and number of segments), there was substantial remodeling within specific branch

Table 1.

Effect of Unilateral 6-OHDA Nigral Lesions on Total Dendritic Length and Number of Segments/MSI Neuron[a]

	6 months		20 months	
	TDL	*TNS*	*TDL*	*TNS*
Contralateral	847 ± 22	38 ± 1	719.3 ± 21	38.0 ± 1.4
Ipsilateral	883 ± 51	39 ± 1	686.2 ± 14	36.7 ± 0.4

[a]Data expressed as mean ± SEM/neuron. There was no significant difference between the data obtained from the ipsilateral vs contralateral striatum for either age group, $P > 0.05$. Abbreviations: TDL: total dendritic length; TNS: total number of segments.

Table 2.

Effect of Unilateral 6-OHDA Nigral Lesions on Average Length of Ordered Segments/MSI Neuron[a]

Order	6 months		20 months	
	Contralateral	*Ipsilateral*	*Contralateral*	*Ipsilateral*
1st	60.8 ± 6.8	61.2 ± 11.6	58.7 ± 5	58.8 ± 9
2nd	196.8 ± 11.8	190.8 ± 31.8	176.0 ± 5.2	165.0 ± 11.3
3rd	278.6 ± 9.9	255.2 ± 20.3	235.6 ± 11.8	219.4 ± 4.1
4th	216.0 ± 9.6	215.2 ± 20.8	151.3 ± 11.6	147.6 ± 14.1
5th	67.4 ± 8.7	123.5 ± 9.6[b]	67.4 ± 5.6	58.2 ± 11.6
6th	25.0 ± 4.8	30.8 ± 4.2	20.8 ± 2.9	16.2 ± 4.2

[a]Data expressed as mean ± SEM/neuron.
[b]Differs from contralateral side, $P < 0.05$.

orders of postsynaptic dendrites ipsilateral to the lesion. Specifically, data from the branch order analysis indicated that there was a selective increase in the length and number of distal (5th and 6th order) but not proximal segments of the dendritic tree for MSI neurons ipsilateral to the lesion in 6-month-old mice. In contrast, there was a consistent but not significant decrease in both the length and number of 5th and 6th ordered segments in the ipsilateral ST of aged (20-month-old) mice. In addition, since terminal segments make up over 85% of all 5th and 6th ordered dendrites, data from our somatopetal analysis found that both the length and number of

Table 3.
Effect of Unilateral 6-OHDA Nigral Lesions on Average Number of Ordered Segments/MSI Neuron[a]

Order	6 months		20 months	
	Contralateral	Ipsilateral	Contralateral	Ipsilateral
1st	5.1 ± 0.28	5.2 ± 0.34	5.6 ± 0.21	5.6 ± 0.40
2nd	9.6 ± 0.33	9.5 ± 0.34	10.1 ± 0.29	9.8 ± 0.42
3rd	11.2 ± 0.48	10.9 ± 0.19	10.8 ± 0.48	10.7 ± 0.58
4th	8.1 ± 0.50	8.2 ± 0.78	7.4 ± 0.33	7.0 ± 0.44
5th	2.7 ± 0.35	4.0 ± 0.38[b]	2.9 ± 0.19	2.5 ± 0.38
6th	0.8 ± 0.12	1.2 ± 0.24	0.9 ± 0.13	0.8 ± 0.09

[a]Data expressed as mean ± SEM/neuron.
[b]Differs from contralateral striatum, $P < 0.05$.

terminal segments for 5th and 6th ordered segments showed a significant increase in the ipsilateral vs contralateral ST of adult but not aged mice.

Data from our spine count analysis are presented in Table 4. We found that there was no significant difference in the linear density of spines along any interval of MSI dendrites between the ipsilateral and contralateral ST of either age group. Similarly, there was no significant difference in the total number of dendritic spines per

Table 4.
Effect of Unilateral 6-OHDA Nigral Lesions on Average Number of Dendritic Spines per 20-μm Interval of Dendrite[a]

Dendritic interval	6 months		20 months	
	Contralateral	Ipsilateral	Contralateral	Ipsilateral
0–20	4.76 ± 0.64	5.32 ± 0.52	6.6 ± 0.87	7.7 ± 0.87
21–40	18.44 ± 0.72	18.04 ± 1.04	22.06 ± 0.82	21.9 ± 0.79
41–60	23.56 ± 0.74	22.26 ± 0.92	26.18 ± 0.80	25.0 ± 1.30
61–80	25.04 ± 0.99	23.16 ± 1.40	25.5 ± 0.87	25.0 ± 1.20
81–100	22.72 ± 1.20	21.6 ± 0.96	23.6 ± 0.60	23.8 ± 1.00

[a]Data expressed as mean ± SEM/20-μm interval. No significant difference between the ipsilateral and contralateral striatum along any interval of the dendrite.

dendrite in the ipsilateral ST compared to the contralateral ST in adult or aged mice.

Data from our study suggests that in adult (6-month-old) mice the loss of modulatory DA input from the SN results in an elongation of distal but not proximal segments of postsynaptic MSI dendrites. These morphological changes reflect an increase in both the length and number of distal but not proximal dendritic segments and are consistent with previous studies that have supported a neurotrophic role for neurotransmitters in the regulation of the size and shape of a target neuron's dendritic architecture.[56,57] However, in contrast to the classic degenerative–regenerative response that has been described in the hippocampus and ST following the loss of glutamatergic input from the cortex,[7,11,12,58,59] the loss of DA fibers results in a net outgrowth of the distal dendrites of MSI neurons. These data suggest that while neurotransmitters may influence the geometry of a target neuron's dendritic arbor, not all neurotransmitter systems have the same influence on morphology. For example, previous in vitro studies have shown that while some neurotransmitters such as serotonin, DA, and high doses of glutamate are known to suppress neuritic elongation and synaptogenesis,[56,57,60,61] others such as somatostatin and nontoxic doses of glutamate can enhance neuritic outgrowth, electrical coupling, and growth cone motility.[56,57,62] In addition, it has been reported[63] that the loss of inhibitory noradrenergic input from the locus ceruleus during the critical period of postnatal development can dramatically affect the normal course of dendritic maturation of neurons in the cortex and hippocampus and lead to the maintenance of a more immature elongated morphology of their dendrites. Our data are consistent with these findings and provide further support for the notion that neurotransmitters serve as important regulatory modulators of neuronal architecture and that the size and shape of a target neuron's dendritic arbor is defined by the summation of neurotransmitter inputs that synapse on an individual dendrite.

Although the specific cellular mechanisms that underlie the remodeling of the dendritic arbor of MSI neurons following DA deafferentation are presently unclear, previous studies suggest that the net effect of dendritic elongation after the DA lesion may, in part, result from the disinhibition of glutamatergic input from the cortex and thalamus. Previous studies have reported that the majority of all DA terminals in the ST synapse on the neck of the dendritic spine of

MSI neurons and are always accompanied by at least one non-DA fiber, which most likely originates from the cortex or thalamus. This unique anatomical arrangement allows for DA fibers to regulate the spread of excitatory activity from the more distally located excitatory input of the corticostriate and thalamostriate pathways[15,16] as well as maintain the physical integrity of individual spines following removal of their DA innervation. In addition, the loss of inhibitory dopaminergic modulation allows for the natural incremental increase of excitatory activity from remaining afferent glutamatergic fibers, which are known to increase intracellular secondary messenger levels such as Ca^{2+} and cAMP and promote dendritic elongation. This hypothesis is consistent with data from previous pharmacologic and electrophysiological studies[64,65] as well as recent in vitro studies by Mattson and colleague,[56,57] who reported that incremental increases of glutamate applied locally to hippocampal target neurons in cell culture can alter intracellular levels of Ca^{2+} and lead to a proliferation of their terminal neurites. They hypothesize that by locally regulating the flow of Ca^{2+} along different regions of the postsynaptic dendrite, neurons can respond to selective changes in presynaptic input following injury-induced deafferentation by modulating dendritic elongation and synaptogenesis. However, there is a delicate balance between the optimum levels of intracellular Ca^{2+} a neuron requires to promote neuritic outgrowth and that which leads to axonal or dendritic regression. Thus, while the plastic response of target neurons to partial deafferentation may be a natural response designed for cell survival, it may also increase its vulnerability to aberrant patterns of reinnervation, chronic elevation of intracellular Ca^{2+}, and lead to cell death.[57]

Our finding that the compensatory response of MSI target neuron dendrites to DA cell loss declines with age suggests that MSI neurons in aged mice have a diminished capacity to remodel their dendritic arbor in response to DA deafferentation. This hypothesis is consistent with previous studies in aged rodents that have reported a reduced capacity of target neurons in the cortex and hippocampus as well as their associated surviving afferent fibers to sprout and reinnervate denervated dendrites following lesions of the entorhinal cortex and/or septohippocampal pathway.[11–13] However, it is important to note that the age-related decline in the plastic response of MSI following the nigrostriatal lesion is not a consistent feature of MSI neurons following deafferentation lesions of other striatal afferent pathways (see next section). Recent studies by Cheng and coworkers[58,59,67] have reported that the capacity of MSI neurons to recover from cortical deafferentation does not decline with age and suggests that while the ability of MSI neurons to remodel their neural networks in response to some forms of deafferentation may decline with age, others remain unchanged. What may account for this difference is currently unknown and requires further investigation. However, these data suggest that while the ST may be able to compensate for changes in the cortical input that naturally occur with normal aging, the lack of an appropriate compensatory response to the excessive dopaminergic deficits associated with PD[18,19] may lead to morphological changes in MSI neurons that contribute to the enhanced severity of functional deficits associated with the progression of the disease as well as the declining efficacy of chronic L-dopa replacement therapy in its treatment.[14]

Effect of Corticostriatal Deafferentation on Dendritic Morphology of Striatal Neurons

To examine the effect of lesion-induced transsynaptic changes in MSI neurons following a deafferentation lesion of the glutamatergic corticostriatal pathway, adult (6-month-old) and aged (25-month-old) mice were decorticated unilaterally by partially removing the skull and carefully aspirating the frontal and part of the parietal cortex using a glass pipe, taking care not to injure the underlying white matter.[58,59] For our study we examined changes in the morphology of MSI target neurons at 3-, 10-, and 30-days postlesion and compared these findings with data taken from intact control rats. These times were chosen based on previous morphological studies of reactive synaptogenesis in the hippocampus following entorhinal cortex lesions and span the time required for the reinnervation of the lesioned site by surviving afferent axons from the contralateral entorhinal cortex, ipsilateral septohippocampal, commissural, and associational pathways.[7,68,69]

We found that in both adult and aged mice, the loss of afferent input from a unilateral corticostriate lesion leads to a transient loss of dendritic spine density on MSI neurons in the ipsilateral ST at 3- and 10-days postlesion but returns to 80% of preoperative levels by 20-days postlesion in adult mice (Table 5). Spine loss occurred in all

Table 5.
Effect of Unilateral Cortical Lesions on Density of Dendritic Spines on MSI Neurons in 6-Month-Old Mice[a]

Dendritic interval	Control	Days postlesion		
		3	10	20
0–20	7.7 ± 1.1	6.4 ± 0.8	3.1 ± 0.6[b]	5.0 ± 0.8
21–40	22.6 ± 1.5	15.6 ± 0.8	10.6 ± 0.8[b]	17.5 ± 1.4
41–60	32.1 ± 1.1	19.3 ± 0.8	16.2 ± 0.9[b]	25.2 ± 0.8
61–80	31.3 ± 1.0	21.1 ± 0.9	19.1 ± 0.9[b]	26.4 ± 1.0
81–100	32.5 ± 1.0	17.1 ± 1.0	17.9 ± 0.8[b]	23.2 ± 1.0

[a]Data expressed as mean ± SEM/20-μm interval.
[b]Maximum spine loss was found at 10-days postlesion ($P < 0.05$) in adult mice and recovered to 80% of preoperative levels by 20-days postlesion.

20-μm linear segments of the spiny dendrite and ranged from 31–47% at 3-days postlesion to 39–53% at 10-days postlesion. Surprisingly, a similar time course of spine loss and regrowth was also found in aged mice (Table 6). Specifically, spine loss occurred along all segments of the spiny dendrite at 3- and 10-days postlesion, ranging from an average of 28% at 3-days postlesion to a maximum of

Table 6.
Effect of Unilateral Cortical Lesions on Density of Dendritic Spines on MSI Neurons in 25-Month-Old Mice[a]

Dendritic interval	Control	Days postlesion		
		3	10	20
0–20	9.0 ± 1.0	6.3 ± 1.0	3.8 ± 0.7[b]	10.3 ± 1.7
21–40	27.5 ± 1.3	16.7 ± 1.4	12.6 ± 0.9[b]	26.6 ± 1.7
41–60	32.9 ± 1.1	24.3 ± 1.5	18.1 ± 1.0[b]	32.2 ± 1.2
61–80	30.3 ± 1.2	21.8 ± 1.0	16.5 ± 0.8[b]	28.2 ± 1.0
81–100	28.3 ± 1.0	20.6 ± 1.3	17.0 ± 1.4[b]	25.6 ± 1.4

[a]Data expressed as mean ± SEM/20-μm interval.
[b]Maximum spine loss was found at 10-days postlesion ($P < 0.05$) in adult mice and is fully recovered to preoperative levels by 20-days postlesion.

47% at 10 days postlesion; however, spine density was fully recovered by 20 days postlesion. In addition, there was no change in the length of striatal dendrites in either adult or aged mice following cortical deafferentation.

In order to determine whether remaining homotypic fibers from the contralateral cortex or heterotypic fibers from the thalamus played a significant role in the induction of spine growth after the cortical lesion, a second lesion was placed in either the contralateral cortex or ipsilateral thalamus 10 days after the first lesion and mice were allowed to survive an additional 15 days (i.e., a total of 25 days after the first lesion) (Table 7). In these cases we found that there was a significant decrease in all segments of the spiny dendrites when compared to similar values obtained at 20 days postlesion in age-matched controls, ranging from 34% to 45% of their normal spine density values. These data are similar to those obtained from mice allowed to survive for 10 days after a unilateral cortical lesion and suggest that a second lesion of the contralateral cortex was effective in preventing the regrowth of dendritic spines after the unilateral cortical lesion. In contrast, spine loss found in the combined cortex and thalamus lesion ranged between 12% and 28% with an average spine loss of 21% of normal control values and was similar to the value obtained at 20-days postlesion in the unilateral cortical lesion group.

Table 7.
Effect of Bilateral Cortical Lesions on Dendritic Spine Density of MSI Neurons of the Striatum[a]

Dendritic interval	Control, No. of Spines	Bilateral lesion		
		No. of Spines	% Change	P value
0–20	7.7 ± 1.1	3.3 ± 0.4	−53	0.001
21–40	22.6 ± 1.5	15.0 ± 0.7	−34	0.001
41–60	32.1 ± 1.1	19.7 ± 0.7	−39	0.001
61–80	31.3 ± 1.0	19.5 ± 0.7	−38	0.001
81–100	32.5 ± 1.0	17.9 ± 0.6	−45	0.001
101–120	29.4 ± 1.0	16.0 ± 0.5	−46	0.001

[a]Data expressed as the mean ± SEM. The lesion of the contralateral striatum was made 10 days after the ipsilateral lesion and effectively prevented the regrowth of dendritic spines.

Data from this study demonstrate that the loss of dendritic spines from striatal MSI neurons following unilateral cortical lesions is a transient phenomenon and that the regrowth of dendritic spines after deafferentation may be attributed to the sprouting of surviving axons from the contralateral cortex. This finding is consistent with data from our previous ultrastructural studies, which found that the newly formed presynaptic terminal have morphological features similar to those of normal cortical afferents and suggests that homotypic fibers from the contralateral cerebral cortex and/or undamaged ipsilateral cerebral cortex are most likely the origin of the newly formed presynaptic terminals. In addition, the finding that the regrowth of dendritic spines after ipsilateral decortication is inhibited by a second lesion placed in the contralateral cortex is in agreement with previous studies by Steward et al.,[70] who found that homotypic fibers from the contralateral entorhinal cortex play an important role in the formation of new synapses following a unilateral entorhinal cortex lesion. However, unlike the formation of new synaptic circuits in the hippocampus, which involves sprouting of surviving presynaptic axons from several afferent pathways, including those from the contralateral entorhinal cortex, septum and commissural/association pathways, the formation of new synaptic circuits in the ST following unilateral cortical lesions is accomplished almost entirely by homotypic neurons from the contralateral cerebral cortex.

Our finding that the recovery of dendritic spine density to preoperative levels in the ST of both adult and aged mice suggests that, unlike the hippocampus, which has been reported to show an age-related delay in the reformation of new synaptic contacts following lesions of the entorhinal cortex,[11,12] the capacity of the ST to remodel its neural circuitry in response to a unilateral lesion of the corticostriatal pathway is not effected by advancing age. Although, the cellular mechanisms that contribute to the preservation of the capacity of the aged ST to restore synaptic connections following a corticostriatal lesion are unclear, previous studies have suggested that several factors affecting both neurons and glia may be involved.[11,12] These include: (1) the ability of reactive glia to remove degenerative debris from the lesion site; and (2) the rate of growth of reactive afferents. While it is difficult to estimate the relative contribution any single factor may play in reactive synaptogenesis, we hypothesize that it is unlikely that the difference in the age-related response to deafferentation lesions in the hippocampus and ST is linked to age-related differences in the basic state of glial hyperactivity between the two regions of the aged brain since previous studies have reported that both in hippocampus[11,12,71,72] and ST[73] glia hypertrophy, in the absence of experimental injury, are characteristic of normal aging. Alternately, we hypothesize that the differential effect of advancing age on the rate of recovery of spine density and new synapse formation in the hippocampus and ST, following glutamatergic deafferentation lesions of the cortex may, more likely, reflect differences in the form of presynaptic sprouting involved in the formation of new synaptic contacts at the lesion site. As outlined previously,[68] two general models of axonal sprouting have been described in the brain based on the origin of the branch point between the newly formed axon and the parent fiber. For example, in collateral sprouting, the formation of new axon collaterals originates along the shaft of the existing axon and grows into a region of the deafferented target that has been previously unoccupied by the parent fiber. Collateral axons typically establish new synaptic contacts at some distance away from the original axon, and this is the principle form of axonal sprouting used by commissural and associational fibers of the hippocampus that invade the middle molecular layer of the dentate gyrus after a unilateral lesion of the entorhinal cortex. In contrast, paraterminal sprouting is characterized by either the enlargement of existing axon terminals, to form multiple presynaptic contacts with adjacent dendritic spines, or the formation of small terminal buds that grow out of parent axon terminals and form synapses with an adjacent dendritic spine or nearby dendrite within a few microns of the original terminal. This form of axonal sprouting is the most common type of sprouting found in the CNS and occurs in regions of the brain where surviving afferent axons already exist in the deafferented target zone such as in the outer molecular layer of the dentate gyrus following a unilateral entorhinal cortex lesion and in the ST following a unilateral cortical lesion.

Based on data from our current study as well as the data of others,[11,12] we have observed that there is an inverse relationship between the type of axonal sprouting required to form new synaptic contacts following neuronal deafferentation and the influence of age on the reinnervation process. Specifically, previous studies by Hoff et al.[11,12] have reported that following an entorhinal cortex lesion, there is a 13-day delay in the "reinnervation index," RI_{50} (the time required after the lesion to reach 50% of the synapses found in control animals), in the middle molecular layer of the dentate gyrus, which is dependent on the collateral sprouting of axons from the commissural/associational pathway, while there was only a 5-day delay in the RI_{50} in the outer layer of the dentate gyrus, which involves both collateral and paraterminal sprouting of existing axons in the terminal field. Conversely, data from our studies suggest that reinnervation of the ST via paraterminal sprouting of homotypic fibers from the contralateral cortex results in no significant delay in the recovery of dendritic spine density to preoperative levels. Although circumstantial, these data suggest that the form of axon sprouting used in the formation of new synaptic contacts following neuronal deafferentation may play some role in the influence of aging on the reinnervation process. However, further studies that examine the RI_{50} in the ST after cortical lesions as well as the involvement of other afferent projection system to the ST will have to be completed before a final conclusion can be reached.

Effect of Striatal Deafferentation on Molecular Markers Related to Neurite Outgrowth (SCG-10 and GAP-43 mRNA)

As a follow-up to our morphological studies, we have initiated studies to examine the molecular events that are involved in synaptic remodeling of the ST following a unilateral lesion of the corticostriatal pathway. In particular, we examined the prevalence of mRNAs for proteins associated with neurite outgrowth in the developing nervous system to determine if the molecular mechanisms that govern neurite outgrowth following neuronal deafferentation in the adult brain are similar to those that regulate the spatial and temporal growth of neural processes during early development. Our initial studies focused on two growth-associated neuronal proteins, SCG-10 and GAP-43, which are known to be highly expressed during the extensive period of developmental synaptogenesis[74,75] and are reported to be integral to neurite outgrowth and new synapse formation in the developing brain. In addition, recent studies have suggested that GAP-43 is closely associated with the growth and regeneration of axonal process in the hippocampus and that the pattern of GAP-43 immunostaining has been reported to change in a time-dependent manner that corresponds to the differential pattern of reinnervation of the dentate gyrus following the unilateral lesion of the entorhinal cortex.

Young adult male Fischer 344 rats (3-months old) were used for these studies and were decorticated unilaterally by partially removing the skull and carefully aspirating the frontal and part of the parietal cortex. By northern blot analysis, we examined changes in the prevalence of mRNA for SCG-10 and GAP-43 at 3-, 10-, and 30-days postlesion in tissue samples from three of the remaining projection pathways to the ST (i.e., contralateral cortex, ipsilateral thalamus, and SN) and compared these findings with data taken from intact control rats. These times were chosen based on our previous morphological data and span the time required for the reinnervation of the lesioned ST by homotypic fibers from the contralateral cortex.[58,59,67]

We found that changes in the prevalence of mRNA for both GAP-43 and SCG-10 are well within the limits of resolution required for northern blot analysis in all brain regions examined and that the temporal sequence of reinnervation of the deafferented ST by homologous fibers from the contralateral cortex are correlated with an increase in prevalence of SCG-10 but not GAP-43 mRNA (Figure 2). Specifically, we found that the prevalence of mRNA for SCG-10 was increased by 13-fold at 3-days postlesion and returned to control levels by 27-days postlesion, a time when most newly formed terminals have reached their targets. In contrast, GAP-43 mRNA prevalence was increased only slightly at 27 days postlesion and was not significantly elevated above the values found in intact controls ($P > 0.05$). In addition, we found that the increase of SCG-10 mRNA following unilateral decortication can be inhibited by a transection of the corpus callosum, which carries the afferent fibers from contralateral cortex (Figure 3). In contrast to the changes found in SCG-10 message in the contralateral cortex, there was no change in the prevalence of mRNA for either SCG-10 or GAP-43 in either the thalamus or SN.

Data from these studies suggest that SCG-10 and GAP-43 mRNA are differentially regulated in the contralateral cortex during synaptic remodeling of the ST following a unilateral lesion of the corticostriatal pathway. In addition, our finding that the maximum increase in SCG-10 mRNA occurs at 3-days postlesion corresponds temporally with the increase in the population of newly formed axon terminals

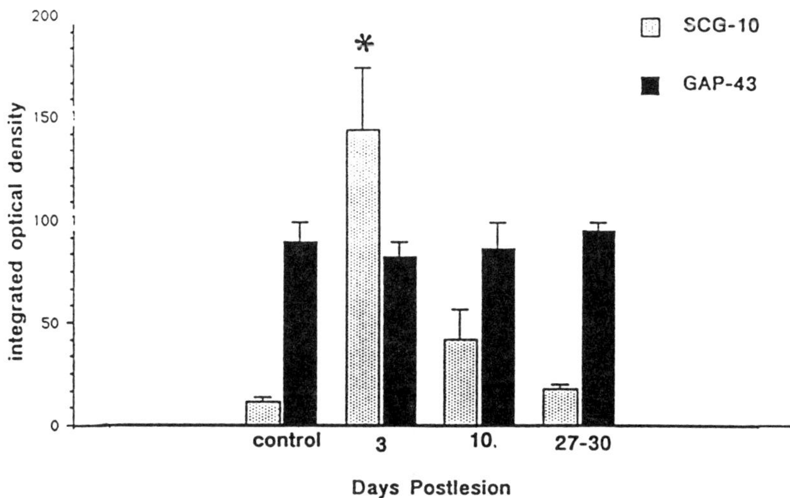

Figure 2.   Effect of a unilateral cortical lesion on the expression of SCG-10 and GAP-43 mRNA in the contralateral cortex. There was a significant increase in SCG-10 message at 3 and 10 days postlesion (* $P<0.01$) that rapidly declined to preoperative levels by 27 days postlesion. In contrast, GAP-43 mRNA was not changed at any postlesion time point examined. MRNA prevalance was quantified by video densitometry using a density wedge and multiple exposures of the autoradiogram to be certain that the signals were in the linear range.

at the lesion site found between 4 and 10 days postlesion in our ultrastructural study[58] and suggests that SCG-10 plays a fundamental role in the sprouting of paraterminal axons from the contralateral cortex. Likewise, the decline in SCG-10 message by 27-days postlesion corresponds to the time when most of the newly formed paraterminal axons have reached their target sites and suggests that without the need to form additional synapses the de novo synthesis of SCG-10 protein may no longer be required.

Although the precise function SCG-10 plays during reactive synaptogenesis in the ST is unknown, previous in vitro studies have reported that the expression of SCG-10 protein is increased in PC12 cells during periods of extensive neurite outgrowth in response to NGF and that, by immunocytochemistry, the protein is concentrated in the axons and growth cones of cultured neurons. In addition, the transient expression of the message during the time course of reactive synaptogenesis and previous biochemcial studies that have

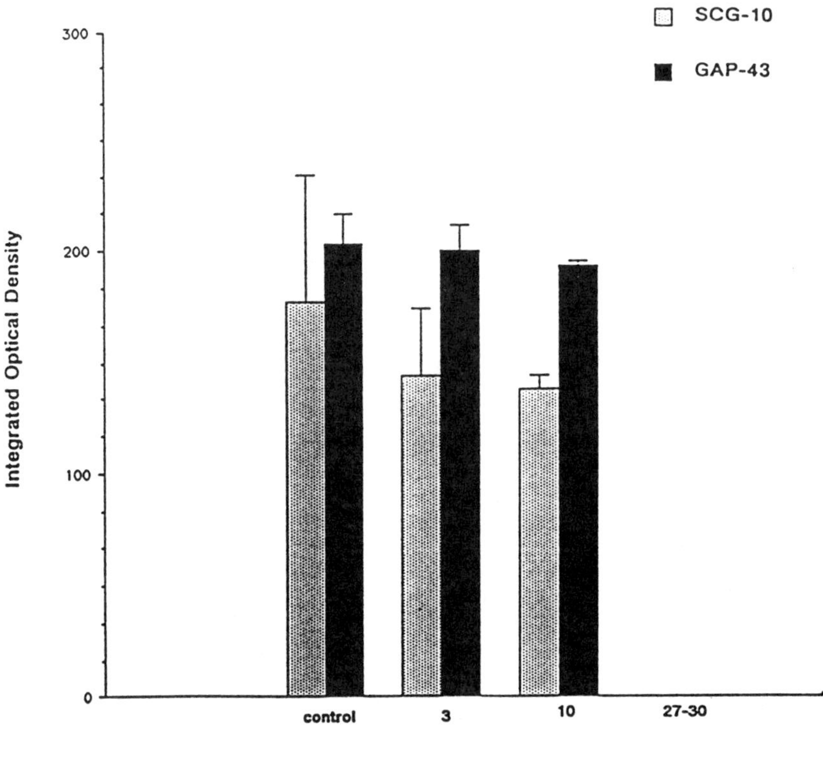

Figure 3.   Effect of corpus collosum transection on SCG-10 and GAP-43 mRNA in the contralateral cortex after a unilateral cortical lesion. We found that the increase in the level of SCG-10 mRNA seen in the contralateral cortex after the unilateral corticostriatal lesion was prevented by transection of the corpus collosum.

characterized the binding of SCG-10 protein with intracellular membranes suggest that SCG-10 may serve as a structure protein during the formation of new neuritic processes. Further studies to evaluate the function of SCG-10 during reactive synaptogenesis in the ST are currently underway. These include in situ hybridization studies to determine the specific population of cortical neurons in the contralateral cortex that respond to unilateral decortication and immunohistochemical studies using antibodies to the SCG-10 to identify the anatomical distribution of the protein in different cell types in the ST as well as to map changes in the pattern of SCG-10 containing synaptic terminals in the deafferented ST.

The finding that SCG-10 and GAP-43 mRNA are differentially regulated in contralateral cortex after a lesion of the ipsilateral corticostriatal pathway was surprising and has led us to hypothesize that, while both SCG-10 and GAP-43 may be part of a general cascade of morphological and molecular events involved in reactive synaptogenesis following brain injury, neurite outgrowth may be differentially regulated in the brain based on the type of axonal sprouting required to form new synaptic contacts at the lesion site, i.e., paraterminal (SCG-10) or collateral (GAP-43) axonal sprouting. Data to support this hypothesis come from current studies in our laboratory of animal models, which employ either paraterminal or collateral forms of axonal sprouting during reactive synaptogenesis. Specifically, we have compared changes in the prevalence of mRNA for SCG-10 and GAP-43 at different times postlesion in the contralateral cortex following a unilateral lesion of the corticostriatal pathway, a model of paraterminal sprouting, with data obtained from the contralateral hippocampus after a combined EC/fimbria-fornix lesion, a model of collateral sprouting. As described previously, data from our current study found that SCG-10 but not GAP-43 mRNA is up-regulated in the contralateral cortex during synaptic remodeling of the deafferented ST and suggests that SCG-10 plays a fundamental role in the sprouting of paraterminal axons from the contralateral cortex. In contrast, preliminary data from our hippocampal study found that following a combined unilateral lesion of both the entorhinal cortex and septohippocampal pathway there was a significant increase in the prevalence of mRNA for GAP-43 but not SCG-10 in the contralateral hippocampus at 14-days postlesion, a time coincident with the sprouting of axon collaterals from the commissural pathway of the inner molecular layer of the dentate gyrus into the middle molecular layer of the deafferented dentate gyrus. In addition, the increase in GAP-43 message by northern blot analysis in the contralateral hippocampus was localized in the CA3 subfield of pyramidal neurons, which form the commissural projection pathway to the contralateral dentate gyrus by in situ hybridization analysis.

Together, data from our studies are consistent with the notion that the induction of both SCG-10 and GAP-43 mRNA are part of the cascade of morphological and molecular events that are involved in reactive synaptogenesis. However, the regulation of SCG-10 and GAP-43 mRNA may be differentially regulated in the brain based on the type of axonal outgrowth required at the lesion site (i.e., paraterminal vs collateral sprouting). Specifically, our data suggest that while the activation of SCG-10 mRNA-related growth mechanisms is required for the type of paraterminal sprouting required to form new synapses on dendritic spines of target neurons that are within a few microns of the original degenerating axon (such as in the ST), GAP-43 mRNA-related mechanisms are involved in the sprouting of axon collaterals in the hippocampus that are needed to form new synaptic contacts at some distance away from the original fiber. This hypothesis is consistent with previous studies that have reported that, in the CNS, injury of a neuron's axon far away from the cell body does not enhance GAP-43 expression in the cell soma,[75–77] whereas the transection of an axon very close to the parent cell body can induce GAP-43 gene expression in the cell body of the transected neuron in order to induce axonal elongation.[78] However, further studies will be needed to test this hypothesis.

Acknowledgments: The 6-OHDA studies reported in this chapter were conducted with the technical assistance of Sally A. Brown, Laurie L. Koek, Barbara Davis, Ph.D. and Walter Fallice, M.D., from the University of Rochester. We would also like to thank Dr. Harry G. Goshgarian from Wayne State University for his assistance with the cortical lesion studies.

References

1. Purvas D, Lichtman JW. 1985. Maintenance and modifiability of synapses. *In* Principles of Neural Development. D Purves, JW Lichtman (eds). Sinauer Associates, Sunderland, MA, pp. 301–328.
2. Purves D, Nja A. 1978. Trophic maintenance of synaptic connections in autonomic ganglia. *In* Neuronal Plasticity. CW Cotman, (ed). Raven Press, New York, pp. 27–47.
3. Black IB. 1978. Regulation of autonomic development. Annu Rev Neurosci 1:183–214.
4. Lichtman JW, Magrassi L, Purves D. 1987. Visualization of neuromuscular junctions over periods of several months in living mice. J Neurosci 7:1215–1222.
5. Purves D, Hadley RD, Voyvodic JT. 1986. Dynamic changes in the dendritic geometry of individual neurons visualized over periods of up to three months in the superior cervical ganglion of living mice. Neuroscience 6:1051–1060.
6. Greenough WT. 1984. Structural correlates of information storage in the mammalian brain: A review and hypothesis. Trends Neurosci 7:229–233.

7. Cotman CW, Anderson KJ. 1988. Synaptic plasticity and functional stabilization in the hippocampal formation: Possible role in Alzheimer's disease. *In* Physiological Basis for Functional Recovery in Neurological Disease. S Waxman (ed). Raven Press, New York, pp. 313–336.
8. Coleman PD, Flood DG. 1986. Dendritic proliferation in the aging brain as acompensatory repair mechanism. Prog Brain Res 70:227–237.
9. Coleman PD, Flood DG. 1987. Neuron numbers and dendritic extent in normal aging and Alzheimer's disease. Neurobiol Aging 8:521–545.
10. Coleman DP, Rogers EK, Flood G. 1990. Neuronal plasticity in normal aging and deficient plasticity in Alzheimer's disease: A proposed intercellular signal cascade. Prog Brain Res 86:75–87.
11. Hoff SF, Scheff SW, Cotman CW. 1982. Lesion-induced synaptogenesis in the dentate gyrus of aged rats: I. Loss and reacquisition of normal synaptic density. J Comp Neurol 205:246–252.
12. Hoff SF, Scheff SW, Cotman CW. 1982. Lesion-induced synaptogenesis in the dentate gyrus of aged rats: II. Demonstration of an impaired clearing response. J Comp Neurol 205:253–259.
13. Scheff SW, Bernardo LS, Cotman CW. 1978. Decrease in adrenergic axon sprouting in the senescent rat. Science 202:775–778.
14. McNeill HT, Brown AS, Rafols AJ, Shoulson I. 1988. Atrophy of medium spiny I striatal dendrites in advanced Parkinson's disease. Brain Res 455:148–152.
15. Freund TF, Powell JF, Smith AD. 1984. Tyrosine hydroxylase-immunoreactive boutons in synaptic contact with identified striatonigral neurons, with particular reference to dendritic spines. Neuroscience 13:1189–1215.
16. Smith AD, Bolam JP. 1990. The neural network of basal ganglia as revealed by the study of synaptic connections of identified neurones. Trends Neurosci 13:259–265.
17. Hornykiewicz O. 1982. Brain neurotransmitter changes in Parkinson's disease. *In* Movement Disorders. CD Marsden, S Fahn (eds). Butterworth, London, pp. 41–58.
18. Hornykiewicz O, Kish JS. 1986. Biochemical pathophysiology of Parkinson's disease. Adv Neurol 45:19–34.
19. Jellinger K. 1986. Overview of morphological changes in Parkinson's disease. Adv Neurol 45:1–18.
20. Taylor A, Saint-Cyr J, Lang A. 1986. Frontal lobe dysfunction in Parkinson's disease, the cortical focus of neostriatal outflow. Brain 109:845–883.
21. Turner B. 1968. Pathology of paralysis agitans. *In* Diseases of the Basal Ganglia. PJ Vinken, GW Bruyn (eds). North Holland, Amsterdam, pp. 212–217.
22. Alexander GE, Crutcher MD. 1990. Functional architecture of basal ganglia circuits: Neural substrates of parallel processing. Trends Neurosci 13:266–271.
23. DeLong MR. 1990. Primate models of movement disorders of basal ganglia origin. Trends Neurosci 13:281–285.
24. Klawans H, Kramer J. 1980. The movement disorders: Diseases of the

basal ganglia. *In* The Science and Practice of Clinical Medicine. NR Rosenberg (ed). Grune and Stratton, New York, Vol. 5, pp. 266–296.

25. Graybiel AM, Ragsdale CW. 1983. Biochemical anatomy of the striatum. *In* Chemical Neuroanatomy. PC Emson, (ed). Raven Press, New York. pp. 427–504.

26. Kemp JM, Powell TPS. 1970. The cortico-striate projection in the monkey. Brain 93:525–546.

27. DiFiglia M, Pasik P, Pasik T. 1976. A Golgi study of neuronal types in the neostriatum of monkeys. Brain Res 114:245–256.

28. Hokfelt T, Ungerstedt U. 1973. Specificity of 6-hydroxydopamine induced degeneration of central monoamine neurons: An electron and fluorescence microscopic study with special reference to intracerebral injection of the nigrostriatal dopamine system. Brain Res 60:269–297.

29. Veening JG, Cornelissen FM, Lieven PAJ. 1980. The topical organization of the afferents to the caudatoputamen of the rat. A horseradish peroxidase study. Neuroscience 5:1253–1268.

30. Arlusion M, Dietl M, Thibault J. 1984. Ultrastructural morphology of dopaminergic nerve terminals and synapses in the striatum of the rat using tyrosine hydroxylase immunocytochemistry: A typographical study. Brain Res Bull 13:269–285.

31. Kubota Y, Inagaki S, Shimada S, Kito S, Eckenstein F, Tohyama M. 1987. Neostriatal cholinergic neurons receive direct synaptic inputs from dopaminergic axons. Brain Res 413:179–184.

32. Gerfen CR. 1989. The neostriatal mosaic: Striatal patch-matrix organization is related to cortical lamination. Science 246:385–388.

33. Kemp JM, Powell TPS. 1971. The termination of fibres from the cerebral cortex and thalamus upon dendritic spines in the caudate nucleus: A study with the Golgi method. Phil Trans R Soc London Ser B 262:429–439.

34. Fonnum F, Storm-Mathisen J, Divac I. 1981. Biochemical evidence for glutamate as neurotransmitter in corticostriatal and corticothalamic fibers in rat brain. Neuroscience 6:863–872.

35. McGeorge AJ, Faull RLM. 1987. The organization and collateralization of corticostriate neurons in the motor sensory cortex of the rat brain. Brain Res 423:318–324.

36. Kemp JM, Powell TPS. 1971. The site of termination of afferent fibers in the caudate nucleus. Phil Trans R Soc London Ser B 262:413–427.

37. Powell TPS, Cowen WM. 1956. A study of thalamostriate relations in the monkey. Brain 79:364–390.

38. Anden NE, Dahlstrom A, Fuxe K, Larsson K, Olson L, Ungerstedt U. 1966. Ascending monoamine neurons to the telencephalon and diencephalon. Acta Physiol Scand 67:313–326.

39. Steinbusch HWM, van der Kooy D, Verhofstad AAJ, Pellegrino A. 1980. Serotonergic and non-serotonergic projections from the nucleus raphe dorsalis to the caudate-putamen complex in the rat, studied by a combined immunofluorescence and fluorescent retrograde axonal labeling technique. Neurosci Lett 19:137–142.

40. Steinbusch HWM, Neiuwenhuys R, Verhofstad AAJ, van der Kooy D.

1981. The nucleus raphe dorsalis of the rat and its projection upon the caudatoputamcn: A combined cytoarchitectonic, immunohistochemical and retrograde transport study. J Physiol (Paris) 77:157–174.

41. Parent A. 1990. Extrinsic connections of the basal ganglia. Trends Neurosci 13:254–271.

42. DiFiglia M, Pasik T, Pasik P. 1980. Ultrustructure of Golgi impregnated and gold-toned spiny and apiny neurons in the monkey neostriatum. J Neurocytol 9:471–492.

43. Preston RJ, McCrea RA, Chang HT, Kitai ST. 1981. Anatomy and physiology of substantia nigra and retrorubral neurons studied by extra and intracellular recording and by horseradish peroxidase labeling. Neuroscience 6:331–344.

44. Kim JS, Bak IJ, Hassler R, Okada Y. 1971. Role of gamma-aminobutyric acid (GABA) in extrapyramidal motor system. 2. Some evidence for the existence of a type of GABA-rich strio-nigral neurons. Exp Brain Res 14:95–104.

45. Ribak CE, Vaughn JE, Roberts E. 1979. The GABA neurons and their axon terminals in rat corpus striatum as demonstrated by GAD immunocytochemistry. J Comp Neurol 187:281–284.

46. Parent A, Smith Y, Arsenault M-Y. 1987. Chemical anatomy of basal gangalia neurons in primates. Adv Behav Biol 32:3–41.

47. DiFiglia M, Aronin N, Martin JB. 1982. Light and electron microscopic localization of immunoreactive leu-enkephalin in the monkey basal ganglia. J Neurosci 2:303–320.

48. Haber SN. 1986. Neurotransmitters in the human and nonhuman primate basal ganglia. Hum Neurobiol 5:159–168.

49. Gale K, Hong J-S, Guidotti A. 1977. Presence of substance P and GABA in separate striatonigral neurons. Brain Res 136:371–375.

50. Hong J-S, Yang HY, Racagni G, Costa E. 1977. Projections of substance-P containing neurons from neostriatum to substantia nigra. Brain Res 122:541–544.

51. Lehmann J, Langer SZ. 1983. The striatal cholinergic interneuron: Synaptic target of dopaminergic terminalis. Neuroscience 10:1105–1120.

52. McNeill TH, Koek LL, Brown SA, Rafols JA. 1990. Quantitative analysis of age-related dendritic changes in medium spiny I (MSI) striatal neurons of C57BL/6N mice. Neurobiol Aging 11:537–550.

53. Marshall FJ, Joyce NJ. 1988. Basal ganglia dopamine receptor autoradiography and age-related movement disorders. Ann NY Acad Sci 515:215–225.

54. Hedreen JC, Chalmers JP. 1972. Neuronal degeneration in rat brain induced by 6-hydroxydopamine: A histological and biochemical study. Brain Res 47:1–36.

55. Hefti F, Melamed E, Wurtman JR. 1980. Partial lesions of the dopaminergic nigrostriatal system in rat brain: Biochemical characterization. Brain Res 195:123–137.

56. Mattson MP, Kater SB. 1987. Calcium regulation of neurite elongation and growth cone motility. J Neurosci 7:4034–4043.

57. Mattson PP. 1988. Neurotransmitters in the regulation of neuronal cytoarchitecture. Brain Res Rev 13:179–212.

58. Cheng H-W. 1989. Dendritic plasticity in aging striatal neurons: Changes induced by deafferentation. Wayne State University, Detroit, MI. PhD thesis.

59. Cheng H-W, Anavi Y, Goshgarian H, McNeill TH, Rafols JA. 1991. Loss and regrowth of striatal spines in adult and aged mice following ipsilateral cortical lesion: A Golgi study. J Comp Neurol (in press).

60. Lankford KL, DeMello FG, Klein WL. 1986. Transient D_1 receptor mediates dopamine inhibition of growth cone motility and neurite outgrowth in a subset of vertebrate CNS neurons. Soc Neurosci Abstr 12:1116.

61. Haydon PG, McCobb DP, Kater SB. 1984. Serotonin selectively inhibits growth cone dynamics and synaptogenesis of specific identified neurons. Science 226:561–564.

62. Bulloch AGM. 1987. Somatostatin enhances neurite outgrowth and electrical coupling of regenerating neurons in *Helisoma*. Brain Res 412:6–17.

63. Maeda T, Tohyama M, Shimizu N. 1974. Modification of postnatal development of neocortex in rat brain with experimental deprivation of locus coeruleus. Brain Res 70:515–520.

64. Brown JR, Arbuthnott GW. 1983. The electrophysiology of dopamine (D_2) receptors: A study of the actions of dopamine on corticostriatal transmission. Neuroscience 10:349–355.

65. Herrling PL, Hull CD. 1980. Iontophoretically applied dopamine depolarizes and hyperpolarizes the membrane of cat caudate neurons. Brain Res 192:441–462.

66. Geddes JW, Monaghan DT, Cotman CW, Lott IT, Kim RC, Chui HC. 1985. Plasticity of hippocampal circuitry in Alzheimer's disease. Science 230:1179–1181.

67. Cheng H-W, Anavi Y, Goshgarian H, McNeill TH, Rafols JA. 1988. Loss and recovery of striatal dendritic spines following lesions in the cerebral cortex of adult and aged mice. Soc Neurosci Abstr 14:1219.

68. Cotman CW, Nadler JV. 1978. Reactive synaptogenesis in the hippocampus. *In* Neuronal Plasticity. CW Cotman (ed). Raven Press, New York, pp. 227–271.

69. Cotman CW, Nieto-Sampedro M, Harris E. 1981. Synapse replacement in the nervous system of adult vertebrates. Physiol Rev 61:684–784.

70. Steward O, Cotman C, Lynch G. 1976. A quantitative autoradiographic and electrophysiological study of the reinnervation of the dentate gyrus by the contralateral entorhinal cortex following ipsilateral entorhinal lesions. Brain Res 114:181–200.

71. Landfield PW, Rose G, Sandles L, Wohlstadter TC, Lynch G. 1977. Patterns of astroglial hypertrophy and neuronal degeneration in the hippocampus of aged memory-deficient rats. J Gerontol 32:3–12.

72. Goss JR, Finch EC, Morgan GD. 1981. Age-related changes in glial fibrillary acidic protein mRNA in the mouse brain. Neurobiol Aging 12:165–170.

73. O'Callaghan PJ, Miller BD. 1990. The concentration of glial fibrillary acidic protein increases with age in the mouse and rat brain. Neurobiol Aging 12:171–174.
74. Stein R, Mori N, Matthews K, Lo L-C, Anderson DJ. 1988. The NGF-inducible SCG10 mRNA encodes a novel membrance-bound protein present in growth cones and abundant in developing neurons. Neuron 1:463–476.
75. Skene JHP. 1989. Axonal growth-associated proteins. Annu Rev Neurosci 12:127–156.
76. Kalil K, Skene JHP. 1986. Elevated synthesis of an axonally transported protein correlates with axon outgrowth in normal and injured pyramidal tracts. J Neurosci 6:2563–2570.
77. Reh TA, Redshaw JD, Bisby MA. 1987. Axons of the pyramidal tract do not increase their transport of growth-associated proteins after axotomy. Mol Brain Res 2:1–6.
78. Lozano AM, Doster SK, Aguayo AJ, Willard MB. 1987. Immunoreactivity to GAP-43 in axotomized and regenerating retinal ganglion cells of adult rats. Abstr Soc Neurosci 13:1389.

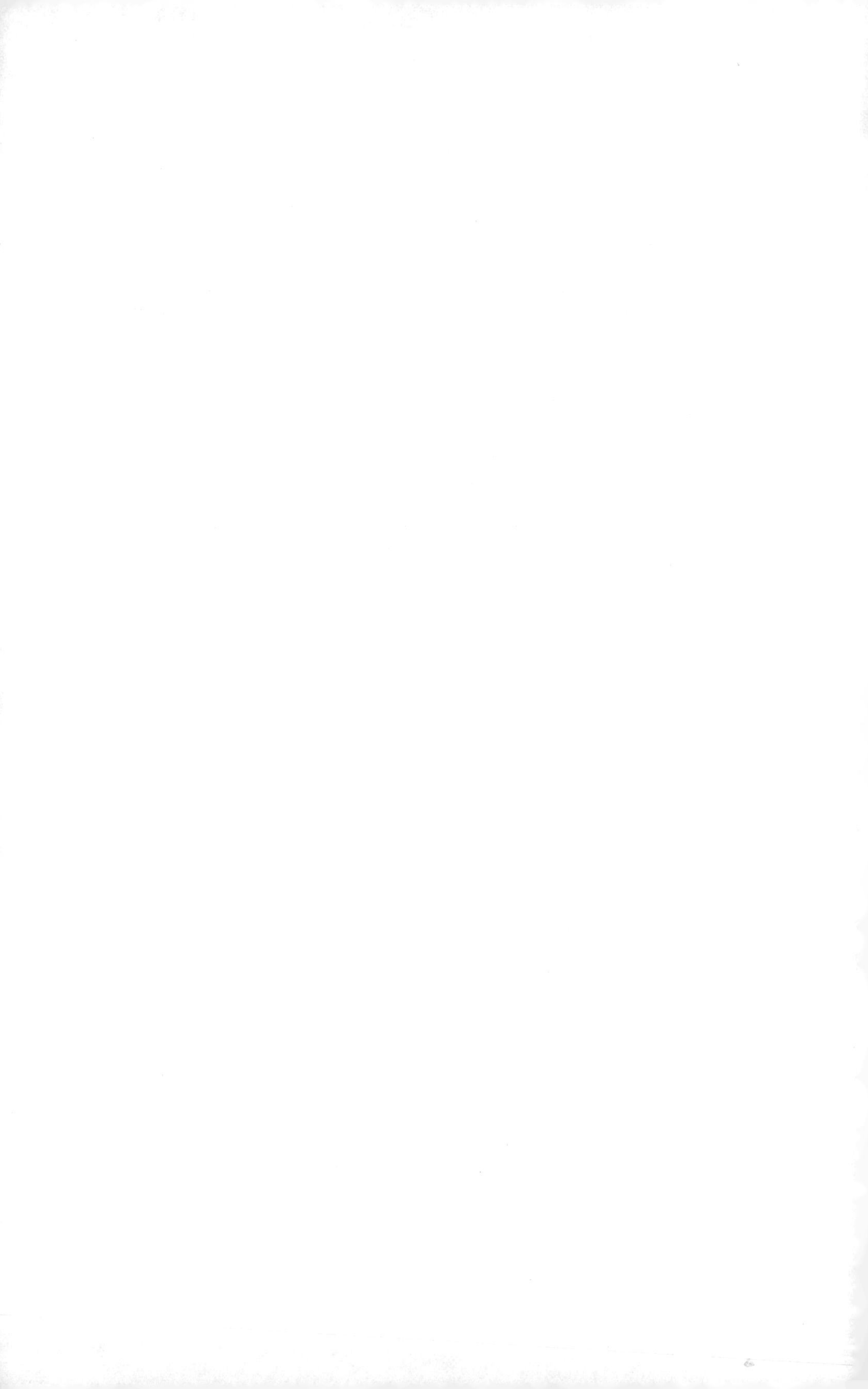

Chapter 20

3-Acetylpyridine-Induced Toxicity of the Nigrostriatal System:
Delayed Degeneration of Dopamine Neurons

*Ariel Y. Deutch, Ann C. Smith,
and Menek Goldstein*

3-Acetylpyridine (3-AP) has been known for over 30 years to induce degeneration of the inferior olivary nucleus.[1] The associated loss of the climbing fiber innervation of the cerebellum was subsequently established.[2,3] In 1974, Desclin and Escubi[3] noted degenerating neurons in the substantia nigra (SN). Subsequent studies confirmed the observation of degeneration in the SN, pars compacta.[4,5] In a recent monograph Balaban[5] reported that 3-AP administration resulted in argyrophilic profiles in both the SN and striatum, suggesting that 3-AP causes lesions in the nigrostriatal dopaminergic (DA) system. Since another pyridine neurotoxin, 1-methyl-4-phenyl-1,2,3,6-tetrahydropyridine (MPTP), causes lesions in the nigrostriatal DA system,[6] the presence of degenerating nigral neurons following 3-AP treatment suggests that two different pyridines, 3-AP and MPTP, might share certain characteristics.

This work was supported by the National Parkinson Foundation Center at Yale University and by the American Parkinson Disease Association.
From Hefti F, and Weiner WJ, (eds.) *Progress in Parkinson's Disease Research—2.* Mount Kisco NY, Futura Publishing Co., Inc., © 1992.

MPTP produces a clinical syndrome virtually indistinguishable from Parkinson's disease (PD)[7–9] and a preferential loss of the nigrostriatal DA neurons.[6,10–14] Although a preliminary communication suggested that MPTP results in cerebellar degeneration,[15] this finding awaits verification. MPTP has been reported to acutely alter glucose utilization in the inferior olive,[16] and the pyridinium metabolite of MPTP, MPP$^+$, is toxic to cerebellar granule cells in vitro.[17] Further studies will be necessary to define the extent of direct and indirect cerebellar pathology after MPTP administration.

3-AP appears to elicit both olivocerebellar and nigrostriatal degeneration.[2,5] The olivocerebellar degeneration observed after 3-AP administration has been well characterized.[2,5,18–24] In contrast, relatively little is known about the effects of 3-AP on nigrostriatal neurons. The combination of olivocerebellar and nigrostriatal lesions induced by 3-AP treatment closely resembles the pathology observed in the olivopontocerebellar atrophies (OPCA) with associated parkinsonism. The OPCAs are marked by a triad of lesions of the inferior olive, basis pontis, and cerebellum;[25–30] accordingly, OPCA patients exhibit classical cerebellar signs.[27,31–33] However, a significant percentage of OPCA patients present with parkinsonian signs,[27,31] and approximately half of the OPCA cases that come to autopsy have significant loss of neurons in the SN.[31]

The striking parallels between the pathology observed in OPCA-associated parkinsonism and 3-AP-treated rats, as well as the possible relationship of 3-AP-induced neurotoxicity and MPTP-induced nigrostriatal lesions, suggest that a broader appreciation of the consequences of 3-AP administration on the mesotelencephalic DA system may offer insights into the mechanisms of degeneration of DA neurons in PD and associated conditions. We have therefore examined the effects of 3-AP administration to rats on central DA function.

Effects of 3-AP on the Striatal Dopamine Innervation

Silver degeneration studies of the effects of 3-AP administration to rats have noted the presence of degenerating somata in the pars compacta of the SN.[3,5] We therefore examined the effects of 3-AP administration to rats on biochemical and anatomical indices of DA function. Animals were treated with the 3-AP–harmaline–

niacinamide protocol originally described by Llinas et al.,[34] with the exception that 85–90 mg/kg of the toxin was administered. Although Llinas et al.[34] suggested that this protocol resulted in selective toxicity to inferior olivary neurons, Balaban[5] reported that there was considerable damage to other central sites; our experiences[35,36] mirror those of Balaban.

Our original examination of the effects of 3-AP was done in animals surviving for 6 weeks after a single injection of the pyridine. These animals exhibited typical signs of cerebellar lesions, including gross ataxia, swaying, and a coarse tremor. Animals sacrificed at this time point had a small but significant decrease in striatal DA concentrations;[35] there was a corresponding decrease in striatal tyrosine hydroxylase (TH) activity. No changes in DA content in the nucleus accumbens or prefrontal cortex were observed. Similarly, concentrations of DA in the SN; (A9 DA cell group) and ventral tegmental area (VTA; A10 DA neurons) were not significantly different in control and 3-AP-treated animals. The lack of effect of 3-AP treatment on DA content in the SN was puzzling in the face of the modest, but significant, decrease in striatal DA levels. We therefore assessed the effects of 3-AP using immunohistochemical methods, staining for TH as a marker of DA neurons

The DA innervation of the striatum, as revealed by the distribution of TH-immunoreactive (TH-ir) fibers, differed in 3-AP-and vehicle-treated rats. Whereas the distribution of TH-ir fibers in the striatum of vehicle-treated animals was grossly homogeneous, without any clear elements of more or less intense staining, the distribution of DA fibers in the striatum of 3-AP-treated animals was clearly heterogeneous, possessing a "patchy" appearance.[36] The patchy nature of the TH-ir fiber distribution was prominent in the dorsolateral striatum, but was not observed in the ventromedial striatum. The DA innervations of the nucleus accumbens, a mesolimbic site, and the anteromedial prefrontal cortex, a mesocortical terminal field, appeared grossly normal.

Two DA innervations of the striatum can be recognized on the basis of developmental and anatomical characteristics.[37–39] The appearance of a patchy appearance of TH-ir fibers in the striatum after 3-AP treatment suggests that one of the two DA innervations was compromised (leading to a lighter appearance), or alternatively that TH protein was increased in one of the two compartments. Since we observed a decrease in striatal TH enzyme activity, the patchy appearance of the striatal DA innervation probably reflects a partial lesion of the nigrostriatal system, preferentially disrupting one of the two striatal DA compartments. Moreover, the distribution of the densely staining TH-ir patches in the dorsolateral striatum, including the subcallosal stria, suggests that the diffuse DA innervation may be the primary target of 3-AP.

The observation that only the dorsolateral striatum exhibited a patchy distribution of TH-ir fibers suggested that the small decrease in striatal DA content seen after 3-AP treatment might actually underestimate the extent of the striatal DA lesion, since we had dissected the entire striatum for the biochemical determinations. In a replication of our original study, we observed that DA levels declined by about 40% in the dorsolateral striatum, but in contrast did not significantly change in the ventromedial striatum.[36] These data suggested that 3-AP preferentially lesioned the DA innervation of the striatal sector subserving sensorimotor integration, the so-called motor striatum.[41–43] Both idiopathic PD and MPTP-induced parkinsonism also preferentially impact on the dorsolateral striatal DA innervation.[12,14,43,44]

Monoamine Oxidase Activity and 3-AP-Induced Neurotoxicity

The neurotoxicity observed after systemic administration of MPTP is due to the formation of the toxic reduced pyridinium MPP$^+$.[45,46] This metabolite is generated by the action of monoamine oxidase, type B (MAO-B);[47,48] the pyridinium then gains access to the DA neuron via the DA transporter.[49] This obligatory dependence of MPTP on MAO-B metabolism was demonstrated by the observation that MAO-B inhibitors, such as deprenyl and pargyline, prevent MPTP-induced nigrostriatal toxicity.[50,51] These studies culminated in clinical trials of deprenyl in PD.[52,53]

The precise mechanisms through which 3-AP results in cell loss are not clear. 3-AP has long been known as an antimetabolite of niacinamide. Pretreatment with niacinamide prevents 3-AP neurotoxicity,[1] and in the protocol used in our investigations, serves to rescue animals from lethal 3-AP effects (see Llinas et al.[34] and Balaban[5]). Indeed, Hicks originally suggested that 3-AP toxicity was an acceleration of niacinamide deficiency.[1] However, it is also possible that a metabolite of 3-AP represents the true neurotoxin, in a fashion analogous to MPP$^+$ being the toxic metabolite of MPTP. In order to determine if 3-AP was a potential substrate for MAO, we assessed the effects of 3-AP on MAO-A and MAO-B activity in vitro and determined if inhibition of MAO-B activity by deprenyl treatment modified 3-AP-induced nigrostriatal toxicity.[36]

3-AP was a potent inhibitor of MAO-B activity in vitro.[36] 3-AP inhibited MAO-B with an IC_{50} of 220 μM; in comparison, MPTP inhibited MAO-B activity (phenylethylamine oxidation) with an IC_{50} of 100 μM.[36] 3-AP was a very weak inhibitor of MAO-A (IC_{50} = 5 mM). While these data suggest that 3-AP may be a substrate for MAO-B, it was not possible to conclude if the pyridine is a substrate for or, alternatively, a competitive inhibitor of MAO-B. In the absence of radiolabeled 3-AP, we therefore examined the effect of deprenyl pretreatment on 3-AP toxicity. Deprenyl did not afford any protection against 3-AP-induced striatal DA depletion.[36] It therefore appears that if 3-AP is an MAO-B substrate, rather than (more likely) an inhibitor of the enzyme, the resultant metabolic product(s) of 3-AP oxidation is not toxic. Thus, 3-AP differs from MPTP in that the latter is critically dependent upon MAO-B for generation of a toxic metabolite, whereas 3-AP is not.

Effects of 3-AP on Midbrain Dopamine Neurons

3-AP treatment of rats results in biochemical and anatomical changes consistent with a partial degeneration of the striatal DA innervation. However, in our biochemical studies of the effects of 3-AP, we did not observe a change in DA concentrations in the SN or VTA. Consistent with this observation, anatomical studies did not reveal any overt changes in the number of midbrain DA neurons in animals sacrificed 6 weeks after 3-AP administration. We were somewhat puzzled by the discrepancy between the events occurring at the cell body level and those observed at the terminal fields. Balaban[5] had noted differences between different strains of rats (albino Sprague-Dawley and pigmented Long-Evans) in susceptibility to 3-AP neurotoxicity. He noted that in certain areas (such as the dorsal raphe) degenerating neurons could be seen in Long-Evans but not Sprague-Dawley rats, although no such difference in susceptibility to 3-AP-induced lesions of the SN was noted. MPTP neurotoxicity is also marked by striking differences in the susceptibility of the nigrostriatal system in different strains of mice: pigmented mice are more susceptible to the toxic actions of MPTP than albino mice.[54,55] Accordingly, we examined the effects of 3-AP administration to albino Sprague-Dawley rats (which were used in our initial studies) and Long-Evans (pigmented) rats; we also examined changes in the nigrostriatal system at various time points after 3-AP treatment.

3-AP resulted in the patchy appearance of striatal TH-ir fibers in both Sprague-Dawley (SD; from Camm Research Institute, Wayne, NJ) and Long-Evans (LE; from Harlan Sprague-Dawley, Indianapolis, IN) rats sacrificed 6 weeks after injection of the pyridine. DA concentrations in the dorsolateral striatum were significantly decreased in the LE rats, although the magnitude of the change was not as great as observed in SD rats (Figure 1). Interestingly, there was also a significant decline in DA content in the nucleus accumbens of

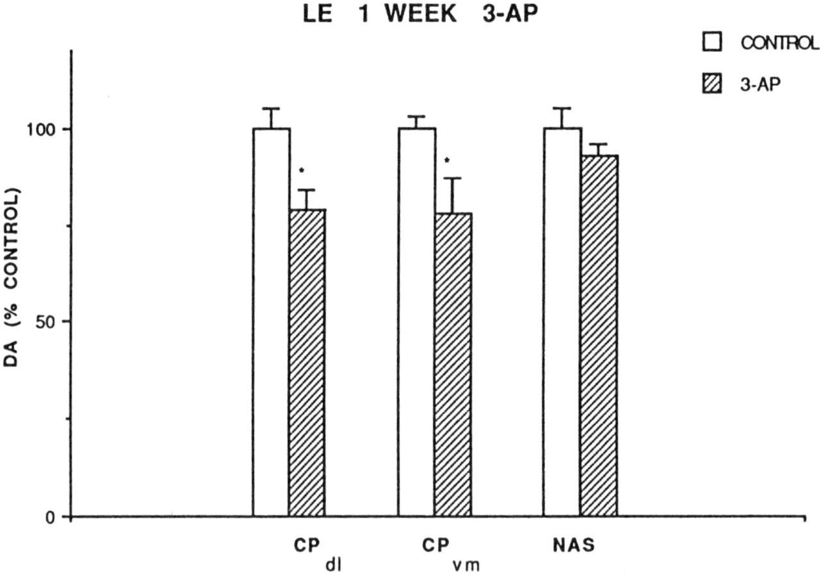

Figure 1. Dopamine concentrations in the dorsolateral (CP_{dl}) and ventromedial (CP_{vm}) and the nucleus accumbens (NAS) in Long-Evans rats 6 weeks after 3-AP treatment. DA levels were significantly decreased in both nigrostriatal sectors. *$P \leq 0.05$.

LE rats, whereas no such change was observed in SD rats (Figure 1). Thus, at 6 weeks after 3-AP treatment, LE rats exhibited the characteristic biochemical and antomical changes in the striatum that we had previously observed in SD rats. In contrast to 3-AP-treated SD rats, in LE rats surviving for 6 weeks also exhibited a small decrease in the number of A9 DA neurons.

We therefore examined the effects of shorter survival periods after 3-AP treatment. The results are shown in Table 1. At 3 weeks after 3-AP treatment, there was no apparent loss of midbrain DA neurons in either strain of rat. In contrast, the number of nigral DA neurons in LE, but not SD, rats treated with 3-AP and sacrificed 1 week later was markedly reduced (Figure 2). The loss of A9 DA neurons was predominantly restricted to the medial half of the substantia nigra. There were a number of very lightly stained TH-ir neurons in the medial nigra (Figure 2B), suggesting that the neurons were either in the process of degenerating or, alternatively, that TH

Table 1.
Temporal Evolution of Alterations in TH-Immunoreactive Neurons and Dopaminergic Innervation of Striatum following 3-AP Treatment of Albino (Sprague-Dawley) or Pigmented (Long-Evans) Rats[a]

| | Time after 3-AP Treatment | | |
	1 Week	3 Weeks	6 Weeks
Substantia nigra			
SD	−	−	−
LE	+ +	−	−/+
Dorsolateral striatum			
SD	−	+	+ +
LE	−/+	+	+ +

[a]Involvement of the dopamine system indicated by presence of pluses (+), ranging from + (mild loss) to + + + (marked degeneration); −/+ indicates that decreases in the number of neurons or the density of striatal innervation observed in some, but not all, treated animals; − indicates no gross alteration in number of substantia nigra neurons or striatal innervation. 3-AP treatment of LE rats results in an early (1 week) loss of TH-ir neurons in the substantia nigra, with recovery to normal by 3 weeks; by 6 weeks after treatment, some (but not all) animals had a small decrease in the number of SN neurons. In contrast, A9 DA neurons in SD rats do not appear affected to 1, 3, or 6 weeks after 3-AP administration.

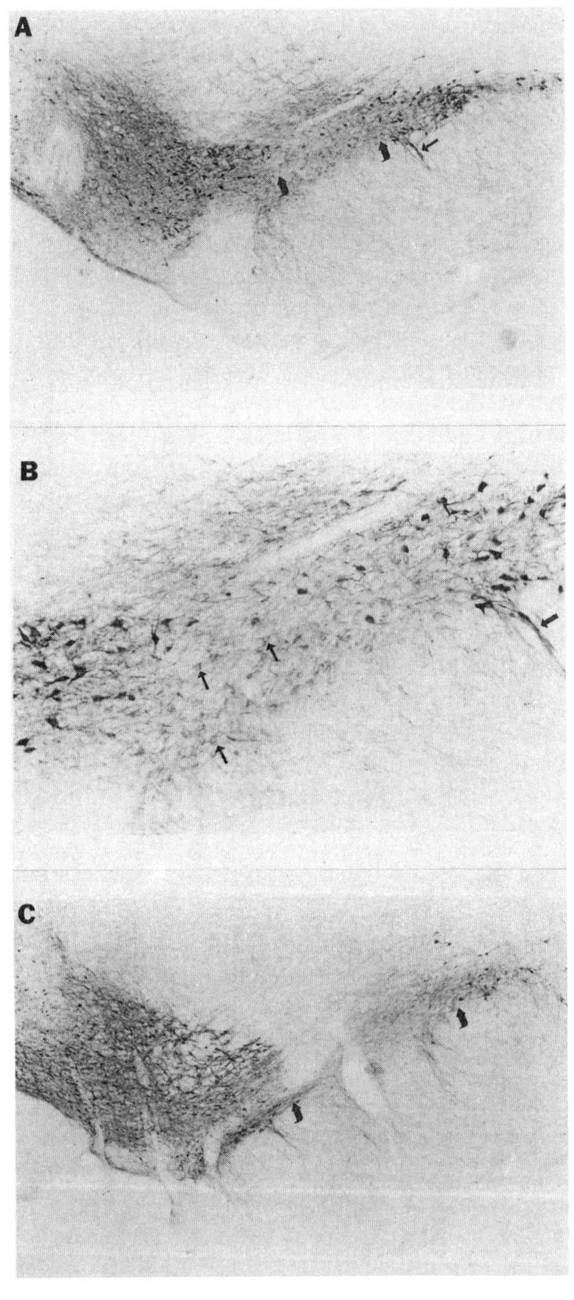

gene expression was decreased. There also appeared to be a slight loss of A10 DA neurons in the VTA in some, but not all, 3-AP-treated animals. In LE and SD rats sacrificed 3 weeks after 3-AP treatment, there was no apparent change in the number of nigral DA neurons, indicating recovery of TH-ir. When examined at 6 weeks after 3-AP treatment, there was a small decrease in the number of DA neurons in the medial SN of LE, but not SD, rats. In the LE rats, some neurons in the medial SN appeared to be atrophied. However, the number of TH-ir neurons in the SN of animals sacrificed after 6 weeks was significantly greater than observed in animals sacrificed 1 week after 3-AP treatment. Six weeks after 3-AP treatment of SD rats, the number of nigral DA neurons in appeared grossly normal.

The loss of TH-ir neurons at 1 week after 3-AP treatment of LE rats suggests that 3-AP may initially act at the cell body level. Since the number of A9 DA neurons appears to be substantially reduced at 1, but not 3, weeks after 3-AP treatment, it is clear that TH immunoreactivity is not a good marker for the neuronal integrity of DA neurons; however, it does reflect the fact that a functional insult to the DA neurons has occurred. The recovery at 3 weeks after 3-AP treatment suggests that the initial treatment may decrease TH gene expression or alter posttranslational processing of TH. This is consistent with the very weakly stained TH-ir neurons we observed in the medial SN at 1 week after 3-AP administration. It is not clear to what degree other factors contribute to the observed decrease in the number of TH-ir neurons, or if the effect is restricted to TH protein.

A discernible decrease in the number of SN DA neurons 1 week after 3-AP treatment was seen only in LE, and not SD (albino) rats. This strain dependency is similar to that seen following MPTP administration to mice.[55] It is not clear to what degree 3-AP-induced

---

Figure 2. Distribution of TH-ir neurons in the ventral mesencephalon of LE rats treated with 3-AP 1 week earlier. There is a large decrease in the number of strongly immunoreactive neurons in the pars compacta of the SN (panels A and C, between curved arrows). The DA neurons in the lateral wing of the SN appear spared. There is no gross loss of DA neurons in the VTA. The area of decreased staining shown in panel A is shown at higher magnification in panel B: a number of very lightly stained TH-ir neurons can be seen (small arrows), which stand in sharp contrast to the densely stained neurons laterally (arrow showing dendritic bundle from densely stained neurons). At more caudal levels (panel C), a similar decrease in staining is observed.

nigrostriatal lesions are manifested in species other than rats. MPTP-induced lesions of the nigrostriatal DA system have been observed in primates, felines, canines, and mice;[6,14,51,55–57] rats are significantly more resistant to the toxin.[59] We have examined the effects of 3-AP administration to both pigmented and albino mice; no disruption of the mouse nigrostriatal DA system was observed following single injections of up to 400 mg/kg in either strain. Hicks[1] reported that in two of 27 animals treated with 3-AP a few large neurons in the SN were necrotic; unfortunately, it is not clear if the animals affected were mice or rats. Other examinations of mice treated with 3-AP have reported lesions of the hippocampus but not SN.[59,60] However, Geller et al.[61] reported lesions of the SN after treatment of mice with another nicotinamide antagonist, 6-aminonicotinamide. Thus, it is not clear to what degree (if any) 3-AP impacts on nigrostriatal DA neurons in the mouse. However, it is clear that 3-AP differs from MPTP in that the former clearly causes lesions in the nigrostriatal DA neurons of rats, whereas the latter is significantly more effective in mice than rats.

The differences between various reports concerning the effects of 3-AP on nigrostriatal DA neurons are reminiscent of the early discrepancies in reports from different laboratories concerning MPTP-induced lesions in mice (see Heikilla and Sonsalla[55]). It seems likely that in order to avoid such discrepancies, careful studies of the treatment parameters, species, and strains of animals studied, and even vendors from whom the animals are obtained will be necessary. The rat is relatively sensitive to 3-AP; this is particularly so in LE-derived rats.

Similarities of Nigrostriatal Lesions in 3-AP- and MPTP-Treated Animals and Weaver Mouse

There are a number of striking similarities between the neurotoxicity of 3-AP and MPTP. These include the findings that the dorsolateral striatal DA innervation is preferentially lesioned by both toxins and the observation that the loss of midbrain DA neurons appears to lag behind terminal field changes. Moreover, the effects of MPTP and 3-AP are manifested to different degrees in different species of animals and in different strains of animals within a given species. There are also differences between the two pyridines. The toxicity of MPTP is dependent upon MAO-B and is prevented by deprenyl pretreatment, whereas 3-AP toxicity is independent of oxidation by MAO-B to a toxic metabolite. In addition, 3-AP causes massive lesions in the olivocerebellar system, but MPTP is not toxic to or only weakly causes lesions in the cerebellar motor system.

3-AP shares with a neurological mutation, the weaver mouse, certain similarities. The weaver mouse exhibits marked cerebellar degeneration.[62,63] In addition, the weaver exhibits a developmentally specific degeneration of the dorsolateral striatal DA innervation,[64–66] and a loss of nigral DA neurons.[67,68] A more restricted disruption of the DA innervation of mesolimbic sites (nucleus accumbens core and lateral olfactory tubercle) has also been reported.[66,68] Thus, the pathology of the weaver mouse is similar to that observed in 3-AP-treated rats. Some of the similarities and differences between MPTP- and 3-AP-lesioned rodents and the weaver mutant mouse are listed in Table 2.

The weaver (*wv*) mutation has recently been localized to a single locus defect.[69,70] The cerebellar degeneration and the DA cell loss seen in the weaver mouse may therefore be related to a single protein. It is intriguing to speculate that 3-AP impacts on the same protein that is altered in the weaver mutant. There are no obvious transmitters in common between DA neurons and the neurons in the cerebellum or olivary complex. A possible exception is neurotensin, which is transiently expressed in early development in the inferior olive[71] and is present in a restricted subset of midbrain DA neurons. There do appear to be small number of DA D_2 receptor sites on the climbing fiber innervation of the cerebellum.[72] However, this also appears to be an unlikely target, since the irreversible alkylation of D_2 receptors by EEDQ is not known to permanently damage DA neurons. Tyrosine hydroxylase has been reported to be transiently expressed between postnatal (P) days P21 and P35 in the cerebellar vermis of mice.[73] In the tottering and leaner mutant mice, Purkinje cells in the vermis continue to express TH throughout adulthood.[73] It remains to be determined if there is an aberrant TH expression in the weaver mouse and to what degree this pattern of TH expression is seen in the rat. However, since not all DA neurons are affected by the weaver gene, and not all midbrain DA neurons degenerate after 3-AP treatment, it would appear unlikely that TH represents a common target. More likely is a protein involved in energy metabolism, which, if involved, would compromise chances for survival of the

Table 2.
Comparison of 3-AP-Treated Rats, MPTP-Treated Primates, and Weaver Mutant Mouse[a]

	3-AP	*MPTP*	*Weaver*
Striatum dopamine system			
Dorsolateral	+ +	+ + +	+ + +
Nucleus accumbens	−/+ [b]	+/+ + [c]	+ [d]
Midbrain Dopamine Neurons			
Substantia nigra	+ +/+ + + [e]	+ + [f]	+ + [g]
Ventral tegmental area	−/+ [b]	+ [c]	−/+
Retrorubral field	−/+ [b,h]	+ + [h]	+ + [i]
Cerebellum	−/+ [j]	? [k]	+ + + [l]
Inferior Olivary Nucleus	+ + +	? [m]	− [n]
Species dependent	Yes	Yes	—
Strain dependent	Yes	Yes	—
Age-related	Yes	Yes	—[o]
MAO-B dependent	No	Yes	—
DA uptake system dependent	?	Yes	—

[a]The table provides a rough estimate of the relative involvement of the nigrostriatal and olivocerebellar system in each of these conditions. Pathological changes (loss of the dopaminergic innervation of the striatum, decreases in numbers of midbrain TH-immunoreactive neurons, loss of cerebellar or inferior olivary neurons) are graded from − (no apparent involvement) to + (mild changes) to + + + (severe pathology). Presence of −/+ indicates variable involvement, seen in some but not all animals or reports. The other footnotes detail specific characteristics.

[b]Loss of dopaminergic innervation observed in some, but not all, treated animals. Conditions necessary for expression not known. LE but not SD rats susceptible.

[c]Observed in animals with overt parkinsonian motor deficits, but not asymptomatic animals.

[d]Mild loss of the DA innervation of the nucleus accumbens core, but not shell.

[e]Early loss of the TH-ir neurons in the medial SN with subsequent recovery. Late (end stage) loss virtually complete.

[f]Similar (but with compressed temporal pattern) to 3-AP (see note e). Prominent ventral tier DA cell loss.

[g]Developmentally specific A9 cell loss, predominantly involving the ventral tier DA neurons.

[h]A8 DA cell loss mainly in the lateral aspects of the retrorubral field.

[i]A8 DA cell loss with dorsoventral thinning.

[j]Alterations in Purkinje cell morphology, but most reports indicate no overt decrease in number of cells.

[k]Single abstract suggesting changes in Purkinje cells; MPP+ toxic to granule cells in vitro.

[l]Virtually complete loss of granule cells in vermis, with less extensive Purkinje cell loss. Less marked granule cell loss in the hemispheres, but with disruption of folial structure present.

[m]No systematic examination and no documented cell loss; changes in local cerebral glucose utilization reported.

[n]No reduction in number of inferior olivary (IO) neurons, but ratio Purkinje cells:IO cells reduced.

[o]Developmentally specific pattern of loss of striatal DA innervation.

neuron. The toxic actions of the MPTP metabolite, MPP$^+$, are thought to occur by interfering with complex I in the mitochondrial electron transport chain;[74] similarly, complex I has been reported to be deficient in PD.[75,76] The effects of 3-AP and the weaver (*wv*) mutation on complex I of the mitochondrial electron transport chain have yet to be determined.

The Temporal Evolution of Nigrostriatal Damage: The Nature of Progressive Lesions

One of the most interesting aspects of 3-AP-induced nigrostriatal degeneration is the progressive nature of the lesion. There appears to be a sequence of events that occurs following 3-AP treatment. On the basis of anatomical studies, 3-AP appears to affect initially DA somata in the SN. There is a subsequent recovery of TH-ir in these DA neurons. Finally, the DA neurons of the SN degenerate, in a relatively slow process, which in some aspects resembles an accelerated senescence.

Our data suggest that 3-AP decreases the number of TH-ir neurons in the SN early after treatment, i.e., at 1 week after 3-AP administration. At this time point we have not observed gross heterogeneities in the distribution of striatal TH-ir fibers. These findings suggest that 3-AP may initially impact at the somatodendritic level. Electrophysiological studies have demonstrated that there is a transient but marked suppression of DA neuron firing shortly after MPTP administration,[77] and that DA levels in both the SN and striatum are substantially decreased 3 hours after MPTP.[77] A number of anatomical investigations have suggested that MPTP results in loss of striatal DA axons without a correspondingly marked reduction in the number of TH-ir perikarya in the SN. However, more extensive analyses of DA markers in animals sacrificed shortly after MPTP administration have revealed that there are early changes in nigral DA neurons that resolve relatively quickly. Electron microscopic studies of SN DA neurons in MPTP-treated mice have shown early (2.5 hours after-MPTP) dilation of the endoplasmic reticulum and have suggested a decrease in the number of mitochondria present;[78] these alterations essentially revert to normal by 10 hours after treatment. Moreover, a marked disruption of astrocytic processes was observed, suggesting compromised blood–brain barrier function occurs shortly after MPTP treatment. Similar electron microscopic analyses of nigral neurons in MPTP-treated dogs illustrate mitochondrial changes (swelling and disruption of christae), which are present at 1 day after MPTP treatment and became more pronounced at 4 days of survival.[79] While these changes are not consistent with the uncoupling of mitochondrial respiration, by 1 day after MPTP treatment, the pathological alterations typically associated with disruption of oxidative energy metabolism may have already occurred.[79]

The transient loss of TH-ir staining in SN DA neurons with subsequent recovery has been reported by a number of investigators.[56,80–84] As previously noted, TH-ir does not appear to serve as a reliable marker for the integrity of the DA neurons, since Nissl-stained sections reveal intact neurons in the pars compacta (see Ricaurte et al.[80]). The transient decrease in TH-ir does, however, appear to reflect injury of DA neurons, which subsequently show evidence of recovery. It is important to recognize that such "recovery" is of TH-ir cellular staining; other parameters of DA function, including TH enzymatic activity, may still be abnormal. Hallman et al.[81] demonstrated that while TH-ir neurons appeared grossly normal after MPTP treatment, DA histofluorescence in nigral neurons was markedly decreased. Mori et al.[83] demonstrated that TH-ir of SN neurons was transiently suppressed after MPTP treatment, but that staining of nigral neurons with DA antibodies was suppressed for a much longer period of time, suggesting TH function was compromised.

These findings suggest that the apparent recovery of nigral DA neurons after MPTP treatment does not adequately represent the functional status of the neuron, which may still be compromised even though TH-ir staining appears grossly normal. There is presumably a similar mechanism operative in animals treated with 3-AP. The latter pyridine results in a delayed neurotoxicity to nigral DA neurons: Balaban[5] noted that by 1 year after 3-AP treatment virtually all of the pars compacta neurons had degenerated. The tempo at which degeneration of nigral DA neurons proceeds thus appears to be relatively slow after the initial insult; it is not clear to what degree this delayed degeneration reflects an acceleration of the normal age-related decrease in DA neurons.

Conclusions

Administration of 3-AP to rats results in nigrostriatal as well as olivocerebellar toxicity. There are several similarities shared between 3-AP and MPTP, as well as distinct differences. The pattern of 3-AP-induced neurotoxicity also resembles to some degree that observed in the Weaver mutant mouse. It will be necessary to determine to what degree the degeneration of DA neurons observed after MPTP and 3-AP treatments is attributable to a common mechanism(s). The definition of the common characteristics shared by 3-AP, MPTP, and the Weaver mutation may offer insights into the mechanisms subserving degeneration of DA neurons.

Additional studies will be required to evaluate the precise characteristics of nigrostriatal degeneration after 3-AP treatment. These studies should include investigations of the biochemical and molecular mechanisms subserving 3-AP-induced neurotoxicity. The neurotoxicity of 3-AP appears to be more widespread than that observed after MPTP treatment. However, the degree to which cerebellar systems are impacted by MPTP and the extent of neuropathology present in animals allowed to survive for long periods (several years) after MPTP treatment remain to be determined. At the present time, 3-AP appears to offer a relatively good animal model for OPCA-associated parkinsonism, whereas MPTP pathology closely resembles the postencephalitic form of parkinsonism. It is important to remember that PD may not be a single entity, but rather reflects the clinical manifestations of primary loss of the nigrostriatal DA system. Thus, different forms of PD (juvenile, postencephalitic, "idiopathic") share in common the degeneration of DA neurons, which may be accomplished through a variety of mechanisms, ranging from toxins to accelerated aging processes. Hence, while 3-AP-induced neurotoxicity may resemble more closely OPCA-associated parkinsonism, it is nonetheless of relevance to PD to focus on the mechanism through which 3-AP results in nigral cell loss. This is particularly true if the slow progression of degeneration in 3-AP-treated animals represents an acceleration of aging.

The neurotoxicity of 3-AP does offer certain advantages over MPTP, which can currently be exploited. Overt symptomatology in PD is not present until striatal DA depletion is extensive. The ability to preserve function in the face of ongoing striatal DA degeneration is thought to reflect the development of compensatory mechanisms.[85–90] The development of therapeutic strategies that enhance or extend the duration over which these compensatory mechanisms are operative potentially offers certain advantages over the available pharmacologic treatments. However, in order to develop such novel therapeutic strategies, it will be necessary to specifically define the various compensatory mechanisms operative and the precise temporal sequence over which these compensatory changes are evoked. Available animal models of PD result in the relatively rapid and extensive depletion of striatal DA stores. For example, 6-hydroxydopamine lesions of the nigrostriatal system typically result in degeneration within a week. MPTP-induced nigrostriatal lesions are present relatively early following treatment, and become maximal within several months. In contrast, 3-AP-induced nigrostriatal degeneration is a process that appears to require considerably more time than MPTP for its full manifestation. The slowly evolving nature of 3-AP-induced DA degeneration may afford investigators a unique opportunity for studying the nature and progression of compensatory mechanisms which prevent overt motor impairment in the initial stages of PD.

Acknowledgments: We are grateful to A. Chistina Grobin for assistance with the biochemical assays and to Drs. J.D. Elsworth and R.H. Roth for helpful discussions.

References

1. Hicks SP. 1955. Pathological effects of antimetabolites. I. Acute lesions in the hypothalamus, peripheral ganglia and adrenal medulla caused by 3-acetylpyridine. Am J Pathol 31:189–197.
2. Desclin JC. 1974. Histological evidence supporting the inferior olive as the major source of cerebellar climbing fibers in the rat. Brain Res 77:365–384.
3. Desclin JC, Escubi J. 1974. Effects of 3-acetylpyridine on the central nervous system of the rat, as demonstrated by silver methods. Brain Res 77:349–364.
4. Butterworth RF, Hamel E, Landreville F, Barbeau A. 1978. Cerebellar ataxia produced by 3-acetyl pyridine in rat. Can J Neurol Sci 5:131–133.
5. Balaban CB. 1985. Central neurotoxic effects of intraperitoneally administered 3-acetylpyridine, harmaline, and niacinamide in Sprague-Dawley and Long-Evans rats: A critical review of central 3-acetylpyridine neurotoxicity. Brain Res Rev 9:21–42.
6. Burns RS, Chieuh CC, Markey SP, Ebert MH, Jacobowitz DM, Kopin IJ. 1983. A primate model of parkinsonism: Selective destruction of

dopamine neurons in the pars compacta of the substantia nigra by *N*-methyl-4-phenyl-1,2,3,6-tetrahydropyridine. Proc Natl Acad Sci USA 80:4546–4550.

7. Langston JW, Ballard P, Tetrud JW, Irwin I. 1983. Chronic parkinsonism in humans due to a product of meperidine-analog synthesis. Science 219:979–980.

8. Burns RS, LeWitt PA, Ebert MH, Pakkenberg H, Kopin IJ. 1985. The clinical syndrome of striatal dopamine deficiency. Parkinsonism induced by 1-methyl-4-phenyl-1,2,3,6-tetrahydropyridine (MPTP). N Engl J Med 312:1418–1421.

9. Ballard PA, Tetrud JW, Langston JW. 1985. Permanent human parkinsonism due to 1-methyl-4-phenyl-1,2,3,6-tetrahydropyridine (MPTP). Neurology 35:949–956.

10. Elsworth JD, Deutch AY, Redmond DE Jr, Sladek JR Jr, Roth RH. 1989. Symptomatic and asymptomatic 1-methyl-4-phenyl-1,2,3,6-tetrahydropyridine (MPTP)-treated primates: Biochemical changes in striatal regions. Neuroscience 33:323–331.

11. Langston JW, Forno LS, Rebert CR, Irwin I. 1984. Selective nigral toxicity after systemic administration of 1-methyl-4-phenyl-1,2,5,6-tetrahydropyridine (MPTP) in the squirrel monkey. Brain Res 292:390–394.

12. German DC, Dubach M, Askari S, Speciale SG, Bowden DM. 1988. 1-Methyl-4-phenyl-1,2,3,6-tetrahydropyridine (MPTP)-induced parkinsonian syndrome in *Macaca fascicularis:* Which midbrain dopaminergic neurons are lost? Neuroscience 24:161–174.

13. Deutch AY, Elsworth JD, Goldstein M, Fuxe K, Redmond DE Jr, Sladek JR Jr, Roth RH. 1986. Preferential vulnerability of A8 dopamine neurons in the primate to the neurotoxin 1-methyl-4-phenyl-1,2,3,6-tetrahydropyridine. Neurosci Lett 68:51–56.

14. Elsworth JD, Deutch AY, Redmond DE Jr, Sladek JR Jr, Roth RH. 1990. MPTP-induced parkinsonism: Relative changes in dopamine concentration in subregions of substantia nigra, ventral tegmental area and retrorubral field of symptomatic and asymptomatic vervet monkeys. Brain Res 513:320–324.

15. Takada M, Sugimoto T, Hattori T. 1988. Cerebellar Purkinje cells: Another neuronal basis of MPTP-induced parkinsonism. Soc Neurosci Abstr 14:1026.

16. Palombo E, Porrino LJ, Bankiewicz KS, Crane AS, Kopin IJ, Sokoloff L. 1988. Administration of MPTP acutely increases glucose utilization in the substantia nigra of primates. Brain Res 453:227.

17. Marini A, Schwartz JP, Kopin I. The neurotoxicity of 1-methyl-4-phenylpyridinium in cultured cerebellar granule cells. J Neurosci 9:3665–3672.

18. Anderson WA, Flumerfelt BA. 1980. A light and electron microscopic study of the effects of 3-acetylpyridine intoxication on the inferior olivary complex and cerebellar cortex. J Comp Neurol 190:157–164.

19. Baetens D, Garcia-Segura LM, Perrelet A. 1982. Effects of climbing fiber destruction on large dendritic spines of Purkinje cells. Exp Brain Res 48:256–262.

20. Denk H, Haider M, Kovac W, Studynka G. 1968. Verhaltenanderung und Neuropathologie bei der 3-Acetylpyridinvergiftung der Ratte. Acta Neuropathol 10:34–44.
21. Desclin JC. 1974. Early terminal degeneration of cerebellar climbing fibers after destruction of the inferior olive in the rat; synaptic relationships in the molecular layer. Anat Embryol 149:87–112.
22. Rossi F, Wiklund L, van der Want JJL, Strata P. 1989. Climbing fiber plasticity in the cerebellum of the adult rat. Eur J Neurosci 1:543–547.
23. Tapia-Arizmendi G, Feria-Velasco A. 1980. Ultrastructural changes induced by 3-acetylpyridine in the central nervous system of adult rats. Arch Invest Med 11:282–294.
24. Van der Want JJL, Wiklund L, Guegan M, Ruigrok T, Voogd J. 1989. Anterograde tracing of the rat olivocerebellar system with phaseolus vulgaris leucoagglutinin (PHA-L). Demonstration of climbing fiber collateral innervation of the cerebellar nuclei. J Comp Neurol 288:1–18.
25. Landis DMD, Rosenberg RN, Landis SC, Schut L, Nyhan WL. 1974. Olivopontocerebellar degeneration. Clinical and ultrastructural abnormalities. Arch Neurol 31:295–307.
26. Koeppen AH, Barron KD. 1984. The neuropathology of olivopontocerebellar atrophy. *In* The Olivopontocerebellar Atrophies. RC Duvoisin, A Plaitakis (eds). Raven Press, New York, pp. 13–38.
27. Berciano J. 1988. Olivopontocerebellar atrophy. *In* Parkinson's Disease and Movement Disorders. J Jankovic, E Tolosa (eds). Baltimore, Urban & Schwarzenberg, pp. 131–151.
28. Bebin EM, Bebin J, Currier RD, Smith EE, Perry TL. 1990. Morphometric studies in dominant olivopontocerebellar atrophy. Comparison of cell losses with amino acid decreases. Arch Neurol 47:188–192.
29. Albin RL, Gilman S. 1990. Autoradiographic localization of inhibitory and excitatory amino acid neurotransmitter receptors in human normal and olivopontocerebellar atrophy cerebellar cortex. Brain Res 522:37–45.
30. Kanazawa I, Kwak S, Sasaki H, Mizusawa H, Muramoto O, Yoshizawa K, Nukina N, Kitamura K, Kurisaki H, Sugita K. 1985. Studies on neurotransmitter markers and neuronal cell density in the cerebellar system in olivopontocerebellar atrophy and cortical cerebellar atrophy. J Neurol Sci 71:193–203.
31. Berciano J. 1982. Olivopontocerebellar atrophy. A review of 117 cases. J Neurol Sci 53:253–272.
32. Duvoisin RC. 1984. An apology and an introduction to the olivopontocerebellar atrophies. *In* The Olivopontocerebellar Atrophies. RC Duvoisin, A Plaitakis (eds). Raven Press, New York, pp 5–12.
33. Duvoisin RC. 1987. The olivopontocerebellar atrophies. *In* Movement Disorders II. CD Marsden, S Fahn, (eds). London, Butterworths, pp 249–269.
34. Llinas R, Walton K, Hillman DE, Sotelo C. 1975. Inferior olive: Its role in motor learning. Science 190:1230–1231.
35. Deutch AY, Rosin DL, Goldstein M, Roth RH. 1989. 3-Acetylpyridine-induced degeneration of the nigrostriatal dopamine system: An animal

model of olivopontocerebellar atrophy-associated parkinsonism. Exp Neurol 105:1–9.

36. Deutch AY, Elsworth JD, Roth RH, Goldstein M. 1990. 3-Acetylpyridine results in degeneration of the extrapyramidal and cerebellar motor systems: Loss of the dorsolateral striatal dopamine innervation. Brain Res 527:96–102.

37. Olson L, Seiger A, Fuxe K. 1972. Heterogeneity of striatal and limbic dopamine innervation: Highly fluorescent islands in developing and adult rats. Brain Res 44:283–288.

38. Graybiel AM. 1984. Correspondence between the dopamine islands and striosomes in the mammalian striatum. Neuroscience 13:1157–1187.

39. Gerfen CR, Herkenham M, Thibault J. 1987. The neostriatal mosaic: II. Patch- and matrix-directed mesostriatal dopaminergic and non-dopaminergic systems. J Neurosci 7:3915–3934.

40. Kunzle H. 1975. Bilateral projections from precentral motor cortex to the putamen and other parts of the basal ganglia. An autoradiographic study in Macacca fascicularis. Brain Res 88:195–209.

41. Pisa M. 1988. Motor functions of the striatum in the rat: Critical role of the lateral region in tongue and forelimb reaching. Neuroscience 24:453–463.

42. Sabol KE, Neill DB, Wage SA, Church W, Justice JB. 1985. Dopamine depletion in striatal subregion disrupts performance of a skilled motor task in the rat. Brain Res 335:33–43.

43. Kish SJ, Shannak K, Hornykiewicz O. 1988. Uneven pattern of dopamine loss in the striatum of patients with Parkinson's disease. N Engl J Med 318:876–880.

44. Piffl C, Bertel O, Schingnitz G, Hornykiewicz O. 1990. Extrastriatal dopamine in symptomatic and asymptomatic rhesus monkeys treated with 1-methyl-4-phenyl-1,2,3,6-tetrahydropyridine (MPTP). Neurochem Int 17:263–270.

45. Chiba K, Trevor A, Castognoli N Jr. 1985. Metabolism of the neurotoxic tertiary amine, MPTP, by monoamine oxidase. Biochem Biophys Res Commun 120:574–578.

46. Yang S-C, Johannessen JN, Markey SP. 1988. Metabolism of [^{14}C]MPTP in mouse and monkey implicates MPP$^+$, and not bound metabolites, as the operative neurotoxin. Chem Res Toxicol 1:228–233.

47. Heikkila RE, Manzino L, Cabbat FS, Duvoisin RC. 1985. Studies on the oxidation of the dopaminergic neurotoxicity of 1-methyl-4-phenyl-1,2,5,6-tetrahydropyridine by monoamine oxidase B. Br J Neurochem 45:1049–1054.

48. Bocchetta A, Piccardi MP, Del Zompo M, Pintus S, Corsini GU. 1985. 1-Methyl-4-phenyl-1,2,3,6-tetrahydropyridine: Correspondence of its binding sites to monoamine oxidase in rat brain, and inhibition of dopamine oxidative deamination in vivo and in vitro. J Neurochem 45:673.

49. Javitch JA, D'Amato RJ, Strittmatter SM, Snyder SH. 1985. Parkinson-ism-inducing neurotoxin N-methyl-4-phenyl-1,2,3,6-tetra-hydropyri-

dine: Uptake of the metabolite N-methyl-4-phenylpyridinium by dopamine neurons explains selective toxicity. Proc Natl Acad Sci USA 82:2173–2177.

50. Heikkila RE, Manzino L, Cabbat FS, Duvoisin RC. 1984. Protection against the dopaminergic neurotoxicity of 1-methyl-4-phenyl-1,2,3,6-tetrahydropyridine by monoamine oxidase inhibitors. Nature 311:467–469.

51. Langston JW, Irwin I, Langston EB, Forno LS. 1984. Pargyline prevents MPTP-induced parkinsonism in primates. Science 225:1480–1482.

52. Tetrud JW, Langston JW. 1989. The effect of deprenyl (selegiline) on the natural history of Parkinson's disease. Science 245:519–522.

53. The Parkinson Study Group. 1989. Effect of deprenyl of the progression of disability in early Parkinson's disease. N Engl J Med 321:1364–1371.

54. Heikilla RE. 1985. Differential neurotoxicity of 1-methyl-4-phenyl-1,2,3,6-tetrahydropyridine (MPTP) in Swiss-Webster mice from different sources. Eur J Pharmacol 117:131–133.

55. Heikilla RE, Sonsalla PK. 1987. The use of the MPTP-treated mouse as an animal model of parkinsonism. Can J Neurol Sci 14:436–440.

56. Schneider JS, Markham CH. 1986. Neurotoxic effects of N-methyl-4-phenyl-1,2,3,6-tetrahydropyridine (MPTP) in the cat. Tyrosine hydroxylase immunohistochemistry. Brain Res 373:258–267.

57. Turner BH, Wilson JS, McKenzie JC, Richtand N. 1988. MPTP produces a pattern of nigrostriatal degeneration which coincides with the mosaic organization of the caudate nucleus. Brain Res 473:60–64.

58. Yurek DM, Deutch AY, Roth RH, Sladek JR Jr. 1989. Morphological, neurochemical, and behavioral characterizations associated with the combined treatment of diethyldithiocarbamate and 1-methyl-4-phenyl-1,2,3,6-tetrahydropyridine. Brain Res 497:250–259.

59. Coggeshall RE, MacLean PD. 1958. Hippocampal lesions following administration of 3-acetylpyridine. Proc Soc Exp Biol Med 98:687–689.

60. Montgomery RL, Christian EL. 1976. Pathologic effects of antimetabolites on the hippocampus of diet controlled mice. Brain Res Bull 1:255–259.

61. Geller LM, Cowen D, Wolf A. 1966. Effect of the antimetabolite, 6-aminonicotinamide, on sound-induced siezures in mice. Exp Neurol 14:86–98.

62. Hirano A, Dembitzer HM. 1973. Cerebellar alterations in the weaver mouse. J Cell Biol 56:478–486.

63. Rakic P, Sidman RL. 1973. Weaver mutant mouse cerebellum: Defective neuronal migration secondary to abnormality of Bergmann glia. Proc Natl Acad Sci USA 70:240–244.

64. Roffler-Tarlov S, Graybiel AM. 1987. The postnatal development of the dopamine-containing innervation of dorsal and ventral striatum. Effects of the weaver gene. J Neurosci 7:2364–2372.

65. Doucet G, Brundin P, Seth S, Murata Y, Strecker RE, Triarhou LC, Ghetti B, Bjorklund A. 1989. Degeneration and graft-induced restoration of dopamine innervation in the weaver mouse neostriatum: A quantitative

radioautographic study of [³H]dopamine uptake. Exp Brain Res 77:552–568.

66. Roffler-Tarlov S, Graybiel AM. 1986. Expression of the weaver gene in dopamine-containing neural systems is dose-dependent and affects both striatal and non-striatal regions. J Neurosci 6:3319–3330.

67. Triarhou LC, Norton J, Ghetti B. 1988. Mesencephalic dopamine cell deficit involves areas A8, A9, and A10 in weaver mutant mice. Exp Brain Res 70:256–265.

68. Graybiel AM, Ohta K, Roffler-Tarlov S. 1990. Patterns of cell and fiber vulnerability in the mesostriatal system of the mutant mouse weaver. I. Gradients and compartments. J Neurosci 10:720–733.

69. Goldowitz D. 1989. The Weaver granuloprival phenotype is due to intrinsic action of the mutant locus in granule cells: Evidence from homozygous Weaver chimeras. Neuron 2:1565–1575.

70. Smeyne RJ, Goldowitz D. 1990. Purkinje cell loss is due to a direct action of the weaver gene in Purkinje cells: Evidence from chimeric mice. Dev Brain Res 52:211–218.

71. Mailleux P, Vanderhaeghen J-J. 1988. Transient neurotensin expression in the human inferior olive during development. Brain Res 456:199–203.

72. Charuchinda C, Supavilai P, Karobath M, Palacios JM. 1987. Dopamine D_2 receptors in rat brain: Autoradiographic visualization using a high-affinity selective agonist ligand. J Neurosci 7:1352–1360.

73. Hess EJ, Wilson MC. 1991. Tottering and leaner mutations perturb transient developmental expression of tyrosine hydroxylase in embryologically distinct Purkinje cells. Neuron 6:123–132.

74. Mizuno Y, Sone N, Saitoh T. 1987. Effects of 1-methyl-4-phenyl-1,2,3,6-tetrahydropyridine and 1-methyl-4-phenyl-pyridinium ion on activities of the enzymes in the electron transport system in mouse brain. J Neurochem 48:1787–1793.

75. Shapira AHV, Cooper JH, Dexter D, Jenner P, Clark JB, Marsden CD. 1989. Mitochondrial complex I deficiency in Parkinson's disease. Lancet 1:1269.

76. Parker WD Jr, Boyson SJ, Parks JK. 1989. Abnormalities of the electron transport chain in idiopathic Parkinson's disease. Ann Neurol 26:719–723.

77. Studer A, Sundstrom E, Jonsson G, Schultz W. 1988. Acute electrophysiological and neurochemical effects of administration of MPTP in mice. Neuropharmacology 27:923–931.

78. Adams JD Jr, Kalivas PW, Miller CA. 1989. The acute histopathology of MPTP in the mouse CNS. Brain Res Bull 23:1–17.

79. Rapisardi SC, Warrington VOP, Wilson JS. 1990. Effects of MPTP on the fine structure of neurons in substantia nigra of dogs. Brain Res 512:147–150.

80. Ricaurte GA, Langston JW, Delanney LE, Irwin I, Peroutka SJ, Forno LS. 1986. Fate of nigrostriatal neurons in young mature mice given 1-methyl-4-phenyl-1,2,3,6-tetrahydropyridine: A neurochemical and morphological reassessment. Brain Res 376:117–124.

81. Hallman H, Lange J, Olson L, Stromberg I, Jonsson G. 1985. Neurochemical and histochemical characterization of neurotoxic effects of 1-methyl-4-phenyl-1,2,3,6-tetrahydropyridine on brain catecholamine neurons in the mouse. J Neurochem 44:117–127.
82. Waters CM, Hunt SP, Jenner P, Marsden CD. 1987. An immunohistochemical study of the acute and long-term effects of 1-methyl-4-phenyl-1,2,3,6-tetrahydropyridine in the marmoset. Neuroscience 23:1025–1039.
83. Mori S, Fujitake J, Kuno S, Sano Y. 1988. Immunohistochemical evaluation of the neurotoxic effects of 1-methyl-4-phenyl-1,2,3,6-tetrahydropyridine (MPTP) on dopaminergic nigrostriatal neurons of young adult mice using dopamine and tyrosine hydroxylase antibodies. Neurosci Lett 90:57–62.
84. Schneider JS, Yuwiler A, Markham CH. 1987. Selective loss of subpopulations of ventral mesencephalic dopaminergic neurons in the monkey following exposure to MPTP. Brain Res 411:144–150.
85. Lloyd KG. 1978. CNS compensation to dopamine neuron loss in Parkinson's disease. *In* Parkinson's Disease. Neurophysiological, Clinical, and Related Aspects. FS Messiha, AD Kenny (eds). New York, Plenum Press, pp 255–266.
86. Agid Y, Javoy F, Glowinski J. 1973. Hyperactivity of DA neurons after partial destruction of nigrostriatal DA system. Nature 245:150–151.
87. Nagatsu T. 1990. Change of tyrosine hydroxylase in the parkinsonian brain and in the brain of MPTP-treated mice as revealed by homospecific TH activity. Neurochem Res 15:425–429.
88. Wolf ME, Zigmond MJ, Kapatos G. 1989. Tyrosine hydroxylase content of residual striatal dopamine nerve terminals following 6-hydroxydopamine administration: A flow cytometric study. J Neurochem 53:879–885.
89. Zigmond MJ, Abercrombie ED, Berger TW, Grace AA, Stricker EM. 1990. Compensations after lesions of central dopaminergic neurons: Some basic and clinical implications. Trends Neurosci 13:290–295.
90. Janson AM, Fuxe K, Goldstein M, Deutch AY. 1991. Hypertrophy of dopamine neurons in the primate following ventromedial mesencephalic tegmentum lesions. Exp Brain Res. 87:232–238.

Chapter 21

Transferrin Receptor Numbers are Altered in Parkinson's Disease and Experimental Dopaminergic Denervation

Deborah C. Mash and William J. Weiner

Parkinson's disease is a progressive neurodegenerative disorder that is characterized by the marked degeneration of nigrostriatal dopaminergic neurons. The pathogenetic event that causes nigral cell degeneration in Parkinson's disease is unknown, although dopaminergic neurons are susceptible to a variety of insults. Considerable interest has been focused on the role of environmental toxins that may lead to the death of nigral dopamine-containing neurons.[1–4] The neuronal complement of dopamine transporters may confer a differential cellular vulnerability resulting from the high-affinity uptake of endogenous or exogenous toxins into the dopaminergic nerve terminal.[5] Selective increases in iron and lipid peroxidation and decreased glutathione oxidizing capacity within the substantia nigra indicate that the disease process may render dopaminergic neurons highly vulnerable to oxidative stress.[6]

From Hefti F, and Weiner WJ, (eds.) *Progress in Parkinson's Disease Research—2.* Mount Kisco NY, Futura Publishing Co., Inc., © 1992.

Iron and Parkinson's Disease

Trace metals have been linked to a diverse number of physiological functions in brain, including neurotransmitter synthesis, release, storage, and binding to dopaminergic receptor recognition sites.[7,8] Several reports have suggested a role for trace metals in the breakdown of neuronal integrity known to occur with normal aging and in neurodegenerative diseases. Alterations in copper for Wilson's disease,[9] aluminum for Alzheimer's disease,[10] and manganese[11] and iron[12-14] for Parkinson's disease have provided support for the hypothesis that trace element derangements in brain may play a role in or contribute to the pathophysiology of these neurodegenerative disorders.

Interest in the role of iron in the cellular pathology of Parkinson's disease was stimulated by an early study of Earle,[15] suggesting an increased content of iron in formalin-fixed tissues and by the results of magnetic resonance imaging.[16] Using X-ray microanalysis, a recent study confirmed that iron is increased in the substantia nigra of patients with Parkinson's disease.[14] Iron determinations within nigral loci were compared between patients with Parkinson's disease and those with progressive supranuclear palsy (PSP). PSP is a parkinsonian syndrome associated with neuronal loss in the substantia nigra without the presence of Lewy bodies. A particular role for iron in the pathophysiology of Parkinson's disease was supported by the finding of strikingly high levels of iron in the Lewy bodies as compared to other mesencephalic areas. The central gray substance, an area devoid of lesions in the disease, did not have increased iron levels. Thus, the increased iron in nigral loci was not likely to have resulted from neuronal death, because it was not observed in PSP.

Environmental toxins or pollutants that are structurally related to the potent dopaminergic neurotoxin, MPTP, may lead to the selective loss of nigral neurons.[1] It has been suggested that the active metabolite of MPTP, MPP$^+$, may kill nigral neurons by free radical-induced lipid peroxidation.[17,18] This cascading neurodegenerative process may continue well into the end-stages of the disease. The cytotoxic events ongoing in the basal ganglia and the substantia nigra may be stimulated by abnormal iron handling, since Fe^{2+} is known to promote oxygen radical formation.[19,20] A general feature of the participation of transition metal ions in radical reactions is that they convert poorly reactive species into more reactive ones. The findings of increased amounts of iron in the parkinsonian brain[12–14] are of interest since hydroxyl radical formation presumably would be enhanced due to the interaction of ferrous iron with hydrogen peroxidase generated by MAO activity[6]. In keeping with this hypothesis, a shift in the iron(II)–iron(III) ratio in favor of iron(III) and the increased levels of ferritin, the iron binding protein, in the substantia nigra in the parkinsonian brain have been reported.[22] Basal lipid peroxidation in the substantia nigra is also increased in Parkinson's disease.[18]

The mechanisms responsible for selective iron accumulation in Parkinson's disease remain to be determined. One possibility is a disease-related dysregulation of iron storage or transport within the putamen and substantia nigra. Transferrin and its receptor mediate the intracellular uptake and transport of iron into neurons and glia.[23] Cellular iron metabolism is self-regulated through iron-dependent changes in the abundance of the iron storage protein ferritin.[24] If the intracellular iron pool is regulated by receptor-mediated ferrotransferrin uptake, then an up-regulation of transferrin receptor number may play a role in the pathogenesis of nigral cell damage in Parkinson's disease.

Transferrin Receptor Regulation in Parkinson's Disease

Regional brain iron concentration varies widely in normal and diseased brain.[25–28] In pathological conditions increased iron deposition is often highest precisely within those brain areas that have normally high iron concentrations. In the human brain, iron content is highest within the extrapyramidal system.[28] However, exactly how iron is transported in the CNS and deposited in high concentrations within discrete brain nuclei, such as the substantia nigra and the putamen, is unknown at present. Iron is normally stored in an inactive form bound to intracellular ferritin or hemosiderin. Transferrin is an 80,000-molecular-weight glycoprotein that functions primarily to transport iron to the cell.[29,30] Transferrin and its receptor are involved in the regulation, intracellular delivery, transport, and subsequent sequestration of iron in brain (Figure 1). Transferrin measurements in rat choroid plexus demonstrate comparable rates of synthesis to those measured in the liver, which is the principal site of

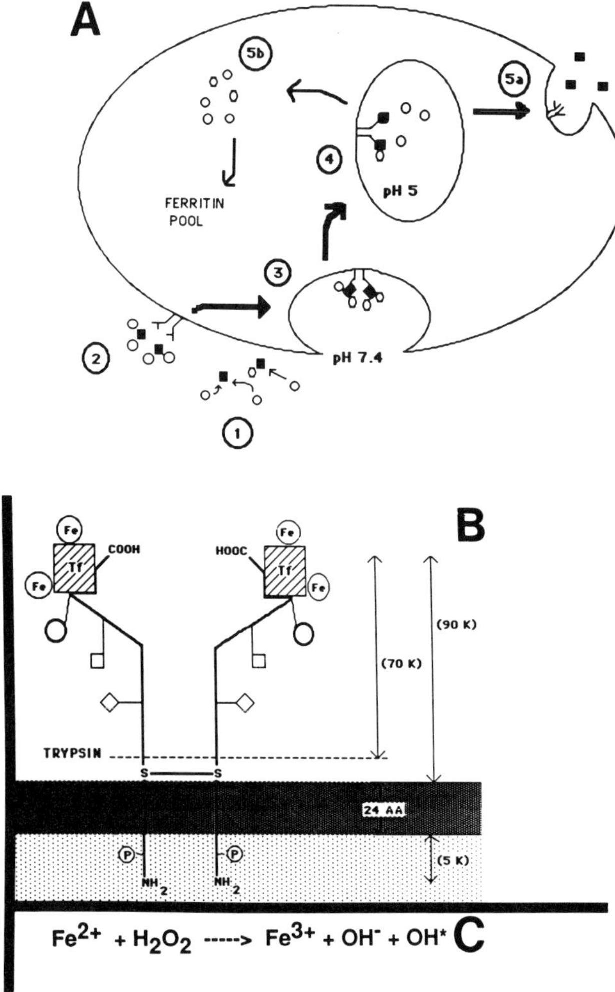

Figure 1. Cellular function of the transferrin receptor and its role in iron uptake. (A) Transferrin is taken up by cells after it binds to its cell surface receptor. The exposure of ferrotransferrin to acidic pH in endosomes results in the rapid dissociation of iron from transferrin. (B) The transferrin receptor is a disulfide linked dimer of 90-kDa glycoprotein subunits capable of binding two transferrin molecules. (C) Abnormal iron handling by receptor-mediated transferrin uptake or a dysregulation in ferritin, the iron storage protein, may lead to the formation of oxyradicals.

plasma transferrin production.[31,32] In addition, transferrin receptors have been demonstrated on endothelial cells of brain capillaries, further suggesting that circulating transferrin gains access to the central nervous system through receptor-mediated transport across the blood–brain barrier. Immunocytochemical localization studies of monoclonal antibodies to rat and human transferrin have demonstrated transferrin-immunopositive oligodendrocytes, astrocytes and neurons.[33]

We have demonstrated that [^{125}I]ferrotransferrin binds with high affinity to striatal membranes in the human brain.[26] The [^{125}I]ferrotransferrin binding site is saturable and displays pharmacologic characteristics that are similar to the transferrin receptor characterized in the rodent brain.[33] The binding affinities (K_d values) for the putamen from control and Parkinson's disease subjects were not significantly different. The affinity constants for the radioligand assayed in the putamen ranged from 2 to 4 nM. Competition binding studies further demonstrate that the affinity of the [^{125}I]ferrotransferrin binding site was not altered in Parkinson's disease. The inhibition constants (IC_{50}) values for ferrotransferrin binding gave a K_i value of 4.5 nM in parkinsonian subjects, which agrees with the affinity constant calculated from the equilibrium binding data. These results demonstrate that the affinity of the iron transport receptor for ferrotransferrin is not altered by the disease process.

Regional assays of the number of transferrin receptors in Parkinson's disease and control subjects demonstrate that the density of transferrin receptors assayed in the putamen was reduced significantly as compared to age-matched subjects.[33] The pattern of dopamine loss in the parkinsonian brain is known to be most severe in the putamen.[35] Previous studies in the primate have demonstrated that the putamen was more responsive to the effects of MPTP, manifesting a greater deficit in dopaminergic markers than in the caudate nuclei.[36] In normal subjects, the density of transferrin receptors was highest in the putamen, with lower numbers of sites assayed in both the globus pallidus and the caudate nucleus (Figure 2). Transferrin receptor densities in the putamen were reduced significantly in idiopathic Parkinson's disease ($P > 0.05$). The reduction in the total number of transferrin receptors assayed in the Parkinson's disease subjects ranged from 20% to 50% of control values. In contrast, the density of transferrin receptors assayed in the head of the caudate nucleus was not significantly different from

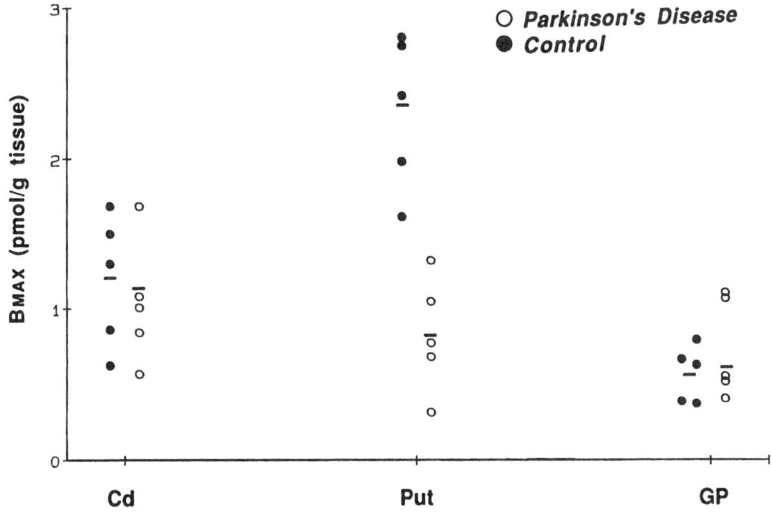

Figure 2. The number of transferrin receptors assayed in the putamen from Parkinson's disease patients was significantly different from nonneurological (control) subjects (Student's *t* test, $P < 0.05$). Cd, caudate; Put, putamen; GP, globus pallidus.

values obtained in age-matched control subjects. These data are in keeping with previous neurochemical observations that demonstrate that in idiopathic Parkinson's disease, the dopamine loss in the putamen was more severely depleted than in the caudate nucleus.[35] In Parkinson's disease, the highest concentrations of dopamine were seen at middle levels of the caudate nucleus taken at the level of the optic chiasm and globus pallidus. This pattern of relative dopamine sparing in the caudate nuclei in Parkinson's disease agrees with the regional assays of transferrin receptor numbers. The density of transferrin receptors assayed in the globus pallidus was unaltered in Parkinson's disease.

Effects of MPTP Treatment on Density of Striatal Transferrin Receptors and Dopamine Transporters

We have demonstrated a marked reduction in the density of both transferrin receptors and [^{3}H] mazindol binding to dopamine transport sites in the mouse striatum 7 days after MPTP treatment.[33] Quantitative densitometric analysis of [125I]ferrotransferrin and [3H] mazindol binding site autoradiograms demonstrated a rapid recovery in [125I]ferrotransferrin binding in the striata of mice sacrificed at later survival times. The time course for the recovery of striatal transferrin receptors preceded the rise in [3H]mazindol binding sites. To establish the time course for the effects of MPTP treatment on the striatal densities of transferrin receptors and [3H]mazindol uptake sites, regional microdensitometric measurements were made within the medial core of the mouse striatum. Transferrin receptors and dopamine uptake site densities (expressed in picomoles per gram of tissue) at different survival times are shown in Figure 3. Region-of-interest microdensitometric measurements of [3H]mazindol binding revealed a 40% depletion in the number of striatal dopaminergic uptake sites at 7 days after MPTP treatment. The number of [3H]mazindol sites was decreased to the same extent up to 28 days after MPTP treatment. At 56 days after MPTP treatment, the number of [3H]mazindol binding sites was increased to near normal levels. The density of transferrin receptors in the mouse striatum were markedly reduced at 7 and 10 days after MPTP treatment. Transferrin receptor number determined at these time points was reduced to 20% of control values. Individual striatal densitometric measurements demonstrated further that the number of transferrin receptors correlated significantly with the density of [3H]mazindol binding sites at 7 and 10 days after MPTP treatment($r = 0.82$, $P < 0.05$). In contrast to the slow recovery in [3H]mazindol binding, the number of striatal transferrin receptors was elevated to approximately 50% of control values at 14 days after MPTP treatment. The binding of [125I]ferrotransferrin to striatal transferrin receptors recovered to ∽90% of control values at the later survival times.

In vitro autoradiography of [125I]ferrotransferrin and [3H]mazindol binding in the MPTP-treated mouse striatum demonstrates a recovery in the density of transferrin receptors and dopamine uptake sites at later survival times. However, the trend toward recovery of striatal [3H]mazindol binding lagged temporally behind the 'normalized' expression of transferrin receptors. In MPTP-treated C57 black mice, dopaminergic parameters are known to show variable rates of recovery, depending upon the dose regimen of MPTP.[37,38] It has been suggested that the recovery in dopaminergic markers following MPTP treatment may result from the collateral sprouting of undam-

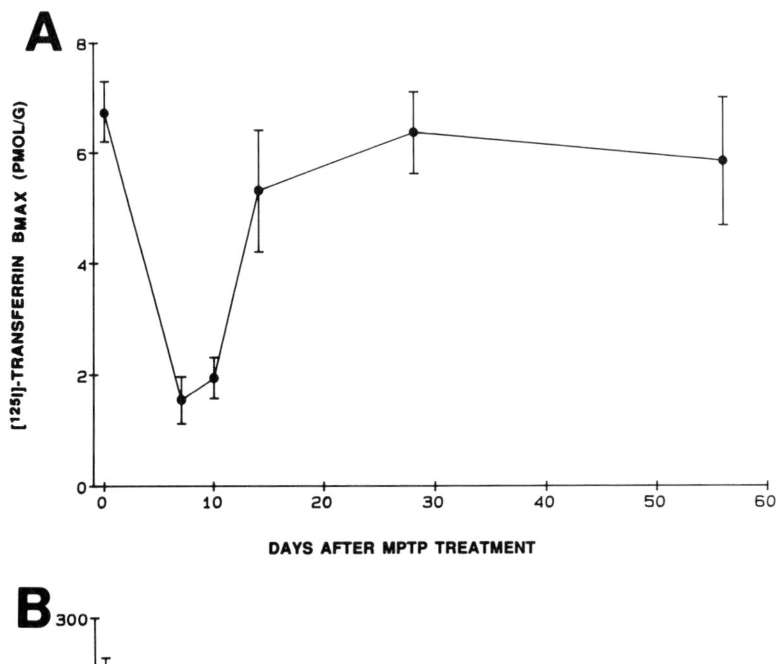

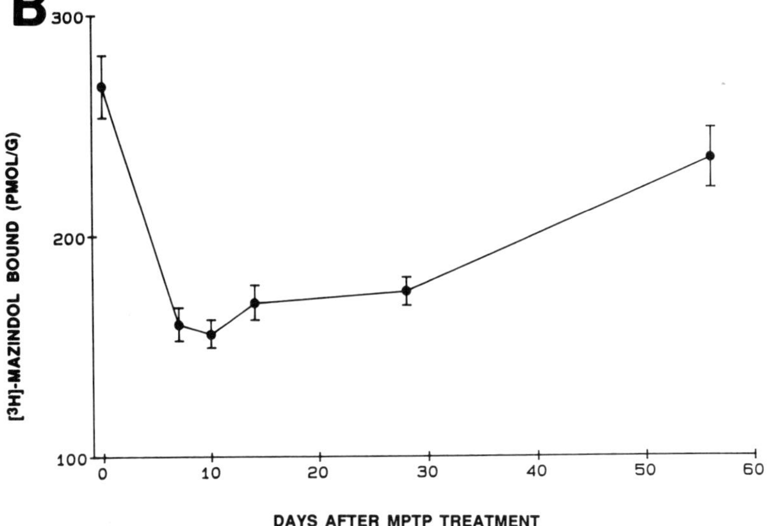

Figure 3. Densitometric analysis of [³H]mazindol binding site and transferrin receptor autoradiograms in the striatum of control and MPTP-treated mice. (A) Time course for the effects of MPTP on the density of transferrin receptors in the mouse striatum. (B) Time course for the effects of MPTP on the density of [³H]mazindol binding site labeling to the striatal dopamine transporter. Mean values were compared to control values using the Student's *t* test.

aged dopaminergic terminals.[39,40] In addition, compensatory changes in dopamine metabolism may account, in part, for the neurochemical recovery observed in some studies. The sustained recovery of transferrin binding observed in the striatum at the later time points may be due to the regenerative sprouting of dopaminergic afferents. The apparent "early" recovery of transferrin receptor densities may result from an up-regulation of transferrin receptor numbers in surviving striatal dopaminergic terminals as a compensatory cellular adaptation to increased striatal metabolic activity.

Functional Implications of Altered Iron Transport in Parkinson's Disease

The active metabolite of MPTP, MPP$^+$, is known to inhibit mitochondrial energy production, with consequent reductions in the levels of cellular ATP. Iron is a major catalytic component of mitochondrial electron transport, and it also serves as a cofactor for several mitochondrial enzymes.[39] The uptake of transferrin-bound iron by neurons involves their receptor-mediated endocytosis and internalization of the transferrin-receptor complex followed by intracellular release, transport, and storage.[29,30] We have previously speculated that the observed heterogeneity in the regional expression of transferrin receptors in the brain may parallel areas that require high basal rates of energy metabolism.[34] The brain derives most of its energy from oxidative metabolism. Since there is a tight coupling between energy metabolism and neuronal activity,[40] regions with high metabolic demands may have correspondingly increased numbers of transferrin receptors on their cell surface in order to facilitate the uptake and intracellular transport of iron. Early compensatory changes in dopaminergic transmission after exposure to MPTP may require enhanced expression of transferrin receptors to facilitate the uptake of iron to meet the increased metabolic demand resulting from striatal dopaminergic denervation.

The release of transferrin-bound iron is known to function also in a number of additional intracellular processes, including to provide iron as a cofactor for monoamine synthesis and degradation. Iron is required as a cofactor for the synthetic enzyme tyrosine hydroxylase and for the mitochondrial enzyme monoamine oxidase. In addition to having the highest MAO activities in brain, the striatum has high metabolic activity, high lipid and oxygen consumption, and an elevated iron content.[11] Taken together, these cellular properties make this brain region highly susceptible to free-radical-induced lipid peroxidation. Iron must exist in a free form as part of the intracellular mobile pool to participate in the formation of oxyradicals.[20] Transferrin receptors are elevated over the substantia nigra in the rat brain[34] and are depleted concomitantly with dopaminergic terminals in the MPTP-treated mouse striatum.[33] Given the iron dependancy for both synthetic and degradative enzyme activities, dopaminergic neurons may express transferrin receptors on their cell surface to facilitate the uptake of iron bound to transferrin.

If the intracellular iron pool is regulated by receptor-mediated ferrotransferrin uptake, then an up-regulation of transferrin receptor number may play a role in the pathogenesis of nigral cell damage in Parkinson's disease. The surviving dopaminergic neurons may increase the number of transferrin receptors in order to meet the increased metabolic demand associated with compensatory changes in dopamine synthesis and turnover. In addition to its metabolic functions, transferrin has growth factor effects.[41] Early in the disease process, dopaminergic neurons attempting to recover function in the denervated parts of the striatum may have increased requirements for receptor-mediated cellular iron uptake and metabolism for repair and regeneration processes. Since the iron storage protein ferritin is not up-regulated in Parkinson's disease,[42] this imbalance could result in an elevated cellular pool of free iron leading to a slow build-up of toxic oxyradicals.

References

1. Kopin IJ, Marker SP. 1988. MPTP toxicity: Implications for research in Parkinson's disease. Annu Rev Neurosci 11:81–96.
2. Langston JW, Ballard P. 1983. Chronic parksinonism in humans due to a product of meperidine-analog synthesis. Science 219:979–981.
3. Michel PP, Dandapani BK, Sanchez-Ramos J, Efange S, Pressman BC, Hefti F. Toxic effects of potential environmental neurotoxins structurally related to 1-methyl-4-phenylpyridinium on cultured rat dopaminergic neurons. J Pharmacol Exp Ther 248:842–850.
4. Snyder SH, D'Amato RJ. 1985. MPTP: A neurotoxin relevant to the pathophysiology of Parkinson's disease. Neurology 36:250–258.
5. Uhl GR. 1990. Parkinson's disease: Neurotransmitters and neurotoxin receptors and their genes. Eur Neurol 30(suppl 1):21–30.

6. Gotz ME, Freyberger A, Riederer P. 1990. Oxidative stress: A role in the pathogenesis of Parkinson's disease. J Neural Transm 29(suppl): 241–249.

7. Tucker DM, Swenson RA, Sanstead HH. Neuropsychological effects of iron deficiency. 1983. *In* Neurobiology of the Trace Elements. IE Dreosit, RM Smith (eds.) Vol. 1(8):269–291.

8. Donaldson J. 1981. The pathophysiology of trace metal: Neurotransmitter interaction in the CNS. Trends Pharmacol Sci 1:75–77.

9. Scheinberg IH, Sternleib I. 1984. Wilson's Disease. WB Saunders, Philadelphia.

10. Birchall JD, Chappell JS. 1988. Aluminum, chemical physiology and Alzheimer's disease. Lancet 2:1008–1010.

11. Donaldson J, Barbeau A. 1985. Manganese neurotoxicity: Possible clues to the etiology of human brain disorders. *In* Neurology and Neurobiology, Vol 15: Metal Ions in Neurology and Psychiatry. S. Gabay, J. Harris, BT Ho (eds). Alan R. Liss, New York, pp 259–285.

12. Dexter D, Carter C, Javoy-Agid F, Agid Y, Lees AJ, Jenner P, Marsden CD. 1987. Increased nigral iron content in the post mortem parkinsonian brain. Lancet 2:1219–1220.

13. Sofic E, Riederer P, Heinsen H, Beckmann H, Reynolds GP, Hebenstreit G, Youdim MBH. 1988. Increased iron(III) and total iron content in post mortem substantia nigra of parkinsonian brain. J Neural Transm 74:199–205.

14. Hirsch EC, Brandel J-P, Galle P, Javoy-Agid F, Agid Y. 1991. Iron and aluminum increase in the substantia nigra of patients with Parkinson's disease: An X-ray microanalysis. J Neurochem 56:446–451.

15. Earle KM. 1968. Studies in Parkinson's disease including X-ray fluorescence spectroscopy of formalin fixed tissue. J Neuropathol Exp Neurol 27:1–14.

16. Rutledge JN, Hilal SK, Silver AJ, Defendini R, Fahn S. 1987. Study of movement disorders and brain iron by MR. Am J Neuroradiol 8: 397–411.

17. Dexter D, Carter C, Agid F, Agid Y, Lees AJ, Jenner P, Marsden CD. 1986. Lipid peroxidation as a cause of nigral cell death in Parkinson's disease. Lancet 2:639–640.

18. Dexter D, Carter C, Wells FR, Javoy-Agid F, Agid Y, Lees AJ, Jenner P, Marsden CD. 1989. Basal lipid peroxidation in substantia nigra is increased in Parkinson's disease. J Neurochem 52:381–389.

19. Halliwell B. 1987. Oxidants and human disease: Some new concepts. Fed Am Soc Exp Biol 892:358–364.

20. Halliwell B, Gutteridge JMC. 1986. Oxygen free radicals and iron in relation to biology and medicine: Some problems and concepts. Mol Aspects Med 8:89–193.

21. Reiderer P, Konradi C, Hebenstreit G, Youdim MBH. 1986. Neurochemical perspectives to the function of monoamine oxidase. Acta Neurol Scand 126:41–45.

22. Riederer P, Sofic E, Wolf-Dieter R, Schmidt B, Reynolds GP, Jellinger K,

Youdim MBH. 1988. Transition metals, ferritin glucathione, and ascorbic acid in parkinsonian brains. J. Neurochem 52:515–520.

23. Swaiman KF, Machen VL. 1986. Iron uptake by mammalian cortical neurons. Ann Neurol 16:66–70.

24. Thiel EC. 1990. Regulation of terratin and transferrin receptor mRNAs. J Biol Chem 265:4771–4774.

25. Norfray JF, Couch JR, Elbe RJ, Good DC, Manyam BV, Patrick JL. 1988. Visualization of brain iron by mid-field MR. Am J Neuroradiol 9:77–82.

26. Dwork AJ, Schon EA, Herbert J. 1988. Nonidentical distribution of transferrin and ferric iron in human brain. Neuroscience 27:333–345.

27. Tennison MB, Bouldin MD, Whaley RA. 1988. Mineralization of the basal ganglia detected by CT in Hallervorden-Spatz syndrome. Neurology 38:154–155.

28. Hock A, Demmel U, Schicha H, Kasperek K, Feinendegen LE. 1975. Trace element concentration in human brain. Brain 98:49–64.

29. Huebers HA, Finch CA. 1987. The physiology of transferrin and transferrin receptors. Physiol Rev 67:520–582.

30. Newman R, Schneider C, Sutherland R, Vodinelich L, Greaves M. 1982. The transferrin receptor. TIBS 7:397–400.

31. Aldred AR, Dickson PE, Marley PD, Schreiber G. 1987. Distribution of transferrin synthesis in brain and other tissues of the rat. J Biol Chem 262:5293–5297.

32. Dickson PW, Aldred AR, Marley PD, Guo-Fen T, Howlett GJ, Schreiber G. 1985. High prealbumin and transferrin mRNA levels in the choroid plexus of rat brain. Biochem Biophys Res Commun 127:890–895.

33. Mash DC, Pablo J, Buck BE, Sanchez-Ramos J, Weiner WJ. 1991. Distribution and number of transferrin receptors in Parkinson's disease and in MPTP-treated mice. Exp Neurol 114:73–81.

34. Mash DC, Pablo J, Flynn DD, Efange SMN, Weiner WJ. 1990. Characterization and localization of transferrin receptors in the rat brain. J Neurochem 55:1972–1979.

35. Kish SJ, Shannak K, Hornykewicz O, 1988. Uneven pattern of dopamine loss in the striatum of patients with idiopathic Parkinson's disease: Pathophysiologic and clinical implications. N Engl J Med 318:876–880.

36. Irwin I, DeLanney LE, Forno LS, Finnegan KT, Di Monte DA, Langston JW. 1990. The evolution of nigrostriatal neurochemical changes in the MPTP-treated squirrel monkey. Brain Res 531:242–252.

37. Sonsalla PK, Heikkila RE. 1986. The influence of dose and dosing interval on MPTP-induced dopaminergic neurotoxicity in mice. Eur J Pharmacol 129:339–345.

38. Ricaurte GA, Langston JW, Delanney LE, Irwin I, Peroutka S, Forno LS. 1986. Fate of nigrostriatal neuronsin young mature mice given 1-methyl-4-phenyl-1,2,3,6-tetrahydropyridine: A neurochemical and morphological reassessment. Brain Res 375:117–124.

39. Youdim MBH. 1985. Brain iron metabolism: Biochemical and behavioral aspects in relation to dopaminergic neurotransmission. *In* Handbook of Neurochemistry, Vol. 10. A. Lajtha (ed). New York. pp 731–757.

40. Sokoloff L. 1981. Localization of functional activity in the central

nervous system by measurement of glucose utilization with radioactive deoxyglucose. J Cereb Blood Flow Metab 1:7–36.

41. Raivich G, Graeber MB, Gehrman J, Kreutzberg GW. 1991. Transferrin receptor expression and iron uptake in the injured and regenerating rat sciatic nerve. Eur J Neurosci 3:919–927.

42. Jenner P, Dexter DT, Schapira AHV, Marsden CD. 1991. Free radical involvement and altered iron metabolism as a cause of Parkinson's disease. *In* The Assessment and Therapy of Parkinson's Disease. CD Marsden, S Fahn (eds). Park Ridge, NJ: Parthenon Publishing, pp 17–30.

5

Weaver Mutant

Chapter 22

The Weaver Mutation:
A Murine Paradigm of Parkinson's Disease

Suzanne K. Roffler-Tarlov

Parkinsonian symptoms occur as a consequence of the death of dopamine-containing neurons. The death of these neurons can result from environmental toxins, from genetic causes, or possibly from combinations of these. For example, a genetic predisposition to the effects of an environmental toxin could be important. Research accomplished during the past decade that has described and analyzed the death of dopamine-containing neurons after the administration of neurotoxins such as 6-hydroxydopamine and 1-methyl-4-phenyl-1,2,5,6-tetrahydropyridine (MPTP) to animals,[1–3] has established firmly the possibility that environmental toxins are likely to play a key role in Parkinson's disease. Davis et al.[4] and Langston et al.[5] have established that MPTP induces parkinsonian symptoms in humans. By contrast, opinion as to the importance of the contribution of heredity to the cause of Parkinson's disease has been cyclic as new information seems to reveal alternately more and then less involvement of genetic factors. Clusters of Parkinson's-like disease that occur in family groups as well as the observation of parkinsonian symptoms that occur within known genetic neurological disorders have suggested a genetic con-

The studies were supported by NIH grant Ns20181 and the Parkinson's Disease Foundation. S.K.R.-T. is the recipient of a Research Scientist Development Award (MH00655).
From Hefti F, and Weiner WJ, (eds.) *Progress in Parkinson's Disease Research—2.* Mount Kisco NY, Futura Publishing Co., Inc., © 1992.

tribution to idiopathic Parkinson's disease.[6,7] Carefully documented family histories and diagnoses later failed to support the hereditary hypothesis and the low concordance rate among monozygotic twins deflated, although never thoroughly demolished, it.[8] Recently, the genetic hypothesis has received a new infusion of support from the discovery of two large kindreds with Parkinson's disease that appear to be inherited with an autosomal dominant pattern.[9] Thus, genetic causes are being examined now with heightened interest.[8,10]

Although genetic involvement in the death of neurons in Parkinson's disease is still debated, it is certain that the viability of mesencephalic dopamine-containing neurons depends upon genetic factors. For example, the extent of vulnerability of dopamine-containing neurons to the administration of MPTP is linked to the genetic background of the animal. That some strains of mice are much more resistant than others has been a consistent finding (refs 11–14 and Heikkila, unpublished observations). Recently, Giovanni et al.[14] showed that an identical dosing schedule for MPTP produced insignificant decrements in striatal dopamine in a Swiss Webster strain, whereas it resulted in a 92% reduction of normal dopamine content in a C57 Bl/6 strain. Several additional mouse strains showed intermediate reductions in dopamine after MPTP administration. Earlier it was reported that among the four mouse strains compared, the C57 Bl/6 was the most sensitive to the neurotoxin, although all strains did suffer massive depletion ranging from 74% in the Swiss Webster to 96% in the C57 Bl/6 strain.[11] However, the same study showed that the most pronounced difference in the toxicity of MPTP between these two strains was with regard to cell death in the mesencephalon. MPTP administration caused destruction of substantial numbers of tyrosine hydroxylase (TH)-positive neurons in the mesencephalon of the C57 Bl/6 mice; whereas no cell death was observed in the mesencephalon of MPTP-treated Swiss Webster mice.

A series of studies point to genetic control of the numbers of TH-positive neurons in the midbrain of normal mice. Measurements of the activity of TH in the striatum and counts of the numbers of TH-positive neurons in the midbrains of two mouse strains have revealed that the activity of the enzyme is correlated with the number of TH-positive cell bodies in the substantia nigra and ventral tegmental area. The numbers of TH-positive mesencephalic neurons were found to be 20–50% fewer in the CBA/J strain than in the Balb/cJ strain.[15,16]

The most compelling illustration of the dependence of viability of dopamine-containing neurons on genetic control is a mutant mouse known as weaver. The weaver mutation offers proof that the dopamine-containing neurons of the midbrain can be destroyed relatively selectively through the action of a gene. This inherited disease bears strong similarities in its pathological alterations to those that follow the administration of several known neurotoxins to animals and to parkinsonism in humans. Like both of the neurotoxins 6-hydroxydopamine and MPTP, weaver destroys dopamine-containing neurons in the midbrain. The effects of weaver are specifically directed toward the dopamine-containing cells among those that contain monoamines,[17,18] and in this selectivity it bears the strongest resemblance to the effects of MPTP among the neurotoxins because the effects of MPTP are also relatively focused on dopamine-containing cells.[7,11,19]

Weaver is a naturally occurring autosomal recessive mutation, one of hundreds of known neurological mutations in mice. It is unique among all those in being the only mutation known to affect dopamine-containing systems. Weaver alters the fate of neurons in at least two areas of the brain. It has been known for several decades that weaver causes the death of large numbers of granule cells in the cerebellum.[20,21] More recently, the discovery was made that a subpopulation of the cerebellar Purkinje cells are also a direct cellular target of the weaver gene.[22] The manifestation of the weaver disease in the cerebellum of the homozygous weaver mice is so striking, easily seen, and takes place in the midst of such a fascinating developmental cascade that attention was focused exclusively on the cerebellum until 1977. In 1977 the report of Lane et al.[23] revealed the surprising puzzle of an effect of the weaver gene upon a neuronal system seemingly unrelated to that in the cerebellum. Lane and colleagues reported the reduction in the concentration of endogenous dopamine in the brain of the weaver mouse. This report was eventually confirmed by a more complete examination[17] demonstrating a massive depletion of dopamine in the striatum of homozygous weaver adults and cell loss in the midbrain. Ann Graybiel and I contributed to the interest in the dopamine-containing system of weaver by finding that the loss of dopamine in the striatum is not uniform.[24] Our reports emphasized that, remarkably, the weaver gene appears to distinguish between the two main functional subdivisions of the dopamine-containing projections that originate in the midbrain as they were described originally.[25,26] The mesolimbic division is relatively spared in homozygous adult weavers; dopamine was found to be retained in the n. accumbens along with all or most of the cells of origin in the ventral tegmental area.[18,24,27–30] In the caudoputamen, the target of the nigrostriatal system, dopamine is reduced by more than 70%, and a corresponding lack of TH-positive cell bodies is found in the substantia nigra.[18,24,28–32] The olfactory tubercle, a target of both mesolimbic and nigrostriatal systems, suffers a 50% reduction of dopamine.[18]

Weaver is a developmental disorder. Dopamine, although present at normal levels at the end of the first postnatal week in homozygous weavers, fails to follow the normal rate and extent of increasing concentrations, so that in adult life the dopamine content of the caudoputamen is little increased in comparison to that present on postnatal day 7.[33] The dopamine content of vulnerable striatal regions in the heterozygous weaver is slightly but significantly affected,[18] without accompanying cell loss in the midbrain.[28,31]

Some time ago, we noted that a number of features are shared by the effects of weaver on the dopamine-containing mesostriatal pathways and the effects of MPTP administration on the same pathways in mice;[34,35] features in common with MPTP-treated primates have been discussed also.[36] These include the massive loss of dopamine in the caudoputamen. For weaver adults the reduction amounts to approximately 70%.[17,18,24] The loss that takes place in MPTP-treated adult mice is approximately the same, i.e., 70–90%. In both cases, the loss of dopamine and its metabolites is permanent.[18,37,38]

One of the most remarkable parallels noted is that both gene and toxin appear to discriminate in their actions between the nigrostriatal pathway and the mesolimbic pathway. Neuronal loss, although not confined to the nigrostriatal system, is strongest there, whereas the mesolimbic path is relatively spared. We have embarked in further studies with Heikkila and collaborators for the purpose of making a direct comparison of the loss that occurs in the homozygous weaver and that which follows the administration of MPTP to normal mice that are on a genetic background that is identical to that of the weavers. That the gene and the toxin affect similar subpopulations of dopamine-containing cells can be seen by the pattern of residual TH-positive cells in the midbrains (Figure 1). Our preliminary results show that most of the neurons spared in both the weaver and an MPTP-treated homozygous normal mouse are in the medially placed

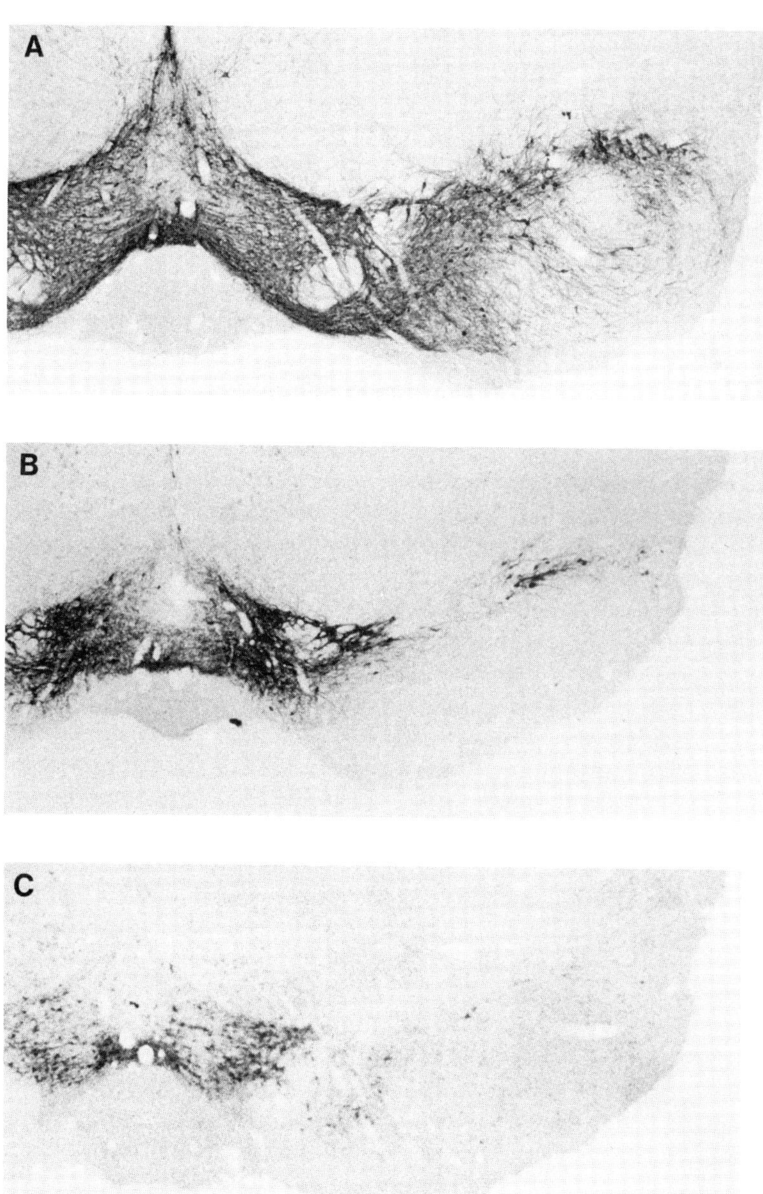

Figure 1. Comparison of patterns of TH-positive neurons in the substantia nigra and ventral tegmental area of an untreated $+/+$ animal (A), an untreated ^{wv}/wv animal (B) and an MPTP-treated $+/+$ animal (C). All mice were adults of the same genetic background: C57 Bl/6J Le-A^{WJ} × CBA/CaGnLef$_1$. The MPTP-treated mouse received two doses of MPTP (15 mg/kg) at 6-hour intervals and was sacrificed 8 days later.

ventral tegmental area. The most severe depletion of TH-positive neurons occurred in the substantia nigra of both animals. There appear to be no ventrally placed TH-positive neurons retained in the substantia nigra of either the weaver (panel B) or the MPTP-treated mouse (panel C, Figure 1).

The similarity in the mesencephalic targets of the mutation and the toxin suggest that there may be a molecular mechanism that links the two. An intriguing possible common denominator could involve glial cells, as they are implicated in the etiology of both disorders. For MPTP-induced toxicity, glial cells are the site at which MPTP is converted by the enzyme monoamine oxidase B (MAO-B) to the true toxic culprit *n*-methyl-4-phenylpyridine (MPP$^+$).[39,40] MPP$^+$ is accumulated in dopamine-containing neurons as a consequence of its affinity for the dopamine transporter.[41] Complicity of glial cells in the cell death that takes place in the weaver's midbrain is unexplored as yet; however, the failure of granule cells to survive in the weaver's cerebellum involves the failure of granule cell apposition to the Bergmann glial guides during the period of granule cell migration. The Bergmann glia are replete with MAO-B.[42]

With the possible involvement of MAO-B activity in the weaver disease in mind, we measured the activity of MAO-A and MAO-B in the three striatal regions of homozygous weavers and homozygous normal mice. Caudoputamen, olfactory tubercle, and n. accumbens were dissected from the brains of three normal and three weaver 7-month-old adults. The tissue was assayed in the laboratory of Richard Heikkila for activity of both MAO-A and MAO-B following a modification[14] of the radioenzymatic assay of White and Stone.[43] The results appear in Table 1. No change in the activity of either enzyme occurred in any of the striatal regions in weaver; thus, compared to normals, alterations in the activity of MAO-B or in the ratio of MAO-B to MAO-A would not seem to be the event that leads to the reduction of dopamine in the weaver's striatum. It is interesting to note that there is approximately twice as much MAO-B activity as MAO-A in both the caudoputamen and the olfactory tubercle. In the n. accumbens, the region in which the weaver's dopamine is spared, there is an even greater ratio of MAO-B to MAO-A (Table 1).

It is possible that the weaver gene holds no mandate for the death of dopamine-containing neurons and cerebellar cells; instead, the action of the gene may put these cells in jeopardy, making them

Table 1.
Activity of MAO-A and MAO-B in Three Striatal Regions of Normal (+/+) and Homozygous Weaver Mice (^{wv}/wv)[a]

| | Activity (nmol/mg protein/hr) | | | | | |
| | MAO-A | | MAO-B | | MAO-B/MAO-A | |
Region	+/+	wv/wv	+/+	wv/wv	+/+	wv/wv
Caudoputamen	15.95 ± .51	17.22 ± 1.5	30.43 ± 1.0	34.63 ± 1.73	1.91	2.01
Olfactory tubercle	18.48 ± 1.26	16.50 ± 1.71	38.11 ± 3.25	34.65 ± 3.01	2.06	2.10
Nucleus accumbens	14.0 ± 2.7	14.76 ± .94	50.33 ± 6.67	53.49 ± .80	3.60	3.62

[a]Enzyme activities were determined using [^{14}C]benzylamine as the substrate for MAO-B and [^{3}H]serotonin as the substrate for MAO-A. Results are expressed as the mean values ± SEM for tissues from three mice. All mice were 7 months old.

vulnerable to intrinsic factors that are safe for normal cells but toxic for the vulnerable sets of weaver neurons. Such a factor could involve oxidation by MAO-B. Because blockade of MAO-B prevents the toxicity of MPTP in mice,[44] we reasoned that inhibition of MAO-B might prevent or delay the death of neurons in the weaver homozygote. Accordingly, we administered deprenyl (2.5 mg/kg, IP) to timed-pregnant females at embryonic (E) day 13 and again at E15. The administration of the deprenyl was continued after the pups were born beginning at postnatal (P) day 4 (the day of birth is P0). Deprenyl was injected IP at a dose of 2.5 mg/kg at 3-day intervals after P4 until the animals were killed at either P21 or P30. In another set of experiments, litters of pups from heterozygous weaver parents were injected at 3-day intervals beginning at P4 also at a dose of 2.5 mg/kg IP. The treated pups were normal homozygotes, weaver heterozygotes, and weaver homozygotes. Treated litters were killed along with untreated litters at 3 or 4 weeks of age. Dopamine was extracted from three striatal regions, the caudoputamen, the olfactory tubercle, and the nucleus accumbens. The results showed that deprenyl administered either before and after birth or only postnatally during the period in which dopamine-containing cells die had no effect on the dopamine content of any of the striatal regions in any of the genetic types. Dopamine content was not retained in the homozygous weaver nor was the content of dopamine influenced by deprenyl administration in either the homozygous normal animals or in the heterozygous weavers.

The behavioral changes that mark the homozygous weaver now can be seen to be attributable to both the damage inflicted by the mutation in the mesostriatal system and in the cerebellum. Treatment of afflicted mice with levodopa ameliorates some of the symptoms characteristic of the adult homozygote. Mice homozygous for the weaver gene are ataxic, have hind-limb weakness, an abnormal grasping reflex, and display tremor, rigidity, and perseverative motor behavior. Unlike patients with Parkinson's disease, weaver mice are hyperkinetic, seemingly unable to inhibit ongoing motor activity. We have seen that low doses of levodopa (100 mg/kg body weight, administered IP) reverse several but not all of these signs for short periods. After levodopa treatment, the weaver's tremor is diminished in amplitude and unchanged in its rhythm. The rigidity of the weaver mice is reduced by L-dopa. Motor perserveration is temporarily abolished by levodopa as is the hyperkinesis characteristic of the weaver. The grasp reflex of the weaver is markedly improved after levodopa. The characteristic ataxia of the weaver mouse seen in walking animals was unchanged by L-dopa treatment, although the treated animals were better able to balance themselves on a rail possibly due to their improved grasp as well as reduced hyperkinesis. Larger doses of L-dopa (400 mg/kg) caused the weaver mice to propel themselves rapidly around the cage; the ataxia was still visible.

An idea that emerges from these studies is that Parkinson's "disease" is a symptom resulting from the death of a specific neuronal system and that the death of these neurons may be caused by one assassin or by a conspiracy among several. Weaver, in which a genetically transmitted early cell death occurs, may provide insight into the cause or causes of Parkinson's disease. We and others are seeking the gene, and studying the involvement of mitochondria. We are examining cultured cells in varied environments and the effects of growth factors on them. The chase continues and one thing is certain: the plot will continue to thicken.

References

1. Zigmond MJ, Berger TW, Grace AA, Stricker EM. 1989. Compensatory responses to nigrostriatal bundle injury. Studies with 6-hydroxydopamine in an animal model of parkinsonism. Mol Chem Neuropathol 10:185–200.
2. Heikkila RE, Hess A, Duvoisin RC. 1984. Dopaminergic neurotoxicity of 1-methyl-4-phenyl-1,2,5,6-tetrahydropyridine in mice. Science 224:1451–1453.
3. Heikkila RE, Sieber BA, Manzino L, Sonsalla PK. 1989. Some features of the nigrostriatal dopaminergic neurotoxin 1-methyl-4-phenyl-1,2,3,6-tetrahydropyridine (MPTP) in the mouse. Mol Chem Neuropathol 10:171.
4. Davis GC, Williams AC, Markey SP, Ebert MH, Caine E, Reichert CM, Kopin I. 1979. Chronic parkinsonism secondary to intravenous injection of meperidine analogues. Psychiatr Res 1:249–254.
5. Langston JW, Ballard PA, Tetrud JW, Irwin I. 1983. Chronic parkinsonism in humans due to a product of meperidine-analog synthesis. Science 219:979–980.
6. Agid Y, Javoy-Agid F, Ruberg M, Pillon B, DuBois B, Duyckaerts C, Hauw JJ, Baron JB, Scatton B. 1986. Progressive supranuclear palsy: Anatomoclinical and biochemical considerations. Adv Neurol 45:191–205.
7. Duvoisin RC. 1986. Genetics of Parkinson's disease. Adv Neurol 45:307–312.

8. Duvoisin RC, Heikkila RE, Nicklas WJ, Hess A. 1986. Dopaminergic neurotoxicity of MPTP in the mouse: A murine model of parkinsonism. *In* Recent Developments In Parkinson's Disease. S Fahn ed. Raven Press, New York.

9. Golbe LI, Di Iorio G, Bonavita V, Miller DC, Duvoisin RC. 1990. A large kindred with autosomal dominant Parkinson's disease. Ann Neurol 27:276–282.

10. Johnson WG, Hodge SE, Duvoisin R. 1990. Twin studies and the genetics of Parkinson's disease—a reappraisal. Mov Disord 5:187–194.

11. Sundstrom E, Stromberg I, Isutsumi T, Alson L, Jonsson G. 1987. Studies on the effect of 1-methyl-4-phenyl-1,2,3,6-tetrahydropyridine (MPTP) on central catecholamine neurons in C57B1/6 mice. Comparison with three other strains of mice. Brain Res 405:26–38.

12. Sonsalla PK, Heikkila RE. 1988. Neurotoxic effects of 1-methyl-4-phenol-1,2,3,6-tetrahydropyridine (MPTP) and methamphetamine in several strains of mice. Prog Neuropsychopharmacol Biol Psychiatry 12:346–384.

13. Jossan SS, Sakurai E, Oreland L. 1989. MPTP toxicity in relation to age, dopamine uptake and MAO-B activity in two rodent species. Pharmacol Toxicol 64:314–318.

14. Giovanni A, Sieber B-A, Heikkila RE, Sonsalla PK. 1991. Correlation between the neostriatal content of the 1-methyl-4-phenylpyridinium species and dopaminergic neurotoxicity following 1-methyl-4-phenyl-1,2,3,6. Tetrahydropyrine administration to several strains of mice. J Pharmacol Exp Ther 257:691–697.

15. Ross RA, Judd AB, Pickel VM, Joh TH, Reis DJ. 1976. Strain-dependent variations in number of midbrain dopaminergic neurones. Nature 264:654–656.

16. Reis DJ, Baker H, Fink JS, Joh TH. 1978. A genetic control of the number of central dopamine neurons in relationship to brain organization, drug responses, and behavior. *In* Catecholamines: Basic and Clinical Frontiers, Vol I. E Usdin, IJ Kopin, J Barchas (eds). Pergamon Press, New York, pp. 23–33.

17. Schmidt MJ, Sawyer BD, Perry KW, Fuller RW, Foreman MM, Ghetti B. 1982. Dopamine deficiency in the weaver mutant mouse. J Neurosci 2:376–380.

18. Roffler-Tarlov S, Graybiel AM. 1986. Expression of the weaver gene in dopamine-containing neural systems is dose-dependent and affects both striatal and nonstriatal regions. J Neurosci 6:3319–3330.

19. Wallace RA, Boldry R, Schmittgen T, Miller D, Uretsky N. 1984. Effect of 1-methyl-4-phenyl-1,2,3,6-tetrahydropyridine (MPTP) on monoamine neurotransmitters in mouse brain and heart. Life Sci 35:285–291..

20. Sidman RL, Green MC, Appel SH. 1965. Catalog of the Neurological Mutants of the Mouse. Harvard University Press, Cambridge, MA pp 66–67.

21. Sidman RL. 1968. Development of interneuronal connections in brains of mutant mice. *In:* Physiological and Biochemical Aspects of Nervous Integration. FD Carlson (ed). Prentice-Hall, Englewood Cliffs, NJ pp 163–193.

22. Smeyne RJ, Goldowitz D. 1990. Purkinje cell loss is due to a direct action of the weaver gene in Purkinje cells: Evidence from chimeric mice. Dev Brain Res 52:211–218.
23. Lane PW, Nadi NS, McBride WJ, Aprison MH, Kusano K. 1977. Content of serotonin, norepinephrine and dopamine in the cerebrum of the "staggerer" "weaver" and "nervous" neurologically mutant mice. J Neurochem 29:349–350.
24. Roffler-Tarlov S, Graybiel AM. 1984. Weaver mutation has differential effects on the dopamine-containing innervation of the limbic and nonlimbic striatum. Nature 307:62–66.
25. Anden NE, Dahlstrom A, Fuxe K, Larsson K, Olson L, Ungerstedt U. 1966. Ascending monoamine neurons to the telencephalon and diencephalon. Acta Physiol Scand 67:313–326.
26. Ungerstedt U. 1971. Stereotaxic mapping of the monoamine pathways in the rat brain. Acta Physiol Scand 197:1–48.
27. Roffler-Tarlov S, Graybiel AM. 1987. The postnatal development of the dopamine-containing innervation of dorsal and ventral striatum: Effects of the weaver gene. J Neurosci 7:2364–2372.
28. Triarhou LC, Norton J, Ghetti B. 1988. Mesencephalic dopamine cell deficit involves areas A8, A9, and A10 in weaver mutant mice. Exp Brain Res 70:256–265.
29. Gupta M, Felten DL, Ghetti B. 1987. Selective loss of monoaminergic neurons in weaver mutant mice--an immunocytochemical study. Brain Res 402:379–381.
30. Graybiel AM, Ohta K, Roffler-Tarlov S. 1990. Patterns of cell and fiber vulnerability in the mesostriatal system of the mutant mouse weaver: I. Gradients and compartments. J Neurosci 10:720–733.
31. Roffler-Tarlov S, Graybiel AM, Martin B, Kauer J. 1987. The mesencephalic dopamine-containing neurons in the weaver mouse. Soc Neurosci Abstr 13:1599.
32. Smith MW III, Cooper TR, Joh TH, Smith DE. 1990. Cell loss and class distribution of TH-I cells in the substantia nigra of the neurological mutant, weaver. Brain Res 510:242–250.
33. Roffler-Tarlov S, Pugatch D, Graybiel AM. 1987. Early effects of the weaver gene on the dopamine-containing innervation of the dorsal striatum. Int Congr Pharmacol 53:308.
34. Roffler-Tarlov S, Graybiel AM. 1988. Genetic and toxin-induced depletion of striatal dopamine. *In* Pharmacology and Functional Regulation of Dopaminergic Neurons. PM Beart, G Woodruff, DM Jackson (eds). Macmillian, New York, pp. 204–210.
35. Roffler-Tarlov S, Pugatch D, Graybiel AM. 1990. Patterns of cell and fiber vulnerability in the mesostriatal system of the mutant mouse weaver. II. High affinity uptake sites for dopamine. J Neurosci 10:734–740.
36. Quinn B, Graybiel AM, Moratalla R, Langston JW, Roffler-Tarlov S, Ohta K. 1990. Patterns of vulnerability of mesostriatal neurons. *In* Alzheimer's and Parkinson Diseases II. M Yoshida (ed). Plenum Press, New York (in press).

37. Ricaurte GA, DeLanney LE, Irwin I, Langston JW. 1987. Older dopaminergic neurons do not recover from the effects of MPTP. Neuropharmacology 26:97–99.
38. Saitoh T, Niijimi K, Mizuno Y. 1987. Long-term effect of 1-methyl-4-phenyl-1,2,3,6-tetrahydropyridine (MPTP) on striatal dopamine content in young and mature mice. J Neurol Sci 77:299–335.
39. Chiba K, Trevor AJ, Castangnola N. 1984. Active uptake of MPP$^+$, a metabolite of MPTP, by brain synaptosomes. Biochem Biophys Res Commun 120:574–578.
40. Markey SP, Johannessen JN, Chiuch CC, Burns RS, Herkenham MA. 1984. Intraneuronal generation of a pyridium metabolite may cause drug-induced parkinsonism. Nature 311:464–467.
41. Javitch JA, D'Amato RJ, Strittmater SM, Snyder SH. 1985. Parkinsonism-inducing neurotoxin n-methyl-4-phenyl-methyl-4-phenylpyridine: Uptake of the metabolite n-methyl-4-phenylpyridine by dopamine neurons explains selective neurotoxicity. Proc Natl Acad Sci USA 82:2173–2177.
42. Levitt P, Pintar JE, Breakefield XO. 1982. Immunocytochemical demonstration of monoamine oxidase B in brain astrocytes and serotonergic neurons. Proc Natl Acad Sci USA 79:6385–6389.
43. White HI, Stone DK. 1964. Species differences in monoamine oxidase-A and -B as revealed by sensitivity to trypsin. Life Sci 36:827–833.
44. Heikkila RE, Manzino L, Cabbat FS, Duvoisin RC. 1984. Protection against the dopaminergic neurotoxicity of 1-methyl-4-phenyl-1,2,5,6-tetrahydropyridine by monoamine oxidase inhibitors. Nature 311:467–469.

Chapter 23

Combined Degeneration of Cerebellar Granule Cells and of Midbrain Dopamine Neurons in the Weaver Mutant Mouse

Bernardino Ghetti and Lazaros C. Triarhou

Degeneration of Nigral Neurons in Genetically Determined Neurological Diseases

The genetic mechanisms that regulate the viability of dopamine (DA) neurons and those involved in the etiology of DA neuron degeneration remain largely unknown. Among disorders of the nigrostriatal DA system, Parkinson's disease is the most frequent. Its etiology remains unclear; however, both environmental and genetic factors have been implicated. Familial cases of Parkinson's disease have been reported and recently a large kindred with autosomal dominant Parkinson disease has been documented clinically and neuropathologically.[1]

In addition to Parkinson's disease, there are neurological conditions in which degeneration of DA neurons appears to be genetically determined. Parkinsonian symptomatology and loss of DA neurons in the substantia nigra are observed in cases of Shy-Drager disease[2-4] and in familial forms of pallidal atrophy,[5,6] olivopontocerebellar atrophy,[7-11] cerebelloolivary atrophy,[12-14]

Supported in part by U.S. Public Health Service grant RO1-NS14426.
From Hefti F, and Weiner WJ, (eds.) *Progress in Parkinson's Disease Research—2*. Mount Kisco NY, Futura Publishing Co., Inc., © 1992.

spinocerebellonigral degeneration,[15,16] Gerstmann-Sträussler-Scheinker disease,[17] and amyotrophic lateral sclerosis.[18–20] Furthermore, loss of neurons in the substantia nigra is observed in cases of familial primary degeneration of the granular layer of the cerebellum, a condition that occurs early in life and is characterized by severe motor incoordination and mental retardation.[21]

In most genetically determined degenerative diseases involving the substantia nigra, loss of mesencephalic DA neurons is concurrent with degenerative events in non-DAergic neuronal groups. This observation suggests that in these conditions a single gene may affect at the same time the viability of different neuronal populations regardless of their transmitter content.

Neurological mutant mice represent an important resource for understanding basic mechanisms of genetically induced aberrations in neural development and of neuronal death.[22] Their usefulness is even greater if one considers the occurrence of homologies between murine and human chromosome segments and genes.[23]

Mesotelencephalic DA deficiency is a part of the neuropathological phenotype in the weaver mutant mouse,[24] which is currently the only laboratory animal where DA cell loss of genetic origin is seen in association with central DA deficiency. In the weaver mouse, similar to human heredodegenerative neurological disorders, there is an involvement of multiple systems; in fact, a primary degeneration of the granule cells of the cerebellum is the other neuropathological manifestation.[22,25] The latter lesion has been better known to neuroscientists, since it was described two decades before the nigrostriatal deficit.

The Weaver Mutant Mouse

The weaver mutation arose in 1961 in mice of the C57BL/6J strain.[26] The mutation has been considered as autosomal recessive; however, the fact that heterozygous animals (*wv/+*) show some mild pathological changes in the cerebellum has led some authors to call the mutation "incomplete dominant."[27] The weaver gene has been localized to mouse chromosome 16, and it has been mapped less than 1 cM proximal to the genes *Ets-2* and *Mx*, in a region that appears to be highly conserved between mouse chromosome 16 and human chromosome 21.[28]

Homozygous weaver mice (*wv/wv*) can be recognized clinically in the second postnatal week by their small size, instability of gait, fine tremor, weakness, and hypotonia. Adult homozygous weaver mutants display a fine rapid tremor of the trunk and extremities, poor limb coordination, instability of gait, toppling over to the sides after several steps, navigational deficits, a hind-paw clasping reflex, and reduced activity in open-field tests.[22,29–33] A behavior not seen in other mutant mice with cerebellar abnormalities is a leaping when the mouse is excited or agitated.[22] Generalized tonic/clonic seizures are observed in *wv/wv* and *wv/+*.

The Weaver Cerebellum

Early studies have documented the neuropathological changes in the cerebellum of weaver mutants.[22,25,34] Degeneration of postmitotic granule cell precursors in the external germinal layer occurs during the first 2 weeks of postnatal life. The earliest detectable mutant phenotype in *wv/wv* and *wv/+* cerebellum is presence of a high number of degenerated neurons in the external germinal layer, suggesting that a degenerative event takes place before the migration of these cells through the molecular layer.[35] The migration of granule cells begins at around postnatal day 4 (P4) in the *+/+* mouse.[36,37]

The *wv/wv* cerebellum can be differentiated from the *wv/+* and *+/+* cerebellum by the amount of cells undergoing degeneration in the external germinal layer as early as P0.[35] The most striking deficit in the adult homozygous weaver cerebellum is the virtual absence of granule cells in the vermis. The adult heterozygous weaver mouse shows an attenuated loss of granule cells in the granular layer; some granule cells, which had not reached the final destination of their migratory path, are scattered in the lower third of the molecular layer.[25] Furthermore, an approximate 50% reduction in the number of vermal Purkinje cells is noted in weaver homozygotes.[38,39] In addition to their being reduced in number, Purkinje cells display a severely altered polarity, with Purkinje cell dendrites frequently oriented toward the depth of the cerebellar cortex.

The Weaver Mesotelencephalic Dopamine Projection System

Studies on the levels of biogenic monoamines in the cerebra of staggerer, nervous, and weaver mutant mice have revealed decreases in DA in adult weaver homozygotes.[40] Subsequent studies showed that there is a 75% DA deficiency in the striatum of *wv/wv* as compared to wild-type controls (+/+), a 77% DA deficiency in frontal cortex, and a 27% DA deficiency in the olfactory tubercle.[24] Serial histological sections through the substantia nigra showed severe neuronal depletion in 6-month-old weaver mutant mice.[24] In all of the studies carried out in our laboratory since 1980, the weaver mutation has been maintained on a B6CBA-*A*$^{w-J}$/*A* hybrid stock, on which homozygous mutants may live for up to 2, and occasionally 2½, years.

Immunohistochemical studies using tyrosine hydroxylase (TH) antisera in 3- to 4-month-old weaver mutant mice showed that immunolabelled neurons of the substantia nigra are substantially reduced in number.[41,42] Subsequent systematic studies of mesencephalic DA neurons in +/+, *wv*/+, and *wv/wv* revealed a 42% decrease of nigral DA neurons in 20-day-old *wv/wv* and no changes in areas A8 and A10 at that age; at 90 days of age, there are losses in all three midbrain DA cell groups, which amount respectively to 56%, 69%, and 26% in areas A8, A9, and A10.[43,44]

Additional studies of weaver mutants at 1 and 2 years of age (Figure 1) have shown that there is an additional neuronal loss in 2-year-old mice. The losses amount to about 60% in area A8, 85% in area A9, and 35% in area A10.[44]

In adult weaver mutant mice, there is a severe loss of DA in the caudoputamen, which is the main target of the nigrostriatal system, whereas DA levels are normal in nucleus accumbens.[45] These findings led investigators to hypothesize that there is a dissociation of *wv* gene effects with a selective sparing of the mesolimbic system.[45,46] However, more recent reports seem to confirm our original results of DA cell losses in areas A8, A9, and A10,[43] even though quantitative data on such losses have not been reported by other investigators.[47]

The neuropathological analysis of the cerebellum in homozygous (*wv/wv*) and heterozygous (*wv*/+) mice has shown that there is a loss of granule cells in both phenotypes and that the degree of cell loss is less severe in *wv*/+.[25] This observation suggests that the weaver gene is partially expressed and induces neuronal degeneration in the *wv*/+ mouse as well. Counts of midbrain DA neurons have not revealed any difference between the cell numbers of +/+ and *wv*/+ mice up to 90 days old; further studies are in progress in older *wv*/+, which may offer additional information on this issue. However, immunocytochemical studies revealed that the dendritic DA projection, which extends from the substantia nigra pars compacta into the pars reticulata, is severely reduced in heterozygotes (*wv*/+).[48] A 60% reduction of dendrites can be detected at 20 days of age, when the number of DA neurons in the substantia nigra does not differ between +/+ and *wv*/+. The dendritic loss is also present in homozygous weaver mice, in which it is slightly more severe than in *wv*/+, probably due to the loss of DA neuron perikarya. Thus, the observation of a severe dendritic alteration in nigral DA neurons provides evidence for weaver gene expression in the substantia nigra of *wv*/+, and it is in line with the idea of a defect in growth and maintenance of neuronal processes.[49]

Degeneration of Dopamine Neurons in Midbrain of Weaver Mutant Mice

From studies of the weaver cerebellum, there is a direct evidence of granule cell degeneration.[25,35] The degeneration begins during or immediately after the last mitotic division of the granule cell precursors and continues in the following 2 weeks. The Purkinje cells are reduced in number; however, the timing of such loss is not known, and direct evidence of Purkinje cell degeneration is not available.

A process of degeneration in the midbrain DA cell groups is inferred from the evidence that DA neurons in the *wv*/*wv* mutant mice are fewer than in +/+ mice at 20 days of age and that their number further declines in *wv*/*wv* by 90 days and later. The precise time of onset of DA neuron degeneration in weaver mice is unknown. In the mouse, neurons of the substantia nigra originate by embryonic day 12.[50] Dopamine neuron degeneration in weaver mice could start during embryonic life or within the first weeks of postnatal life. It is conceivable that there is a time interval between the onset of DA cell loss and the manifestation of neurological signs. Such signs do appear when a critical number of synapses, dendrites, and nerve cell perikarya have been lost. In addition to the instability of gait, a fine tremor, possibly related to the DA deficiency, is detectable in *wv*/*wv* mutant mice as early as during the second postnatal week. By 20 days of age, 42% of the DA neurons are lost in the substantia nigra. It is of interest to note that the information currently available indicates that in humans, parkinsonian signs are correlated with 80% loss of nigral neurons.[51,52] So far, quantitative data have not been reported in weaver mice younger than 20 days of age.

The pathological features of nigral neuron degeneration have been studied by light and electron microscopy. In 12-, 16-, and 20-day-old weaver mutants, degenerating cells can be found in 1-μm thick, Epon-embedded sections. In any microscopic field of the substantia nigra and of the ventral tegmental area, the majority of neurons show normal cytoplasm and nucleus. In particular, no intranuclear or intracytoplasmic inclusions are observed, and Lewy bodies, the typical cellular lesions observed in Parkinson's disease, are not seen in the nigral neurons of the weaver midbrain. Occasionally, osmiophilic intracytoplasmic material is observed; however, it is not possible to determine whether this represents an abnormality of the cytoplasm.

Nerve cells in various stages of degeneration are found (Figure 2a,b). Pyknosis of the nucleus is one of the first detectable changes. The cytoplasm shows a reduction in the number of cisterns of rough endoplasmic reticulum. Ribosomes are sparsely distributed in the cytoplasm. Glial processes surround the degenerating cells. In more advanced stages of degeneration, the nucleus and cytoplasm are severely deformed and osmiophilic. Degenerating dendritic processes are often found in the neuropil (Figure 3). Some dendrites contain osmiophilic material and vesicular structures; others are entirely osmiophilic, even though they are still in synaptic contact with presynaptic axon terminals. In several instances, degenerating cell processes are completely surrounded by glial cytoplasm, and it is not possible to recognize whether they are remnants of dendrites or axons.

Changes in Target Areas of Midbrain Dopamine Neurons in Weaver Mutant Mice

The density of DA fibers, studied by means of catecholamine histofluorescence and TH and DA immunocytochemistry, is substantially reduced in dorsal striatum but not in nucleus accumbens.[45,53,54] Using a radioautographic technique of [³H]DA uptake by striatal slices, it was found that the remaining striatal DA fibers

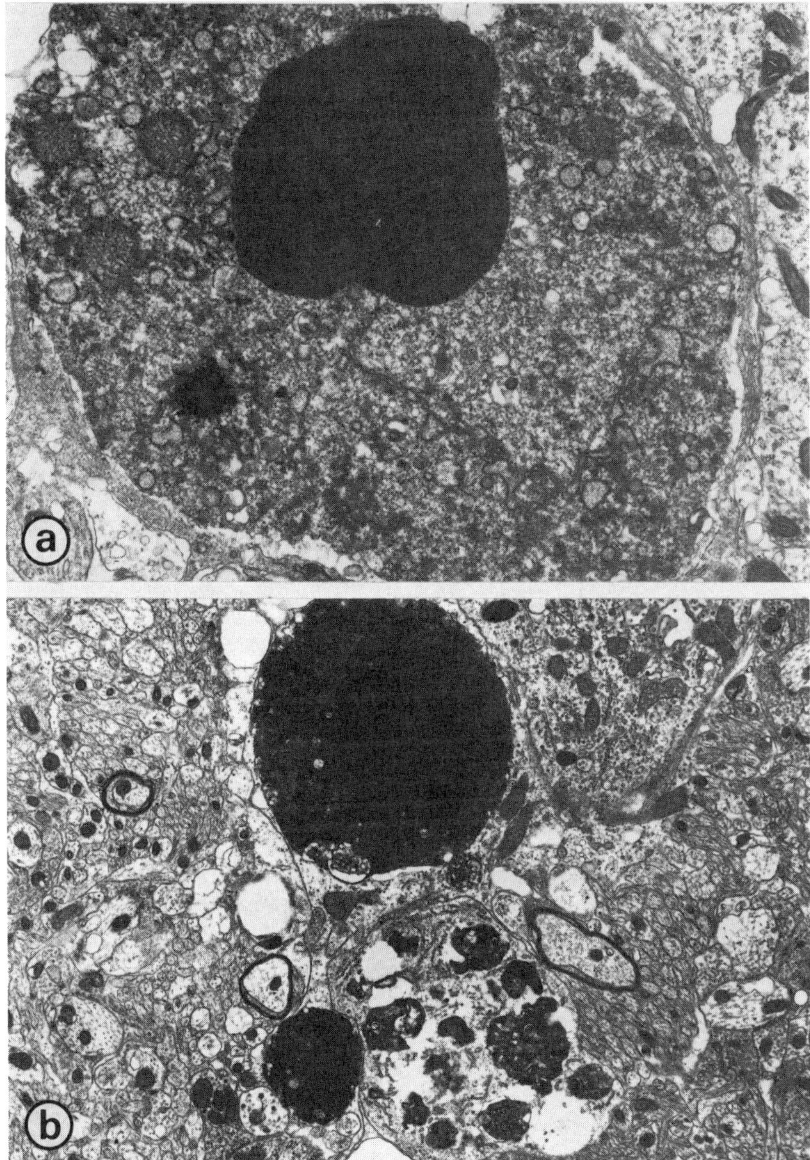

Figure 2. Degenerating nerve cells in the substantia nigra of a 16- (a) and a 20-day-old (b) weaver mutant mouse.

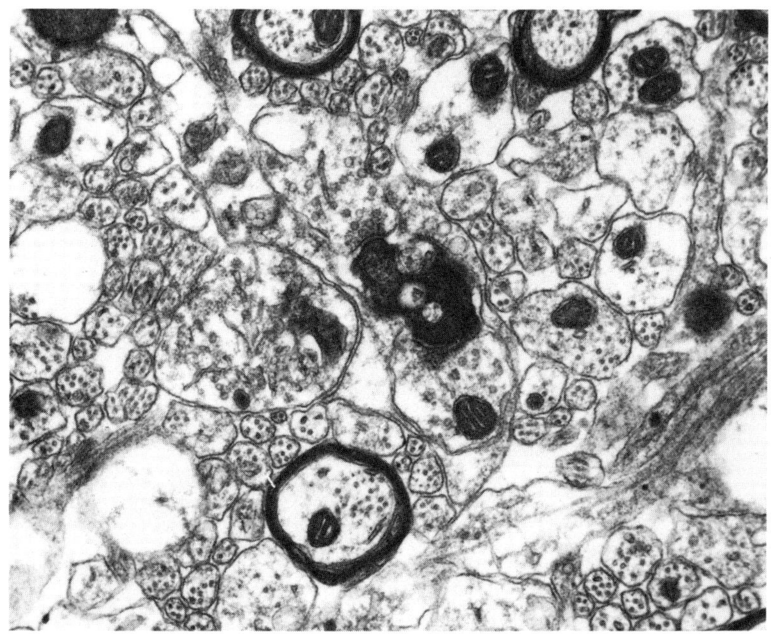

Figure 3. Dendrites of the weaver substantia nigra in advanced stages of degeneration.

display defective characteristics of DA uptake and storage; further, DA axons of the nucleus accumbens, where DA content does not differ from normal, also display features of deficient uptake and storage of DA.[54] In agreement with these findings, biochemical studies on the high-affinity uptake of [^{3}H]DA by synaptosomal preparations of striatum have shown defective DA uptake in both dorsal striatum and nucleus accumbens.[55]

Studies carried out by electron microscopy showed that striatal DA afferents establish an inadequate synaptic connectivity on resident striatal neurons.[53] DA axon terminals in the weaver striatum are fewer in number, and only 53% of them appear to establish junctional synaptic relationships with their target neurons, as opposed to 85–90% in controls. Moreover, there is an increase in the incidence of axosomatic contacts made by incoming DA fibers. Such axosomatic contacts are commonly seen during the early ontogeny of the nigrostriatal anlage and their persistence in adult weaver mice may indicate immaturity of synaptic connectivity.

At this time information on the structure of neurons of the caudoputamen in weaver mutants is lacking. As often occurs in degenerative neurogenetic diseases, neuronal loss due to transneuronal degeneration or atrophy (secondary) of the cells synaptically related to neurons—targets of the mutation—might take place in weaver mutants. Since in most cases transneuronal cell death proceeds slowly, it is possible that secondary losses would be best detectable and measurable in old rather than young weaver mutants.

DA D_2 receptor binding is increased in the striatum of 5- to 6-month-old weaver mutant mice.[56] This may occur in response to the loss of DA neurons in the midbrain and the decrease in DA content in the striatum of homozygous mutants. When specific [^{3}H]spiperone binding was measured in the dorsolateral, dorsomedial, and ventrolateral striatum and in the nucleus accumbens of *wv/wv*, *wv/+*, and *+/+* mice at 20 days and 1, 3, 6, 9, and 12 months of age, the difference in specific binding in dorsolateral striatum between *wv/wv* and *+/+* mice was significantly greater at 6 months than the difference at 1 month and at 12 months of age.[57] DA D_1 receptor binding is unchanged in the weaver.[58]

Among other target areas of the midbrain DAergic pathways, the frontal and cingulate cortex of weaver mice reveal a substantial reduction in the density of TH-immunoreactive fibers,[59] consistent with the DA deficiency in frontal cortex, as found by neurochemical methods.[24]

Conclusions

There are three main considerations regarding the significance of the weaver disease as a model particularly suitable for dissecting out mechanisms of DA neuron degeneration.

1. Animal models that have the typical cellular, neuroanatomical, and behavioral changes characteristic of idiopathic (sporadic) or familial Parkinson's disease are not available. So far, most models of Parkinson's disease and of parkinsonism have been defined and used as such on the basis of an anatomical lesion of the substantia nigra with neuronal loss, regardless of the modality of its induction,

whether electrolytic or neurotoxic. Degeneration and loss of nigral neurons, loss of DAergic synapses, DA deficiency, and increase of DA D_2 receptors are all observed in a consistent manner in weaver mice. Thus, such natural disease fits well among models of parkinsonism, and it may be useful not only in elucidating the cause of the weaver condition and accompanying effects of nigrostriatal DA deficiency and of postsynaptic adaptive mechanisms, but also in understanding general biological principles pertinent to nigrostriatal degeneration.

2. DA neurons of the substantia nigra are at risk in a variety of genetic neurodegenerative disorders.[1–21] Combined involvement of DAergic and other neuronal systems may give rise to a variety of clinical pictures. In each disorder a single genetic mutation presumably results in the degeneration of specific neuronal subsets. Molecular links between subsets of neurons may be predicted on the basis of the neuropathological phenotypes observed in those genetic disorders, which are characterized by a deficit of multiple neuronal systems, not connected synaptically. Thus, in the weaver mutant mouse failures of neuronal migration, of neural process elongation and maintenance, as well as cell death in two populations of neurons, which are not connected synaptically with each other, are most likely part of a chain of events initiated by a single faulty gene. The concept of an intrinsic action of the weaver gene in granule cells and DA neurons is supported by studies with normal and weaver chimeras (ref. 60, and personal communication from Dr. Dan Goldowitz). In order to make progress in our understanding of how the constellation of genes regulates the neuronal network, this natural disease of the laboratory mouse offers "a window" to be used in the search for a putative molecular link between midbrain DA neurons and cerebellar granule cells.

3. The *wv* locus is located in a region of the mouse genome homologous to the human genome. Whether a gene similar to *wv* exists in humans and induces a neurological disease remains to be determined.

References

1. Golbe LI, Di Iorio G, Bonavita V, Miller DC, Duvoisin RC. 1990. A large kindred with autosomal dominant Parkinson's disease. Ann Neurol 27:276–282.
2. Shy GM, Drager GA. 1960. A neurological syndrome associated with

orthostatic hypotension. A clinical–pathologic study. Arch Neurol 2: 511–527.

3. Oppenheimer DR. 1983. Neuropathology of progressive autonomic failure. *In* Autonomic Failure. R Bannister (ed). Oxford University Press, Oxford, pp 267–283.

4. Oppenheimer DR. 1984. Disease of the basal ganglia, cerebellum and motor neurons. *In* Greenfield's Neuropathology, 4th ed. JH Adams, JAN Corsellis, LW Duchen (eds). Arnold, London, pp 699–747.

5. Jellinger K. 1969. Degeneration and exogenous lesions of the pallidum and striatum. *In* Handbook of Clinical Neurology, Vol 6, Disease of the Basal Ganglia. PJ Vinken, GW Bruyn (eds). North Holland, Amsterdam, pp 632–643.

6. Mayer JM, Mikol J, Haguenau M, Dellanave J, Pepin B. 1986. Familial juvenile parkinsonism with multiple systems degenerations. A clinico-pathological study. J Neurol Sci 72:91–101.

7. Berciano J. 1982. Olivopontocerebellar atrophy. A review of 117 cases. J Neurol Sci 53:253–272.

8. Bonduelle M, Escourolle R, Bouygues P, Lormeau G, Gray F. 1976. Atrophie olivo-ponto-cérébelleuse familiale avec myoclonies. Les limites de la dyssynergie cérébelleuse myoclonique. (Syndrome de Ramsay-Hunt). Rev Neurol (Paris) 132:113–124.

9. Rondot P, de Recondo J, Davous P, Vedrenne C. 1983. Menzel's hereditary ataxia with slow eye movement and myoclonus. A clinico-pathological study. J Neurol Sci 61:65–80.

10. Rosenberg RN. 1984. Joseph disease: An autosomal dominant motor system degeneration. Adv Neurol 41:179–193.

11. Continho P, Guimaraes A, Scaravilli F. 1982. The pathology of Machado-Joseph disease. Report of a possible homozygous case. Acta Neuropathol (Berlin) 58:48–54.

12. Guillain G, Garcin R, Bertrand I. 1931. Sur un syndrome cérébelleux précéde d'un état hypertonique. Rev Neurol (Paris) 1:565–575.

13. Bogaert L Van, Borremans P. 1947. Sur une atrophie cerebelleuse corticale avec debut de sclerose axiale et atteinte des noyaux gris centraux. Troubles mentaux. Lipomatose symetrique. J Belge Neurol Psychiatr 47:249–267.

14. Carter HR, Sukuvajana C. 1956. Familial cerebello-olivary degeneration with late development of rigidity and dementia. Neurology 6:876–884.

15. Castaigne P, Cambier J, Cathala HP, Augustin P. 1961. Association chez plusieurs malades d'une même fratrie d'une maladie de Freidreich et d'un syndrome parkinsonien. Rev Neurol (Paris) 105:452–454.

16. Garcin R, Raverdy P, Delthil S, Man HX, Chimenes H. 1961. Sur une affection hérédofamiliale associant cataracte, atrophie optique, signes extrapyramidaux et certains stigmates de la maladie de Friedreich. Rev Neurol (Paris) 104:373–379.

17. Ghetti B, Tagliavini F, Masters CL, Beyreuther K, Giaccone G, Verga L, Farlow MR, Conneally PM, Dlouhy SR, Azzarelli B, Bugiani O. 1989. Gerstmann-Sträussler-Scheinker disease: II. Neurofibrillary tangles and

plaques with PrP-amyloid coexist in an affected family. Neurology 39: 1453–1461.

18. Bogaert L Van, Radermecker MA. 1954. Scléroses latérales amyotrophiques typiques et paralysies agitantes héréditaires dans une même famille avec une forme de passage possible entre les deux affections. Monatsschr Psychiat U Neurol 127:185–203.

19. Haberlandt WF. 1964. Amyotrophische Lateralsklerose. Fischer, Stuttgart.

20. Bonduelle M, Bouygues P, Escourolle R, Lormeau G. 1968. Évolution simultanée d'une sclérose latérale amyotrophique, d'un syndrome parkinsonien et d'une démence progressive (A propos de deux observations anatomo-cliniques. Essai d'interprétation). J Neurol Sci 6:315–332.

21. Ferrer I, Sirvent J, Manresa JM, Galofré E, Fernández-Alvarez E, and Pineda M. 1987. Primary degeneration of the granular layer of the cerebellum (Normal type). A Golgi study. Acta Neuropathol (Berlin) 75: 203–208.

22. Sidman RL, Green MC, Appel SH. 1965. Catalog of the Neurological Mutants of the Mouse. Harvard University Press, Cambridge, MA, pp 66–67.

23. Lyon MF, Searle AG. 1989. Genetic variants and strains of the laboratory mouse. *In* The International Committee on Standardized Genetics Nomenclature for Mice, 2nd ed. Oxford University Press, New York.

24. Schmidt MJ, Sawyer BD, Perry KW, Fuller RW, Foreman MM, Ghetti B. 1982. Dopamine deficiency in the weaver mutant mouse. J Neurosci 2: 376–380.

25. Rakic P, Sidman RL. 1973. Sequence of developmental abnormalities leading to granule cell deficit in cerebellar cortex of weaver mutant mice. J Comp Neurol 152:103–132.

26. Lane PW. 1964. Mouse News Letter 30:32.

27. Sotelo C. 1980. Mutant mice and the formation of cerebellar circuitry. TINS 3:33–36.

28. Reeves RH, Crowley MR, Lorenzon N, Pavan WJ, Smeyne RJ, Goldowitz D. 1989. The mouse neurological mutant weaver maps within the region of chromosome 16 that is homologous to human chromosome 21. Genomics 5:522–526.

29. Lalonde R. 1986. Acquired immobility response in weaver mutant mice. Exp Neurol 94:808–811.

30. Lalonde R. 1987. Motor abnormalities in weaver mutant mice. Exp Brain Res 65:479–481.

31. Lalonde R, Botez MI. 1986. Navigational deficits in weaver mutant mice. Brain Res 398:175–177.

32. Lalonde R. 1986. Delayed spontaneous alternation in weaver mutant mice. Brain Res 398:178–180.

33. Triarhou LC, Ghetti B. 1987. Neuroanatomical substrate of behavioural impairment in weaver mutant mice. Exp Brain Res 68:434–436.

34. Sidman RL. 1968. Development of interneuronal connections in brains of mutant mice. *In* Physiological and Biochemical Aspects of Nervous

Integration. FD Carlson (ed). Prentice-Hall, Englewood Cliffs, NJ, pp 163–193.

35. Smeyne RJ, Goldowitz D. 1990. Development and death of external granular layer cells in the weaver mouse cerebellum: A quantitative study. J Neurosci 9:1608–1620.

36. Miale I, Sidman RL. 1961. An autoradiographic analysis of histogenesis in the mouse cerebellum. Exp Neurol 4:277–296.

37. Fujita S. 1967. Quantitiative analysis of cell proliferation and differentiation in the cortex of the postnatal mouse cerebellum. J Cell Biol 32:277–287.

38. Blatt GJ, Eisenman LM. 1985. A qualitative and quantitative light microscopic study of the inferior olivary complex of normal, reeler, and weaver mutant mice. J Comp Neurol 232:117–128.

39. Smeyne RJ, Goldowitz D. 1990. Purkinje cell loss is due to a direct action of the weaver gene in Purkinje cells: Evidence from chimeric mice. Dev Brain Res 52:211–218.

40. Lane JD, Nadi NS, McBride WJ, Aprison MH, Kusano K. 1977. Contents of serotonin, norepinephrine and dopamine in the cerebrum of the "staggerer," "weaver" and "nervous" neurologically mutant mice. J Neurochem 29:349–350.

41. Triarhou LC, Low WC, Ghetti B. 1986. Transplantation of ventral mesencephalic anlagen to hosts with genetic nigrostriatal dopamine deficiency. Proc Natl Acad Sci USA 83:8789–8793.

42. Gupta M, Felten DL, Ghetti B. 1987. Selective loss of monoaminergic neurons in weaver mutant mice—an immunocytochemical study. Brain Res 402:379–382.

43. Triarhou LC, Norton J, Ghetti B. 1988. Mesencephalic dopamine cell deficit involves areas A8, A9 and A10 in weaver mutant mice. Exp Brain Res 70:256–265.

44. Ghetti B, Triarhou LC. 1990. Profile of mesencephalic dopamine neuron loss in weaver mutant mice during life-span. Soc Neurosci Abst 6:1138.

45. Roffler-Tarlov S, Graybiel AM. 1984. Weaver mutation has differential effects on the dopamine-containing innervation of the limbic and nonlimbic striatum. Nature 307:62–66.

46. Roffler-Tarlov S, Graybiel AM. 1986. Expression of the weaver gene in dopamine-containing neural systems is dose-dependent and affects both striatal and nonstriatal regions. J Neurosci 6:3319–3330.

47. Graybiel AM, Ohta K, Roffler-Tarlov S. 1990. Patterns of cell and fiber vulnerability in the mesostriatal system of the mutant mouse weaver. I. Gradients and compartments. J Neurosci 10:720–733.

48. Triarhou LC, Ghetti B. 1989. The dendritic dopamine projection of the substantia nigra: Phenotypic denominator of weaver gene action in hetero- and homozygosity. Brain Res 501:373–381.

49. Willinger M, Haaksma C. 1985. Cytoplasmic morphology of weaver (*wv*) mouse cerebellar neurons at the culture substratum. J Neurosci Res 13:163–182.

50. Taber Pierce E. 1973. Time of origin of neurons in the brain stem of the mouse. Prog Brain Res 40:53–65.

51. Bernheimer H, Birkmayer W, Hornykiewicz O, Jellinger K, Seitelberger F. 1973. Brain dopamine and the syndromes of Parkinson and Huntington. Clinical, morphological and neurochemical correlations. J Neurol Sci 20:415–455.
52. Mann DMA, Yates PO. 1983. Possible role of neuromelanin in the pathogenesis of Parkinson's disease. Mech Ageing Dev 21:193–203.
53. Triarhou LC, Norton J, Ghetti B. 1988. Synaptic connectivity of tyrosine hydroxylase immunoreactive nerve terminals in the striatum of normal, heterozygous and homozygous weaver mutant mice. J Neurocytol 17: 221–232.
54. Doucet G, Brundin P, Seth S, Murata Y, Strecker RE, Triarhou LC, Ghetti B, Björklund A. 1989. Degeneration and graft-induced restoration of dopamine innervation in the weaver mouse neostriatum: A quantitative radioautographic study of [^{3}H] dopamine uptake. Exp Brain Res 77: 552–568.
55. Roffler-Tarlov S, Pugatch D, Graybiel AM. 1990. Patterns of cell and fiber vulnerability in the mesostriatal system of the mutant mouse weaver. II. High affinity uptake sites for dopamine. J Neurosci 10:734–740.
56. Kaseda Y, Ghetti B, Low WC, Richter JA, Simon JR. 1987. Dopamine D-2 receptors increase in the dorsolateral striatum of weaver mutant mice. Brain Res 422:178–181.
57. Kaseda Y, Ghetti B, Low WC, Norton J, Brittain H, Triarhou LC, Richter JA, Simon JR. 1990. Age-related changes in striatal dopamine D-2 receptor binding in weaver mutant mice and effects of ventral mesencephalic grafts. Exp Brain Res 83:1–8.
58. Ohta K, Graybiel AM, Roffler-Tarlov S. 1989. Dopamine D-1 binding sites in the striatum of the mutant mouse weaver. Neuroscience 28:69–82.
59. Triarhou LC, Low WC, Ghetti B. 1988. Layer-specific innervation of the dopamine-deficient frontal cortex in weaver mutant mice by grafted mesencephalic dopaminergic neurones. Cell Tissue Res 254:11–15.
60. Goldowitz D. 1989. The weaver granuloprival phenotype is due to intrinsic action of the mutant locus in granule cells: Evidence from homozygous weaver chimeras. Neuron 2:1565–1575.

Chapter 24

The Weaver Mutant Mouse as a Model for Intrastriatal Grafting of Fetal Dopamine Neurons

Lazaros C. Triarhou, Walter C. Low, Guy Doucet, Patrik Brundin, Anders Björklund, and Bernardino Ghetti

Weaver mutant mice are characterized by neuropathological alterations in two neural systems associated with motor function, the cerebellar cortex,[1] and the mesotelencephalic dopamine (DA) projection system.[2] The cellular aspects of neuronal degeneration are discussed in detail in Chapter 23 of this volume. Concerning the genetically determined degeneration of DA neurons in the substantia nigra (SN), the magnitude of cell loss reaches about 70% at 3 months of age,[3] and it is associated with a 75% reduction in striatal DA concentration.[2] The extent of nigrostriatal involvement reoccurs consistently in the mutants. In that respect, weaver homozygotes offer a valuable experimental model for neural transplantation studies, in which the ability of grafted DA neurons to survive and become integrated with the host neuronal circuitry can be studied in the framework of a natural disease.

The authors wish to acknowledge grant support from U.S. Public Health Service (R29-NS29283, RO1-NS14426, PO1-NS27613), Swedish Medicial Research Council (04X-3874), and Fonds de la recherche en santé du Québec.
From Hefti F, and Weiner WJ, (eds.) *Progress in Parkinson's Disease Research—2.* Mount Kisco NY, Futura Publishing Co., Inc., © 1992.

Our goal has been to reconstruct the damaged circuitry in the neurogenetic disease through replacement of degenerated neurons by intracerebral transplantation of fetal ventral mesencephalic neurons. Cellular mechanisms of graft action are extensively studied in two other animal models of DA deficiency, induced chemically by the neurotoxins 6-hydroxydopamine (6-OHDA) and methylphenyltetrahydropyridine (MPTP).[4–7] A natural model of DA neuron degeneration is a valuable complement to the chemical models; the uniqueness of the weaver lies on the fact that the mesostriatal DA depletion is progressive, taking place over several months, and incomplete, in contrast with the acute degeneration induced in toxic models. Thus, neural transplantation studies in the weaver can address specific aspects of graft integration with the chronic pathological CNS. In this chapter we report on histochemical properties and behavioral effects of unilateral and bilateral transplantations of fetal DA-containing neurons to the mutant striatum.

Methodological Issues

It is generally thought that the optimal developmental stage to harvest embryonic neurons for neural grafting is around the cessation of mitotic divisions by the corresponding neuroblasts. Neurons in the mouse SN originate by embryonic day (E) 12.[8] To prepare mesencephalic grafts of dissociated cell suspensions we have used E12 donor tissue. For grafting solid pieces of donor tissue we have used slightly older animals (E14–E15); in that case the embryonic brain yields firmer chunks of tissue, which can be grafted intact.

Donor mesencephalic tissue can be implanted into the striatum of the recipient animals in several different ways (cf. ref. 9 and Figure 1): (1) solid grafts can be inserted stereotaxically into the lateral cerebral ventricle, adjacent to the caudate-putamen complex of the host; (2) solid grafts can be placed into a neocortical cavity, which is prepared in advance by aspiration of the cortex overlying the dorsal neostriatum, according to the delayed-cavity transplantation protocol;[10] or (3) donor tissue can be made into a cell suspension by gentle enzymatic dissociation and grafted by stereotaxic surgery directly into the striatal parenchyma.[11]

In our studies so far we have used adult weaver mutant mice (2–4 months old at the time of grafting) as recipients of fetal

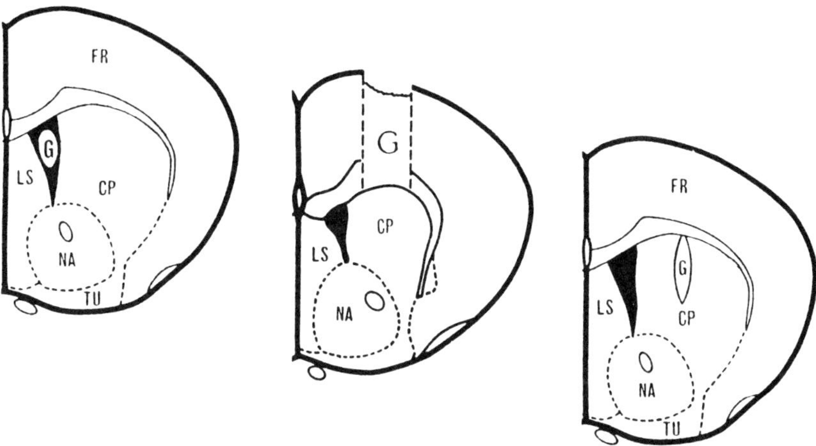

Figure 1. Schematic drawing of the methods for graft placement into the striatum. Left: Graft in the lateral cerebral ventricle. Center: Graft in a preformed cortical cavity. Right: Intrastriatal cell suspension. Abbreviations: G, graft; CP, caudate-putamen; FR, frontal cortex; LS, lateral septum; NA, nucleus accumbens; TU, olfactory tubercle.

mesencephalic tissue. We have followed all of the above approaches, i.e., solid intraventricular grafts,[12] solid grafts into a neocortical cavity[13–17] and intrastriatal cell suspensions.[18,19] The choice of a particular technique may depend on specific demands of experimental design; nevertheless, cell suspension grafts have usually yielded a higher survival rate than solid grafts (>90% vs ~50%).

Structural and Temporal Parameters of Graft Survival and Outgrowth

Histological evidence for survival of grafted DA neurons in the mutant brain has been obtained from experiments with both solid and cell suspension grafts. Immunopositivity for tyrosine hydroxylase (TH) (Figure 2A,B) and immunonegativity for DA β-hydroxylase,[12] or immunopositivity directly for DA,[18] were taken as evidence for the DAergic nature of grafted cells. Surviving transplants contain on the average between 200 and 1200 DA neurons.

The average DA deficiency in the adult weaver striatum amounts to 75%;[2] nigrostriatal DA axons in the dorsolateral and dorsomedial

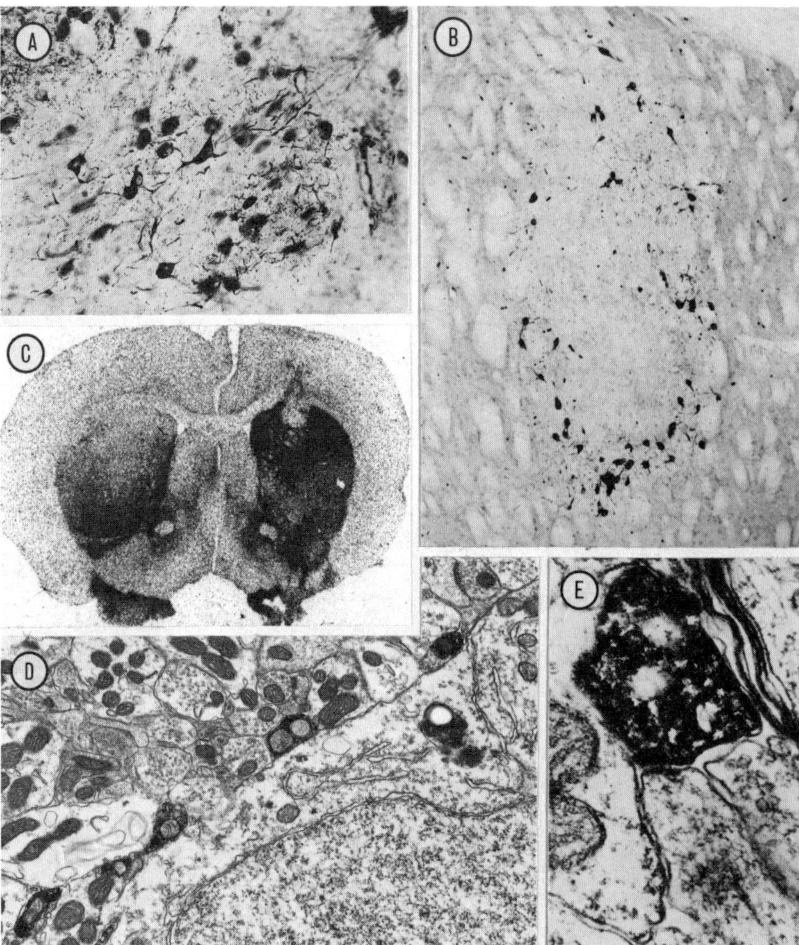

Figure 2. (A) Tyrosine hydroxylase immunoreactive neurons in a solid graft that was placed into a neocortical cavity. Reproduced from ref. 13. (B) Tyrosine hydroxylase immunoreactivity in a cell suspension graft implanted into the striatal parenchyma; original unpublished micrograph. (C) Autoradiography of [^{3}H]dopamine uptake in the case of a cell suspension graft to the right striatum. Reproduced from ref. 18. (D,E) Electron microscopic localization of tyrosine hydroxylase immunoreactivity in the striatum of grafted weaver mutants, showing innervation of unlabeled neuronal elements of the host by immunopositive axon terminals. (D) Reproduced from ref. 15. (E) original unpublished micrograph.

aspects of the caudate-putamen are reduced to an even greater extent: TH or DA immunoreactive fibers are very scarce in those areas.[15,18] The use of a quantitative radioautographic technique of [³H]DA uptake revealed an almost complete absence of DA axons in the dorsal aspect of the weaver neostriatum and an increasing density of DA innervation towards ventral areas (Figure 2C, left hemisphere); the remaining neostriatum was overlaid by diffuse silver grains, suggesting a deficient DA uptake and storage mechanism in residual DA fibers.[18]

Reinnervation of the caudate-putamen complex by TH immunoreactive fibers is observed to a depth of 250 μm at 1 month after grafting;[12] at longer survival times of 4.5 months, the depth of reinnervation extends to about 1000 μm.[13]

Weaver mice with DA cell suspension grafts display, in contrast to the intrinsic neostriatal DA innervation, graft-derived DA fibers with the normal, clustered type of varicosity labeling after uptake of [³H]DA.[18] Computerized image analysis of silver grain density in film radioautographs showed a mean DA reinnervation of neostriatal tissue surrounding the graft of about 20%, in some cases up to 80%, of the density seen in wild-type mice, with a gradual decrease with distance up to 1000–1400 μm away from the graft (Figure 2C, right hemisphere). These data show that a quantitatively significant DA reinnervation of the weaver neostriatum can be provided by fetal mesencephalic grafts and that these DA fibers become functional, at least with respect to DA uptake and storage mechanisms, in a neostriatal environment where intrinsic weaver DA axons are biochemically deficient.

Grafted DA neurons and the resulting fiber outgrowth are sustained over periods of time when the intrinsic nigrostriatal system of the weaver mutant has considerably declined. However, preliminary observations on long-term weaver mice, 9 months after transplantation, suggest that the graft-derived DA fiber outgrowth may be reduced in the affected striatum with time, in spite of good survival of grafted DA neurons.[18]

Specificity of Graft Host Interconnections

Both in normal and weaver striatum, junctional contacts formed by TH immunoreactive nerve terminals are predominantly of the symmetrical type. It was estimated that about 90% of the contacts are junctional in normal striatum, whereas only 50% of the few remaining axons in the weaver striatum display a junctional membrane specialization at 20 days of age,[20] the latter proportion declining further to about one-fourth of the normal value at 8.5 months of age.[15]

Following DA neuron transplantation (Figures 2D and 2E), the incidence of junctional contacts is returned to normal values (91%);[15] further, the profile of the newly established synaptic connectivity resembles the normal situation in regard to subcellular domains of host striatal neurons that are synaptically invested by graft-derived DA axons. Thus, the majority of contacts in the reinnervated striatum (84%) are made with dendritic shafts and spines, which is the case in the normal situation (92% in wild-type animals).

Preliminary evidence further indicates that, during striatal reinnervation by the graft, the compartmentalization that characterizes the normal mesostriatal projection is preserved, i.e., a subset of nigral DA neurons immunoreactive for 28-kDa Ca^{2+}-binding protein (CaBP) innervate neurons of the striatal matrix, which are also CaBP-immunoreactive.[16]

It is suggested, therefore, that in repopulating the denervated weaver striatum, graft-derived DA afferents display a connectional selectivity, i.e., they establish relationships preferentially with those postsynaptic loci that are normally innervated by DA nerve terminals. In this context, it is possible that DA fibers originating in the grafts invest postsynaptic sites that had either been vacated from the intrinsic DA input or had never received such an input.

Cellular Mechanisms of Graft Action

Previous studies in rats have shown that it is possible to establish a terminal axonal network in the DA-denervated striatum by intracerebral grafting of fetal mesencephalic tissue.[21,22] The transplant-derived innervation leads to release of DA in the striatum as determined by methods of in vivo microdialysis[23] and in vivo voltammetry.[24] DA fibers from grafts were found to form synaptic connections with striatal neurons of the host in rats with 6-OHDA lesions[25,26] and in weaver mutants (described under the preceding heading).

The increase in DA D_2 receptor binding, which is induced by 6-OHDA treatment in rats, can be normalized by nigral transplants.[27]

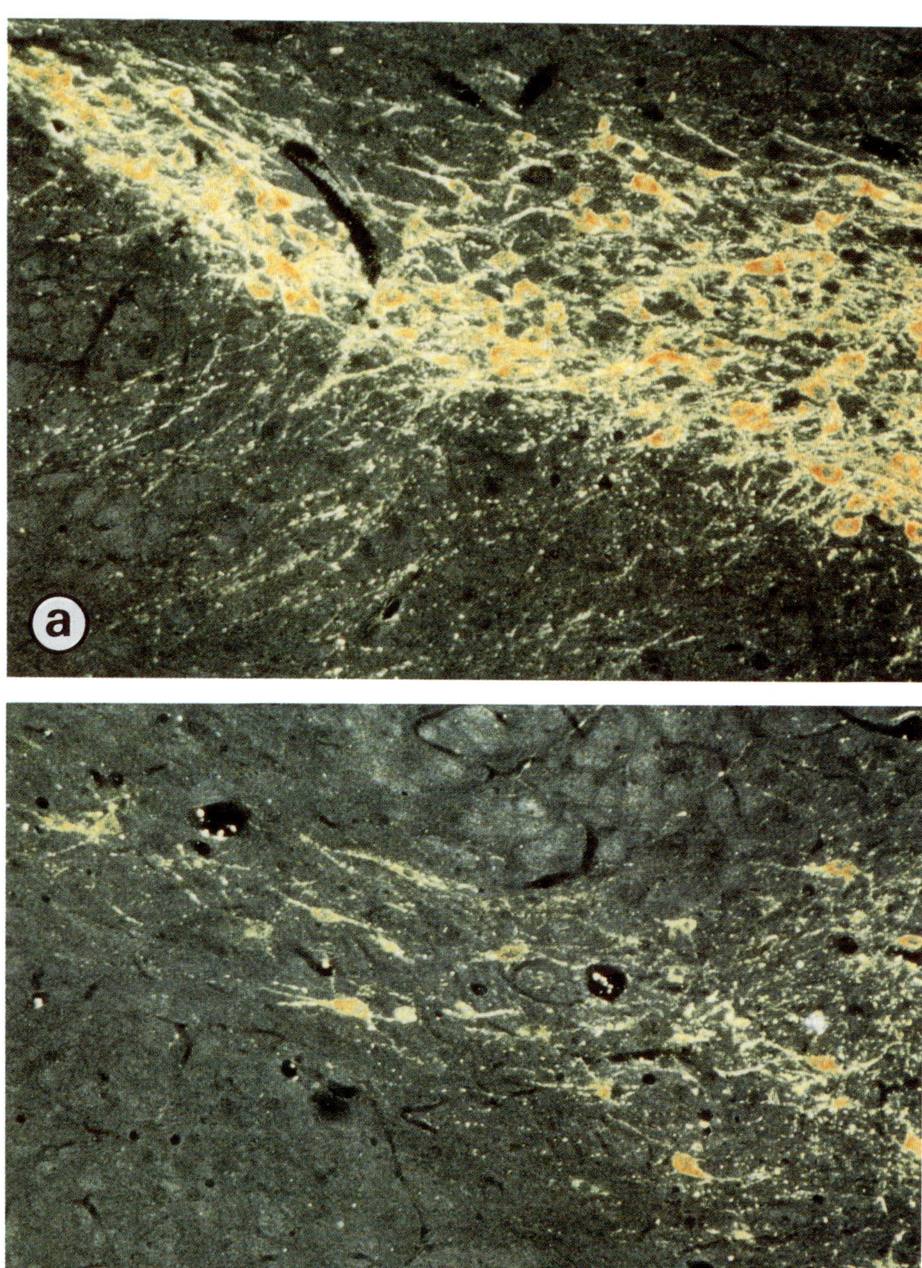

Figure 1. TH immunoreactive neurons in the substantia nigra of a $+/+$ mouse (a) and a *wv/wv* mouse (b). The age of both animals is two years. The cellular deficit at this age amounts to about 85%.

In weaver mutant mice, DA-containing grafts appear to prevent or reverse the 20–30% increase in DA D_2 receptor binding that is observed in the dorsolateral striatal quadrant of nongrafted mutants at 6 months of age.[17]

The precise mechanisms by which grafts may promote functional recovery in experimental animals are only partially understood, and it has been suggested that a multitude of trophic, neurohumoral, and synaptic mechanisms may be responsible.[4]

In one study, remnant DA neurons of the SN were removed ipsilaterally to the graft by local (intranigral) injection of 6-OHDA prior to histological processing, in order to selectively study graft-derived fibers.[19] In that case, TH immunoreactive fibers were found in the host dorsolateral striatum after removal of the ipsilateral SN. Considering that the SN is the only source of endogenous DA supply to this region, it was concluded that such fibers originate in the graft. That experiment provided direct evidence for innervation of the host striatum by graft-derived afferents rather than by fibers belonging to the host and being in some way stimulated by the graft, a mechanism that has been suggested in the case of adrenal medullary grafts to the striatum of MPTP-treated mice.[7]

Normally, the striatum receives only axons of DA neurons from the SN, while DA dendrites are confined to the SN.[28] When a mesencephalic cell suspension is placed intrastriatally, then grafted DA neurons, in addition to axons, extend dendrites into the recipient striatum.[19] The ratio of the incidence of TH immunoreactive axons over that of TH immunoreactive dendrites in the reinnervated striatum is 2:1 in the area proximal to the graft (0–500 μm away) and 20:1 in the area distal to the graft (500–1000 μm away). This effect brings up a difference between the graft-derived innervation and the normal striatal DA supply. DA dendrites of the SN pars reticulata represent one of the brain areas where dendritic release of neurotransmitter has been demonstrated.[29,30] It has been suggested that the dendritic release of DA may contribute, in conjunction with the synaptic input of DA nerve terminals, to the functional effects of the grafts.[19]

Extent and Limits of Functional Recovery

Behavioral studies in the weaver mutant mouse have disclosed a number of locomotor, spatial orientation, and memory deficits;[31–34] some of those deficits are not seen in other mutants with cerebellar lesions only,[35] whereas others are known to be altered by drugs that interfere with catecholamine function[36] or even to be induced by 6-OHDA lesions of the mesostriatal DA projection in normal animals.[32,37] We would expect that behaviors of weaver mutants that are catecholamine-mediated may be improved following bilateral intrastriatal grafting of ventral mesencephalic grafts.

Previous studies in rodents have shown that unilateral destruction of the nigrostriatal pathway by 6-OHDA results in a spontaneous rotational bias to the side ipsilateral to the lesion.[38] With time, spontaneous rotational behavior subsides, but it can still be induced pharmacologically; amphetamine, an agent that releases DA from presynaptic terminals, causes a rotational bias to the side ipsilateral to the lesion.[39] Reinnervation of the chemically denervated striatum by grafted DA neurons has been shown to rectify the rotational bias displayed by animals with unilateral lesions.[11,40,41]

Normal and unoperated weaver mutant mice do not display any substantial preference for either side following administration of amphetamine, beyond the normal variation observed among individual animals. In weaver mutants with DA-containing grafts to the right striatum (solid[14] or cell suspensions[18,19]), amphetamine elicits a significant rotational bias toward the left side. Rotating mice still manifest signs of the superimposed cerebellar ataxia.

The effect of unilateral DA grafts on amphetamine-induced rotations in weaver mice parallels in a way that of rats with bilateral 6-OHDA lesions and unilateral DA-containing grafts;[42] in both situations a circling bias is displayed toward the side contralateral to the graft, which, relative to the grafted replenished side appears as the side of a lesion.

Weaver mice display instability of gait, poor coordination of the limbs, and a fine rapid tremor of the trunk and extremities.[43] The hind-limbs assume an abducted and extended position and the body is lowered to the surface of the ground. Affected animals topple over to the side after every few steps and move their limbs rapidly in an attempt to right themselves. The tremor of the extremities is particularly noticeable when animals fall and try to right themselves. The behavioral syndrome is probably underlain by both the cerebellar and nigrostriatal deficits.[37] One might assume, for example, that intention tremor would have a cerebellar basis, while resting tremor would be due to the pathology of the basal ganglia. Thus, the weaver mouse presents a model in which one may attempt to dissect out ataxic from parkinsonian components of the behavioral phenotype. One way of going about this is by means of neural transplantation. Whereas until now there is no evidence supporting the behavioral correction of cerebellar ataxia following neural grafting, there is ample evidence that in rodents fetal grafts of SN are capable of functionally correcting behaviors associated with experimental DA deficiency.

Weaver mice with bilateral grafts move about, toppling over to the side about 70% fewer times than nonoperated mutants.[16] Moreover, the extremities appear flexed rather than hyperextended, and animals are able to sustain their body in a raised relief, contrasting with the lowered, widened stance of nongrafted mutants. Despite this apparent neurological improvement, tremor and a certain gait instability are still present.

In equilibrium tests, animals are placed on a horizontal wooden bar suspended above the floor.[44] The ability of normal mice to stay on the bar exceeds 3 minutes. Unoperated weaver mice fall off the bar within several seconds after their placement on it. Weaver mutants with bilateral nigral transplants are able to stay on the bar for 2.5 times longer on the average than nonoperated mutants.[16] Occasionally, a grafted mouse may make a 180° turn on the bar without falling off; in such instances, mice secure their position by wrapping the tail around the bar.

The cerebellar component of the behavioral phenotype is a common denominator among the various experimental groups. In a sense, bilateral replacement of striatal DA would render the weaver mutant from combined parkinsonian/ataxic to ataxic only. This is a problem that cannot be avoided, but it is overridden by the benefits of using the mutant striatum as a vector for the analysis of donor tissue growth inside the pathological brain.

In conclusion, these findings indicate that the critical neuronal machinery of the striatum needed to respond appropriately to DA release must be present in weaver and that neural grafting is a viable approach for studying DAergic function in this spontaneous neurodegenerative disorder of the mesostriatal DA projection system.

References

1. Rakic P, Sidman RL. 1973. Sequence of developmental abnormalities leading to granule cell deficit in cerebellar cortex of weaver mutant mice. J Comp Neurol 152:103–132.

2. Schmidt MJ, Sawyer BD, Perry KW, Fuller RW, Foreman MM, Ghetti B. 1982. Dopamine deficiency in the weaver mutant mouse. J Neurosci 2: 376–380.

3. Triarhou LC, Norton J, Ghetti B. 1988. Mesencephalic dopamine cell deficit involves areas A8, A9 and A10 in weaver mutant mice. Exp Brain Res 70:256–265.

4. Björklund A, Lindvall O, Isacson O, Brundin P, Wictorin K, Strecker RE, Clarke DJ, Dunnett SB. 1987. Mechanisms of action of intracerebral neural implants: Studies on nigral and striatal grafts to the lesioned striatum. Trends Neurosci 10:509–516.

5. Brundin P, Björklund A. 1987. Survival, growth and function of dopaminergic neurons grafted to the brain. Prog Brain Res 71:293–308.

6. Redmond DE, Roth RH, Elsworth JD, Sladek JR, Collier TJ, Deutsch AY, Haber S. 1986. Foetal neuronal grafts in monkeys given methylphenyltetrahydropyridine. Lancet 1:1125–1127.

7. Bohn MC, Cupit L, Marciano F, Gash DM. 1987. Adrenal medulla grafts enhance recovery of striatal dopaminergic fibers. Science 237:913–916.

8. Taber Pierce E. 1973. Time of origin of neurons in the brain stem of the mouse. Prog Brain Res 40:53–65.

9. Olson L. 1985. On the use of transplants to counteract the symptoms of Parkinson's disease: Background, experimental models, and possible clinical applications. *In* Synaptic Plasticity. CW Cotman (ed) Guilford, New York, pp 485–505.

10. Stenevi U, Björklund A, Svendgaard N-A. 1976. Transplantation of central and peripheral monoamine neurons to the adult rat brain: Techniques and conditions for survival. Brain Res 114:1–20.

11. Björklund A, Schmidt RH, Stenevi U. 1980. Functional reinnervation of the neostriatum in the adult rat by use of intraparenchymal grafting of dissociated cell suspensions from the substantia nigra. Cell Tissue Res 212:39–45.

12. Triarhou LC, Low WC, Ghetti B. 1986. Transplantation of ventral mesencephalic anlagen to hosts with genetic nigrostriatal dopamine deficiency. Proc Natl Acad Sci USA 83:8789–8793.

13. Triarhou LC, Low WC, Ghetti B. 1987. Synaptic investment of striatal cellular domains by grafted dopamine neurons in weaver mutant mice. Naturwissenschaften 74:591–593.

14. Low WC, Triarhou LC, Kaseda Y, Norton J, Ghetti B. 1987. Functional innervation of the striatum by ventral mesencephalic grafts in mice with inherited nigrostriatal dopamine deficiency. Brain Res 435:315–321.

15. Triarhou LC, Low WC, Norton J, Ghetti B. 1988. Reinstatement of synaptic connectivity in the striatum of weaver mutant mice following transplantation of ventral mesencephalic anlagen. J Neurocytol 17:233–243.

16. Triarhou LC, Low WC, Ghetti B. 1990. Dopamine neurone grafting to the weaver mouse neostriatum. Prog Brain Res 82:187–195.

17. Kaseda Y, Ghetti B, Low WC, Norton J, Brittain, Triarhou LC, Richter JA, Simon JR. 1990. Age-related changes in striatal dopamine D-2 receptor binding in weaver mice and effects of ventral mesencephalic grafts. Exp Brain Res 83:1–8.

18. Doucet G, Brundin P, Seth S, Murata Y, Strecker RE, Triarhou LC, Ghetti B, Björklund A. 1989. Degeneration and graft-induced restoration of dopamine innervation in the weaver mouse neostriatum: A quantitative radio-autographic study of [³H]dopamine uptake. Exp Brain Res 77:552–568.
19. Triarhou LC, Brundin P, Doucet G, Norton J, Björklund A, Ghetti B. 1990. Intrastriatal implants of mesencephalic cell suspensions in weaver mutant mice: Ultrastructural relationships of dopaminergic dendrites and axons issued from the graft. Exp Brain Res 79:3–17.
20. Triarhou LC, Norton J, Ghetti B. 1988. Synaptic connectivity of tyrosine hydroxylase immunoreactive nerve terminals in the striatum of normal, heterozygous and homozygous weaver mutant mice. J Neurocytol 17:221–232.
21. Björklund A, Stenevi U. 1979. Reconstruction of the nigrostriatal pathway by intracerebral nigral transplants. Brain Res 177:555–560.
22. Perlow MJ, Freed WJ, Hoffer BJ, Seiger Å, Olson L, Wyatt RJ. 1979. Brain grafts reduce motor abnormalities produced by destruction of nigrostriatal dopamine system. Science 204:643–647.
23. Strecker RE, Sharp T, Brundin P, Zetterström T, Ungerstedt U, Björklund A. 1987. Autoregulation of dopamine release and metabolism by intrastriatal nigral grafts as revealed by intracerebral dialysis. Neuroscience 22: 169–178.
24. Rose G, Gerhardt G, Strömberg I, Olson L, Hoffer B. 1985. Monoamine release from dopamine-depleted rat caudate nucleus reinnervated by substantia nigra transplants: An in vivo electrochemical study. Brain Res 341:92–100.
25. Freund TF, Bolam JP, Björklund A, Stenevi U, Dunnett SB, Powell JF, Smith AD. 1985. Efferent synaptic connections of grafted dopaminergic neurons reinnervating the host neostriatum: A tyrosine hydroxylase immunocytochemical study. J Neurosci 5:603–616.
26. Mahalik TJ, Finger TE, Strömberg I, Olson L. 1985. Substantia nigra transplants into denervated striatum of the rat: Ultrastructure of graft and host interconnections. J Comp Neurol 240:60–70.
27. Freed WJ, Ko GN, Niehoff DL, Kuhar MJ, Hoffer BJ, Olson L, Cannon-Spoor HE, Morihisa JM, Wyatt RJ. 1983. Normalization of spiroperidol binding in the denervated rat striatum by homologous grafts of substantia nigra. Science 222:937–939.
28. Björklund A, Lindvall O. 1984. Dopamine-containing systems in the CNS. *In* Handbook of Chemical Neuroanatomy, Vol 2. A Björklund, T Hökfelt (eds). Elsevier, Amsterdam, pp 55–122.
29. Björklund A, Lindvall O. 1975. Dopamine in dendrites of substantia nigra neurons: Suggestions for a role in dendritic terminals. Brain Res 83:531–537.
30. Chéramy A, Leviel V, Glowinski J. 1981. Dendritic release of dopamine in the substantia nigra. Nature 289:537–542.
31. Lalonde R. 1986. Acquired immobility response in weaver mutant mice. Exp Neurol 94:808–811.
32. Lalonde R. 1987. Motor abnormalities in weaver mutant mice. Exp Brain Res 65:479–481.

33. Lalonde R, Botez MI. 1986. Navigational deficits in weaver mutant mice. Brain Res 398:175–177.
34. Lalonde R. 1986. Delayed spontaneous alternation in weaver mutant mice. Brain Res 398:178–180.
35. Lalonde R, Botez MI. 1985. Exploration of a hole-board matrix in nervous mice. Brain Res 343:356–359.
36. Porsolt RD, Bertin A, Blavet N, Deniel M, Jalfre M. 1979. Immobility induced by forced swimming in rats: Effects of agents which modify central catecholamine and serotonin activity. Eur J Pharmacol 57:201–210.
37. Triarhou LC, Ghetti B. 1987. Neuroanatomical substrate of behavioural impairment in weaver mutant mice. Exp Brain Res 68:434–436.
38. Ungerstedt U. 1971. Striatal dopamine release after amphetamine or nerve degeneration revealed by rotational behaviour. Acta Physiol Scand 367(suppl):49–68.
39. Marshall JF, Ungerstedt U. 1977. Supersensitivity to apomorphine following destruction of the ascending dopamine neurons: Quantification using the rotational model. Eur J Pharmacol 41:361–367.
40. Dunnett SB, Björklund A, Stenevi U, Iversen SD. 1981. Behavioural recovery following transplantation of substantia nigra in rats subjected to 6-OHDA lesions of the nigrostriatal dopamine pathway. I. Unilateral lesions. Brain Res 215:147–161.
41. Brundin P, Isacson O, Gage FH, Prochiantz A, Björklund A. 1986. The rotating 6-hydroxydopamine-lesioned mouse as a model for assessing functional effects of neuronal grafting. Brain Res 366:346–349.
42. Dunnett SB, Björklund A, Stenevi U, Iversen SD. 1981. Behavioural recovery following transplantation of substantia nigra in rats subjected to 6-OHDA lesions of the nigrostriatal dopamine pathway. I. Bilateral lesions. Brain Res 229:457–470.
43. Sidman RL, Green MC, Appel SH. 1965. Catalog of the neurological mutants of the mouse. Harvard University Press, Cambridge, MA pp 66–67.
44. Bureš J, Burešová O. Huston JP. 1976. Techniques and Basic Experiments for the Study of Brain and Behavior. Elsevier/North-Holland Biomedical Press, Amsterdam.

6

Trophic Factors for Dopaminergic Neurons

Chapter 25

Study of Dopaminergic Neuronal Differentiation and Survival by Use of Three-Dimensional Reaggregate Tissue Culture and Monoclonal Hybrid Cell Lines

Alfred Heller, Lisa Won, Hyung Choi, Bruce Wainer, and Philip C. Hoffmann

Since the demonstration by Ehringer and Hornykiewicz in 1960[1] of a marked reduction in the levels of dopamine in the basal ganglia of parkinsonian patients at autopsy, interest has been focused on the degeneration of dopaminergic neurons of the nigrostriatal projection as an essential feature of the pathogenesis of this disease. Neuronal survival in the peripheral and central nervous systems is dependent on cell differentiation and the establishment of functional connections with appropriate target cells.[2] In the case of the dopaminergic neurons of the pars compacta of the substantia nigra, major axonal synaptic connections are formed with telencephalic structures including the basal ganglia, limbic, and neocortical structures.[3] The mechanisms that determine whether a given set of neurons can

From Hefti F, and Weiner WJ, (eds.) *Progress in Parkinson's Disease Research—2.* Mount Kisco NY, Futura Publishing Co., Inc., © 1992.

function as dopaminergic targets and the role of such cells in providing trophic influences for dopaminergic neuronal survival is, however, as yet unclear. Given the precedent provided by the death of peripheral sensory and sympathetic neurons when they are deprived of nerve growth factor (NGF),[4] and the role of this factor in septal cholinergic neuronal survival,[5] it seems entirely possible that loss of similar trophic factors for central dopaminergic neurons may be at least one of the causes for the degeneration of dopaminergic neurons in Parkinson's disease. The recent findings of trophic effects of brain-derived neurotrophic factor (BDNF) on dopaminergic neurons in culture is, of course, of interest in this regard.[6,7]

Analysis of the interdependence of dopaminergic neurons and their target cells in the intact brain presents formidable experimental barriers. The use of tissue culture for such studies provides a means of simplifying the experimental system so as to make it more amenable for analysis. Among the culture systems available, the rotation-mediated reaggregate tissue culture system first described by Moscona and Moscona[8] and later applied by DeLong and Sidman,[9] Seeds,[10] and Garber and Moscona[11] to cells of the central nervous system has proved to be a particularly useful approach to the examination of cell–cell interactions involved in neuronal differentiation and survival. In this system, embryonic brain regions are dissected and dissociated with trypsin and mechanical shearing forces into single-cell suspensions (Figure 1). All of the neuronal processes are removed by this treatment.[12] The suspended cells (typically $7.5–15 \times 10^6$ in number) are placed in culture medium in flasks which are rotated at 70–80 revolutions per minute at 37°C in an incubator. The vortex in the medium that results from the rotation produces cellular collisions. As a consequence, the cells begin to adhere to one another causing the formation of cellular reaggregates during the next 24 hours in culture.[13] The neurons thereafter resume their differentiation within the reaggregates. As many as 500–700 such reaggregates may be formed depending upon the number of cells originally added to each flask. The reaggregates are reasonably uniform in shape, approximating spheres of roughly 300 μm in diameter (Figure 2). These reaggregates provide three-dimensional structures in which the developing neurons and glia from specific areas of brain can interact with respect to cell–cell associations, process formation, and the establishment of synaptic connections with appropriate target cells. The cellular composition of the

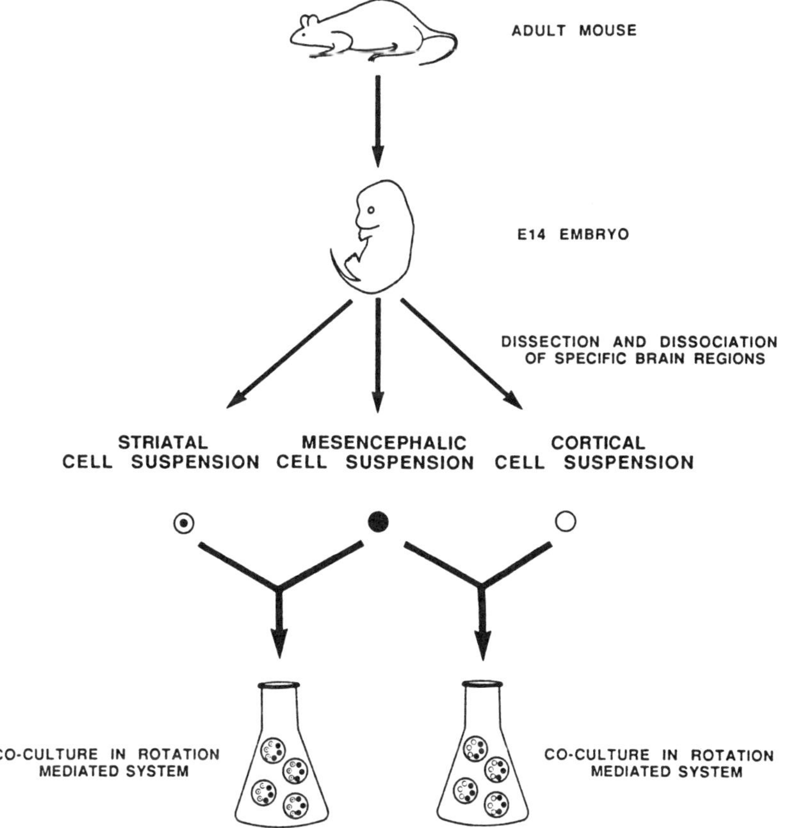

Figure 1.   Schematic illustration of the preparation of reaggregates from specific embryonic brain regions.

reaggregates can be varied almost at will, depending on the needs of the particular experiment. The only limitation on the method is the necessity to obtain cells from the embryonic brain at times that are in close proximity to the birth dates of the neurons of interest in order to obtain successful reaggregation. Two or more dissociated cell suspensions stemming from different brain regions can be mixed with the result being the formation of reaggregates of the cells from a variety of brain regions with or without specific connectivities (Figure 1). For example, reaggregates can be constituted from (1)

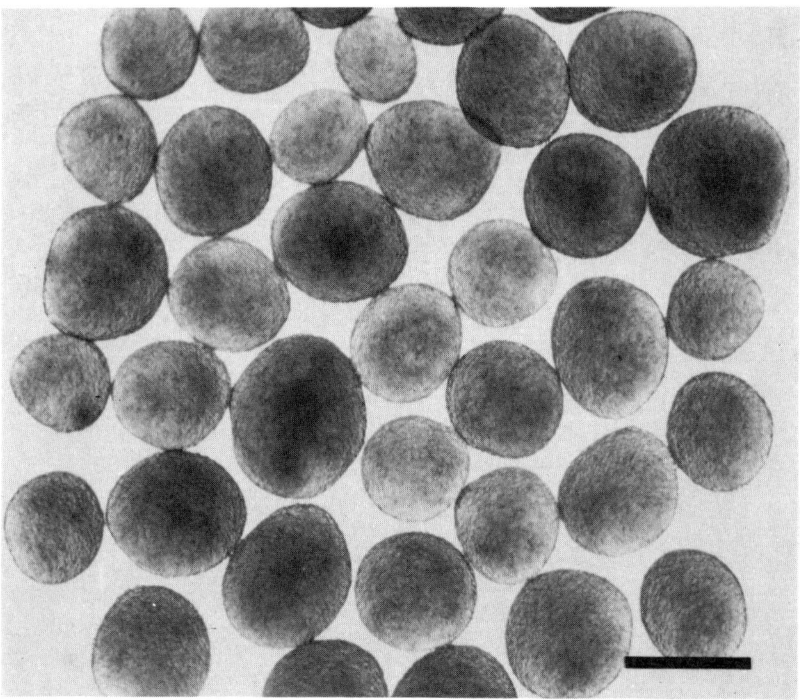

Figure 2.   Photomicrograph of RMT-CS reaggregates after 3 weeks in culture. Calibration bar = 300 μm.

cells from a region of the brain containing a neurochemically identified population of neurons and (2) cells prepared from an area that is normally innervated by these neurons. Such combinations are particularly useful for studying the cellular interactions that occur during development and the nature of trophic relationships between neurons and their target cells. On the other hand, one can reaggregate the neurochemically identified neurons with dissociated cells from brain areas with which they are not normally in synaptic contact. In the case of dopaminergic neurons, reaggregates consisting of cells from the rostral mesencephalon (the area containing dopaminergic neurons) with cells from the corpus striatum (the area containing target cells for the dopaminergic neurons) can be compared to reaggregates of rostral mesencephalic cells with tectal cells (an area of the brain with which dopaminergic neurons do not make synaptic contact, i.e., a nontarget area).

The rotation-mediated reaggregation of dopamine-containing cells from the rostral mesencephalic tegmentum (RMT) with cells from one of their target areas, the corpus striatum (CS), results in reaggregates (RMT-CS) that represent a model of the innervation of CS by dopaminergic cells of the substantia nigra. Such reaggregates can be maintained in culture for extended periods of time of up to at least 3 months. Since the cells within such reaggregates show a remarkable recapitulation of the normal neurochemical and morphological development seen in vivo within the intact embryonic and neonatal brain,[14] the approach provides a useful model system for the examination of those factors that determine neuron-to-neuron connectivity and the role of such synaptic connections in cell differentiation and survival.

Among the fundamental issues to be resolved with regard to the differentiation and survival of dopaminergic neurons are questions of the underlying cellular and molecular mechanisms that result in cell–cell recognition, including the association of cells of like lineage into nuclear groups and the ability of neuronal processes, particularly axons, to make synaptic contact with appropriate target cells. Additional information on the mechanisms by which target cells influence neuronal differentiation and survival is obviously essential to an understanding of normal development as well as dysfunction in a variety of disease states which involve cell death. Examination of the differentiation of dopaminergic neurons within the three-dimensional reaggregate system has provided a number of interesting clues to understanding these complex processes. This flexible cell culture system is amenable to appropriate experimental manipulation for the possible resolution of a number of these issues.

The three-dimensional character of the reaggregate system provides an environment in which the cultured cells can migrate and form normal cell–cell associations. In such reaggregate systems, cells of like lineage will form clusters, a phenomenon that has been demonstrated with a variety of cell types.[11,15–18] In initial experiments with dopaminergic neurons visualized by catecholamine-induced histofluorescence, it was observed by Levitt et al.[19] in reaggregates of mesencephalic cells that by 24 hours in culture the fluorescent cells appeared to be evenly distributed in sections obtained from such reaggregates. By two days in culture, however, such fluorescent cells were observed as small clusters which, over the next 24 hours, formed bands of fluorescent cells. A subsequent quantitative study by Hemmendinger et al.[20] using reaggregates of RMT cells alone or of these cells in combination with target cells of the CS or of the frontal cortex (FCx) or with nontarget cells of the tectum, confirmed these initial observations. In this study, it was shown that the dopaminergic neurons were spatially clustered following 3, 7, or 12 days in culture. Moreover, such "sorting out" or clustering by the embryonic dopaminergic neurons occurred in the presence of either target or nontarget cells.[20] This capacity of dopaminergic neurons to sort out or cluster by migration within the cell mass of the reaggregate demonstrates that dopaminergic neurons within the reaggregates retain an essential property of neurons of like lineage, i.e., the ability to associate with one another and form nuclear groupings. Since the embryonic morphological architecture was destroyed during cell dissociation and the phenomenon occurs even in the absence of appropriate target cells, these studies on dopaminergic cell association provide direct evidence that the requisite information for migration, cell association, and nuclear formation by cells of like lineage in the developing brain is contained within the cells themselves and is not dependent on the presence of appropriate axonal synaptic connections or the prior formation of a normal brain cytoarchitecture.

While the migration and clustering of dopaminergic neurons within the reaggregate culture system is not dependent on the presence of target or nontarget cells, many other features of the morphological and neurochemical development of these neurons are apparently regulated by trophic influences from target areas such as the CS. The formation of axonal processes,[21] the development of appropriate synaptic connections,[22] and dopaminergic cell survival[23] are dependent on the presence of target cells in the reaggregate. When reaggregates are prepared from cells of the RMT with cells of the tectum, the dopaminergic cells extend thick dendritic processes, but no obvious axonal arborizations (Figure 3A). On the other hand, in the presence of cells of the CS or FCx (anatomical subdivisions of the brain receiving extensive dopaminergic innervation), the dopaminergic neurons form a dense plexus of dopaminergic axons extending some distance away from the dopaminergic cell bodies into the neuropil of the reaggregate (Figures 3B and 3C). At 7 days in culture, it is necessary to "load" the dopaminergic cells with exogenous dopamine in order that they contain sufficient dopamine to allow the cell bodies as well as the punctuate pericellular axons to be visualized with Falck-Hillarp fluorescence histochemistry. However, by 14–21 days in culture, the dopaminergic neurons, synthesize and retain sufficient endogenous dopamine to allow them to be visualized by the histofluorescent procedure without the addition of exogenous dopamine.[14] This is the result of an almost fivefold increase in the dopamine content of these cells as determined by high-performance liquid chromatography (HPLC) in the 14-day cultures as compared to 7-day cultures and a 23-fold increase by 21 days in culture.[14]

This neurochemical index of the increasing development of the dopaminergic neurons in the cocultures is paralleled by the increasing morphological development of the pericellular axonal fluorescent patterns. The ability of the developing dopaminergic neurons to take up and store exogenous dopamine increases with elapsing time in culture, such that it is enhanced 12-fold after 21 days in culture compared to that which occurs in 3-day cultures. Moreover, the 14- and 21-day-old cocultures are much more sensitive to the monoamine-depleting effects of either reserpine or 6-hydroxydopamine, agents which require neuronal uptake and storage mechanisms in order to produce their pharmacologic effects. Taken collectively, these results strongly suggest that with increasing time in culture, the immature dopaminergic neurons develop the systems necessary for uptake and storage of exogenous dopamine just as they do in the normal intact developing brain.[14]

The pattern of axonal development in 3-week-old RMT-CS and RMT-FCx reaggregates is shown in Figure 3. In the RMT-FCx reaggregates it is possible to more easily discern single axons with beaded varicosities coursing through the neuropil (Figure 3C) than in RMT-CS reaggregates (Figure 3B). It is of considerable interest that the dopaminergic axonal patterns within the two types of reaggregates mimic those that are found in the CS and FCx in situ (see ref. 21 for a visual comparison of the reaggregate patterns with the in situ patterns). It is clear from these studies that the presence of cells from target areas (CS or FCx) is required in order for dopaminergic neurons to fully express their normal phenotypic development of axonal arborization and neuronal connectivity, i.e., there is a trophic relationship between dopaminergic neurons and cells from their target areas.

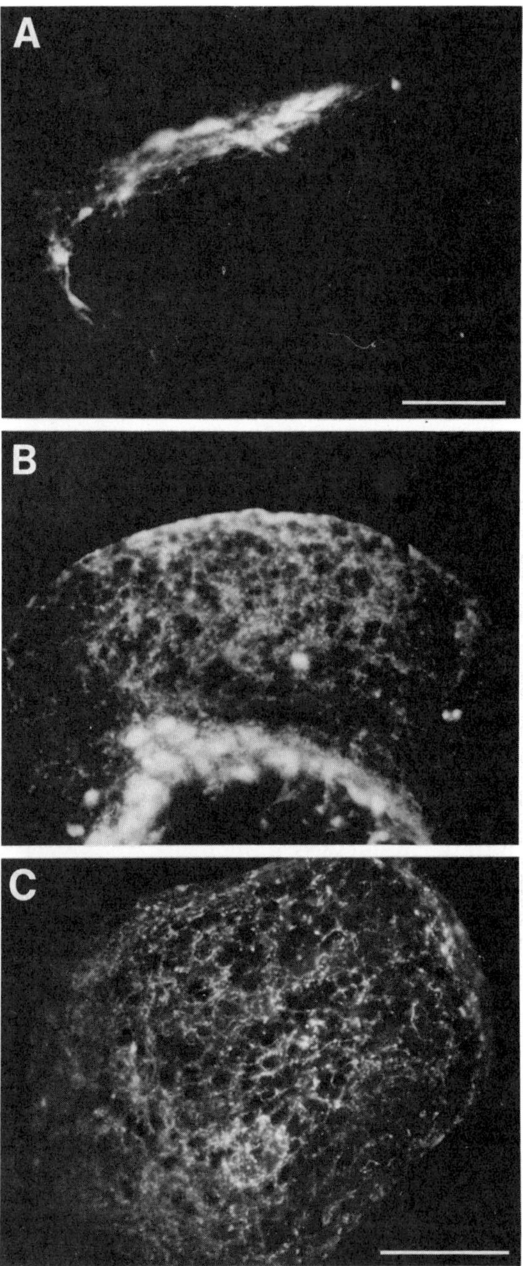

Ultrastructural studies have demonstrated that the development of axonal processes by dopaminergic neurons results in the formation of synaptic connections with appropriate target cells. A correlated light and electron microscopic study utilizing an antibody to tyrosine hydroxylase (TH) as a marker for dopaminergic neurons demonstrates the existence of such synapses.[22] Histological sections from 21-day-old RMT-CS reaggregates were first stained by the peroxidase–antiperoxidase technique[24] to visualize TH-immunoreactive neurons. As is the case when such neurons are revealed by catecholamine-induced histofluorescence, immunoreactive perikarya are found to be clustered as the result of the sorting out process (Figure 4). The morphological features of these reaggregate TH-immunoreactive neurons are very similar to those described for these neurons when they develop in situ. The dopaminergic cell bodies are ovoid, multipolar, and approximately 20 μm in diameter. At the ultrastructural level, their perikarya contain an eccentrically located nucleus and abundant cytoplasm. These dopaminergic neurons receive synaptic input from at least two types of axonal boutons: those yielding symmetrical synaptic specializations and those demonstrating asymmetrical synaptic specializations. On the other hand, TH-immunoreactive boutons form typical symmetrical synaptic specializations with nonimmunoreactive perikarya, dendritic shafts, and dendritic spines.[22]

In order to ascertain the neurochemical nature of the synaptic target cells, an antibody against DARPP-32 (a dopamine and adenosine 3′,5′-monophosphate-regulated phosphoprotein) was used as a marker for the visualization of striatal dopaminoceptive neurons.[25] The method of Levey et al.,[26] utilizing sequential staining, can be used to localize two antigens in the same section, thus allowing the demonstration of dopaminergic neurons (TH-immunoreactive cells) and their target cells (DARPP-32-immunoreactive

---

Figure 3. Photomicrographs of sections through 3-week-old reaggregates processed by the Falck-Hillarp histofluorescence technique. (A) An RMT-tectal reaggregate containing clustered fluorescent cell bodies (on the lower aspect of the photomicrograph) which lack extensive fiber proliferation. (B) An RMT-CS reaggregate containing clustered fluorescent cell bodies at the lower aspect of the section and dense patches of punctate fluorescence. (C) RMT-FCx reaggregate containing thin fluorescent fibers bearing varicosities. Calibration bars: A and B, 50 μm; C, 80 μm.

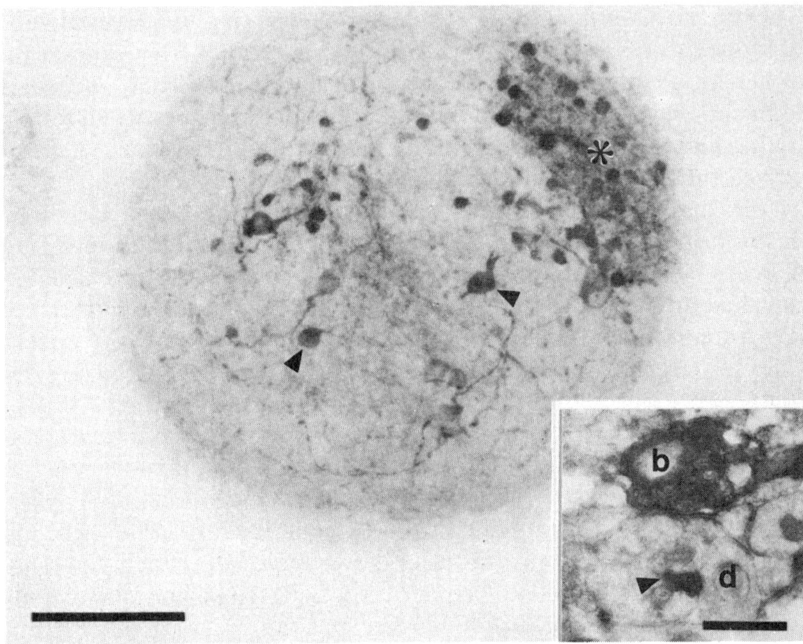

Figure 4. Black and white photomicrograph of a 50-μm section through a 21-day-old RMT-CS reaggregate that was double labeled for TH and DARPP-32 immunoreactivity. The arrowheads point out some of the larger TH-positive cell bodies. Note the cluster of smaller, darker DARPP-32-positive cell bodies (asterisk). The granular immunoreactivity that surrounds these DARPP-32 cell bodies is associated with TH-positive axons and DARPP-32 axons and dendrites. Calibration bar = 100 μm. An electron micrograph of such an area is shown in the inset. A TH-immunoreactive bouton (b) is shown making synaptic contact with a DARPP-32-immunoreactive dendrite (d). The TH immunoreactivity can be distinguished by its dark, diffuse reaction product, while the DARPP-32 reaction product consists of crystals (arrowhead). Calibration bar = 0.5 μm.

cells) in the same histological section. TH immunoreactivity is first revealed with diaminobenzidine, which yields a brown, diffuse reaction product. Following incubation with the primary antibody directed against DARPP-32, DARPP-32 structures are visualized with benzidine dihydrochloride, which yields a blue, granular reaction product. Although a maximal appreciation of the results requires inspection of the published color photomicrograph in which one can readily distinguish the two-colored reaction products,[22]

Figure 4, a black and white print of a similar color photomicrograph, illustrates the principle morphological findings. The larger cell bodies present in the center of the field (arrow heads) are TH-immunoreactive. These cells are ovoid, multipolar, and roughly 20 μm in diameter. They are seen to extend long, beaded processes throughout the neuropil. The small, very dark cell bodies (asterisk) present in the upper right of the field of view are DARPP-32-immunoreactive cells. These cell bodies are roughly 9–15 μm in diameter and are round or oval in shape. The observed clustering of DARPP-32 cell bodies represents, yet again, an example of the phenomenon of cell sorting that has been consistently observed as embryonic neurons develop within reaggregates. The diffuse, punctate reaction product that surrounds these DARPP-32-labeled cell bodies is a mixture of TH-immunoreactive terminals and DARPP-32-labeled processes, suggesting a close association of TH-containing axons with DARPP-32-labeled cells. Electron microscopic observation of TH-positive boutons in such DARPP-32 neuronal clusters shows that synapses are indeed formed between the dopaminergic axons and DARPP-32-containing neurons[22] (inset in Figure 4).

The synaptic connections between dopaminergic neurons and their target cells in the reaggregate system not only appear similar to those formed in the intact brain, but such synaptic connections also appear to be functional in terms of dopamine release. The dopaminergic neurons respond to appropriate stimuli that normally evoke dopamine release.[27] This property has been assessed in RMT-CS reaggregates after 17–22 days in culture. Following incubation with [³H]dopamine to label the transmitter pool in the dopaminergic neurons, reaggregates were superfused over a period of 2 hours and fractions of the superfusate collected and counted for radioactivity. Spontaneous release of [³H]dopamine occurs at the rate of roughly 1% of that stored in the tissue every 2 minutes. The spontaneous release of radioactivity from the reaggregates is reduced by 40% when tetrodotoxin is superfused. Since tetrodotoxin is known to block voltage-dependent sodium channels, this finding suggests the existence of spontaneous electrical activity within the developing dopaminergic neurons. Exposure to graded concentrations of extracellular potassium, which results in neuronal depolarization, increases the release of radioactivity in a potassium concentration-dependent fashion. The depolarization-induced release of [³H]dopamine requires the presence of extracellular calcium, suggesting the involvement of voltage-dependent calcium channels in the release process. The compound, *d*-amphetamine, known to induce dopamine release in vivo, produces release of [³H]dopamine from the RMT-CS reaggregates in a dose-dependent manner. Finally, the neuropeptide, substance P, an agonist at tachykinin receptors known to be present on dopaminergic cell bodies within the mesencephalon,[28] is capable of increasing the release of [³H]dopamine twofold when superfused onto the reaggregates.[27]

An additional feature of this target cell-dependent development and maintenance of axonal processes is its importance for dopaminergic cell survival.[23] After 7 days in culture, RMT-CS reaggregates contain roughly 3–4 times as many dopaminergic neurons as visualized by histofluorescence as are found in reaggregates of RMT cells, alone or in RMT-tectal reaggregates. Similarly, there is a target cell-dependent effect of FCx cells on the survival of mesencephalic dopaminergic neurons, although the effect is quantitatively less, with enhanced survival on the order of 1.5-fold.[23]

The intensity of catecholamine-induced histofluorescence is dependent upon the concentration of catecholamine present in the neurons and, if the concentration falls below a certain level, the neurons are no longer visible as histofluorescent structures.[29] Thus, the possibility exists that the apparent comparative difference in the numbers of dopaminergic cell bodies resulted from a reduction of catecholamine concentration rather than an actual loss of catecholamine-containing cell bodies. Therefore, these experiments were extended to 13 days in culture and the dopaminergic neurons were visualized by an alternative procedure, TH immunocytochemistry. In addition, dopamine levels in the reaggregates were assayed by HPLC in parallel. For these experiments, cell numbers were estimated by counting neurochemically identified cells in a sample of histological sections. The volume of these sections as well as the total volume of reaggregate tissue contained within a given flask was obtained as previously described.[30] From these data, the total number of neurochemically identified cells contained within experimental groups can be compared with each other. The results (Table 1) show that there is roughly a 60% reduction in the number of TH-positive cells in RMT-tectal flasks (dopaminergic cells with nontarget cells) when they are compared to the number of such cells in RMT-CS flasks (dopaminergic cells with target cells). The target cell-dependent effect on cell

Table 1.

Comparison of Number of Tyrosine-Hydroxylase (TH)-Positive Cells and Dopamine Levels in Reaggregates of Mesencephalic Cells with Target Cells of Corpus Striatum (RMT-CS) or with Nontarget Cells of Tectum (RMT-Tectal)[a]

	TH-positive cells/flask[b]	Dopamine (ng/mg protein)[c]
RMT-CS	30,372 ± 4,765	8.7 ± 0.2
RMT-tectal	12,206 ± 920	2.9 ± 0.2

[a]RMT-CS and RMT-tectal reaggregates were cultured for 13 days and then harvested for TH immunocytochemistry and analysis of their endogenous dopamine levels. The values represent the mean ± standard error of the mean; $N = 4$.
[b]TH-positive cells/flask were estimated by the method of Heller et al.[30] Cells/flask in the RMT-CS reaggregates were significantly different from cells/flask in the RMT-tectal reaggregates; $P \leq 0.001$ by the statistical model described in Heller et al.[30]
[c]Endogenous dopamine levels were determined by high-performance liquid chromatography.[14] Endogenous dopamine levels in RMT-CS reaggregates were significantly different from those in the RMT-tectal reaggregates; $P \leq 0.001$ by a two-tailed t-test.

survival is therefore observed when either TH immunocytochemistry or catecholamine-induced histofluorescence is used to visualize the dopaminergic neurons. Moreover, endogenous dopamine levels in non-target-cell-containing reaggregates (RMT-tectal) are also reduced by approximately 59%, in parallel with the reduction in dopaminergic neurons. Thus, the presence of target cells results in an apparent increase in survival of dopaminergic neurons, suggesting that the target cells provide a trophic influence to the dopaminergic neurons. The loss or reduction of such a trophic influence could well play a role in the death of dopaminergic neurons, which is involved in the pathogenesis of Parkinson's disease.

The relationship between dopaminergic neurons and their target cells of the CS appears to be reciprocal; the target cells providing trophic factor(s) necessary for the differentiation and survival of dopaminergic neurons and the synaptic connections of dopaminergic neurons with striatal cells apparently providing modulatory influences for the striatal cells. It has been demonstrated by radioactive ligand binding assays that both D_1 and D_2 dopaminergic receptors are present in RMT-CS reaggregates. In a preliminary study, Perry et al.[31] showed that there was a potential interaction of presynaptic dopaminergic neurons with striatal target neurons. This interaction was assessed by preparing RMT-CS, RMT-tectal, and CS, alone, reaggregates. After 21 days in culture, the density of D-1 binding sites was determined by labeling membrane preparations from these reaggregates with [^{125}I]SCH-23982, a D-1 selective antagonist. The RMT-CS reaggregates expressed twice as many D-1 binding sites as did CS reaggregates and five times as many as did RMT-tectal reaggregates. These results suggest that receptor expression in the target cells may be influenced by interactions with their developing presynaptic counterparts.

Collectively, studies of both pre- and postsynaptic markers at the neurochemical and morphological level strongly suggest that embryonic dopaminergic neurons and their target cells in the striatum can be dissociated to yield single-cell suspensions that lack any of the embryonic brain structure and then recombined in vitro to form reaggregates in which the neurons reassociate with one another in an appropriate fashion, continue to differentiate with the elaboration of axons and dendrites, establish appropriate synaptic connections, and begin to function as neuronal systems.

While not directly relevant to the issue of dopaminergic cell survival and Parkinson's disease, it should be noted that this recapitulation of normal neuronal development within rotation-mediated reaggregates is not restricted to mesencephalic dopaminergic neurons and their target cells. Analogous experiments have examined cholinergic cells derived from the septum and their interactions with their target cells of the hippocampus, cerebellum being used as a source of dissociated, nontarget cells.[32] The results of these experiments reveal the same target cell-dependent developmental events that are observed with the dopaminergic neurons and their target cells, namely, (1) hippocampal cell-dependent process formation by the developing septal neurons, which is not present in septal cerebellar reaggregates; and (2) marked enhancement of septal cholinergic cell survival in reaggregates containing the hippocampal target cells as compared to septal cells reaggregated by themselves, or in the presence of the nontarget cerebellar cells. Ultrastructural observations confirm that cholinergic septal neurons degenerate in the absence of their hippocampal target cells.[33]

The fact that dopaminergic neurons in reaggregate culture are capable, in the presence of target cells, of forming appropriate synaptic connections with such cells provides an opportunity to examine the nature of the signals involved in axonal target recognition. Such experiments were conducted by presenting the dopaminergic cells of the RMT simultaneously with both target (CS) cells and nontarget (tectal) cells in the same reaggregates and observing the pattern of axonal proliferation within the reaggregate tissue.[34] Such analysis requires the ability to distinguish target from nontarget cells within the reaggregates. To this end, dissociated RMT cells containing dopaminergic neurons and dissociated nontarget tectal cells were incubated with wheat germ agglutinin that had been conjugated to the fluorescent dye, rhodamine. These cells were then combined with nondyed CS cells and allowed to reaggregate. The resulting "triple" reaggregates were cultured for 9 days, harvested, and processed for catecholamine-induced histofluorescence. Again in this case, cell sorting was observed in that nontarget cells revealed by their red, rhodamine fluorescence became segregated from the nondyed CS target cells. One could discern within the histological sections discrete areas consisting of either target cells (nondyed) or nontarget cells (red-dyed) along with the greenish histofluorescent dopaminergic cell bodies and their processes. In order to distinguish axonal from dendritic processes, the size of the dopaminergic neuronal dendritic fields was assessed with RMT-tectal reaggregates in which axonal proliferation is at a minimum. After the subtraction of dopaminergic dendritic fluorescence, 85% of the presumed axonal fibers in the triple reaggregates are confined to the striatal target cell areas. Examination of other RMT-CS-tectal reaggregates cultured for only 4 days revealed dopaminergic neurons with short processes confined to the vicinity of the cell bodies from which they arise. After an additional 2 days (6 days of culture), 71% of the axons are still confined to the nondyed, target cell-containing area, despite the fact that these processes extended themselves further away from the cell bodies. These results[34] provide direct evidence that the mechanisms resulting in restriction of dopaminergic processes to target-cell-containing areas occur as the result of specific interactions between the outgrowing dopaminergic axons and their cellular environment. The distribution of dopaminergic axons suggests that easily diffusable factors are probably not involved in the restriction of dopaminergic fibers to the target cell areas, since there is very little ingrowth of dopaminergic processes into nontarget-cell-containing areas that are immediately adjacent to the process-containing target cell areas. In addition, these findings raise the interesting possibility that nontarget cells may be capable of actively excluding inappropriate innervation.

Examination of the developmental potential of dopaminergic neurons in the three-dimensional reaggregate culture system has provided a number of insights into the cellular interactions involved in these developmental events. Moreover, a number of inferences can be drawn from these findings as to the molecular mechanisms underlying cell–cell recognition, synaptic connectivity, and neuronal survival. However, an unraveling of the molecular mechanisms involved requires a further simplification of the system and a more reductionist approach. As relatively simple and useful as three-dimensional reaggregate culture of dopaminergic neurons has proven, we are nevertheless still dealing with these neurons in a highly complex system. In an area such as the mesencephalon, the dopaminergic neurons comprise only 0.5–1.0% of the total neuronal population, and even this subpopulation is made up of a complex of neurons that are topographically arranged in terms of their axonal projections to a wide diversity of subdivisions of the brain. A similar complexity exists in terms of populations of neurons in the brain areas innervated by the dopaminergic neurons, such as the CS.[35] This problem of heterogeneity of neuronal cell types is considerable even without taking into account the known effects of glia from different brain regions on dopaminergic neuronal differentiation.[36] In addition, primary cells are probably not the optimal source of material from which to define and isolate trophic factors. This reservation is based upon at least three considerations. First, there is an obvious limitation on the amount of tissue that can be obtained from a given area of the embryonic brain. Second, there is good reason to believe that only very small amounts of trophic factors are likely to be present in such brain areas.[37] Finally, as noted above, even a circumscribed brain area is very heterogenous in terms of the number of cell types present within it, the most obvious example being the coexistence of neurons and glial cells. Given this reservation, it seems reasonable to attempt to circumvent these limitations by developing cell lines that would express the dopaminergic or striatal neuronal phenotypes. Such cell lines could yield virtually unlimited amounts of homogenous cells for investigations into the detailed cellular and molecular events that regulate and maintain nigrostriatal cell differentiation, and phenotypic expression and survival, processes which apparently fail in Parkinson's disease.

The technique of somatic cell fusion has been utilized in our laboratory to produce monoclonal hybrid neuronal cell lines. This technique was first applied to the production of hybrid cell lines from both embryonically derived[38] and neonatally derived[39] septal cholinergic neurons, as well as cell lines derived from hippocampal cells that produce NGF.[40] More recently, this approach has been used for the production of catecholamine-producing cell lines derived from embryonic mesencephalon[41] and striatal lines bearing both D-1 and D_2 receptors.[42] For the purpose of producing catecholamine-containing cell lines, mesencephalic cells were dissociated with trypsin and then suspended in culture medium containing phytohemagglutinin. This suspension of primary brain cells was then layered over a carpet of cells (70% confluent) of a hypoxanthine phosphoribosyltransferase (HPRT) deficient neuroblastoma cell line (N18TG2). In order to promote cell fusions, the cells were exposed to polyethylene glycol for 1 minute. After washing, the cells were incubated overnight. The medium was then changed to one containing hypoxanthine, aminopterin, and thymidine. Such a medium selects against the HPRT-deficient neuroblastoma parent cells, while allowing hybrid cells that have acquired the HPRT gene from the primary cell parent to survive and multiply. Colonies of growing hybrid cells were subcloned by a modified single-cell plating technique[43] to generate monoclonal cell lines.

Cell lines derived from the mesencephalon were screened for catecholamine content. Catecholamine content is a suitable screen for detecting the desired hybrid cells because the neuroblastoma parent has nondetectable endogenous levels of catecholamines. Fifty-two monoclonal hybrid cell lines were obtained. One of these (MN9D) contains high endogenous levels of dopamine (105 ng/mg protein), one (MN9H) contains high endogenous levels of the immediate precursor of dopamine, L-dopa (186 ng/mg protein), and one (MN9X) contains no detectable level of catecholamine.[41] MN9D cells also contain norepinephrine, but only at one third the level of dopamine. On the other hand, the level of norepinephrine in MN9H cells is roughly equivalent to their dopamine content. Both catecholamine-positive cell lines release L-dopa and dopamine into the culture medium. MN9D cells when treated with 1 mM n-butyrate for 7 days extend long neurite-like processes (Figure 5). The endogenous catecholamine level in such differentiated cells is sufficiently high to allow for the catecholamine-induced histofluorescent

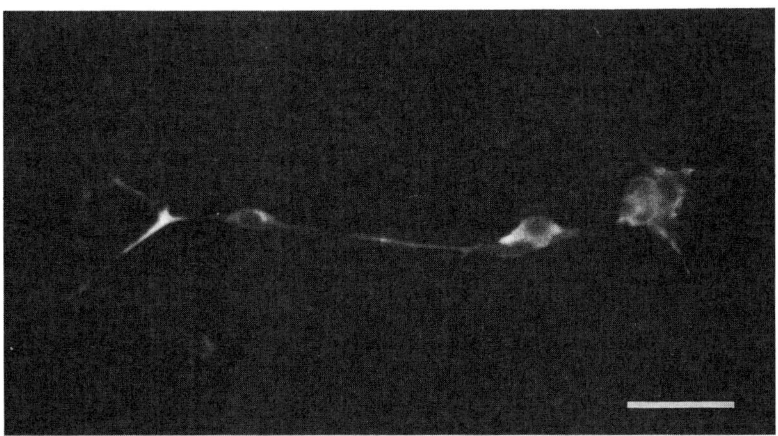

Figure 5.   A photomicrograph of MN9D cells treated with 1 mM *n*-butyrate in monolayer culture for 7 days. Note the long neurites. The cells synthesize and retain sufficient catecholamine to be visualized by Falck-Hillarp histofluorescence. Calibration bar = 50 μm.

visualization of the cell bodies as well as the processes (Figure 5). Chromosomal analysis shows that both of these hybrid cell lines (MN9D and MN9H) possess a larger number of chromosomes than the neuroblastoma parent, although not as many as would result from a one-to-one fusion of the primary brain cell parent with the neuroblastoma parent. When MN9D and MN9H cell lines were again subcloned, the resultant cells possessed identical endogenous catecholamine levels as the cells from which they were cloned, demonstrating their monoclonal nature.[41]

The hybrid cell lines can also be distinguished from the neuroblastoma parents morphologically. Typically, they are approximately two times as large as the neuroblastoma cells and they undergo mitosis at a slower rate. The hybrid cells' neurochemical and morphological properties appear to be stable for months. Moreover, they can be frozen and stored. After thawing, they resume their growth and show no alteration in their catecholamine levels or in their morphology. The phenomenon of cell aggregation, a property of embryonic cells, can be used to further substantiate the fact that the hybrid cells possess traits acquired from the embryonic primary brain cell parent. Specifically, dissociated single-cell suspensions of (1) the parent neuroblastoma, (2) PC-12 cells derived from a pheochromocytoma, and (3) the hybrid cell lines were placed in the rotation-mediated reaggregation system for 24 hours. Both hybrid cell lines formed cellular aggregates, but neither the parent neuroblastoma cells nor the PC-12 cells aggregated. This result indicates that the hybrid cell lines must have acquired the property of aggregation from the embryonic primary brain cell parents. The neuronal character of the hybrid cell lines is also demonstrated by their expression of neurofilament protein subunits NF150 and NF200. These subunits, characteristic of neurons, can be demonstrated immunocytochemically, both in a perinuclear location and in the neurite-like processes. On the other hand, there is no detectable labeling of the hybrid cells with a monoclonal antibody directed against glial fibrillary acidic protein, strongly suggesting that there was no glial component in their parentage.[41]

The MN9D hybrid cells also show a fundamental property of excitable cells, the generation of depolarization-induced action potentials measured under whole-cell, current-clamp conditions. The underlying voltage-dependent sodium currents can be measured under voltage-clamp conditions. Some of the electrophysiological properties of dopaminergic neurons studied in vivo or in slice preparations in vitro are not present in the MN9D cells. Since these properties are derived from voltage-dependent calcium channels and calcium-sensitive ion channels in proximal axonal segments, their absence in the MN9D cells may be the result of: (1) calcium buffering in the EGTA-containing recording pipet, or (2) the absence of neuronal processes on the MN9D cells from which the recordings were obtained. On the other hand, the whole-cell sodium currents can not be distinguished on the basis of their activation and inactivation properties from the sodium currents through rodent brain sodium channels.[41]

Finally, the MN9D cells are much more sensitive to the monoamine-depleting effects of the active metabolite, MPP$^+$, of the dopaminergic neurotoxin, N-methyl-4-phenyl-1,2,3,6-tetrahydropyridine, than are PC-12 cells. Depletion of the endogenous dopamine levels of the two cell lines by roughly 40% required 24 hours of exposure to 1 μM MPP$^+$ in the case of the MN9D cells, but 100 μM MPP$^+$ (two orders of magnitude greater) in the case of the PC-12 cells. This result strongly suggests that the MN9D cells more closely resemble primary dopaminergic neurons of the central nervous system than do PC-12 cells, despite the fact that both cell lines are able to synthesize and store dopamine.[41]

While the monoclonal hybrid dopaminergic cell lines demonstrate a number of interesting properties, their usefulness for the study at the cellular and molecular level of trophic interactions between dopaminergic cells and their neuronal targets in the striatum depends on the ability of such hybrid cells to interact with other neurons and to distinguish between target and nontarget cellular elements. In a preliminary study, it has been possible to show that the MN9D dopaminergic cell line is indeed capable of responding in a differential fashion to the presence of nontarget as opposed to target cells.[44] In these experiments, 2000 MN9D dopamine-containing hybrid cells were aggregated with 8 million dissociated CS, FCx, tectal, or thalamic cells in the rotation-mediated reaggregate system. The reaggregates were exposed to 1 mM *n*-butyrate during days 2–7 in culture to suppress the overgrowth of the MN9D cells. At the end of 7 days in culture, the reaggregates were processed for: (1) chromatographic determination of endogenous dopamine levels, (2) histological observation following cresyl violet staining, and (3) catecholamine-induced histofluorescence. The MN9D hybrid cells show markedly (10- to 20-fold) higher endogenous levels of dopamine in the presence of target cells (CS or FCx) as compared to such levels in reaggregates containing nontarget cells (tectum or thalamus). Sections stained with cresyl violet allow one to distinguish the larger MN9D hybrid cells from the smaller primary brain cells in the reaggregates. Inspection of these stained sections and cell counting following dissociation of the reaggregates revealed that there is no difference in the number of MN9D hybrid cells in the various reaggregate types. On the other hand, only in reaggregates containing target cells does one find brightly fluorescent MN9D hybrid cells. Thus, it is apparent that MN9D hybrid cells responded differentially to the two different cellular environments (target or nontarget) to which they were exposed.

The MN9D cells aggregated (1) only with one another or (2) with target cells having essentially identical levels of endogenous dopamine. However, when MN9D cells are aggregated in the presence of nontarget cells as described above, a reduction in dopamine levels and histofluorescence is observed (Choi et al., unpublished observations). These data suggest that target cells play a permissive role in the expression of the dopaminergic phenotype by MN9D cells and that there is an active inhibition of this phenotype by the nontarget cells. The differential response of MN9D cells to the presence of target and nontarget tissue suggests that such a cell line may be a model appropriate for the study of cellular and molecular mechanisms involved in examining both positive and negative trophic interactions.

Studies of dopaminergic neurons and their interactions with target cells utilizing the three-dimensional reaggregate system has provided information with regard to a number of important issues concerning the normal development and differentiation of dopaminergic neurons that may be pertinent to our understanding of the failure of dopaminergic function, which is at least a major component in the pathogenesis of Parkinson's disease. Use of the reaggregate system involves the complete dissociation of the cells of interest and stripping of their neuronal processes, as well as destruction of their cytoarchitectural relationships. Despite this, it is clear that dopaminergic cells in the proper cellular environment are capable, within this system, of undergoing extensive differentiation and establishing, or reestablishing, appropriate cellular relationships with their neighboring cells and target neurons. Given these findings, it seems reasonable to suggest that information necessary for the formation of dopaminergic nuclear groups, neuronal differentiation, and selective innervation of target cells is contained within the cells themselves and does not require the morphological substrate of the intact brain. At least some of the factors involved in axonal recognition and synapse formation with target cells appear to be nondiffusable. In order to facilitate the examination of the molecular mechanisms underlying dopaminergic differentiation, dopaminergic monoclonal hybrid cells have been generated. The finding that primary, brain nontarget cells can suppress the dopaminergic phenotype of the hybrid MN9D cells raises the possibility that similar nontarget effects on developing dopaminergic neurons may occur in vivo. Such effects could account for the inability of dopaminergic axons to innervate nontarget areas of the developing brain.

Acknowledgments: The authors wish to acknowledge the valuable technical assistance of Eligia Buhay, Nancy Bubula, Francis Karapas, Christine Martin, Sandy Nelson and Steve Price. Dr. Barbara Heller, Department of Mathematics, Illinois Institute of Technology provided the statistical procedures utilized in this research and a critical review of the manuscript.

References

1. Ehringer H, Hornykiewicz O. 1960. Verteilung von Noradrenalin und Dopamin (3-Hydroxtyramin) im Gehirn des Menschen und ihr Verhalten bei Erkrankungen des Extrapyramidalen Systems. Klin Wochenschr 38:1236–1239.
2. Oppenheim RW. 1991. Cell death during development of the nervous system. Annu Rev Neurosci 14:453–501.
3. Bjorklund A, Lindvall O. 1984. Dopamine-containing systems in the CNS. *In* Handbook of Chemical Neuroanatomy, Vol. 2. A Bjorklund, T Hokfelt, eds. Elsevier, Amsterdam, p 55–122.
4. Levi-Montalcini R. 1966. The nerve growth factor: its mode of action on sensory and sympathetic nerve cells. Harvey Lect 60:217–259.
5. Hefti F. 1986. Nerve growth factor (NGF) promotes survival of septal cholinergic neurons after fimbrial transections. J Neurosci 6:2155–2162.
6. Hyman C, Hofer M, Barde Y-A, Juhasz M, Yancopoulos GD, Squinto SP, Lindsay RM. 1991. BDNF is a neurotrophic factor for dopaminergic neurons of the substantia nigra. Nature 350:230–232.
7. Knusel B, Winslow JW, Rosenthal A, Burton LE, Seid DP, Nikolics K, Hefti F. 1991. Promotion of central cholinergic and dopaminergic neuron differentiation by brain-derived neurotrophic factor but not neurotrophin 3. Proc Natl Acad Sci USA, 88:961–965.
8. Moscona A, Moscona H. 1952. The disassociation and aggregation of cells from organ rudiments of the early chick embryo. J Anat 86:287–301.
9. DeLong GR, Sidman RL. 1970. Alignment defect of reaggregating cells in cultures of developing brains of reeler mutant mice. Dev Biol 22:584–599.
10. Seeds NW. 1971. Biochemical differentiation in reaggregating brain cell culture. Proc Natl Acad Sci USA 73:1858–1861.
11. Garber BB, Moscona AA. 1972. Reconstruction of brain tissue from cell suspensions: I. Aggregation patterns of cells dissociated from different regions of the developing brain. Dev Biol 27:217–234.
12. Garber BB, Huttenlocher PR, Larramendi LHM. 1980. Self-assembly of cortical plate cells in vitro within embyronic mouse cerebral aggregates, golgi and electron microscopic analysis. Brain Res 201:255–278.
13. Monroy A, Moscona AA. 1979. Introductory Concepts in Developmental Biology. University of Chicago Press, Chicago.
14. Kotake C, Hoffmann PC, Heller A. 1982. The biochemical and morphological development of differentiating dopamine neurons co-aggregated with their target cells of the corpus striatum in vitro. J Neurosci 2:1307–1315.
15. Wilson HV. 1907. On some phenomena of coalescence and regeneration in sponges. J Exp Zool 5:245–258.
16. Wilson HV, Penney JT. 1930. The regeneration of sponges (*Microciana*) from dissociated cells. J Exp Zool 56:73–147.
17. Townes PL, Holtfreter J. 1955. Directed movements and selective adhesion of embryonic amphibian cells. J Exp Zool 128:53–118.
18. Moscona AA. 1956. Development of heterotypic combinations of

dissociated embryonic chick cells. Proc Soc Exp Biol Med 92:410–416.

19. Levitt P, Moore RY, Garber BB. 1976. Selective cell association of catecholamine neurons in brain aggregates in vitro. Brain Res 111:311–320.

20. Hemmendinger LM, Garber BB, Hoffmann PC, Heller A. 1981. Selective association of embryonic murine mesencephalic dopamine neurons in vitro. Brain Res 222:417–422.

21. Hemmendinger LM, Garber BB, Hoffmann PC, Heller A. 1981. Target neuron-specific process formation by embryonic mesencephalic dopamine neurons in vitro. Proc Natl Acad Sci USA 78:1264–1268.

22. Won L, Price S, Wainer BH, Hoffmann PC, Bolam JP, Greengard P, Heller A. 1989. Correlated light and electron microscopic study of dopaminergic neurons and their synaptic junctions with DARPP-32-containing cells in three-dimensional reaggregate tissue culture. J Comp Neurol 289:165–177.

23. Hoffmann PC, Hemmendinger LM, Kotake C, Heller A. 1983. Enhanced dopamine cell survival in reaggregates containing telencephalic target cells. Brain Res 274:275–281.

24. Sternberger LA. 1979. The unlabeled antibody peroxidase–antiperoxidase (PAP) method. *In* Immunocytochemistry, John Wiley & Sons, New York, pp 104–169.

25. Ouimet CC, Greengard P. 1990. Distribution of DARPP-32 in the basal ganglia: An electron microscopic study. J Neurocytol 19:39–52.

26. Levey A, Bolam JP, Rye D, Hallanger A, De Muth R, Mesulam M, Wainer BH. 1986. A light and electron microscopic procedure for sequential double antigen localization using diaminobenzidine and benzidine dihydrochloride. J Histochem Cytochem 35:1449–1457.

27. Shalaby I, Kotake C, Hoffmann PC, Heller A. 1983. Release of dopamine from coaggregate cultures of mesencephalic tegmentum and corpus striatum. J Neurosci 3:1565–1571.

28. Mantyh PW, Maggio JE, Hunt SP. 1984. The autoradiographic distribution of kassinin and substance K binding sites is different from the distribution of substance P binding sites in rat brain. Eur J Pharmacol 102:361–364.

29. Fuxe K, Hokfelt T, Jonsson G, Ungerstedt U. 1970. Fluorescence microscopy in neuroanatomy. *In* Contemporary Research Methods in Neuroanatomy. WJH Nauta, SOE Ebbesson (eds). Springer-Verlag, Berlin.

30. Heller A, Kontur P, Hoffmann P, Heller B. 1988. Quantitation of neurochemically identified neurons in reaggregate tissue cultures. J Neurosci Methods 25:83–90.

31. Perry BD, Wainwright MW, Won L, Heller A, Hoffmann P. 1990. The influence of dopamine neurons on D-1-dopamine receptor binding site development in three dimensional reaggregate tissue culture. Soc Neurosci Abstr 16:646.

32. Hsiang J, Wainer BH, Shalaby IA, Hoffmann PC, Heller A, Heller B. 1987. Neurotrophic effects of hippocampal target cells on developing septal cholinergic neurons in culture. Neuroscience 21:333–343.

33. Hsiang J, Price SD, Heller A, Hoffmann PC, Wainer BH. 1988. Ultrastructural evidence for hippocampal target cell-mediated trophic effects on septal cholinergic neurons in reaggregating cell cultures. Neuroscience 26:417–431.
34. Won L, Heller A, Hoffmann PC. 1989. Selective association of dopamine axons with their striatal target cells in vitro. Dev Brain Res 74:93–100.
35. Graybiel A, Ragsdale CW Jr. 1983. Biochemical anatomy of the striatum. *In* Chemical Neuroanatomy. PC Emson ed. Raven Press, New York, pp 427–504.
36. Denis-Donini S, Glowinski J, Prochiantz A. 1984. Glial heterogeneity may define the three-dimensional shape of mouse mesencephalic neurones. Nature 307:641–643.
37. Barde Y-A. 1988. What, if anything, is a neurotrophic factor? TINS 11:343–346.
38. Hammond DN, Wainer BH, Tonsgard JH, Heller A. 1986. Neuronal properties of clonal hybrid cell lines derived from central cholinergic neurons. Science 234:1237–1240.
39. Lee HJ, Hammond DN, Large TH, Wainer BH. 1990. Immortalized young adult neurons from the septal region: Generation and characterization. Dev Brain Res 52:219–228.
40. Lee HJ, Hammond DN, Large TH, Roback JD, Sim JA, Brown DA, Otten UH, Wainer BH. 1990. Neuronal properties and trophic activities of immortalized hippocampal cells from embryonic and young adult mice. J Neurosci 10:1779–1787.
41. Choi HK, Won LA, Kontur PJ, Hammond DN, Fox AP, Wainer BH, Hoffmann PC, Heller A. 1992. Immortalization of embryonic mesencephalic dopaminergic neurons by somatic cell fusion. Brain Res (in press).
42. Wainwright MW, Perry BD, Kontur P, Heller A. 1990. Expression of D-1-dopamine receptor binding sites in an immortalized murine corpus striatum cell line. Soc Neurosci Abstr 16:646.
43. Puck TT, Marcus PI, Cieciura SJ. 1956. Clonal growth of mammalian cells in vitro. J Exp Med 103:273–284.
44. Choi HK, Won LA, Heller A. 1990. The dopamine content of immortalized hybrid neurons is dependent on the presence of target tissue. Soc Neurosci Abstr 16:996.

Chapter 26

Neuronal Specificities of the Neurotrophins: Therapeutic Potential in Neurodegenerative Diseases?

Ron M. Lindsay, Ralph F. Alderson, Beth Friedman, Carolyn Hyman, Nancy Y. Ip, Mark E. Furth, Peter C. Maisonpierre, Stephen P. Squinto, and George D. Yancopoulos

The recent molecular cloning of brain-derived neurotrophic factor (BDNF) and neurotrophin-3 (NT-3) has established the existence of an NGF-related family of neurotrophic factors—the neurotrophins.[1-4] The availability of recombinant BDNF and NT-3 has allowed the initiation of a broad in vitro study of the neuronal specificity of each of these factors. Using primary cultures of developing CNS neurons from various brain regions, we have established that BDNF: (1) promotes the survival and phenotypic differentiation of rat septal cholinergic neurons,[5] a property consistent with the discovery of high levels of BDNF expression within the hippocampus;[6-8] and (2) promotes the survival of rat nigral dopaminergic neurons and protects these neurons from the dopaminergic neurotoxins 6-hydroxydopamine and MPTP.[9] Thus the neurotrophic

From Hefti F, and Weiner WJ, (eds.) *Progress in Parkinson's Disease Research—2.* Mount Kisco NY, Futura Publishing Co., Inc., © 1992.

effects of BDNF towards neuronal populations known to degenerate in two of the major human neurodegenerative diseases—Alzheimer's and Parkinson's disease—provokes the question of whether any of the novel neurotrophic factors may have therapeutic potential in halting the progression or even ameliorating the symptoms of devastating neurological disorders.

Until recently, NGF was the only fully characterized neurotrophic factor that had been shown both in vitro and in vivo to be essential for the survival of specific populations of neurons during development and to be important for maintenance of the differentiated phenotype of mature neurons.[10–12] The most widely known action of NGF is the role of this prototypical neurotrophic factor as a survival factor for developing sympathetic and neural crest-derived sensory neurons. It is now clear that NGF is not only a neurotrophic factor for peripheral neurons—in vitro and in vivo studies have shown survival promoting effects of NGF towards cholinergic neurons of the basal forebrain,[13–18] a role consistent with the demonstration of high levels of NGF mRNA in the targets of these neurons—the hippocampus and cortex.[19–21] Furthermore the actions of NGF are not confined to development. Although mature neurons may no longer require NGF as a survival factor, it has been shown, for example, that NGF is essential for maintenance of the fully differentiated phenotype of adult sensory neurons.[22,23]

Therapeutic Potential of NGF?

Findings that have indicated that NGF is not only a trophic factor for developing neurons but is also vital as a maintenance factor and/or regulator of the function of mature neurons have prompted a great deal of interest and speculation in the possible involvement and therapeutic use of neurotrophic factors in degenerative diseases.[24] Clearly much of this speculation has been driven by the finding that cholinergic neurons of the basal forebrain, one of several populations of neurons that degenerate in Alzheimer's disease, are responsive to NGF.[13–18] It has now been demonstrated both in rats and primates that axotomy-induced degeneration of cholinergic neurons of the septum can be reversed by intraventricular infusion of NGF.[16,17,25,26] Although caution should be exercised in drawing any conclusions from such animal studies regarding the possible efficacy of NGF in

Alzheimer's disease, these studies have been instrumental in advancing the notion that neurotrophic factors in general may have enormous therapeutic potential for the treatment of neurodegenerative diseases. While it is clear that rapid degeneration of cholinergic neurons following an acute insult such as axotomy is not at all representative of the slow progressive loss of many different types of neurons during the long course of Alzheimer's disease, the clear demonstration that intraventricular infusion of a protein growth factor can rescue degenerating neurons is in itself an important new principle.

Neuronal Specificity of NGF

The specificity of NGF has been shown to be limited to sympathetic neurons, certain neural crest-derived sensory neurons, and cholinergic neurons of the basal forebrain. Thus the lack of effect of NGF on many different types of neurons has long predicted the existence of other neurotrophic factors with different neuronal specificities. Although a number of distinct and potent neurotrophic activities have been described, purification and molecular characterization of these molecules has been hampered by their extremely low abundance.[27] The low abundance has also severely limited characterization of the neuronal specificities of these activities either in tissue culture or animal studies. The cloning of three novel neurotrophic factors in the last 2 years—brain-derived neurotrophic factor (BDNF), neurotrophin-3 (NT-3), and ciliary neurotrophic factor (CNTF) has opened a new era in the biology of neurotrophic factors.[1–4,28,29]

Brain-Derived Neurotrophic Factor (BDNF)

BDNF was first described as a neurotrophic factor with survival-promoting effects on dorsal root ganglion (DRG) sensory neurons.[30–32] Although this action of BDNF was similar to that of NGF towards DRG neurons, NGF-neutralizing antibodies did not block BDNF activity. Using sensory neurons as a bioassay Barde et al.[31] first purified BDNF from pig brain. A clear indication that BDNF had distinct neuronal specificity(s) from NGF was established when it was shown that BDNF could support the survival of sensory neurons of the neural placode-derived nodose ganglion, neurons which are refractory to NGF.[33–35] It has since been established that BDNF supports the survival of other placode-derived sensory neurons,[36] none of which respond to NGF. The recent cloning of BDNF has allowed the production of recombinant BDNF, which in turn is permitting detailed characterization of the biological actions of BDNF, especially its neuronal specifity, and has also led directly to the discovery of a completely novel neurotrophic factor— neurotrophin-3 (NT-3).[2–4]

Effects of BDNF on Survival and Phenotypic Expression of Septal Cholinergic Neurons in Culture

NGF promotes survival and differentiation of developing forebrain cholinergic neurons.[13–15] Intraventricular infusion of NGF in adult rats or monkeys can prevent the atrophy and loss of phenotypic makers of septal cholinergic neurons that normally result from axotomy of the septohippocampal pathway following a fimbria–fornix lesion.[16,17,25,26] These studies are interesting not only because they provide a clear indication that neurotrophic factors can act to sustain the survival of mature neurons that would otherwise rapidly degenerate as a consequence of axotomy, but specifically because basal forebrain cholinergic neurons have been identified as one of the major neuronal populations that degenerate in Alzheimer's disease.

The homology of BDNF (see below) to NGF prompted us to investigate whether or not BDNF might also influence the survival or phenotypic differentiation of cholinergic neurons cultured from the embryonic rat basal forebrain. Using a histochemical stain for acetylcholinesterase (AChE) and antibodies to choline acetyltransferase (ChAT) to identify cholinergic neurons, we have established that BDNF has similar effects to NGF in increasing the survival of septal cholinergic neurons in vitro.[5] After 12 days in culture there were 2.4-fold more AChE-positive cells in BDNF-treated cultures as compared to controls. As observed with NGF, the greatest effects of BDNF on cholinergic neuron survival were seen at low cell densities.[5,14] Although there were some clear differences in the dose–response curves to NGF and BDNF, we found that effects of BDNF on the expression of phenotypic markers in septal cultures were broadly similar to NGF.[5] BDNF-induced increases in ChAT activity, AChE activity, high-affinity, sodium-dependent choline uptake, and the number of NGF-receptor immunopositive cells were essentially of the same magnitude (two- to threefold) as previously reported following NGF treatment.

Whereas there were no additive or synergistic effects of NGF and BDNF in terms of survival of AChE-positive cells, indicating that both growth factors probably act upon the same neuronal population, BDNF and NGF clearly act synergistically in stimulating maximal expression of ChAT activity.[5] Although it is not immediately obvious as to why these cholinergic neurons should be responsive to two members of the neurotrophin family, it is noteworthy that BDNF mRNA is as abundant as NGF mRNA in the adult hippocampus,[6–8] the target field of septal cholinergic neurons. NT-3 levels are also exceptionally high in the developing and adult hipppocampus.[6] It will be interesting to determine whether or not this third member of the neurotrophin family has any effect upon the survival or differentiated phenotype of septal cholinergic neurons.

Effects of BDNF on Survival of Nigral Dopaminergic Neurons in Culture

As yet there have been no reports of a fully characterized growth factor having direct neurotrophic action towards dopaminergic neurons of the developing or mature substantia nigra. NGF has no effect upon the survival of nigral dopaminergic neurons. There have been some reports of effects of basic fibroblast growth factor (bFGF) on these neurons,[37,38] but it now appears that the effects of bFGF may be indirect, possibly mediated through effects of bFGF on glial cells rather than through direct action on nigral dopaminergic neurons.[37]

Using cultures of ventral mesencephalon derived from E14 rat embryo brain, we have now established that BDNF is a neurotrophic factor for dopamine neurons of the developing substantia nigra.[9] When established from E14 brain and maintained in serum-free, chemically defined medium, mesencephalic cultures were found to be essentially free of nonneuronal cells, especially astrocytes and fibroblasts. Under these conditions, there is a progressive loss of dopaminergic neurons after the first 1 or 2 days in culture. Using antibodies to the enzyme tyrosine hydroxylase (TH) to identify dopaminergic neurons, BDNF treatment was found to enhance the survival of TH$^+$ cells, such that after 8 days the number of TH$^+$ cells was fivefold higher in BDNF-treated cultures as compared to controls.[9] Delaying the addition of BDNF to these cultures for several days greatly diminished the effect of BDNF on sustaining the number of TH$^+$ cells. This clearly suggests that BDNF is required to sustain the survival of developing nigral dopaminergic neurons, as opposed to simply up-regulating TH expression to levels detectable by immunocytochemistry. In agreement with earlier studies, NGF did not enhance the survival of TH$^+$ cells. Similarly, we found little or no effect of bFGF or ciliary neurotrophic factor (CNTF) on these cells.

In tissue culture and in vivo, nigral dopaminergic neurons have been shown to be susceptible to the neurotoxic effects of both 6-OH-dopamine and MPP$^+$ (1-methyl-4-phenylpyridinium, the active metabolite of MPTP). These two neurotoxins have thus found wide use as the basis of rodent and primate models of Parkinson's disease.[39] We have established that BDNF not only enhances the survival of dopaminergic neurons in culture but also protects these neurons against the neurotoxicity of MPP$^+$.[9] In the absence of BDNF, there was an 80% loss of TH$^+$ neurons in cultures that were exposed to MPP$^+$ for 48 hours. Neither bFGF nor NGF treatment induced any resistance to the toxicity of MPP$^+$, but pretreatment of cultures with BDNF greatly reduced the loss of TH$^+$ neurons after 48 hours of exposure to MPP$^+$. Not only was BDNF treatment found to protect dopaminergic neurons against MPP$^+$, but also against 6-OH-dopamine toxicity, as measured by a reduced loss of TH$^+$ neurons or dopamine uptake.

The finding that BDNF enhances the survival of developing nigral dopaminergic neurons in culture and protects these neurons to a large degree from the neurotoxicity of MPP^{+}[9] is of particular interest in terms of a possible novel therapeutic approach to the treatment of Parkinson's disease. There is no doubt that progressive degeneration and loss of nigral dopaminergic neurons is the major pathology associated with Parkinson's disease, although there is no clear understanding as to the underlying cause of the specific loss of these neurons. It is likely, by analogy to known effects of NGF, that a neurotrophic factor such as BDNF, which enhances the survival of dopaminergic neurons during development, may also be involved in the maintenance of these neurons in the adult. Thus pharmacologic doses of BDNF may rescue mature dopaminergic neurons from the insult(s) that leads to their progressive loss in parkinsonism. The fact that 6-OH-dopamine and MPTP treatment of rodents and nonhuman primates provide well-established animal models of parkinsonism[39] will allow testing of this hypothesis in the near future.

Discovery of a Third Member of the NGF Family— Neurotrophin-3 (NT-3)

Molecular cloning of BDNF has established that NGF and BDNF are members of a gene family. Although similarities in the physico-chemical properties of NGF and BDNF (similar monomer molecular size of 12–14kDa, highly basic proteins of pI 9–10) had suggested possible homologies, only upon cloning was it clear that sequences of the two mature proteins were highly homologous (>55% identity). The striking structural similarity of BDNF to NGF immediately suggested that other members of an even larger NGF-related family might exist. Employing polymerase chain reaction (PCR) methodology to amplify novel related sequences with oligonucleotide primers corresponding to several of the most highly conserved regions of NGF and BDNF, Maisonpierre et al.[2] and Hohn et al.[3] simultaneously discovered a third member of the NGF family, a gene that encodes a neurotrophic factor now known as neurotrophin-3 (NT-3). The same gene has now been cloned by other groups,[4] and has in one instance been referred to as hippocampal-derived neurotrophic factor (HDNF).[40] As with NGF and BDNF, NT-3 is generated from a pre-pro NT-3 species, which yields a mature protein of 119 amino acids.[2] Mature NT-3 from the rat shares 57% amino acid identity with rat NGF and 58% amino acid identity with rat BDNF. The six cysteine residues that form three disulfide bridges in NGF are completely conserved among all three neurotrophins, and the regions of greatest homology between NT-3 and either NGF or BDNF are mostly localized around these cysteine residues.[2] NT-3 and BDNF have now been cloned from a variety of vertebrate species. Remarkably there is 100% conservation of the amino acid sequence of NT-3 and BDNF among all mammalian species examined (human, rat, mouse, pig) to date.[41] Such a degree of sequence conversation is virtually unprecedented among protein families.

Neurotrophic Properties of NT-3 towards PNS Neurons: Comparison with NGF and BDNF

To compare the biological activity of NT-3 to the known neuronal specificities of NGF and BDNF towards PNS neurons, recombinant rat NT-3, BDNF, and NGF have been assayed for neurite promoting activity in both explant and dissociated, neuron-enriched cultures of chick embryo dorsal root ganglion (DRG) sensory neurons. NGF and BDNF both promote fiber outgrowth from explants of E8 chick embryo DRG, with BDNF being less potent than NGF. NT-3 was found to be equipotent with NGF in promoting fiber outgrowth from E8 chick DRG explants. In dissociated neuron-enriched cultures, NT-3 promoted survival of 50–60% of E8 DRG neurons,[2] an effect greater than that of BDNF (30–40%) but similar to that of NGF. Thus each of the three neurotrophins exerts a neurotrophic action towards a significant proportion of chick DRG neurons. Given that each factor alone can sustain the survival of 30–60% of E8 DRG neurons, it is likely that there is some overlap in their specificities towards subtypes of DRG neurons.

Whereas NGF and BDNF both promote fiber outgrowth from explants of chick DRG, NGF alone promotes survival and neurite outgrowth from sympathetic neurons either in explant or dissociated neuron-enriched cultures.[34] Conversely, BDNF, but not NGF, promotes survival and neurite outgrowth of neural placode-derived sensory neurons, such as those of the nodose ganglion.[33–36] NT-3 promoted neurite outgrowth from both neural-crest (DRG) and neural placode-derived (nodose:NG) sensory neurons. The effect of NT-3 towards NG neurons was found to be more potent than BDNF, and separate experiments indicate that the effects of BDNF and NT-3 are additive,[3] suggesting that each factor acts upon different sub-populations of NG neurons. In addition to effects upon sensory neurons, NT-3 produced limited fiber outgrowth from explants of sympathetic neurons. The effects of NT-3 on sympathetic neurons were found to be very small compared to NGF, but consistent with effects upon a small population of sympathetic neurons. BDNF has no effect upon explants of paravertebral sympathetic chain ganglia.

Conclusion

The postulated role of neurotrophic factors in development of the nervous system, maintenance and regulation of the function of mature neurons, and regeneration of injured neurons is based largely on our understanding of the biology of NGF. The wealth of information on NGF and the paucity of data on other neurotrophic factors until recently is undoubtedly due to there being a rich biochemical source of NGF (in the mouse salivary gland) versus extremely low abundance of other neurotrophic factors. The recent cloning of BDNF, NT-3, and CNTF and the likelihood of other neurotrophic molecules being cloned in the near future opens the door to producing these rare molecules by recombinant techniques. The more widespread availability of these proteins, and antibodies and probes to detect their sites and levels of synthesis etc., should soon demonstrate the importance of novel neurotrophic factors, molecules related to and distinct from NGF. As greater understanding of the neuronal specificity of novel neurotrophic factors emerges, the potential utility of such molecules as therapeutic agents will increase. It has already been proposed that there is a rational basis to assess NGF in the treatment of neurodegenerative disease such as Alzheimer's and in the treatment of certain peripheral neuropathies. Based on the specificity of BDNF for nigral dopaminergic neurons as well as forebrain cholinergic neurons, BDNF may prove to have even greater therapeutic potential than NGF. Animal studies to assess this potential are in progress.

References

1. Leibrock J, Lottspeich F, Hohn A, Hengerer B, Masiakowski P, Thoenen H, Barde Y-A. 1989. Molecular cloning and expression of brain-derived neurotrophic factor. Nature 341:149–152.
2. Maisonpierre PC, Belluscio L, Squinto S, Ip NY, Furth ME, Lindsay RM, Yancopoulos GD. 1990. Neurotrophin-3: A neurotrophic factor related to NGF and BDNF. Science 247:1446–1451.
3. Hohn A, Leibrock J, Bailey K, Barde Y-A. 1990. Identification and characterization of a novel member of the nerve growth factor/brain-derived neurotrophic factor family. Nature 344:339–341.
4. Rosenthal A, Goeddel DV, Nguyen T, Lewis M, Shih A, Laramee GR, Nikolics K, Winslow JW. 1990. Primary structure and biological activity of a novel human neurotrophic factor. Neuron 4:767–773.

5. Alderson RF, Alterman AL, Barde Y-A, Lindsay RM. 1990. Brain-derived neurotrophic factor increases survival and differentiated functions of rat septal cholinergic neurons in culture. Neuron 5:297–306.
6. Maisonpierre PC, Belluscio L, Friedman B, Alderson R, Wiegand SJ, Furth ME, Lindsay RM, Yancopoulos GD. 1990. NT-3, BDNF and NGF in the developing rat nervous system: Parallel as well as reciprocal patterns of expression. Neuron 5:501–509.
7. Hofer M, Pagliusi SR, Hohn A, Leibrock J, Barde Y-A. 1990. Regional distribution of brain-derived neurotrophic factor in the adult mouse brain. EMBO J 8:2459–2464.
8. Phillips HS, Hains JM, Laramee GR, Rosenthal A, Winslow JW. 1990. Widespread expression of BDNF but not NT-3 by target areas of basal forebrain cholinergic neurons. Science 250:290–294.
9. Hyman C, Hofer M, Barde Y-A, Juhasz M, Yancopoulos GD, Squinto SP, Lindsay RM. 1991. BDNF is a neurotrophic factor for dopaminergic neurons of the substantia nigra. Nature 350:230–232.
10. Levi-Montalcini R, Angeletti PU. 1968. Nerve growth factor. Physiol Rev 48:534–569.
11. Thoenen H, Barde Y-A. 1980. Physiology of nerve growth factor. Physiol Rev 60:1284–1335.
12. Lindsay RM. 1988. The role of neurotrophic growth factors in development, maintenance and regeneration of sensory neurons. *In* The Making of the Nervous System. J Parnavelas, CD Stern, RV Stirling (eds). Oxford University Press, New York pp 148–165.
13. Hefti F, Hartikka J, Eckenstein F, Gnahn H, Heumann R, Schwab M. 1985. Nerve growth factor (NGF) increases choline acetyltransferase but not survival or fiber outgrowth of cultured fetal septal cholinergic neurons. Neuroscience 14:55–68.
14. Hartikka J, Hefti F. 1988. Development of septal cholinergic neurons in culture: Plating density and glial cells modulate effects of NGF on survival and expression of transmitter-specific enzymes. J Neurosci 8:2967–2985.
15. Hatanaka H, Tsukui H, Nihonmatsu I. 1988. Development change in the nerve growth factor action from induction of choline acetyltransferase to promotion of cell survival in cultured basal forebrain neurons from postnatal rat. Dev Brain Res 39:88–95.
16. Hefti F. 1986. Nerve growth factor promotes survival of septal cholinergic neurons after fimbrial transections. J Neurosci 6:2155–2161.
17. Williams LR, Varon S, Peterson G, Wictorin K, Fischer W, Björklund A, Gage FH. 1986. Continuous infusion of nerve growth factor prevents basal forebrain neuronal death after fimbria fornix transection. Proc Natl Acad Sci USA 83:9231–9235.
18. Whittemore SR, Seiger A. 1987. The expression, localization and functional significance of β nerve growth factor in the central nervous sytem. Brain Res Rev 12:439–464.
19. Shelton DL, Reichardt LF. 1986. Studies on the expression of β nerve growth factor (NGF) gene in the central nervous system: Level and regional distribution of NGF mRNA suggest that NGF functions as a

trophic factor for several distinct populations of neurons. Proc Natl Acad Sci USA 83:2714–2718.

20. Auburger G, Heumann R, Hellweg R, Korsching S, Thoenen H. 1987. Developmental changes in nerve growth factor and its mRNA in the rat hippocampus: Comparison with choline acetyltransferase. Devel Biol 120:322–328.

21. Whittemore SR, Ebendal T, Larkfors L, Olson L, Seiger A, Stromberg I, Persson H. 1986. Developmental and regional expression of β nerve growth factor messenger RNA and protein in the rat central nervous system. Proc Natl Acad Sci USA 83:817–821.

22. Lindsay RM. 1988. Nerve growth factors (NGF, BDNF) enhance axonal regeneration but are not required for survival of adult sensory neurons. J Neurosci 8:2394–2405.

23. Lindsay RM, Harmar AJ. 1989. Nerve growth factor regulates expression of neuropeptide genes in adult sensory neurones. Nature 337:362–364.

24. Hefti F, Hartikka J, Knusel B. 1989. Function of neurotrophic factors in the adult and aging brain and their possible use in the treatment of neurodegenerative diseases. Neurobiol Aging 10:515–533.

25. Koliatsos VE, Nauta HJ, Clatterbuck RE, Holtzman DM, Mobley WC, Price DL. 1990. Mouse nerve growth factor prevents degeneration of axotomized basal forebrain cholinergic neurons in the monkey. J Neurosci 10:3801–3813.

26. Tuszynski MH, U HS, Amaral DG, Gage FH. 1990. Nerve growth factor infusion in the primate brain reduces lesion-induced cholinergic neuronal degeneration. J Neurosci 10:3604–3614.

27. Barde Y-A. 1989. Trophic factors and neuronal survival. Neuron 2:1525–1534.

28. Lin L-FH, Mismer D, Lile JD, Armes LG, Butler ET III, Collins F. 1989. Purification, cloning and expression of ciliary neurotrophic factor (CNTF). Science 246:1023–1025.

29. Stöckli KA, Lottspeich F, Sendtner M, Masiakowski P, Carroll P, Götz R, Lindholm D, Thoenen H. 1989. Molecular cloning, expression and regional distribution of rat ciliary neurotrophic factor. Nature 342:920–923.

30. Barde YA, Edgar D, Thoenen H. 1980. Sensory neurons in culture: changing requirements for survival factors during embryonic development. Proc Natl Acad Sci USA 77:1199–1203.

31. Barde Y-A, Edgar D, Thoenen H. 1982. Purification of a new neurotrophic factor from mammalian brain. EMBO J 1:533–549.

32. Barde Y-A, Davies AM, Johnson JE, Lindsay RM, Thoenen H. 1987. Brain derived neurotrophic factor. Prog Brain Res 71:185–189.

33. Lindsay RM, Thoenen H, Barde YA. 1985. Placode and neural crest-derived sensory neurons are responsive at early developmental stages to brain-derived neurotrophic factor (BDNF). Dev Biol 112:319–328.

34. Lindsay RM, Barde Y-A, Davies AM, Rohrer H. 1985. Differences and similarities in the neurotrophic requirements of sensory neurons derived from neural crest and neural placode. J Cell Sci Suppl 3: 115–129.

35. Lindsay RM, Rohrer H. 1985. Placodal sensory neurons in culture: Nodose ganglion neurons are unresponsive to NGF, lack NGF receptors but are supported by a liver-derived neurotrophic factor. Dev Biol 112:30–48.
36. Davies AM, Thoenen H, Barde Y-A. 1986. The response of chick sensory neurons to brain-derived neurotrophic factor. J Neurosci 6:1897–1904.
37. Knusel B, Michel PP, Schwaber JS, Hefti F. 1990. Selective and nonselective stimulation of central cholinergic and dopaminergic development in vitro by nerve growth factor, basic fibroblast growth factor, epidermal growth factor, insulin and the insulin-like growth factors I and II. J Neurosci 10:558–570.
38. Otto D, Unsicker K. 1990. Basic FGF reverses chemical and morphological deficits in the nigrostriatal system of MPTP-treated mice. J Neurosci 10:1912–1921.
39. Zigmond MJ, Stricker EM. 1989. Animal models of Parkinsonism using selective neurotoxins: Clinical and basic implications. Int Rev Neurobiol 31:1–79.
40. Ernfors P, Ibanez CF, Ebendal T, Olson L, Persson H. 1990. Molecular cloning and neurotrophic activities of a protein with structural similarities to nerve growth factor: Developmental and topographical expression in the brain. Proc Natl Acad Sci USA 87:5454–5458.
41. Yancopoulos GD, Maisonpierre PC, Ip NY, Aldrich TH, Belluscio L, Boulton TG, Cobb MH, Squinto SP, Furth ME. 1991. Neurotrophic factors, their receptors and the signal transduction pathways they activate. Cold Spring Harbor Symp Quant Biol 55:(in press).

Chapter 27

Brain-Derived Neurotrophic Factor (BDNF) Stimulation of Dopaminergic Neuron Differentiation

Beat Knüsel, Klaus D. Beck, John W. Winslow, Louis E. Burton, Karoly Nikolics, and Franz F. Hefti

Neurotrophic Factors and Neurodegenerative Diseases

Normal development and adult function of neurons is regulated by minute amounts of soluble proteins, commonly called neurotrophic factors. With possible clinical relevance, such factors have been implicated in various degenerative diseases of the nervous system, including Parkinson's disease. Nerve growth factor (NGF) is the first and best characterized neurotrophic factor and serves as the paradigm for the more recently discovered similar molecules, BDNF and neurotrophin-3 (NT-3). Other factors with suggested neurotrophic actions include basic fibroblast growth factor (bFGF), epidermal growth factor (EGF), insulin and the insulin like growth factors I and II, i.e., proteins that were previously identified and characterized based on biological effects on non-neuronal cells.[1,2]

From Hefti F, and Weiner WJ, (eds.) *Progress in Parkinson's Disease Research—2*. Mount Kisco NY, Futura Publishing Co., Inc., © 1992.

The Neurotrophins NGF, BDNF, and NT-3

NGF, a small, basic protein, was originally purified from mouse salivery glands and found to be necessary for normal developmental growth and differentiation of peripheral sympathetic and sensory neurons, and it remains important for the maintenance of normal function of these cells during adult life.[3] In the brain the cholinergic neurons of the basal forebrain express NGF receptors,[4–6] and NGF increases the activity of choline acetyltransferase (ChAT) and acetylcholinesterase (AChE) in these neurons in culture and in vivo.[7–9] Parallel increases of levels of ChAT activity, NGF, and NGF mRNA support the view that NGF is involved in the establishment of the cholinergic septohippocampal projection.[10] In accordance with this model, NGF protein is synthesized in the target areas of cholinergic neurons and has been shown to be retrogradely transported to the basal forebrain in the adult rat.[3,11]

BDNF was purified from pig brain using survival of chick sensory neurons as a bioassay and was found to be, like NGF, a small, basic protein.[12] Amino acid and nucleotide sequences of BDNF show extensive homology with NGF.[13–16] Purification and cloning of BDNF led to the discovery of NT-3, an additional protein related to NGF and BDNF, by several research groups using polymerase chain reaction (PCR) techniques.[15,17–20] Rat, mouse, and human amino acid sequences for NT-3 are identical and share 57% and 58% identities with rat NGF and BDNF, respectively. The family of proteins which includes NGF, BDNF, and NT-3 is now referred to as the *neurotrophins*.

Messenger RNA for BDNF is found predominantly in the central nervous system (CNS).[13,19,21] This is very different from the distribution of NGF mRNA, which is found in many non-CNS tissues.[22,23] The relatively high abundance of BDNF mRNA in the CNS suggests the presence of considerably higher levels of BDNF than NGF in the brain.[13] Levels of BDNF mRNA in the brain are developmentally regulated.[24] Maximal concentrations in the adult brain were found in the hippocampus, particularly in CA2 and CA3 neurons, and in cortical areas,[16,21,24] but BDNF is also found in striatum (Denton and Hefti, unpublished observations). These findings suggest that BDNF plays a role in the function of various populations of CNS neurons and, possibly, nonneuronal cells.

NT-3 mRNA is found in brain as well as in many peripheral organs.[18,19,21,24] In the adult rat brain, NT-3 mRNA is highly localized to hippocampal CA1 and CA2 pyramidal neurons.[16,21] However, during early development high levels are expressed in cerebellum. Both in cerebellum and in hippocampus NT-3 levels seem to peak during periods of maximal developmental growth of these structures and then to decline to lower adult levels.[24]

The analysis of possible cellular targets of BDNF and NT-3 is still at an early stage. In the peripheral nervous system of the chick, BDNF supports the survival of subpopulations of sensory neurons.[25,26] Another system in which BDNF is known to play a role are the retinal ganglion neurons. Most E17 rat ganglion neurons can be rescued in culture by the addition of BDNF,[27] without affecting the total number of cells or neurons in the ganglion. In this system the effects of BDNF are not limited to the prenatal period since in adult rat retinal explants BDNF acts as a trophic factor and supports both the survival of rat retinal ganglion neurons and increases the rate of axonal elongation.[28] Recently, the cholinergic neurons of the basal forebrain have been shown to be stimulated by BDNF.[29,30] Interestingly, maximal responsiveness of these neurons occurs for BDNF at a different time of development in vitro then for NGF.[30] It was also found that the development of the NGF-unresponsive GABAergic neurons of the basal forebrain and of the dopaminergic neurons of the mesencephalon are stimulated by BDNF (see below).[30] Dopaminergic stimulation by this protein as described in more detail has also been demonstrated in another recent study.[31]

NT-3 supports the survival of chick sympathetic neurons and of subpopulations of sensory neurons.[17–20] No NT-3 responsive cell populations in the CNS have been reported yet. In initial studies. NT-3 did not seem to trophically affect forebrain cholinergic or mesencephalic dopaminergic neurons.[30] More recent experiments, however, showed a stimulatory effect of high concentrations of NT-3 on basal forebrain cholinergic neurons (unpublished data). Additivity studies, however, suggest that NT-3 at such high concentrations might stimulate the NGF receptor.

Indirect Evidence for Existence of Trophic Factors Acting on Dopaminergic Neurons

Several earlier studies provided indirect evidence for the existence of neurotrophic factors acting on mesencephalic dopaminergic neurons. Heller and collaborators found that survival and biochemical differentiation of dopaminergic cells in cultures of aggregated neurons was increased when dopaminergic neurons were cocultured with cells from the corpus striatum. In such cocultures the number of dopaminergic neurons, the density of the neurites, and the evoked release of dopamine were higher than in cultures containing only nigral neurons.[31] The fact that cocultures with cells from areas other than the striatum failed to be similarly effective suggested that striatal cells exert a selective trophic influence on dopaminergic cells. Similar effects of striatal cells on dopaminergic neurons were described by Prochiantz and collaborators, who used cultures of dissociated neurons.[32] The trophic effect of striatal cells in these cultures required cell–cell contact between nigral and striatal neurons. Isolated membranes from striatal tissue were equally effective as living striatal cells. These findings were taken to suggest that a membrane-bound molecule expressed by striatal target cells mediates the trophic actions on dopaminergic neurons. Tomozawa and Appel[33] reported the partial purification of a peptide isolated from striatal tissue that promoted survival and differentiation of dopaminergic neurons in cultures of dissociated nigral cells. Dal Toso et al.[34] characterized a small protein producing similar trophic effects. However, this molecule was later found to probably be identical to bFGF.[35] Valdes et al.[36] reported the initial purification of a 55-kDa protein stimulating dopamine synthesis of cultured mesencephalic neurons. Together, these findings suggested the existence of one or more factors able to promote survival, function, and neurite elongation of dopaminergic neurons.

Actions of Trophic Factors on Mesencephalic Dopaminergic Neurons In Vitro

Trophic actions of characterized growth factors on dopaminergic neurons of the substantia nigra were assessed in our laboratory using previously established cell culture systems.[37,38] Cultures were prepared from fetal Wistar rats of embryonic age E15–16. Ventral mesencephalon was dissected to include the dopaminergic nuclei A8, A9 (substantia nigra), and A10 (ventral tegmental area) but not the noradrenergic locus ceruleus. The tissue was dispersed into a suspension of individual cells by gentle mechanical trituration without using enzymes. The dissociated cells were grown in 24-well plates, precoated with polyethyleneimine, in modified L15 medium containing various amino acids, vitamins, antibiotics, glucose, and bicarbonate. Routinely 5% horse serum and 0.5% fetal calf serum were present but in some experiments serum was replaced by the serum-free N2 additions of Bottenstein and Sato.[39] Plating densities were 2–4 × 10^5 cells/cm². Of these cells 0.5–1% were dopaminergic as established by immunocytochemical staining for the catecholaminergic marker enzyme tyrosine hydroxylas (TH). After 5–12 days in vitro, cultures were taken for measurement of dopamine uptake rate, for TH immunocytochemistry, or for biochemical determination of TH activity. Growth factors were present in the cultures as indicated in the results.

In initial experiments basic fibroblast growth factor (bFGF), epidermal growth factor (EGF), transforming growth factor alpha (TGF-α), insulin, IGF-I, and IGF-II were found to promote dopaminergic differentiation in culture in a dose-dependent manner (Figure 1). bFGF has been shown to affect various populations of neurons and neuron like cells. It supports survival and subsequent fiber outgrowth of dissociated rodent fetal neurons in culture.[40,41] Basic FGF promotes survival and differentiation of cholinergic neurons of the rat basal forebrain and, in addition to its effects on neurons, has also a profound mitogenic effect on glial cells.[38,42] Insulin, IGF-I, and IGF-II are involved in the regulation of metabolism and cellular growth of many tissues. The three proteins exhibit overlapping specificities for receptors.[43] There is abundant evidence for the existence of insulin and IGF receptors in the brain, and the IGFs have been shown to be synthesized in the brain.[44] The function of insulin and IGFs in the CNS is not clear, despite findings that they stimulate survival and neurite outgrowth in cultured central and peripheral neurons.[45,46] Besides their actions on mesencephalic dopaminergic neurons, insulin, IGF-I, and IGF-II also promote the biochemical differentiation of septal and pontine cholinergic neurons.[38] The similarity of effects on different neuronal populations suggests that insulin and the IGFs act rather nonselectively on all or most neurons during development. The growth factors of this related family, therefore, seem unlikely candidates as target-derived, neuron-population-specific neurotrophic factors. Nevertheless, their time-and site-specific presence might be required for normal early CNS development, and their function during this time might be different from later, more general, stimulating influences on many biochemical parameters. EGF and TGF-α are potent mitogens for several cell types.

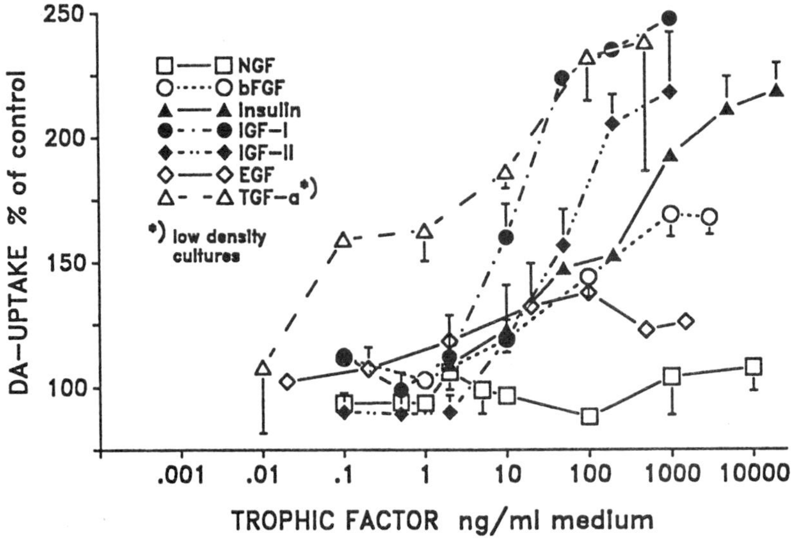

Figure 1. Dose–response curves for effects of growth factors on dopaminergic cells of ventral mesencephalon in culture. Results show dopamine uptake. Cultures of dissociated fetal rat brain cells (E16/E17) were grown for 1 week in the continuous presence or absence (control) of growth factors in modified L-15 medium with serum. Normal plating density was 0.8×10^6, for TGF-α 0.3×10^6 cells per 16-mm well. Each symbol represents the mean of 4–8 individual cultures and bars show standard errors. Error bars were omitted where they would have appeared smaller than the symbol.

EGF was found to enhance survival and neurite growth of cultured subneocortical and cerebellar neurons of the neonatal rat brain.[47] EGF and EGF receptor immunoreactivity were demonstrated in the rat brain.[48] TGF-α, which shows structural homology to EGF, is present in several brain areas and is synthesized in cell bodies of selected rat forebrain regions, among them the striatum.[49,50] TGF-α mRNA has been shown to occur rather selectively in the dopaminergic target area, the corpus striatum,[51] a fact that calls for attention since TGF-α in our experiments very efficiently promoted dopmaine uptake of mesencephalic cultures (Figure 1). It was found, however, that the effect of TGF-α completely depends on plating density and possibly on mitogenic activity of noneuronal cells in the cultures. At densities of 0.4×10^6 cells/cm^2, at which many other growth factors stimulate dopaminergic differentiation, or in the presence of mitogenic inhibitors, no effect of TGF-α on dopamine uptake in mesencephalic cultures was observed (data not shown). These findings suggest that the trophic action of TGF-α represents an indirect response and is mediated by other neurons or nonneuronal cells.

Recently, recombinant NGF, BDNF, and NT-3 became available in sufficient quantities to be tested for trophic actions on cultured cells. Production of recombinant human BDNF and NT-3 and their use in such studies are described in a recent publication.[30] We were able to confirm that NGF does not stimulate dopaminergic development in our mesencephalic cultures, even at concentrations up to 10 μg/ml medium (Figure 1), in corroboration of earlier results by other authors.[52] Similarly, NT-3, which was tested at maximal concentration of 1 μg/ml did not increase dopaminergic differentiation (Figure 2). In contrast, the third presently known member of the family of the neurotrophins, BDNF, when added to the medium of mesencephalic cultures resulted

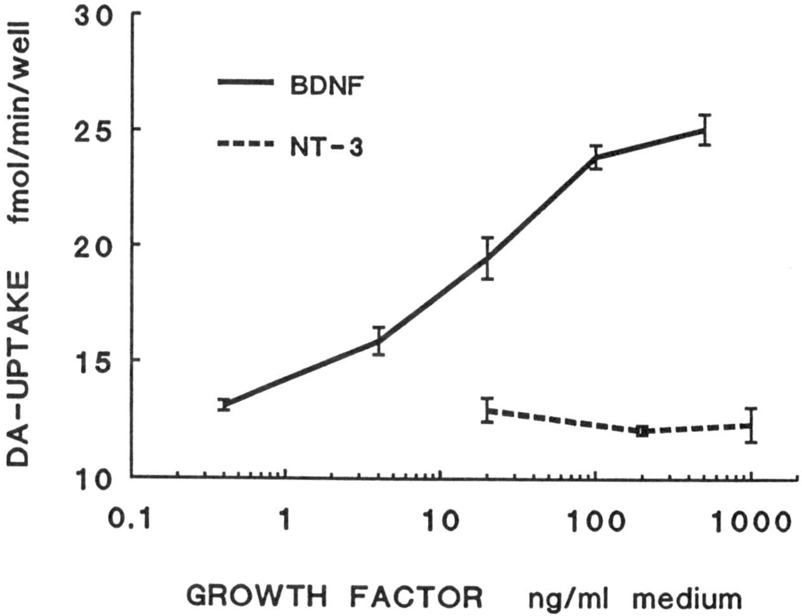

Figure 2. Dopamine uptake in cultures of ventral mesencephalon was elevated by BDNF but not by NT-3. Cultures were grown for 7 days in L15 medium with 5% horse and 0.5% fetal bovine serum. Recombinant human BDNF or NT-3 were produced in transfected human kidney embryo-carcinoma cells and were added to the culture medium 2 days after plating and with a medium change after 5 days in vitro. Graph shows mean ± standard error (N = 4).

in marked elevation of dopamine uptake in a dose-dependent manner. Maximal stimulation was achieved at approximately 100 ng/ml (Figure 2). The potency of the same preparation of BDNF on basal forebrain cholinergic neurons was identical.[30] After 6 days in vitro and treatment with BDNF during days 2–6, the increase in dopamine uptake reached approximately 100% over control. No differences were observed in the response of dopaminergic neurons to BDNF whether the cultures were grown in serum-free or serum-containing medium.

Detailed Characterization of Trophic Effects of BDNF on Mesencephalic Cells

The effect of BDNF on mesencephalic dopaminergic neurons was compared to its effect on the cholinergic neurons of the basal forebrain. The responsiveness of the cholinergic neurons to BDNF in vitro is a function of the developmental stage. There is a gradual decline of responsiveness during development of the cultures to both BDNF and bFGF, and this decreasing responsiveness contrasts with the increasing responsiveness to NGF.[30,38] As opposed to the observations on cholinergic neurons, where BDNF produced about threefold elevations of ChAT activity after only 2 days of exposure when treated early during development in vitro,[30] maximal relative increase of dopamine uptake was observed only after longer exposure times (Figure 3). The mesencephalic dopaminergic neurons, therefore, do not show an initial fast response to BDNF as occurs in basal forebrain cholinergic neurons.

In basal forebrain cultures BDNF treatment slightly increases total cell density and the density of cholinergic neurons.[30] Corresponding observations were made also in mesencephalic cultures. To quantitate this effect, we performed cell counts on fixed cultures which were immunostained for the precursor synthesizing enzyme tyrosine hydroxylase (TH). Counted were total number of cells and number of TH positive (TH^+) cells (Table 1). We found that the increase in total cell number by treatment with BDNF was rather modest and insufficient to explain the increased dopamine uptake. The relative increase in the number of TH^+ neurons, although greater than the increase in total cells, was still considerably smaller than the extent of the stimulation of dopamine uptake. BDNF treatment also enhanced the activity of the TH enzyme (Figure 4). Surprisingly, this

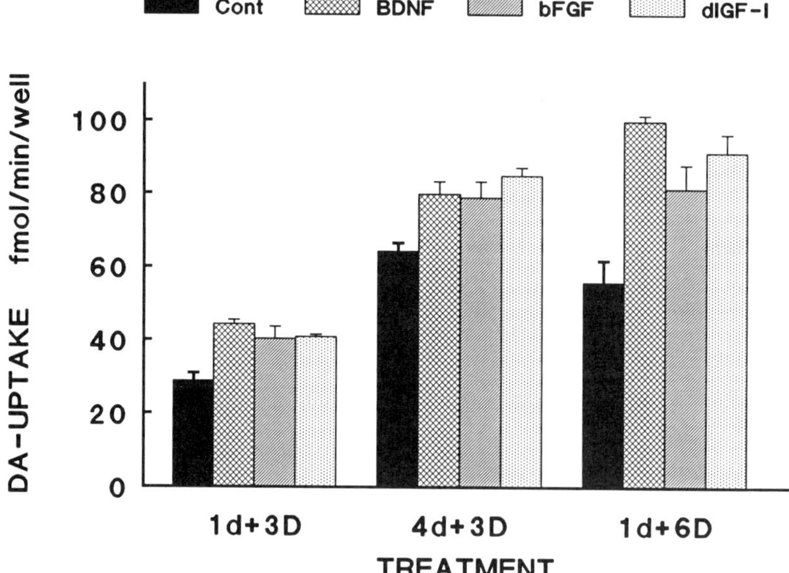

Figure 3.   Maximal increase of dopamine uptake in mesencephalic cultures is observed only after extended treatment with BDNF, bFGF, or des-(1-3)-IGF-I. The mesencephalic dopaminergic neurons lack the initial fast response to BDNF or bFGF as observed in basal forebrain cholinergic neurons.[30] 1d + 3D: 1 day delay, followed by 3 days of treatment; assay after 4 days in vitro. 4d + 3D: 4 days delay, followed by 3 days of treatment; assay after 7 days in vitro. 1d + 6D: 1 day delay, followed by 6 days of treatment; assay after 7 days in vitro.

Table 1.
BDNF Elevates Number of Dopaminergic Cells and Uptake Rate for [^{3}H]Dopamine[a]

Treatment	TH$^+$ cells per well	Total cells per well	DA uptake (fmol/min/well)
Control	948 ± 43	95,844 ± 7,634	17.5 ± 0.1
BDNF (100 ng/ml)	1275 ± 76[*b]	103,161 ± 8,299	34.0 ± 1.0**
% change by BDNF	+ 34.5	+ 7.6	+ 94.3

[a]Embryonic age E15 mesencephalic cultures were grown for 7 days in L15 medium with 5% horse and 0.5% fetal bovine serum. Recombinant human BDNF was added to the culture medium 2 days after plating and with a medium change after 5 days in vitro. The table gives means ± standard error.
[b]*$P < 0.01$; **$P < 0.001$ (Student's t test). $N = 4$.

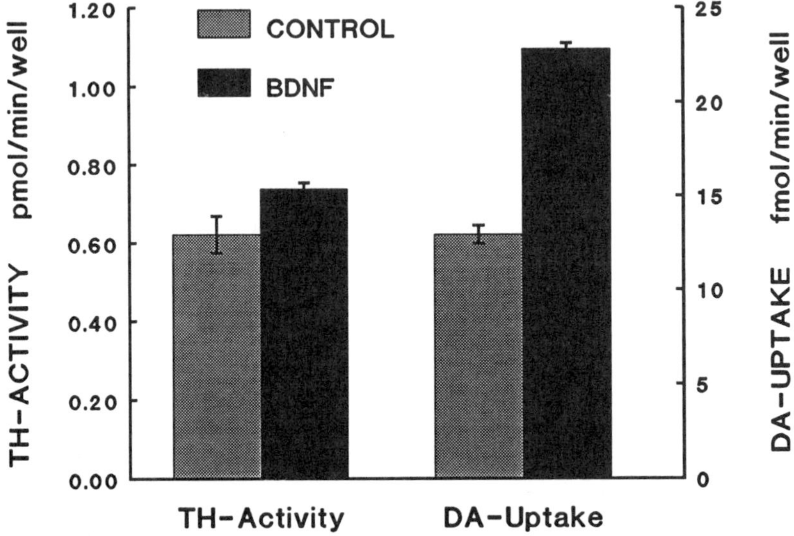

Figure 4. BDNF treatment of mesencephalic cultures is more effective on dopamine uptake than on TH activity. Cultures were grown for 7 days and treated from 2 days after plating. Results for dopamine uptake and TH activity are from parallel cultures.

effect was small, comparable to the effect of BDNF on total protein levels (Table 2). We conclude: (1) that BDNF treatment promotes survival and biochemical differentiation of dopaminergic neurons in culture, and (2) that individual parameters reflecting dopaminergic differentiation are affected to varying degrees.

BDNF Protection against MPP⁺ Toxicity

The neurotoxin 1-methyl-4-phenyl-1,2,3,6-tetrahydropyridine (MPTP) and its active metabolie 1-methyl-4-phenylpyridinium (MPP⁺) selectively destroy dopaminergic neurons and induce park-insonism in vivo. MPP⁺ toxicity in mesencephalic cultures has been extensively studied in our laboratory.[37] We used this model to test for possible protective effects of trophic factors against degeneration of dopaminergic neurons. In initial experiments the cultures were treated with growth factors for 3–5 days and then, in continued

Table 2.
Total Protein Mass in Cultures is Increased by BDNF and bFGF

Treatment	Protein (μg/well)
Control	133.9 $\pm$ 4.2
BDNF	174.2 $\pm$ 5.3*
bFGF	196.5 $\pm$ 6.3*

*$P < 0.01$ (Student's t test). $N = 4$. Cultures were grown as for Table 1.

presence of the growth factors, with 1μM MPP$^+$ for 1 day. The cultures were assayed for dopamine uptake immediately after treatment. No protection against dopaminergic toxicity of MPP$^+$ was evident under these experimental conditions (Table 3). In a second series of experiments, MPP$^+$ treatment was with 0.5 μM only but in absence of growth factors and was followed by a recovery period of 3 days under control conditions without growth factor or MPP$^+$. Using this experimental paradigm, we found that BDNF and bFGF pretreatment resulted in a modest acceleration of the recovery of dopaminergic cells from MPP$^+$ injury. However, such an effect was

Table 3.
Growth Factors BDNF and bFGF Accelerate Recovery of Dopaminergic Cells from MPP$^+$ Injury

Growth factor	No MPP$^+$	With MPP$^+$	% remaining
1.0 μM MPP$^+$, 1 day			
Control	24.4 $\pm$ 0.7	2.5 $\pm$ 0.1	10.1
BDNF	45.8 $\pm$ 1.9	3.3 $\pm$ 0.1	7.2
0.5 μM MPP$^+$, 1 day, followed by 3 days without treatment			
Control	60.3 $\pm$ 1.2	26.6 $\pm$ 0.8	44.1
BDNF	58.6 $\pm$ 5.2	46.3 $\pm$ 1.0*	79.0
bFGF	63.4 $\pm$ 5.3	35.9 $\pm$ 2.2*	55.9

Cultures were grown in presence or absence (control) of growth factors for 5 days and then treated, either in continued presence of the growth factors with 1 μM MPP$^+$ or without growth factors with 0.5 μM MPP$^+$, for 1 day. The cultures were assayed for dopamine uptake either immediately after treatment or after a recovery period of 3 days under control conditions without growth factors and MPP$^+$.*$p<0.01$.

only evident with submaximal MPP$^+$ concentrations, resulting in approximately 50% reduction of dopamine uptake in control cultures without growth factors. The exact nature of the protective effects of bFGF and BDNF needs to be established. It seems interesting that the recovery period appeared to be essential for the observation of a protective effect. This suggests a long-lasting priming of dopaminergic neurons by BDNF, which allowed them to recover from an insult faster than untreated neurons. It cannot be excluded, however, that MPP$^+$ protection might be the result of an indirect effect, since both effective growth factors result in increased number of cells in our cultures.

Cholinergic and Dopaminergic Response to BDNF Seem to be Mediated by Identical or Similar Receptors

The molecular identity of neurotrophin receptors remains poorly understood. Binding studies with iodinated BDNF resulted in characterization of high- and low-affinity receptors on chick dorsal root ganglion cells with affinities of 1.7×10^{-11} M and 1.3×10^{-9} M, respectively, similar to the two characterized receptors for NGF. Indeed, since BDNF binds to the low-affinity NGF receptor with similar affinity as NGF,[53] a hypothesis can be entertained that an identical low-affinity receptor protein is part of the high-affinity receptors for NGF and BDNF and possibly also NT-3. The receptors, according to this model, could gain their specificity by association with another protein. However, recently it has been shown that the *trk* protooncogene is expressed in PC12 pheochromocytoma cells and is closely linked to NGF action in these cells.[54] It is particularly interesting that a related gene, *trkB*, is expressed in the nervous system.[55] The molecular structure of *trk* suggests an intracellular protein kinase domain, a membrane spanning part, and a large extracellular domain, a structure reminiscent of several membrane spanning protein kinase growth factor receptors, e.g., the receptors for EGF, bFGF, and insulin.[56–59] It is tempting to speculate that a family of *trk* genes might have evolved in parallel with the neurotrophins to code for their specific receptors. With this speculation in mind, a group of compounds that have been shown to selectively inhibit the NGF response in different systems might warrant special interest. Originally it was observed that K–252a, an alkaloid-like compound of microbial origin, reversibly and selectively inhibits the NGF-induced morphological transformation of proliferating PC12 pheochromocytoma cells into neuron like cells. Also in PC12 cells the NGF-stimulated, but not the bFGF or EGF-stimulated, phosphorylation of selected proteins is inhibited.[60–65] Later, inhibition of NGF actions in cells of the mammalian peripheral nervous system in primary cultures was found by several investigators.[62,66,67] K-252a inhibits NGF actions without interfering with the binding of the trophic factor to its receptor,[61] but inhibition of NGF actions by K-252a and similar compounds is believed to occur at a very early step after receptor binding, possibly at the transducing element of the NGF high-affinity receptor, since all cellular and biochemical effects seem to be abolished. We found in a recent study that K-252a and two structurally related protein kinase inhibitors, K-252b and staurosporine, completely and selectively inhibit the NGF mediated activity increase of the cholinergic marker enzyme ChAT in cultures of rat basal forebrain cells.[68] The neurotrophic actions of bFGF and insulin in this culture system and in cultures of ventral mesencephalon are not affected. We subsequently found that K-252b, an inhibitor with almost no toxicity in our cultures, abolishes neurotrophic actions on cholinergic neurons by all three neurotrophins NGF, BDNF and NT-3, but not by bFGF (Figure 5A). K-252b also inhibited the response to BDNF in mesencephalic cultures, while the effect of bFGF in the same experiment was only slightly reduced (Figure 5B). These results imply that in basal forebrain cultures, the actions of BDNF and NT-3 involve mechanisms very similar to those of NGF and, in particular, that BDNF effects on central cholinergic and on dopaminergic neurons are mediated by receptor mechanisms which are very similar or identical.

Conclusions

In cell culture experiments various growth factors have been shown to stimulate dopaminergic function of mesencephalic cells.[35,38] These factors are bFGF, EGF, insulin, and the insulin-related growth factors IGF-I and IGF-II. We now add evidence that BDNF is a particularly potent and efficient trophic factor for mesencephalic dopaminergic neurons. Surprisingly, the effects of BDNF on brain cells in culture are in many ways similar to the effects

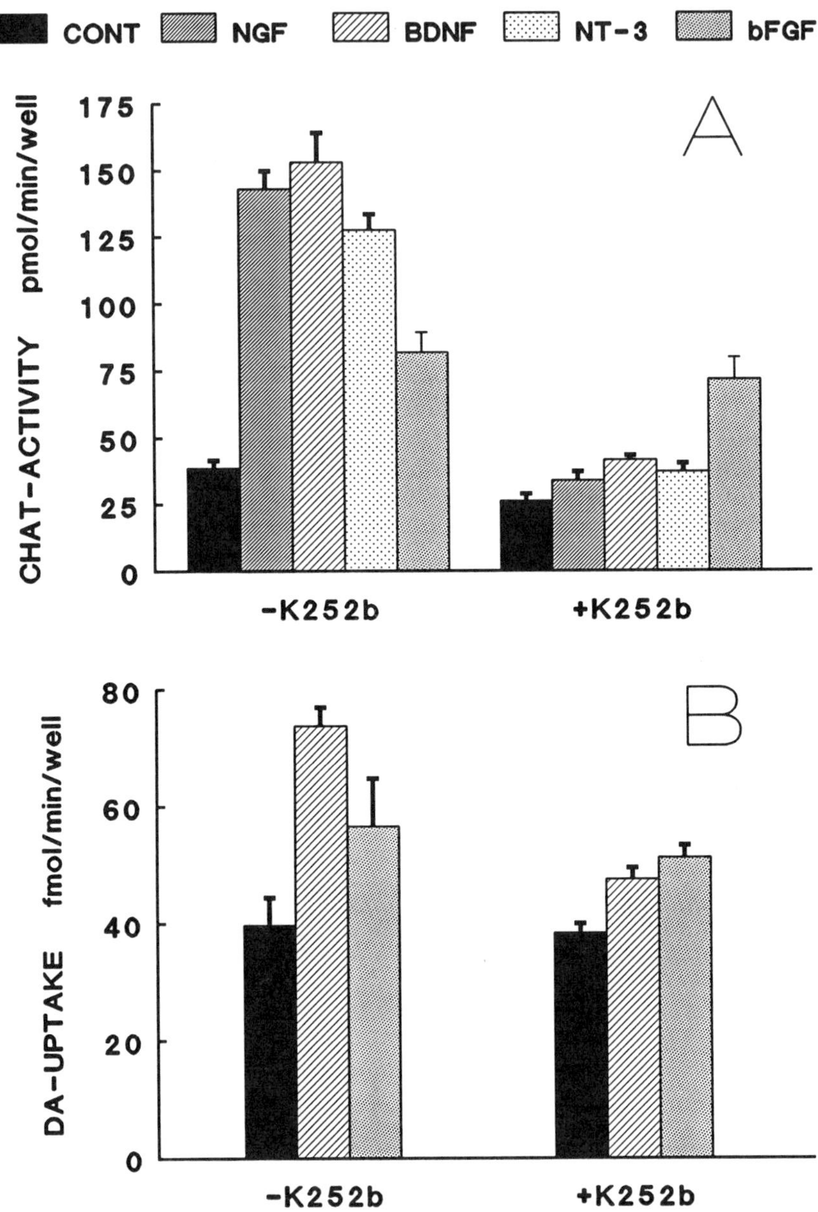

Figure 5. Inhibition of trophic factor action by the protein kinase inhibitor K-252b. (A): ChAT activity in basal forebrain cultures. (B): Dopamine uptake in ventral mesencephalic cultures. Cultures were grown for 7 days and treatment was for 5 days from day 2 of culture. Concentration of K-252b was 2.5 μM. Concentrations of growth factors were: NGF, 50 ng/ml; BDNF, 100 ng/ml; NT-3, 1.5 μg/ml; bFGF, 1 μg/ml.

of bFGF.[30,38] Both elevate ChAT activity and GABA uptake in basal forebrain cultures, dopamine uptake in mesencephalic cultures, and protein levels in all culture types. These results indicate effects of BDNF and bFGF on a spectrum of cells in the brain, a situation that is very different from NGF whose only clearly established actions in the brain are its effects on the cholinergic neurons of basal forebrain and the striatum. bFGF lacks a signal peptide typical for released proteins, and it has been questioned whether this protein plays a physiological role as a neurotrophic factor. Instead, it has been proposed that bFGF may act as an "injury factor" released in events involving cellular destruction.[69] Our finding that the spectrum of neurotrophic responses produced by BDNF and bFGF are similar suggests the possibility that bFGF released after injury further stimulates biological responses normally produced by BDNF.

While several growth factors stimulate dopaminergic differentiation in vitro, current interest focuses on BDNF because of the following reasons: (1) BDNF is a potent enhancer of dopaminergic differentiation in culture; (2) The sequence for BDNF codes for a signal peptide indicating that it might be released from producing cells in the intact brain and under physiological conditions;[13–16] (3) BDNF is heterogeneously distributed in the adult brain. While mRNA for BDNF in the adult rat is less abundant in the striatum than in many other brain areas, e.g., the hippocampus, its level is still considerably higher than that of NGF mRNA;[14,70,71] (4) BDNF administration in vivo can prevent naturally occurring neuronal cell death[25,26,72] and in vitro promotes the survival of dopaminergic neurons. The demonstration, therefore, of BDNF effects on central dopaminergic neurons, as outlined in this chapter, raises hope for new approaches to the treatment of Parkinson's disease.

References

1. Hefti F, Hartikka J, Knusel B. 1989. Function of neurotrophic factors in the adult and aging brain and their possible use in the treatment of neurodegenerative disease. Neurobiol Aging 10:515–533.
2. Hefti F, Denton TL, Knusel B, Lapchak PA. 1991. Neurotrophic factors: What are they and what are they doing? In Neurotrophic Factors. SE Loughlin, JH Fallon (eds). Academic Press, New York (in press).
3. Thoenen H, Bandtlow C, Heumann R. 1987. The physiological function

of nerve growth factor in the central nervous system: Comparison with the periphery. Rev Physiol Biochem Pharmacol 109:145–178.

4. Richardson PM, Verge Issa VMK, Riopelle RJ. 1986. Distribution of neuronal receptors for nerve growth factor in the rat. J Neurosci 6:2312–2321.

5. Yan O, Johnson EM. 1988. An immunohistochemical study of the nerve growth factor receptor in developing rats. J Neurosci 8:3481–3498.

6. Riopelle RJ, Richardson PM, Verge VMK. 1987. Distribution and characteristics of nerve growth factor binding on cholinergic neurons of rat and monkey forebrain. J Neurochem Res 12:923–928.

7. Gnahn H, Hefti F, Heumann R, Schwab M, Thoenen H. 1983. NGF-mediated increase of choline acetyltransferase (ChAT) in the neonatal forebrain: Evidence for a physiological role of NGF in the brain? Dev Brain Res 9:45–52.

8. Hefti F, Hartikka J, Eckenstein F, Gnahn H, Heumann R, Schwab M. 1985. Nerve growth factor (NGF) increases choline acetyltransferase but not survival or fiber outgrowth of cultured fetal septal cholinergic neurons. Neuroscience 14:55–68.

9. Mobley WC, Rutkowski JL, Tennekoon GI, Buchanan K, Johnston MV. 1985. Choline acetyltransferase activity in striatum of neonatal rats increased by nerve growth factor. Science 229:284–287.

10. Large TH, Bodary SC, Clegg DO, Weskamp G, Otten U, Reichardt LF. 1986. Nerve growth factor gene expression in the developing rat brain. Science 234:352–355.

11. Whittemore SR, Seigar A. 1987. The expression, localization and functional significance of beta-nerve growth factor in the central nervous system. Brain Res Rev 12:439–464.

12. Barde YA, Edgar D, Thoenen H. 1982. Purification of a new neurotrophic factor from mammalian brain. EMBO J 1:549–553.

13. Leibrock J, Lottspeich F, Hohn A, Hofer M, Hengerer B, Masiakowski P, Thoenen H, Barde YA. 1989. Molecular cloning and expression of brain-derived neurotrophic factor. Nature 341:149–152.

14. Hofer M, Pagliusi SR, Hohn A, Leibrock J, Barde YA. 1990. Regional distribution of brain-derived neurotrophic factor mRNA in the adult mouse brain. EMBO J 9:2459–2464.

15. Jones KR, Reichardt LF. 1990. Molecular cloning of a human gene that is a member of the nerve growth factor family. Proc Natl Acad Sci USA 87:8060–8064.

16. Phillips HS, Hains JM, Laramee GR, Rosenthal A, Winslow JW. 1990. Widespread expression of BDNF but not NT3 by target areas of basal forebrain cholinergic neurons. Science 250:290–294.

17. Ernfors P, Ibanez CF, Ebendal T, Olson L, Persson H. 1990. Molecular cloning and neurotrophic activities of a protein with structural similarities to nerve growth factor: Developmental and topographical expression in the brain. Proc Natl Acad Sci USA 87:5454–5458.

18. Hohn A, Leibrock J, Bailey K, Barde YA. 1990. Identification and characterization of a novel member of the nerve growth factor/brain-derived neurotrophic factor family. Nature 344:339–341.

19. Maisonpierre PC, Belluscio L, Squinto S, Ip NY, Furth ME, Lindsay RM, Yancopoulos GD. 1990. Neurotrophin-3: A neurotrophic factor related to NGF and BDNF. Science 247:1446–1451.
20. Rosenthal A, Goeddel DV, Nguyen T, Lewis M, Shih A, Laramee GR, Nikolics K, Winslow JW. 1990. Primary structure and biological activity of a novel human neurotrophic factor. Neuron 4:767–773.
21. Ernfors P, Wetmore C, Olson L, Persson H. 1990. Identification of cells in rat brain and peripheral tissues expressing mRNA for members of the nerve growth factor family. Neuron 5:511–526.
22. Heumann R, Schwab M, Merkl R, Thoenen H. 1984. Nerve growth factor-mediated induction of choline acetyltransferase in PC12 cells: Evaluation of the site of action of nerve growth factor and the involvement of lysosomal degradation products of nerve growth factor. J Neurosci 4:3039–3050.
23. Shelton DL, Reichardt LF. 1984. Expression of the β-nerve growth factor gene correlates with the density of sympathetic innervation in effector organs. Proc Natl Acad Sci USA 81:7951–7955.
24. Maisonpierre PC, Belluscio L, Friedman B, Alderson RF, Wiegand SJ, Furth ME, Lindsay RM, Yancopoulos GD. 1990. NT-3, BDNF, and NGF in the developing rat nervous system: Parallel as well as reciprocal patterns of expression. Neuron 5:501–509.
25. Lindsay RM, Thoenen H, Barde YA. 1985. Placode and neural crest-derived sensory neurons are responsive at early developmental stages to brain-derived neurotrophic factor. Dev. Biol 112:319–328.
26. Ernsberger U, Rohrer H. 1988. Neuronal precursor cells in chick dorsal root ganglia: Differentiation and survival in vitro. Dev Biol 126:420–432.
27. Johnson D, Lanahan A, Buck CR, Sehgal A, Morgan C, Mercer E, Bothwell M, Chao M. 1986. Expression and structure of the human NGF receptor. Cell 47:545–554.
28. Thanos S, Bahr M, Barde YA, Vanselow J. 1989. Survival and axonal elongation of adult rat retinal ganglion cells. In vitro effects of lesioned sciatic nerve and brain derived neurotrophic factor. Eur J Neurosci 1:19–26.
29. Alderson RF, Alterman AL, Barde YA, Lindsay RM. 1990. Brain-derived neurotrophic factor increases survival and differentiated functions of rat septal cholinergic neurons in culture. Neuron 5:297–306.
30. Knusel B, Winslow JW, Rosenthal A, Burton LE, Seid DP, Nikolics K, Hefti F. 1991. Promotion of central cholinergic and dopaminergic neuron differentiation by brain-derived neurotrophic factor but not neurotrophin-3. Proc Natl Acad Sci USA 88:961–965.
31. Hyman C, Hofer M, Barde YA, Juhasz M, Yancopoulos GD, Squinto SP, Lindsay RM. 1991. BDNF is a neurotrophic factor for dopaminergic neurons of the substantia nigra. Nature 350:230–232.
31. Shalaby IA, Kotake C, Hoffmann PC, Hellelr A. 1983. A release of dopamine from coaggregate cultures of mesencephalic tegmentum and corpus striatum. J Neurosci 3:1565–1571.
32. Denis-Donini S, Glowinski J, Prochiantz A. 1983. Specific influence of

striatal target neurons on the in vitro outgrowth of mesencephalic dopaminergic neurites: A morphological quantitative study. J Neurosci 3:2292–2299.

33. Tomozawa Y, Appel SH. 1986. Soluble striatal extracts enhance development of mesencephalic dopaminergic neurons in vitro. Brain Res 399:111–124.

34. Dal Toso R, Giorgi O, Soranzo C, Kirschner G, Ferrari G, Favaron M, Benvegnu D. 1988. Development and survival of neurons in dissociated fetal mesencephalic serum-free cell cultures: I. Effects of cell density and of an adult mammalian striatal-derived neuronotrophic factor (SDNF). J Neurosci 8:733–745.

35. Ferrari G, Minozzi MC, Toffano G, Leon A, Skaper SD. 1989. Basic fibroblast growth factor promotes the survival and development of mesencephalic neurons in culture. Dev Biol 133:140–147.

36. Valdes HB, Nonner D, Rulli D, Gralnik L, Barrett JN. 1988. Trophic effects of striatal proteins on central dopaminergic neurons in culture. *In* Progress in Parkinson Research. F Hefti, WJ Weiner (eds). Raven Press, New York, pp 163–172.

37. Michel PP, Dandapani BK, Knusel B, Sanchez-Ramos J, Hefti F. 1989. Toxicity of 1-methyl-4-phenylpyridinium for rat dopaminergic neurons in culture: Selectivity and irreversibility. J Neurochem 54:1102–1109.

38. Knüsel B, Michel PP, Schwaber JS, Hefti F. 1990. Selective and nonselective stimulation of central cholinergic and dopaminergic development in vitro by nerve growth factor, basic fibroblast growth factor, epidermal growth factor, insulin and the insulin-like growth factors I and II. J Neurosci 10:558–570.

39. Bottenstein JE, Sato GH. 1979. Growth of a rat neuroblastoma cell line in serum-free supplemented medium. Proc Natl Acad Sci USA 76:514–519.

40. Morrison RS, Sharma A, DeVellis J, Bradshaw RA. 1986. Basic fibroblast growth factor supports the survival of cerebral cortical neurons in primary culture. Proc Natl Acad Sci USA 83:7537–7541.

41. Walicke P, Cowan WM, Ueno N, Baird A, Guillemin R. 1986. Fibroblast growth factor promotes survival of dissociated hippocampal neurons and enhances neurite extension. Proc Natl Acad Sci USA 83:3012–3016.

42. Grothe C, Otto D, Unsicker K. 1989. Basic fibroblast growth factor promotes in vitro survival and cholinergic development of rat septal neurons: Comparison with the effects of nerve growth factor. Neuroscience 31:649–661.

43. Rechler MM, Nissley SP. 1985. The nature and regulation of the receptors for insulin-like growth factors. Annu Rev Physiol 47:425–442.

44. Baskin DG, Wilcox BJ, Figlewicz DP, Dorsa DM. 1988. Insulin and insulin-like growth factors in the CNS. Trends Neurosci 11:107–111.

45. Aizenman Y, Weischsel ME Jr, De Vellis J. 1986. Changes in insulin and transferrin requirements of pure brain neuronal cultures during embryonic development. Proc Natl Acad Sci USA 83:2263–2266.

46. Recio-Pinto E, Rechter MM, Ishii DN. 1986. Effects of insulin, insulin-like growth factor-II and nerve growth factor on neurite formation and

survival in cultured sympathetic and sensory neurons. J Neurosci 6:1211–1219.

47. Morrison RS, Kornblum HJ, Leslie FM, Bradshaw RA. 1987. Trophic stimulation of cultured neurons from neonatal rat brain by epidermal growth factor. Science 238:72–75.

48. Fallon JH, Seroogy KB, Loughlin SE, Morrison RS, Bradshaw RA, Knauer DJ, Cunningham DD. 1984. Epidermal growth factor immunoreactive material in the central nervous system: Localization and development. Science 224:1107–1109.

49. Code RA, Seroogy KB, Fallon JH. 1987. Some transforming growth factor-alpha connections and their colocalization with enkephalin in the rat central nervous system. Brain Res 421:401–405.

50. Derynck R. 1988. Transforming growth factor alpha. Cell 54:593–595.

51. Wilcox JN, Derynck R. 1988. Localization of cells synthesizing transforming growth factor-alpha mRNA in the mouse brain. J Neurosci 8:1901–1904.

52. Dreyfus CF, Peterson ER, Crain SM. 1980. Failure of nerve growth factor to affect fetal mouse brain catecholaminergic neurons in culture. Brain Res 194:540–547.

53. Rodriguez-Tebar A, Dechant G, Barde YA. 1990. Binding of brain-derived neurotrophic factor to the nerve growth factor receptor. Neuron 4:487–492.

54. Kaplan DR, Martin-Zanca D, Parada LF. 1991. Tyrosine phosphorylation and tyrosine kinase activity of the *trk* proto-oncogene product induced by NGF. Nature 350:158–160.

55. Klein R, Martin-Zanca D, Barbacid M, Parada LF. 1990. Expression of the tyrosine kinase receptor gene *trKB* is confined to the murine embryonic and adult nervous system. Development 109:845–850.

56. Ullrich A, Coussens L, Hayflick JS, Dull TJ, Gray A, Tam AW, Lee J, Yarden Y, Libermann TA, Schlessinger J, Downward J, Mayes ELV, Whittle N, Waterfiled MD, Seeburg PH. 1984. Human epidermal growth factor receptor cDNA sequence and aberrant expression of the amplified gene in A431 epidermoid carcinoma cells. Nature 309:418–424.

57. Carpenter G, King L, Cohen S. 1978. Epidermal growth factor stimulates phosphorylation in membrane preparations in vitro. Nature 276:409–410.

58. Carpenter G, Cohen S. 1990. Epidermal growth factor. J Biol Chem 265:7709–7712.

59. Ushiro H, Cohen S. 1980. Identification of phosphotyrosine as a product of epidermal growth factor-activated protein kinase in A-431 cell membranes. J Biol Chem 255:8363–8365.

60. Kase H, Iwahashi K, Nakanishi S, Matsuda Y, Yamada K, Takahashi M, Murakata C, Sato A, Kaneko M. 1987. K-252 compounds, novel and potent inhibitors of protein kinase C and cyclic nucleotide-dependent protein kinases. Biochm Biophys Res Commun 142:436–440.

61. Koizumi S, Contreras ML, Matsuda Y, Hama T, Lazarovici P, Guroff G. 1988. K-252a: A specific inhibitor of the action of nerve growth factor on PC12 cells. J Neurosci 8:715–721.

62. Matsuda Y, Fukuda J. 1988. Inhibition by K-252a, a new inhibitor of protein kinase, of nerve growth factor-induced neurite outgrowth of chick embryo dorsal root ganglion cells. Neurosci Lett 87:11–17.
63. Hashimoto S. 1988. K-252a, a potent protein kinase inhibitor blocks nerve growth factor-induced neurite outgrowth and changes in the phosphorylation of proteins in PC12h cells. J Cell Biol 107:1531–1539.
64. Smith DS, King CS, Pearson E, Gittinger CK, Landreth G. 1989. Selective inhibition of nerve growth factor-stimulated protein kinases by K-252a and 5′-S-methyladenosine in PC12 cells. J Neurochem 53:800–806.
65. Sano M, Nishiyama K, Kitajima S. 1990. A nerve growth factor-dependent protein kinase that phosphorylates microtubule-associated proteins in vitro: Possible involvement of its activity in the outgrowth of neurites from PC12 cells. J Neurochem 55:427–435.
66. Doherty P, Walsh FS. 1989. K-252a specifically inhibits the survival and morphological differentiation of NGF-dependent neurons in primary cultures of human dorsal root ganglia. Neurosci Lett 96:1–6.
67. Borasio GD. 1990. Differential effects of the protein kinase inhibitor K-252a on the in vitro survival of chick embryonic neurons. Neurosci Lett 108:207–212.
68. Knusel B, Hefti F. 1991. K-252b is a selective and non-toxic inhibitor of nerve growth factor action on cultured brain neurons. J Neurochem 57(3):955–962.
69. Barde YA. 1988. What, if anything, is a neurotrophic factor? Trends Neurosci 11:343–346.
70. Shelton DL, Reichardt LF. 1986. Studies on the expression of the beta nerve growth factor (NGF) gene in the central nervous system: Level and regional distribution of NGF mRNA suggest that NGF functions as a trophic factor for several distinct populations of neurons. Proc Natl Acad Sci USA 83:2714–2718.
71. Korsching S, Auburger G, Heumann R, Scott J, Thoenen H. 1985. Levels of nerve growth factor and its mRNA in the central nervous system of the rat correlate with cholinergic innervation. EMBO J 4:1389–1393.
72. Hofer MM, Barde YA. 1988. Brain-derived neurotrophic factor prevents neuronal death in vivo. Nature 331:261–262.

7

Transplantation

Chapter 28

Human Fetal Mesencephalic Grafts:
Target-Directed Outgrowth and Dopamine Release in Rat Host

Ingrid Strömberg, Per Almqvist, Craig van Horne,
Marc Bygdeman, Lars Olson, Barry Hoffer,
and Greg Gerhardt

Grafting catecholamine-rich tissue to patients with severe Parkinson's disease as a tool to counteract the symptoms of the disease has been tried on an experimental basis, but has yet not become a routine therapeutic technique. Initially, the adrenal medulla was used as a source of catecholamine-rich tissue.[1–6] Recently, long-lasting effects of adrenal autograft has been obtained by supporting the grafts with infusion of nerve growth factor for several weeks postoperatively.[7] The second approach currently undergoing clinical trails employs human fetal mesencephalic tissue.[8–13] Several attempts to improve the efficacy of the grafting techniques have been presented, such as using thinner implantation cannulas to obtain better cell survival,[14] and cryopreservation of tissue to investigate viability of the cells before implantation.[15] To improve the clinical results, however, more

This study was supported by Swedish Medical Research Council 08868 and 03185, USPHS grants NS-09199, and the Lars Hierta, Palle Ferb, Harald and Greta Jeansson, and the Karolinska Institute Foundations.
From Hefti F, and Weiner WJ, (eds.) *Progress in Parkinson's Disease Research—2.* Mount Kisco NY, Futura Publishing Co., Inc., © 1992.

information is needed from animal research. From rodent experiments it has been shown that human fetal tissue survives grafting in the animal model of Parkinson's disease[16,17] and can compensate behavior deficiency.[16–20] When attempting to transfer these results into clinical trials, several problems remain, such as how a complete vs incomplete denervation status of the target areas influences graft survival and nerve fiber outgrowth. Both caudate nucleus and putamen have been targets for implantations.[6,21] The degree of denervation is more pronounced in putamen than in the caudate nucleus.[22] If outgrowth and graft survival is influenced by the degree of dopamine denervation of the host, then it becomes important not only to select where to do an implant, but also to select patients in an "optimal" stage of the disease, regarding the loss of dopamine terminals, when planning grafting therapy.

One advantage of using human fetal tissue in xenografting to rats is that the human fetal neurons appear to grow for longer distances than what is seen in rat allograft experiments.[23–25] It has been shown that human fetal tissue can reinnervate the total volume of a rat caudate nucleus.[20,24] Furthermore, the use of xenografting makes it possible to distinguish the graft and graft-derived nerve fibers from host by using human-specific immunohistochemical markers.[20,25–27] Thus, it should be possible to detect graft-derived nerve terminals in intact host striatal tissue.

In this study, partly presented elsewhere,[19,24] we have examined growth from human fetal mesencephalic tissue placed either into the lateral ventricle or into cingulate cortex of unilaterally denervated rats as well as dopamine release in grafted striata. Previous data have shown that dopamine can be released in striata, reinnervated by human mesencephalic grafts.[27,28] Here we will present data on the time course of extracellular dopamine after potassium-evoked release and relate this to the efficiency of dopamine in graft-reinnervated striata.

Materials and Methods

Recipient Animals and Behavior

Female Sprague-Dawley rats were used as transplant recipients. Stereotaxic injections of 6-hydroxydopamine (6-OHDA; 8 μg/4 μl in

Ringer's solution containing 0.2 mg/ml ascorbic acid) into the medial forebrain bundle were performed unilaterally. The completeness of the denervations was tested by challenging the rats with low doses (0.05 mg/kg, SC) of apomorphine and registering the turning behavior.[29] Rats repeatedly showing the characteristic two peaks rotational pattern[30] and rotating a minimum of 500 turns over 60 minutes after the apomorphine injection were selected for transplantation. After grafting, rotational behavior was tested monthly. All recipients received daily injections, 6 days per week, of cyclosporin A (Sandoz, 10 mg/kg, or day before injection-free day 15 mg/kg) and vibramycin (Pfizer, 2 mg/kg) IP from the day prior to grafting, in order to minimize graft rejection.

Transplantation Procedure

Human fetal ventral mesencephalic tissue was dissected from first-trimester abortions. Women, admitted for elective abortions and with no prior knowledge of this study, were informed both orally and in writing of the goals of the study, and they gave their consent. Anonymity was strictly maintained. The abortions were routinely performed with low vacuum aspiration. The study was approved by the regional ethical committee of the Karolinska Institute and all experiments confirmed to guidelines of the Swedish Medical Association and the U.S. Public Health Service.

Ventral mesencephalic tissue was grafted as solid tissue pieces. Each piece contained dopamine-rich tissue from one side of the brain stem. These tissue pieces were identified under a stereomicroscope in brain-stem fragments using the pontine and mesencephalic flexures as landmarks. The transplantations were performed stereotaxically under halothane anesthesia. The grafts were placed either into the lateral ventricle ipsilateral to the dopamine denervation or into cingulate cortex in contrast with corpus callosum (Figure 1).

Immunohistochemistry

For immunohistochemical evaluations, rats were perfused with Ca^{2+}-free Tyrode's solution followed by 4% paraformaldehyde in 0.1 M phosphate buffer. After postfixation in the same fixative, the brains were rinsed in 10% sucrose before sectioning for indirect

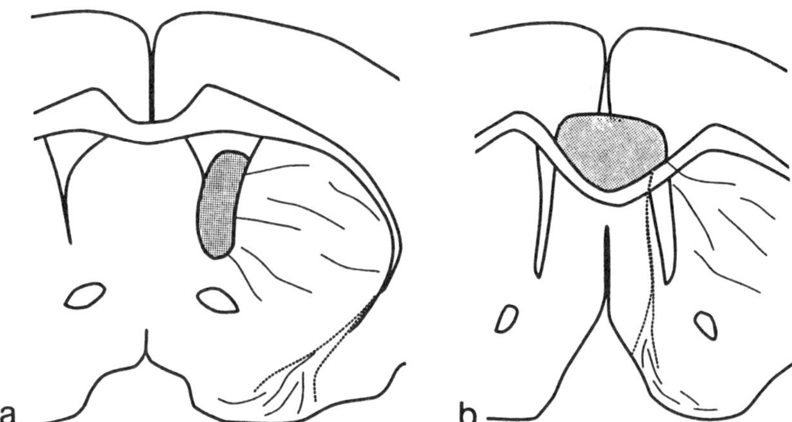

Figure 1. Camera lucida drawings from coronal sections showing the placements of the grafts (shaded areas) placed intraventricularly (a) or in the cingulate cortex (b). The dotted lines show graft-derived nerve fiber bundles. The thin solid lines demonstrate nerve fiber outgrowth from the grafts. Only the lesioned striatum was innervated by the transplants. Graft-derived nerve fibers were also seen in ventral parts of striatum. TH immunohistochemistry within the transplant and outgrowing nerve fibers was also positive to antibodies against human specific Thy-1. From ref. 24.

immunohistochemistry.[31] Sections were rinsed in 0.1 M phosphate buffer saline (PBS) before incubation in antibodies against tyrosine hydroxylase (TH; Pel Freeze, Clinical Systems Division, Wisconsin) diluted 1:100, or human specific Thy-1[32] diluted 1:100 in PBS containing 0.3% Triton for 48 hours. After rinsing in PBS, the sections were then incubated in fluorescein isothiocyanate-conjugated secondary antibodies, rinsed, and mounted in 90% glycerine in phosphate buffer containing 0.1% *p*-phenylenediamine as an antifading agent.[33] Antibody-based detection methods do not permit absolute chemical identification of antigens and the data should be interpreted accordingly.

In Vivo Electrochemistry

In vivo electrochemical measurements employed a high-speed (5-Hz) chronoamperometric recording system (IVEC-5; Medical Systems Corp.). Rats were anesthetized with chloral hydrate, intubated, and placed in a stereotaxic frame. Nafion-coated multiple carbon-fiber working electrodes were characterized for sensitivity and selectivity.[34] The electrodes showed good sensitivity to dopamine and serotonin, while being insensitive to ascorbic acid, DOPAC, 5-HIAA and uric acid. Square-wave pulses of 0.0 to +0.55 volts, with respect to an Ag–AgCl reference electrode implanted remote from the recording site, were applied to the working electrode for 0.20 seconds. The resulting oxidation and reduction currents were digitally integrated. Local application of potassium solution (120 mM KCl and 2.5 mM $CaCl_2$), performed from micropipets by using pressure ejection, were used to induce transmitter release.

Results

Xenografts Counteract Behavioral Deficits

Reduction in apomorphine-induced rotations were first observed at 2 months postgrafting. No differences in the graft-induced reductions of turning behavior were seen between animals with grafts placed in cingulate cortex and those with grafts in the lateral ventricle. The reduced amount of turning was mainly due to a shorter duration of turning behavior. Consequently, the second of the two peaks seen before transplantation was reduced. This second peak in apomorphine-induced turning behavior had totally disappeared at the end of the testing period (Figure 2).

Axonal Outgrowth is Target-Specific

Immunohistochemical evaluations were performed at 1.5 months and 5–7 months postgrafting. TH-immunoreactive neurons were found in all grafts. The graft-host interface was well fused both when the transplant was placed in the ventricle and when it was located in the cingulate cortex. When the graft was placed in the ventricle, TH-positive neurons had migrated across the ependymal lining into host striatum (Figure 3a and b). Such migration was never observed across a graft–septum or a graft–cortex interface.

The grafts had reinnervated the lesioned striata in all animals except for one rat, where the graft survival time was 1.5 months

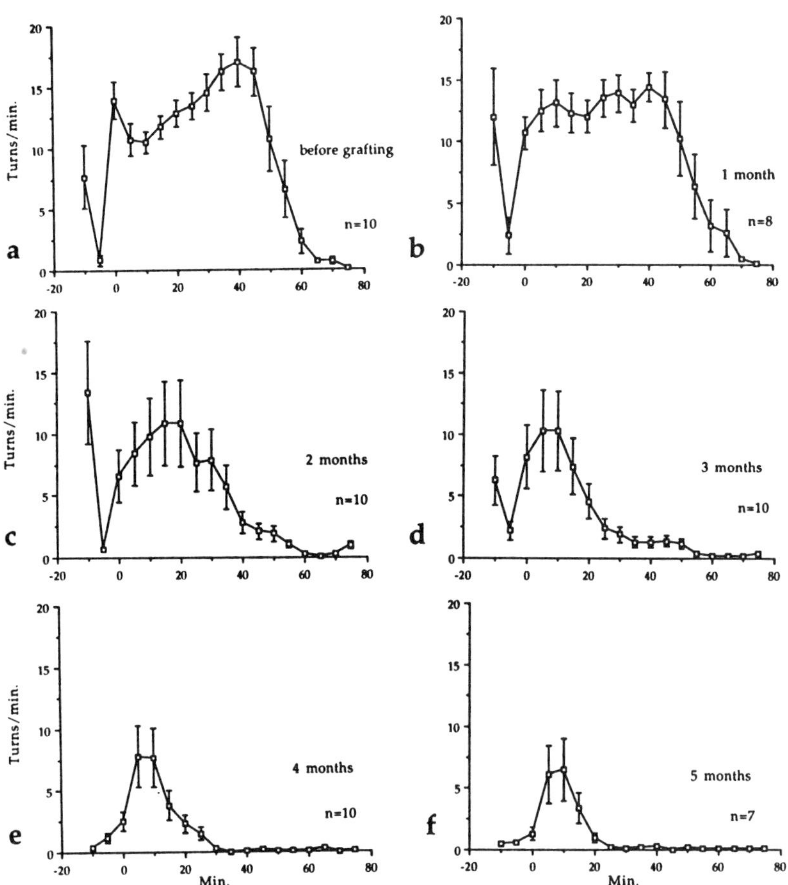

Figure 2. Apomorphine-induced turning behavior of all rats grafted with human fetal mesencephalic tissue. Rotational behavior prior to grafting (a). Rotations at monthly intervals (b–f) up to 5 months (f) after grafting. Each graph shows the number of turns/min (± SEM) vs time. Apomorphine was injected at time 0. At 2 months after grafting a reduction of the number of turns is pronounced. This reduction becomes more marked with time, and at 5 months after transplantation only a part of the first two peaks seen prior to grafting remains. n = number of rats tested. Partly from ref. 19.

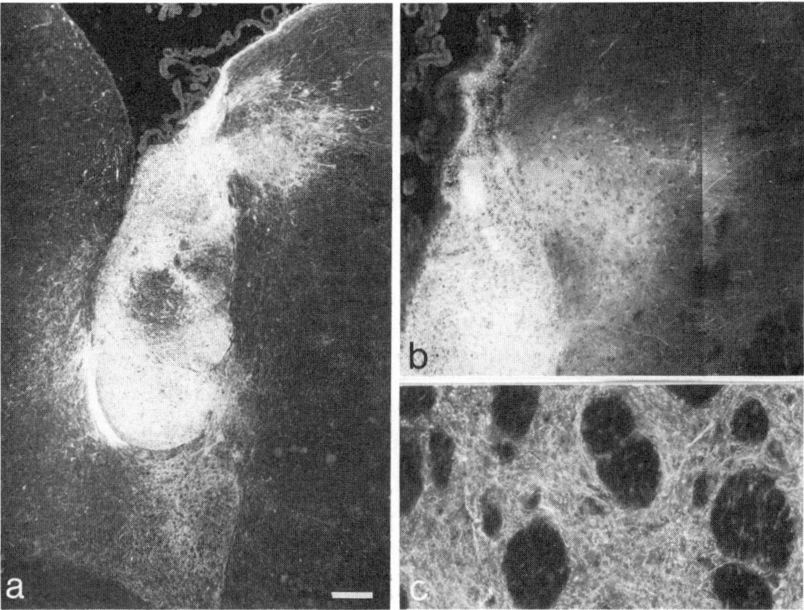

Figure 3. Intraventricular human fetal graft 1.5 months after grafting (a and b). TH positivity is seen within the graft. The graft is densely populated with TH-positive neurons (a). At 1.5 months after grafting most of the host striatum is still noninnervated, but TH-positive neurons have migrated into host striatal tissue (a). Thy-1 immunoreactivity (b) at the graft–host interface shows that the TH-positive cells in (a) also are Thy-1-immunoreactive. Six months after grafting, a relatively high density of TH-immunoreactive nerve fibers had reinnervated host striatum (c). Here is shown center parts of host striatum. (a) is reproduced from ref. 24. Scale bars: a = 200 μm, b = 100 μm, and c = 50 μm.

(Figure 3). When the graft was placed in cingulate cortex, TH-positive fibers had penetrated through corpus callosum and then invaded the lesioned striatum. The TH-positive fiber bundles that penetrated corpus callosum, as well as the grafts, were Thy-1-immunoreactive (Figure 4a). Furthermore, Thy-1-positive fibers were only observed in the lesioned striata, indicating that graft-derived nerve fibers only had grown into the dopamine-depleted side (Figure 1). There was no detectable difference in nerve fiber density between striata reinnervated by grafts placed in the ventricle and grafts in cortex. The nerve fiber density was high throughout the total volume of striatum (Figure 3c), although it was less dense

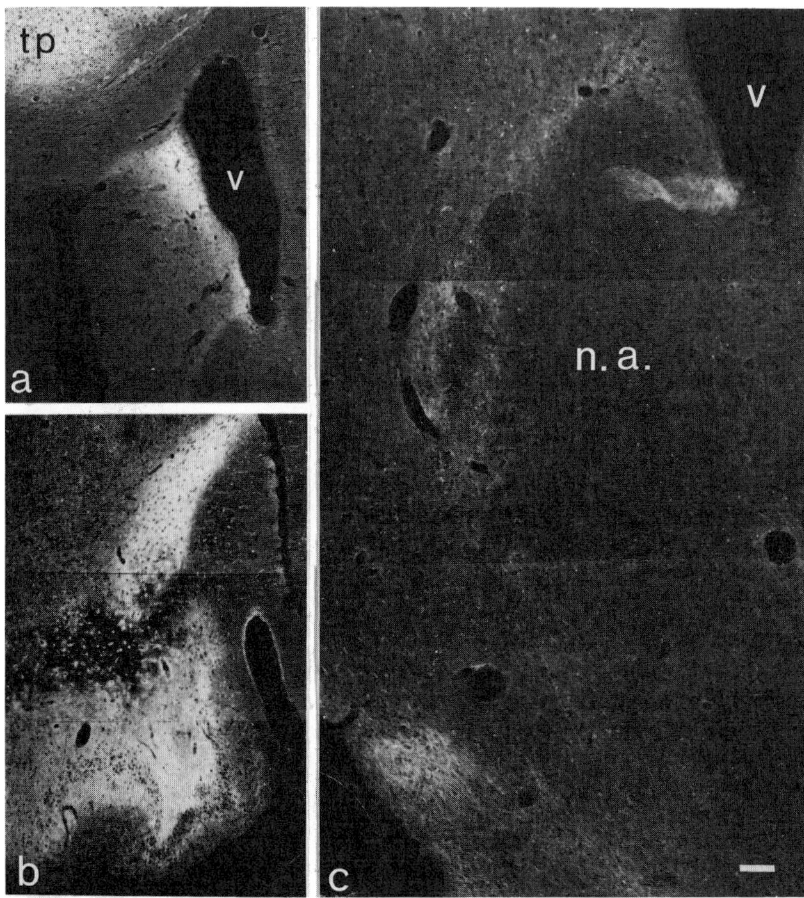

Figure 4. Thy-1-immunoreactivity from a rat with an human fetal mesencephalic transplant (tp) placed in cingulate cortex 5 months after grafting. A Thy-1-positive fiber bundle is seen medial to the ventricle (v) running in a dorsoventral direction. (c) This fiber bundle avoided the area of nucleus accumbens (n.a.). Another Thy-1-positive fiber bundle was formed as a continuation of lateral parts of corpus callosum before arborization in ventral parts of striatum (b). (b) is reproduced from ref. 24. Scale bars: a = 200 μm, b = 100 μm, c = 75 μm.

further away from the graft, i.e., in the lateral parts of striatum, close to the lateral corpus callosum.

Thick nerve fiber bundles penetrated from the graft into host septal areas, when the graft was placed in the ventricle (Figure 3a). These fiber bundles followed the surface of the transplants until it reached the striatum. TH-positive nerve fibers were found in septum to a density that is seen in normal septal areas and thus were much less dense than that found in reinnervated striata. There was a complete overlap between human specific Thy-1 immunoreactivity and the TH-positive nerve fibers. The graft-derived nerve terminals in septal areas did not reach longer than 500 μm from the transplant.

Globus pallidus was totally devoid of graft-derived fibers and appeared negative with respect to TH immunoreactivity. In cases when the intraventricularly placed graft was attached to globus pallidus, TH- and Thy-1-immunoreactive fiber bundles followed the graft–host interface until they reached striatum and arborized.

When the human mesencephalic tissue was placed in cingulate cortex, TH-immunoreactive nerve fibers reinnervated only cortical areas close to the graft. A high density of TH-positive nerve fibers within the transplant and an abrupt delineation between host cortex and the grafted tissue was observed.

The TH- and Thy-1-positive nerve fiber bundles that penetrated corpus callosum from the human mesencephalic grafts placed in cortex often followed the medial parts of the lateral ventricle in a dorsoventral direction (Figure 4a). In some cases, these bundles could be followed on the medial surface of nucleus accumbens, leaving the neuropil of this nucleus totally Thy-1-negative (Figure 4c). Another type of newly formed fiber bundle in dorsoventral direction was seen laterally as a continuation of the lateroventral aspects of corpus callosum (Figure 4b). All these fiber bundles were only found ipsilateral to the 6-OHDA lesions.

In ventral limbic areas, the olfactory tubercle and ventral pallidum, dense TH-positive fiber networks were observed. No difference in nerve fiber density in ventral limbic areas was observed between animals with intraventricularly placed grafts and rats with transplants placed in cingulate cortex. In adjacent sections, Thy-1 immunoreactivity completely overlapped TH-positive fiber networks on the lesioned side (Figure 4b), leaving the control side Thy-1-negative.

Release of Dopamine in Graft-Reinnervated Striatum

Using local applications of potassium, dopamine-like responses were recorded, as suggested by the ratio between reduction and oxidation current responses. The average response in control striata was 2.65 ± 0.17 μM. In ungrafted, 6-OHDA-lesioned striata the average amplitude was 0.35 ± 0.06 μM, while following grafting of human fetal dopamine neurons, the potassium-induced response was clearly increased to 1.52 ± 0.15 μM. Areas close to the graft, with a presumably more dense innervation, showed amplitudes close to what was observed in the control side (Figure 5a). The reduction to oxidation current suggested that the response seen in 6-OHDA-lesioned striata contained higher amounts of serotonin than was seen in control and graft-reinnervated striata.

Interestingly, in remote areas of innervated territory, where histochemical data suggest fewer nerve terminals, the time course of the dopamine-like signals recorded by the in vivo chronoamperometry was much more prolonged. The rise time to reach the maximal amplitude also was increased when recording from less densely reinnervated areas (Figure 5b).

Discussion

Taken together, the behavioral, histochemical, and in vivo electrochemical data presented above clearly demonstrate the efficacy of the human-to-rat dopaminergic xenografts. It is shown that the fetal dopaminergic neurons do not grow indiscriminately to all surrounding areas, but grow in a highly target-specific manner. From rat allograft studies, it has been suggested that fetal brain tissue may express low target specificity. Thus, locus ceruleus neurons have been reported to produce dopamine and reduce amphetamine-induced turning behavior when grafted to 6-OHDA-lesioned recipients.[35] However, as shown here, the dopamine neurons appear to grow only into areas that are dopamine-depleted. Moreover, it has been shown that human locus ceruleus grafts implanted into 6-OHDA-lesioned striata of immunosuppressed rats survives grafting, but at 3 months postgrafting fail to form nerve terminals reinnervating host striatum.[36] This is not because human locus ceruleus neurons are incapable of forming nerve fibers at this stage,

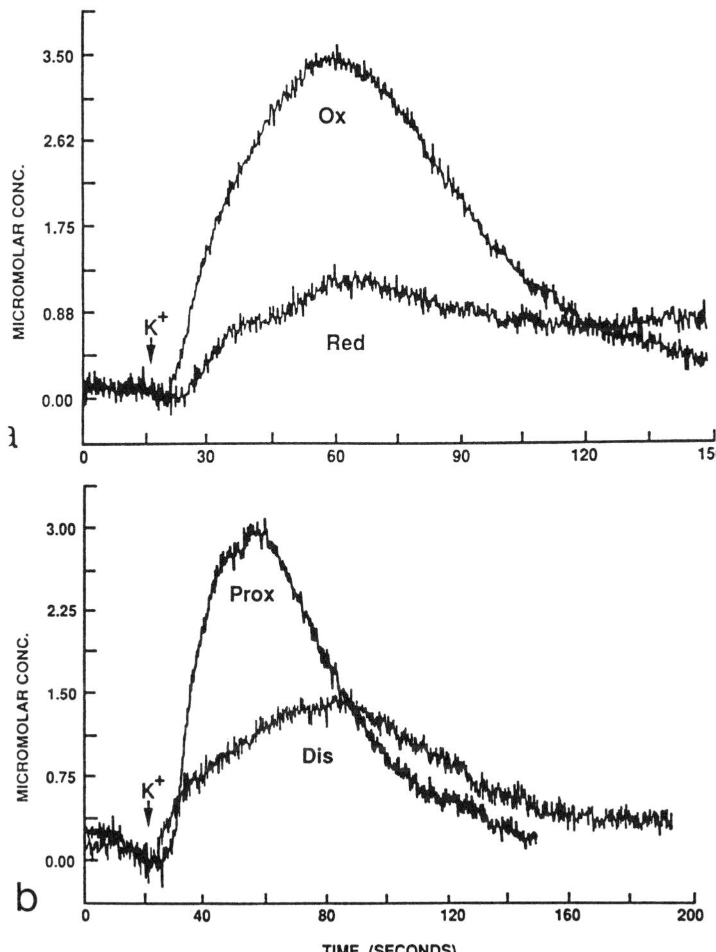

Figure 5. High-speed in vivo electrochemical recordings of potassium-evoked overflow of monoamines in striatum close to a human fetal mesencephalic graft (a). The Ox curve represents the oxidation current signal and the Red curve is the simultaneous reduction current signal. Examples of recording sites are shown proximal (Prox) and distal (Dis) to the graft in graft-reinnervated striatum (b). Recordings from sites distal to the graft show longer duration and longer rise time. From ref. 19.

since they readily form nerve fibers if grafted to the anterior chamber of the eye, where nerve fibers extend into host iris as soon as 13 days in oculo.[37] Thus, it seems as if human fetal catecholamine neurons express a very specific direction of the outgrowing fibers from graft to host only into appropriate target areas, depending on what type of neurons that have been grafted.

The rotational behavior was improved as early as 2 months after grafting. This is earlier than seen before.[16,20] The apomorphine-induced rotations, however, are not reduced as completely as has been reported for rotations induced by amphetamine.[16] The noncomplete correction of apomorphine-induced rotational behavior might be due to fewer implants dopaminergic neurons or less viability to form nerve terminals, but as these rotations are reduced earlier than noted in amphetamine-induced rotations, this is probably not the case. More likely is that the grafts are unable to compensate for all deficits caused by a 6-OHDA-induced dopamine depletion.

The electrochemical data in the present study show that dopamine released from the dopamine nerve terminals under normal circumstances is efficiently cleared from the extracellular space, probably by reuptake into the terminals. This gives the electrochemical signal a typical fast time course. However, in sparsely innervated areas, the amplitude of the release was much smaller, while the duration of the electrochemical signal was much longer, suggesting the presence of dopamine in the extracellular space for longer time periods. These findings suggest that dopamine released from the graft-derived nerve terminals may diffuse to reach a larger volume of host striatum than the reinnervated area. Thus, the effects of the grafts may be more widespread than earlier thought, making efficient use of extracellular diffusion pathways in a mode recently referred to as volume transmission.[38]

The finding that the grafts extend fibers only into denervated striatum as opposed to intact, as seen with Thy-1 immunoreactivity, suggests that a dopamine-depleted striatum has a stronger influence on a fetal graft than an intact striatum. A dopamine-denervated striatum might produce increased levels of a putative dopaminotrophic factor that influences the direction of the growth. In rat allograft studies, dopamine neurons grafted to intact animals show both outgrowing fibers and reduce behavioral deficits induced later by lesioning the host dopaminergic system.[39,40] However, these implantations were performed on neonates at a time when striatum has incomplete dopamine innervation.[41,42] This means that the grafted neurons can compete with host nigral neurons for noninnervated areas. Furthermore, a suggested dopaminotrophic factor might be expressed at increased levels before complete innervation occurs, just as the levels of nerve growth factor are higher in neonates than in adults.[43]

Taken together, these results show that dopamine released in reinnervated striata has a prolonged extracellular half-life, suggesting that the grafts might be more efficient than indicated by the density and extent of innervation. Furthermore, graft-derived dopaminergic nerve terminals exhibit highly specific outgrowth patterns in rat host and reinnervate only dopamine-depleted areas that normally are targets for nigral neurons.

References

1. Backlund E-O, Granberg P-O, Hamberger B, Knutsson E, Mårtensson A, Sedvall G, Seiger Å, Olson L. 1985. Transplantation of adrenal medullary tissue to striatum in parkinsonism. First clinical trials. J Neurosurg 62: 169–173.
2. Backay R, Herring C. 1989. Central nervous sytem grafting in the treatment of parkinsonism. Stereotact Funct Neurosurg 53:1–20.
3. Goetz CG, Olanow CW, Koller WC, Penn RD, Cahill D, Moratz R, Stebbins G, Tanner CM, Klawans HL, Shannon KM, Comella CL, Witt T, Cox C. 1989. Multicenter study of autologeous adrenal medullary transplantation to the corpus striatum in patients with advanced Parkinson's disease. N Engl J Med 320:337–341.
4. Jiao S, Zhang W, Cao J, Zhang A, Wang H, Ding M, Zhang Z, Sun J, Sun Y, Shi M. 1988. Study of adrenal medullary tissue transplantation to striatum in parkinsonism. *In:* Transplantation into the Mammalian CNS. Progress in Brain Research, DM Gash, JR Sladek Jr, (eds). Elsevier Vol. 78, pp. 575–580.
5. Lopez-Lozano JJ, Abascal J, Bravo G, CPH Neural Transplantation Group. 1990. A year follow-up of autoimplants of perfused adrenal medulla into parkinsonian patients. *In:* Neuronal Transplantation: From Molecular Basis to Clinical Application. Progress in Brain Research. SB Dunnett, S-J Richards, (eds). Elsevier Vol. 82, 657–663.
6. Madrazo I, Drücker-Colin R, Martinez-Marta J, Torres C, Becerril JJ. 1989. Open microsurgical autograft of adrenal medulla to the right caudate nucleus in Parkinson's disease: A report of two cases. N Engl J Med 316:831–834.
7. Olson L, Backlund E-O, Ebendal T, Freedman R, Hamberger B, Hansson P, Hoffer B, Lindblom U, Meyerson B, Strömberg I, Sydow O, Seiger Å. 1991. Intraputaminal infusion of nerve growth factor to support adrenal

medullary autografts in Parkinson's disease. One-year follow-up of first clinical trial. Arch Neurol 48(4):373–381.

8. Freed CR, Breeze RE, Rosenberg NL, Schneck SA, Wells TH, Barrett JN, Grafton ST, Mazziotta JC, Eidelberg D, Rottenberg DA. 1990. Therapeutic effects of fetal dopamine cells transplanted in a patient with Parkinson's disease. *In:* Neuronal Transplantation: From Molecular Basis to Clinical Application. Progress in Brain Research. SB Dunnett, S-J Richards, (eds). Elsevier, Vol. 82, pp 715–721.

9. Hitchcock ER, Kenny BG, Clough CG, Hughes RC, Henderson BTH, Detta A. 1990. Stereotactic implatation of foetal mesencephalon (STIM): The UK experience. *In:* Neuronal Transplantation: From Molecular Basis to Clinical Application. Progress in Brain Research. SB Dunnett, S-J Richards, (eds). Elsevier, Vol. 82, pp. 723–728.

10. Lindvall O, Rehncrona S, Gustavii B, Brundin P, Åstedt B, Widner H, Lindholm T, Björklund A, Leenders KL, Rothwell JC, Frackowiak R, Marsden CD, Johnels B, Steg G, Freedman R, Hoffer BJ, Seiger Å, Strömberg I, Bygdeman M, Olson L. 1988. Fetal dopamine-rich mesencephalic grafts in Parkinson's disease. Lancet 2:1443.

11. Lindvall O, Rehncrona S, Brundin P, Gustavii B, Åstedt B, Widner H, Lindholm T, Björklund A, Leenders KL, Rothwell JC, Frackowiak R, Marsden CD, Johnels B, Steg G, Freedman R, Hoffer BJ, Seiger Å, Bygdeman M, Strömberg I, Olson. 1989. Human fetal dopamine neurons into striatum in two patients with severe Parkinson's disease. A detailed account of methodology and a 6-month follow-up. Arch Neurol 46:615–631.

12. Lindvall O, Brundin P, Widner H, Rehncrona S, Gustavii B, Frackowiak R, Leenders KL, Sawle G, Rothwell JC, Marsden CD, Björklund A. 1990. Grafts of fetal dopamine neurons survive and improve motor function in Parkinson's disease. Science 247:574–577.

13. Madrazo I, Leon V, Torres C, Auilera MC, Varela G, Alvarez F, Fraga A, Drücker-Colin R. Ostrosky F, Skurovich M, Franco R. 1988. Transplantation of fetal substantia nigra and adrenal medulla to caudate nucleus in two patients with Parkinson's disease. N Engl J Med 318:51.

14. Brundin P, Björklund A, Lindvall O. 1990. Practical aspects of the use of human fetal brain tissue for intracerebral grafting. *In:* Neuronal Transplantation: From Molecular Basis to Clinical Application. Elsevier, Progress in Brain Research. SB Dunnett, S-J Richards, (eds). Vol. 82, 707–714.

15. Redmond DE, Naftolin F, Collier TJ, Leranth C, Robbins RJ, Sladek CD, Roth RH, Sladek JR Jr. 1988. Cryopreservation, culture and transplantation of human fetal mesencephalic tissue into monkeys. Science 242:768–771.

16. Brundin P, Nilsson O, Strecker R, Lindvall O, Åstedt B, Björklund A. 1986. Behavioural effects of human fetal dopamine neurons grafted in a rat model of Parkinson's disease. Exp Brain Res 65:235–240.

17. Strömberg I, Bygdeman M, Goldstein M, Seiger Å, Olson L. 1986. Human fetal substantia nigra grafted to the dopaminc-denervated

striatum of immunosuppressed rats: Evidence for functional reinnervation. Neurosci Lett 71:271–276.

18. Clarke DJ, Brundin P, Strecker RE, Nilsson OG, Björklund A, Lindvall O. 1988. Human fetal dopamine neurons grafted in a rat model of Parkinson's disease: Ultrastructural evidence for synapse formation using tyrosine hydroxylase immunoctyochemistry. Exp Brain Res 73:115–126.

19. Strömberg I, van Horne C, Bygdeman M, Weiner N, Gerhardt GA. 1991. Function of intraventricular human mesencephalic xenografts in immunosuppressed rats: An electrophysiological and neurochemical analysis. Exp Neurol 112(2):140–152.

20. van Horne C, Mahalik T, Hoffer B, Bygdeman M, Almqvist P, Stieg P, Seiger Å, Olson L, Strömberg I. 1990. Behavioral and electrophysiological correlates of human mesencephalic dopaminergic xenograft function in the rat striatum. Brain Res Bull 25:325–334.

21. Lindvall O, Backlund E-O, Farde L, Sedvall G, Freedman R, Hoffer B, Nobin A, Seiger Å, Olson L. 1987. Transplantation in Parkinson's disease: Two cases of adrenal medullary grafts to the putamen. Ann Neurol 22:457–468.

22. Kish SJ, Shannak K, Hornykiewicz O. 1988. Uneven pattern of dopamine loss in the striatum of patients with idiopathic Parkinson's disease. Pathophysiologic and clinical implications. N Engl J Med 318:876–880.

23. Strömberg I, Gerhardt G, van Horne C, Bygdeman M, Olson L, Hoffer B. 1991. Electrophysiological and in vivo electrochemical recordings in rats with intraventricular human xenografts. In Eric K. Ferntröm Symposium. Intracerebral Transplantation in Movement Disorders-Experimental Basis and Clinical Experiences. O Lindvall (ed). Elsevier, Amsterdam, (in press).

24. Strömberg I, Bygdeman M, Almqvist P. 1991. Target specific outgrowth from human mesencephalic tissue grafted to cortex or ventricle of immunosuppressed rats. J Comp Neurol.

25. Wictorin K, Brundin P, Gustavii B, Lindvall O, Björklund A. 1990. Reformation of long pathways in adult rat central nervous system by human forebrain neuroblasts. Nature 347:556–558.

26. Strömberg I, Almqvist P, Bygdeman M, Finger TE, Gerhardt GA, Granholm A-C, Mahalik TJ, Seiger Å, Hoffer BJ, Olson L. 1988. Intracerebral xenografts of human mesencephalic tissue into athymic rats: Histochemical and in vivo electrochemical studies. Proc Natl Acad Sci USA 85:8331–8434.

27. Strömberg I, Almqvist P, Bygdeman M, Finger TE, Gerhardt GA, Granholm A-C, Mahalik TJ, Seiger Å, Olson L, Hoffer BJ. 1989. Human fetal mesencephalic tissues grafted to dopamine-denervated striatum of athymic rats: Light- and electron-microscopical histochemistry and in vivo chronoamperometric studies. J Neurosci 9:614–624.

28. Brundin P, Strecker RE, Widner H, Clarke DJ, Nilsson OG, Åstedt B, Lindvall O, Björklund A. 1988. Human fetal dopamine neurons grafted

in a rat model of Parkinson's disease: Immunological aspects, spontaneous and drug-induced behaviour, and dopamine release. Exp Brain Res 70:192–208.

29. Ungerstedt U, Arbuthnott G. 1970. Quantitative recording of rotational behaviour in rats after 6-hydroxydopamine lesions of the nigrostriatal dopamine system. Brain Res 24:485–493.

30. Understedt U, Herrera-Marschitz M. 1981. Behavioural pharmacology of dopamine receptor mechanisms. *In* Chemical Neurotransmission: 75 Years. L Stjärne, P Hedqvist, H Lagerkrantz, A Wennmalm (eds). Academic Press, New York, pp 481–494.

31. Coons AH. 1958. Fluorescent antibody methods. *In* General Cytochemical Methods. F Danielli (ed). Academic Press, New York, pp 399–422.

32. Berglund E, Almqvist P, Lindroos H, Carlsson S, Stigbrand T. 1987. Antigenic pattern of human brain glycoproteins as described by monocolonal antibodies. J Neurochem 48:809–815.

33. Johnson D, de C Nogueira-Araujo G. 1981. A simple method of reducing the fading of immunofluorescence during microscopy. J Immunol Methods 43:349–350.

34. Gerhardt GA, Oke AF, Nagy G, Moghaddam B, Adams RN. 1984. Nafion-coated electrodes with high selectivity for CNS electrochemistry. Brain Res 190:390–395.

35. Nishino H, Hatashitani M, Ishida Y, Hida H, Makino T, Sakurai T, Furuyama F, Isobe Y, Sato H. 1990. Phenotypic plastisity of locus coeruleus noradrenaergic neurons after transplantation into the dopamine-depleted caudate in the rat. Prog Brain Res 82:515–521.

36. Seiger Å, Bygdeman M, Goldstein M, Almqvist P, Hoffer B, Strömberg I, Olson L. 1988. Human fetal catecholamine-containing tissues grafted intraocularly and intracranially to immuno-compromised rodent hosts. Prog Brain Res 78:449–455.

37. Olson L, Strömberg I, Bygdeman M, Granholm A-C, Hoffer B, Freedman R, Seiger Å. 1987. Human fetal tissues grafted to rodent hosts: structural and functional observations of brain, adrenal and heart tissues in oculo. Exp Brain Res 67:163–178.

38. Fuxe K, Agnati LF, Härfstrand A, Cintra A, Aronsson M, Zoli M, Gustavsson J-Å. 1988. Principles for the hormone regulation of wiring transmission and volume transmission in the central nervous system. Curr Top Neuroendocrinal 8:1–53.

39. Rogers DC, Martel FL, Dunnett SB. 1990. Nigral grafts in neonatal rats protect from aphagia induced by subsequent adult 6-OHDA lesions: The importance of striatal location. Exp Brain Res 80:172–176.

40. Snyder-Keller AM, Carder RK, Lund RD. 1989. Development of dopamine innervation and turning behavior in dopamine-depleted infant rats receiving unilateral nigral transplants. Neuroscience 30:779–794.

41. Olson L, Seiger Å, Fuxe K. 1972. Heterogeneity of striatal and limbic dopamine innervation: Highly fluorescent islands in developing and adult rats. Brain Res 44:283–288.

42. Voorn P, Karlsbeek A, Jorritsma-Byham B, Groenewegen HJ. 1988. The

pre- and postnatal development of the dopaminergic cell groups in the ventral mesencephalon and the dopaminergic innervation of the striatum of the rat. Neuroscience 25:857–887.

43. Whittemore SC, Ebendal T, Lärkfors L, Olson L, Seiger Å, Strömberg I, Persson H. 1986. Developmental and regional expression of β-nerve growth factor messenger RNA and protein in the rat central nervous system. Proc Natl Acad Sci USA 83:817–821.

Chapter 29

Fetal Tissue Implants Improve Parkinsonian Signs in Patients with the On–Off Phenomenon

Curt R. Freed, Neil L. Rosenberg, Stuart A. Schneck, and Robert E. Breeze

Experiments in animal models of Parkinson's disease have shown that fetal mesencephalic dopamine neurons placed into the striatum of adult animals can survive and grow neural processes. Changes in behavioral responses to amphetamine and apomorphine have been seen.[1-8] Fetal cells from an early gestational age are best for transplant; for humans, this is tissue from a first trimester fetus.[9,10] Because of the success in the animal studies, fetal tissue has been implanted into patients with Parkinson's disease. Techniques used for these transplants have shown considerable variability, with most investigators using stereotaxic implants rather than open procedures. There is still no agreement on whether caudate or putamen should receive the implants, on the number of fetuses necessary for successful transplant, on the use of immunosuppressants, or on the techniques for cell preservation and tissue injection.[11-16] Since Kish et al. have demonstrated that the most severe dopamine depletion in Parkinson's disease is in the putamen, it is reasonable that the putamen should be a primary focus for tissue implant.[17]

Only three detailed descriptions of human fetal transplant

From Hefti F, and Weiner WJ, (eds.) *Progress in Parkinson's Disease Research—2.* Mount Kisco NY, Futura Publishing Co., Inc., © 1992.

operations are published. The first by Lindvall et al. described two patients in whom there was little clinical improvement following the implant of fetal tissue into one site in caudate and two in putamen on one side of brain.[14] In that experiment performed in 1987, the patients showed clinical deterioration for several weeks after the implant. One possible shortcoming of those experiments was the use of a large implantation cannula (2.5 mm diameter). A second problem may have been cell death caused by holding tissue in unbuffered normal saline at room temperature.

For our human transplant experiments, we have used techniques which we have found effective in monkey experiments.[5] In those experiments, small cannulae (0.8 mm) were associated with good transplant survival. We used multiple needle passes in the monkey. A total of five needle tracks were spaced 3 mm apart in the anterior posterior dimension with two tracks in caudate and three in putamen on one side of the brain. Using methods for cell preservation devised by Kawamoto and Barrett,[18] we found that good transplant results were obtained with cell preservation in chilled Ringer's or phosphate-buffered saline. Adapting these techniques to man in an operation we performed in 1988, we found that a 1.5-mm cannula was necessary to provide the stiffness to accurately target the caudate and putamen from the working distance dictated by the BRW stereotaxic apparatus. We spaced cannula tracks 4 mm apart in caudate and putamen. Using these methods, we have reported on the improvement in motor performance in one patient 6 months[13] and 12 months[15] after fetal tissue implant. We now report results in three patients we have operated upon.

The third report is by Lindvall et al.[16] of an operation performed in 1989 in which they described positive results 5 months after surgery in a patient who received tissue from multiple embryos implanted unilaterally in putamen. They attributed the improvement in outcome in this experiment compared to their 1987 experiments to their use of a smaller cannula (1.0 mm) and chilled buffered saline for cell preservation.

Methods

The first patient was a 52-year-old man with a 20-year history of Parkinson's disease treated with multiple drugs taken every 2½ hours while awake (sinemet, bromocriptine, amantadine, and trihexyphenidyl). The patient had considerable variation in his motor performance over a time course of hours. Walking was particularly difficult especially before the first morning dose of drugs. He had freezing spells which affected him about 30% of the day. The patient was classified as Hoehn and Yahr stage 4 because of his difficulty walking. The patient had had the same neurologist for 17 years and had careful titration of drugs during that time. For the study, the patient was examined by another neurologist at frequent intervals using the Unified Parkinson's Disease Rating Scale (version 3.0)[19] Most examinations were done before and 1 hour after drug administration.

Patient 2 was a 62-year-old man with a 20-year history of Parkinson's disease treated with sinemet four times per day. That patient had undergone bilateral lesions of the thalamus 1 year prior to the fetal implant. The patient had never had on–off episodes but had suffered most from tremor. The thalamic lesions reduced the tremor but made bradykinesia and handwriting worse. A drug effect could be demonstrated in the second patient by taking the patient off drugs for 1 day and comparing the patient's movement during a day on drugs with the day off drugs. There was an approximately 20% reduction in movement speed off drugs.

We have devised a home-based computer system to permit daily self-testing by patients in their own homes. This apparatus measures reaction times, the speed of hand movements on each side of the body, and walking speed. The tests are done before and 1 hour after the first dose of drugs in the morning.[15] This testing scheme is particularly useful for patients suffering from the on–off phenomenon. Such patients are usually off before the first dose of drugs, and therefore this testing method provides a clear discrimination of drug effect on a daily basis. One day a week, the patients performed these tests every hour for 15 hours a day while awake.

In the first patient, a preoperative 6-L-[18F]fluorodopa positron emission tomographic study was performed at Memorial Hospital in New York. Because this instrument went out of service prior to the postoperative scan, a postoperative PET scan was done at UCLA in Los Angeles 9 months after transplantation.

Tissue for the transplants was obtained from therapeutic abortions. The transplant protocol and consent forms for parkinson patients and for the donors of the fetal tissue were approved by the University of Colorado Health Sciences Center Institutional Review Board for the protection of human subjects.

Human fetal brain tissue of about 7 and 8 weeks of gestation (Carnegie stages 19–23)[20] was recovered from routine suction abortion. Informed consent from the mother was obtained only after the abortion was finished. Sterile collection apparatus was used; otherwise, there was no change in the standard abortion procedure. The patient and the tissue donor were unknown to each other, and the woman was not paid.

We developed whole mount tyrosine hydroxylase immunocytochemical techniques to demonstrate surface landmarks for dissecting human fetal dopamine cells from fragments of mesencephalon. This technique provided clear landmarks to dissect a block of tissue 2 × 4 × 1 mm from the rostral half of the ventral mesencephalon, which contained most of the mesencephalic dopamine cells. For patient 1, the tissue was disrupted by trituration with a fire-polished glass Pasteur pipet and 400 μl of cold isotonic phosphate/bicarbonate-buffered saline with glucose (pH 7.2). The total volume of the tissue suspension was about 400 μl. Aliquots of 40 μl for each transplant track were placed in individual sterile tubes. Using acridine orange and ethidium bromide, we found that cell viability averaged 85% in each vial. The time between tissue acquisition and placement in the brain was about 12 hours and during that time, the tissue was kept at 8°C.

In the second and third patients, we used a somewhat modified technique. In an effort to improve the ability to distribute fetal tissue homogeneously without the additional tissue trauma of trituration, we developed a technique for extruding fetal tissue through a tapered glass extruder as shown in Figure 1. In experiments in rats, this technique has produced good graft survival. Mesencephalic tissue from 8-week gestation embryos was extruded through a narrow bore glass cannula, yielding a strand of fetal tissue with a length of approximately 15 cm, and 1.0-cm aliquots of this tissue were then used for each transplant track.

For all three patients, we matched the ABO group of the patient to the fetal tissue using anti-A and anti-B monoclonal antibodies directed against sections of the fetal torso.

The risk of viral transmission from the maternal donor to the patient was reduced by serological investigations for HIV I, hepatitis B, cytomegalovirus, and syphilis. These studies were all done in the hours prior to transplantation. We estimated the risk of herpes

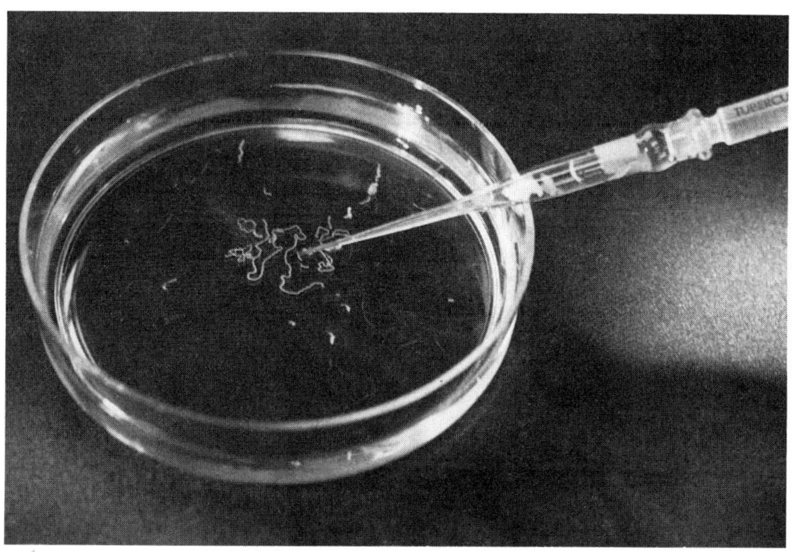

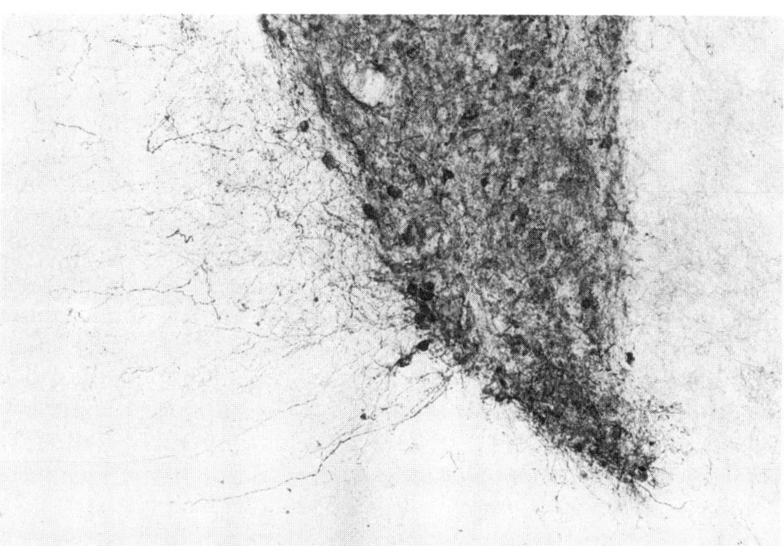

Figure 1. *Top:* Extrusion of fetal tissue by glass capillary tube. To provide homogeneous aliquots of fetal mesencephalic tissue, we have extruded the tissue using the device shown in the figure. Segments of this extruded tissue can then be reaspirated into a needle for injection into the brain. This column of tissue provides a better tissue plug for retransplant than does a suspension and can be given in measured quantities. *Bottom:* Human fetal mesencephalic dopamine tissue plugs implanted in 6-hydroxydopamine lesioned rat striatum. The rat was immunosuppressed with cyclosporine 10 mg/kg per day. Fiber outgrowth demonstrated by tyrosine hydroxylase immunocytochemistry is that which has occurred within 30 days following implantation.

transmission at 1 in 500. The risk of bacterial infection was reduced by washing the fetal tissue fragments through 12 wells of buffer.

The need for immunosuppression after fetal tissue implants into brain is uncertain. Therefore, we are using immunosuppressants only in every other transplant patient. The first and third patients were not immunosuppressed; the second was. In the first patient, fetal tissue was implanted on the right side of brain in an effort to improve motor performance on the left side, which had always been worse than the right. In the second patient, fetal tissue was implanted in the left side of brain with the hope that the implant might improve the patient's handwriting, which was an important disability in his job as an attorney. The third patient received implants bilaterally in the putamen.

Surgery was performed stereotaxically using CT guided coordinates. In the first patient, the transplant cannula was a 19-gauge needle (1.0 mm OD) inside a 17-gauge guide cannula. The 17-gauge guide cannula had an outer diameter of 1.5 mm. In the second patient, we used a combination guide cannula of 17 gauge leading into brain but stopping above the striatum. A second, 22-gauge needle passed into the caudate or putamen. The outer diameter of the 22-gauge cannula was 0.7 mm. Patients were awake during surgery and were sedated as needed with intravenous midazolam in addition to local anesthesia in the scalp. An anterior approach was used in all instances with trajectories aimed to avoid the posterior limb of the internal capsule. There were no postoperative complications. No patient had a fever during the postoperative period. The immuno-suppressed patient was given a loading dose of 15 mg/kg intravenous cyclosporine, 1 g intravenous methylprednisolone, and azathioprine. The azathioprine was discontinued as soon as therapeutic levels of cyclosporine were reached 2 days after starting the cyclosporine (>150 ng/ml whole blood).

There were no complications of surgery. The first patient complained of headache on the day after surgery, probably because of subdural air following incision of the dura. The second and third patients were asymptomatic after surgery. The first two patients spent 1 day in the intensive care unit for observation and were then transferred to ward beds. The third patient was returned to his hospital room from the recovery room. Patients 1 and 3 were discharged on the third hospital day; the second spent 5 days in the hospital during a taper of high-dose prednisone.

Results

We have published detailed transplant results in the first patient at 1 year.[15] This report focuses on the months after that time. The 3-month interval from 12 to 15 months was important because we decided to try to optimize drug therapy beginning at 12 months. At that time, the MAO-B inhibitor deprenyl was started, which led to an increase in dystonia and freezing episodes. We decided that this clinical deterioration was likely due to dopamine agonist overdose and so we reduced doses of sinemet, bromocriptine, amantadine, and trihexyphenidyl. As shown in Figure 2, this reduction in drug dosing

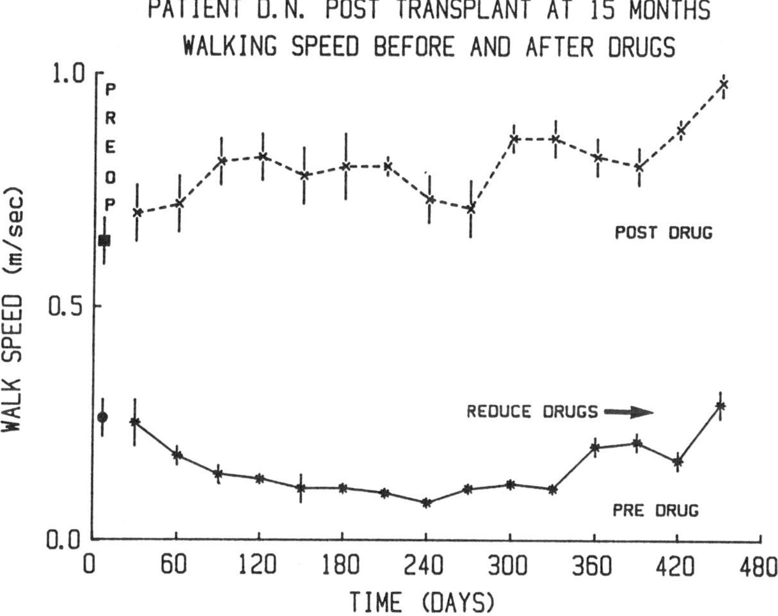

Figure 2. Walking speed before and 1 hour after the first dose of drugs in the morning. The speed is in meters per second. Average preoperative walking speeds are shown in the means at the left-hand margin. Walking speed 1 hour after drugs improved after transplant, while the ability to walk before the first dose of drugs declined substantially. When drugs were reduced beginning at 1 year, there was an increase in walking speed both before and after drugs. Walking speed after drugs increased 53% to 1 m/sec, a normal walking speed. Before drugs, walking speed improved from a depressed level to 12% greater than preoperatively.

led to an increase in walking speed before and after the first morning dose of drugs. In the first 12 months after surgery, walking speed before the morning dose of drugs had systematically declined and was 40% slower than preoperatively. One interpretation of this observation is that the transplant had grown and reduced dopamine receptor supersensitivity postsynaptically. Assuming that walking before the first morning dose of drugs is helped by receptor supersensitivity, it is reasonable to assume that reducing dopamine agonist therapy might restore supersensitivity. While this is a hypothetical suggestion at this time, we found that a 44% reduction in sinemet (from 900 to 500 mg/day) and a 43% cut in bromocriptine (from 17.5 to 10 mg/day) was associated with a dramatic improvement in walking speed both before and after drugs. With the reduction in drug dosing at 15 months, the ability to walk before the first morning dose of drugs was improved to 12% faster than preoperatively and speed after drugs increased 53% to 1 m/sec, a normal walking speed.

The transplant has led to a more predictable response to the first morning dose of drugs. As shown in Figure 3, there was a highly significant increase in the probability of a good response to drugs 1 hour after the first morning dose of drugs. A good response was defined as the ability to walk faster than 0.5 m/sec. On a monthly basis, this response rate has been 100% at 14 and 15 months.

Finger speed in our conditional reaction time–movement paradigm showed a tendency toward slower speeds before the first morning dose of drugs at 15 months compared to 12 months (Figure 4). Drug responses were maintained. Because of greater improvement in the left hand than the right, left and right hand speeds have become the same following surgery. These speeds are normal.

The speed of rapid alternating movements in the left hand, the side opposite to the implant, has shown an interesting response, as shown in Figure 5. The speed has improved 41% before the first morning dose of drugs and has become equivalent to the speed of the right hand. However, the left hand has shown a reduced response to drugs. On inspection of video tapes done by the patient at home, we found that the left hand becomes dyskinetic on drugs and therefore loses precision, which affects rapid alternating movements. The finger speed (shown above in Figure 4) is preserved for the left hand since precision is less important for the single movement of the finger tested in that task.

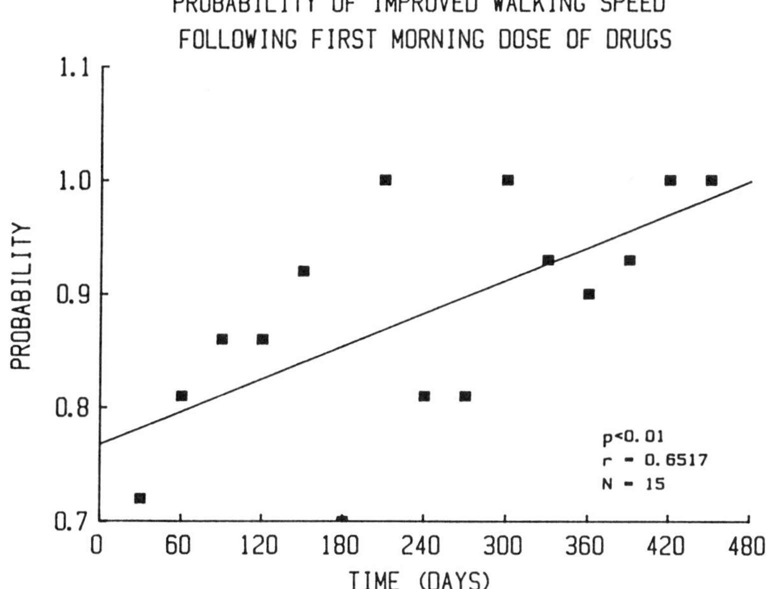

Figure 3.   Probability of improved walking speed following the first morning dose of drugs. Prior to surgery and in the early weeks after surgery, the patient responded to drugs just over 70% of the time. The response is to the first morning dose of drugs following an all-night period off drugs. With 30 days per month recorded, 1 day without a drug response would reduce the walking speed to > 0.5 m/sec. The response at 14 and 15 months has been 100%. Regression analysis showed $r = 0.65$, $P < 0.01$.

Both the clinical neurologic exam and the patient's reports have paralleled these computer findings. In addition to responses inventoried by the Unified Parkinson's Disease Rating Scale, the patient also reported relief of chronic constipation 1 month after surgery. He has regained the ability to whistle. Fluorodopa PET scanning done 9 months postoperatively was limited in its interpretability because the preoperative scan was not done on the same scanner. Nonetheless, in two of three cuts showing caudate and putamen, there was apparently greater uptake of the [^{18}F]dopa on the transplanted side of brain. Table 1 shows the changes in drug doses 15 months after surgery compared with the preoperative doses.

The second patient, now 1 year after surgery, showed no change in clinical state despite the fact that the patient was immunosup-

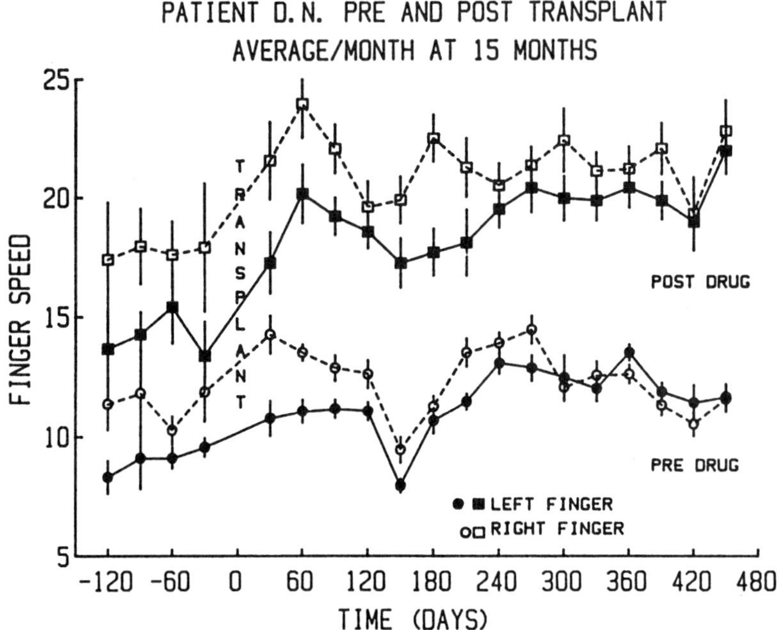

Figure 4.   Finger speed before and after the first dose of drugs in the morning. Finger speed is measured in centimeters per second. The reduction in drugs that occurred at 1 year was associated with some reduction in predrug motor performance, particularly in the right hand (open symbols/dashed lines). In fact, right-hand performance predrug returned to a level seen before the implant operation. The postdrug movement speed in both hands was maintained, and both hands were similar in speed. Reaction time (not shown) was unaffected by Parkinson's disease, the hand being used, or the transplant.

pressed and the cannula used for the transplant in the second patient was smaller than for the first patient. Figure 6 shows results of rapid alternating movement testing in this patient. There was no change in speed in either hand during the 12 months after surgery.

There were important differences in the clinical picture of the first and second patients. The second patient had a much less dramatic response to drugs. In order to see a drug effect, comparisons of movement speed during a day off drugs were compared to a day on drugs. The reduction in walking speed off drugs was only about 20%. The patient had also undergone bilateral lesions of the thalamus.

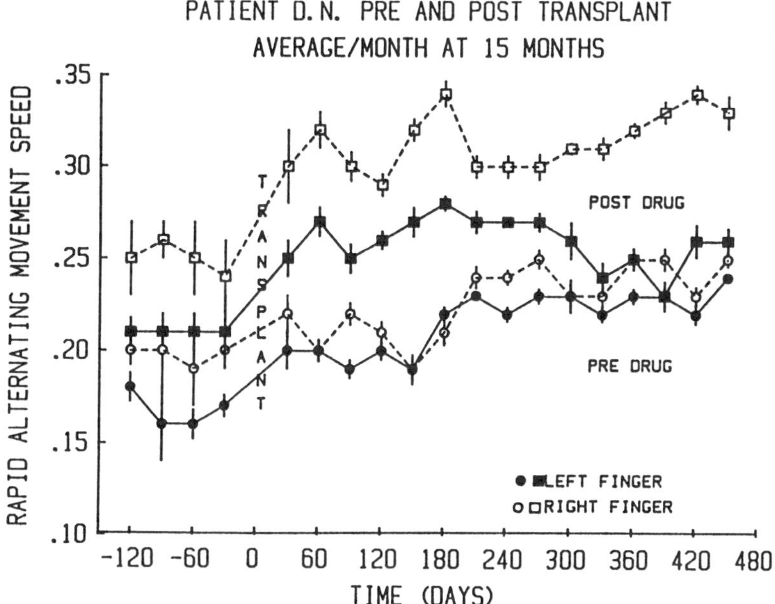

Figure 5. Speed of rapid alternating movements before and after the first morning dose of drugs. Rapid alternating movements improved in both the left and right hand compared to preoperative values. In the left hand, however, the speed of rapid alternating movements was not much enhanced by drug administration. The reason for this was a tendency toward a dyskinetic response in the left hand 1 hour after drugs. This dyskinetic response was not present in the right hand.

Table 1.
Medication Changes in Patient 1 Fifteen Months after Fetal Tissue Implant

Medication (mg/day)	Pretransplant	Posttransplant	% Change
L-Dopa (sinemet)	900	500	−44
Bromocriptine	17.5	10	−43
Trihexyphenidyl	8	6	−25
Amantadine	300	200	−33
Deprenyl	0	10	

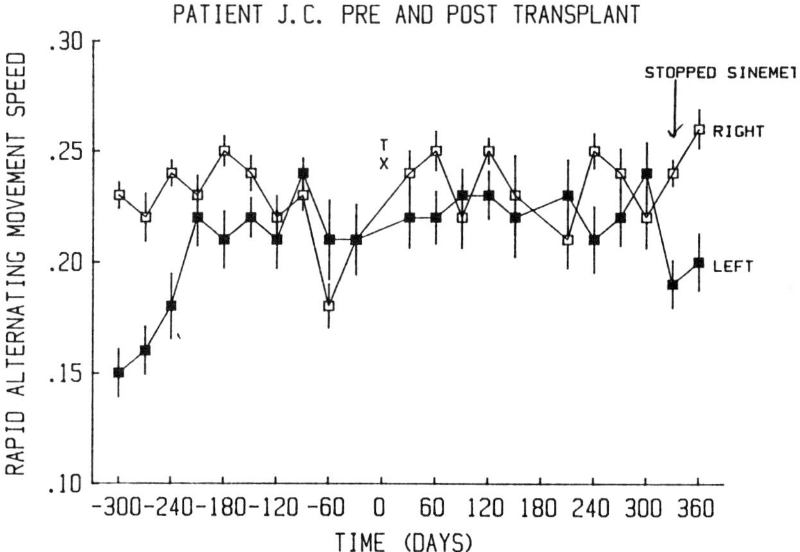

Figure 6.   Speed of rapid alternating movements in patient 2 before and after fetal tissue implant in left caudate and putamen. There was no improvement in finger speed in either hand after surgery.

While relieving tremor, these operations were associated with a worsening of handwriting and the patient believes that they may have made bradykinesia worse. The patient has had chronic constipation, which has persisted following surgery. He is also impotent. One year after surgery, all sinemet therapy was discontinued with no clinical deterioration measured by computer testing. Immunosuppression with cyclosporine was also stopped at 1 year followed by tapering of prednisone dose over 2 months without change in clinical parkinsonian status.

A third patient with signs of the on–off phenomenon similar to patient 1 has been operated on with implants into the putamen bilaterally. Seven injections into each putamen were performed. Five months after surgery, the patient has improved movement before his first dose of drugs in the morning, and both examining neurologists and the patient have been impressed with improvement in the smoothness of motor control. A plot of the percent on time is shown in Figure 7.

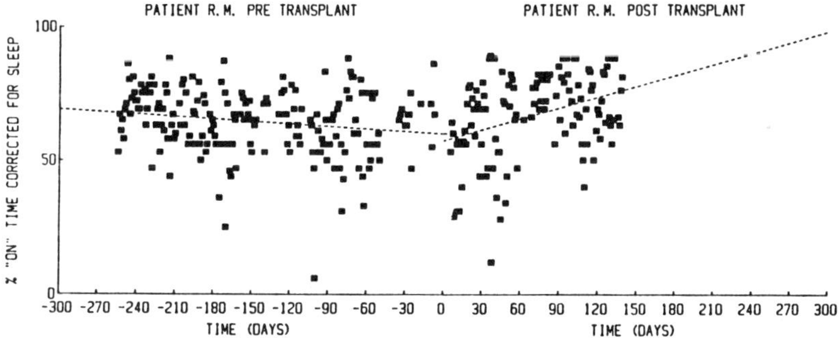

Figure 7. Fraction of time spent on by patient 3 before and after surgery. Tissue was implanted bilaterally in putamen. The downward trend preoperatively has reversed in the months postoperatively.

Discussion

We have found clinical improvement in parkinson state in two patients with the on–off phenomenon 5 and 15 months after surgery. In a third patient, who has a less dramatic response to drugs, there has been no objective change in the parkinsonian condition.

In the first patient, we found that a reduction in drug dose 1 year after surgery led to further improvement in clinical state, particularly in the ability to walk before the first morning dose of drugs as well as an improved walking speed after drug administration. The probability of responding to the first dose of drugs with an increase in walking speed has been 100% in the last 2 months. We would make the suggestion that diminished receptor supersensitivity might have been responsible for the reduction in walking speed before the first morning dose of drugs, which we had seen for the first 12 months after tissue implantation. Reduction of drugs at 12 months may have restored receptor supersensitivity.

Our home-based computer testing system has demonstrated its value both for seeing the initial transplant response and for following drug manipulations. We believe that this sort of system is likely to have value for many parkinson patients, particularly when efforts are underway to optimize drugs. Two tests, one of rapid alternating movements and the other measuring the speed of a single finger movement, demonstrate that these tests have independent usefulness. The test of finger speed alone showed improvement on the side of brain contralateral to the transplant both before and after the first morning dose of drugs. By contrast, the test of rapid alternating movements showed an improvement in predrug performance but a relative loss of drug response. Because the patient also has a television camera in his home, we could see that the reason for the loss in speed of rapid alternating movements was dyskinesias in the left hand associated with drug administration. These objective observations matched the patient's report of a tendency for the side opposite to the transplant to have more dyskinetic activity following drug administration than the other side of the body.

In our second patient, followed for 12 months after surgery, we saw little in the way of objective motor improvement as measured by computer testing. This patient had had bilateral thalamotomies but also demonstrated no fluctuations in motor activity, which could be related to single doses of L-dopa.

The third patient who has the on–off phenomenon appears to be having a symmetrical and significant response to fetal cell implants placed bilaterally in putamen. Based on these three patients, we would suggest that the most likely patient to respond to fetal tissue implant is one who has a dramatic and easily demonstrated response to L-dopa on a dose-by-dose basis. Because this transplant procedure is associated with some risk, we believe it should be reserved for patients who are still responding to drugs, but who have problems with excess movements, freezing spells, and severe bradykinesia off drugs. Because our first and third patients seem to have had a therapeutic response to the transplant even without immunosuppression, we think it is possible that patients will not require immunosuppression to get a transplant effect. However, we will continue to immunosuppress every other patient to see the relative response in the immunosuppressed and nonimmunosuppressed patient groups.

Changes in autonomic function have also been seen in these patients. As do many patients with Parkinson's disease, our patients suffered from chronic constipation. In the first and third patients, the constipation has resolved. Constipation in the second patient did not improve. We suggest that a systematic inventory of autonomic signs be made prior to transplant to see the effect of fetal tissue implant on cardiovascular, bowel, bladder, and sexual function.

Many centers are now pursuing fetal tissue implants for

Parkinson's disease,[11–16] so that the value of this treatment should become evident in the next few years. These studies should answer such questions as which patient gets a good response to transplant. Is a patient with severe on–off phenomenon more likely to respond to transplant than a patient with only a wearing-off response to drug therapy? Does immunosuppression improve transplant effects? How much clinical improvement needs to be seen to justify the costs and risks of fetal implant surgery? Can patients be cured of Parkinson's disease or must we be satisfied with rolling back the clock to a time in the course of the disease when the drug response was more satisfactory? The exciting era of brain repair is underway, and these answers should be forthcoming.

Acknowledgments: We thank Robert E. Stanton, the late Charles E. Stanton, Denver, Colorado, and the National Parkinson Foundation for their generous support of this research.

References

1. Bjorklund A, Stenevi U. 1979. Reconstruction of the nigrostriatal dopamine pathway by intracerebral nigral transplants. Brain Res 177:555–560.
2. Perlow MJ, Freed WJ, Hoffer BJ, Seiger A, Olson L, Wyatt RJ. 1979. Brain grafts reduce motor abnormalities produced by destruction of nigrostriatal dopamine system. Science 204:643–647.
3. Bakay RAE, Barrow DL, Schiff A, Fiandanca MS. 1985. Biochemical and behavioral correction of MPTP Parkinson-like syndrome by fetal cell transplantation. Appl Neurophysiol 48:358–361.
4. Redmond DE, Sladek JR, Roth RH, Collier TJ, Elsworth JD, Deutsch AY, Haber S. 1986. Fetal neural grafts in monkeys given methylphenyltetrahydropyridine. Lancet 1:1125–1127.
5. Freed CR, Richard JB, Sabol KE, Reite ML. 1988. Fetal substantia nigra transplants lead to dopamine cell replacement and behavioral improvement in Bonnet monkeys with MPTP-induced Parkinsonism. *In* Pharmacology and Functional Regulation of Dopaminergic Neurons. PM Beart, G Woodruff, DM Jackson, (eds). New York, Macmillan, pp 353–360.
6. Dunnett SB, Bjorklund A, Schmidt RH, Steveni U, Iversen SD. 1984. Intracerebral grafting of neuronal cell suspensions, IV. Behavioral recovery in rats with unilateral 6-OHDA lesions following implantation of nigral cell suspensions in different forebrain sites. Acta Physiol Scand 522(suppl):29–37.
7. Dunnett SB, Whishaw IQ, Jones GH, Isacson O. 1986. Effects of dopamine-rich grafts on conditioned rotation in rats with unilateral 6-hydroxydopamine lesions. Neurosci Lett 68:127–133.

8. Richards JB, Freed CR. 1987. Effects of fetal substantia nigra transplants on lesion-induced deficits in trained circling behavior. Soc Neurosci Abstr 13:831.

9. Brundin P, Nilsson OG, Strecker RE, Lindvall O, Astedt B, Bjorklund A. 1986. Behavioral effects of human fetal dopamine neurons grafted in a rat model of Parkinson's disease. Brain Res 65:235–240.

10. Stromberg I, Bygdeman M, Goldstein M, Seiger A, Olson L. 1986. Human fetal substantia nigra grafted to the dopamine-denervated striatum of immunosuppressed rats: Evidence for functional reinnervation. Neurosci Lett 71:271–276.

11. Madrazo I, Leon V, Torres C, Aguilera C, Varela G, Alvarez F, Fraga A, Drucker-Collin R, Ostrosky R, Skurovich M, Franco R. 1988. Transplantation of fetal substantia nigra and adrenal medulla to the caudate nucleus in two patients with Parkinson's disease. N Engl J Med 318:51.

12. Hitchcock ER, Clough C, Hughes R, Kenny B. 1988. Embryos and Parkinson's disease. Lancet 1:1274.

13. Freed CR, Breeze RE, Rosenberg NL, Barrett JN, Rottenberg DA. 1989. Transplant of human fetal dopamine cells in a patient with Parkinson's disease. Clin Res 37:517A.

14. Lindvall O, Rehncrona S, Brundin P, Gustavii B, Astedt B, Widner H, Lindholm T, Bjorklund A, Leenders KL, Rothwell JC, Frackowiak R, Marsden CD, Johnels B, Steg G, Freedman R, Hoffer BJ, Seiger A, Bygdeman M, Stromberg T, Olson L. 1989. Human fetal dopamine neurons grafted into the striatum in two patients with severe Parkinson's disease. Arch Neurol 46:615–631.

15. Freed CR, Breeze RE, Rosenberg NL, Schneck SA, Wells TH, Barrett JN, Grafton ST, Huang SC, Eidelberg D, Rottenberg DA. 1990. Transplantation of human fetal dopamine cells for Parkinson's disease: Results at 1 year. Arch Neurol 47:505–512.

16. Lindvall O, Brundin P, Widner H, Rehncrona S, Gustavii B, Frackowiak R, Leenders KL, Sawle G, Rothwell JC, Marsden CD, Bjorklund A. 1990. Grafts of fetal dopamine neurons survive and improve motor function in Parkinson's disease. Science 247:574–577.

17. Kish SJ, Shannak K, Hornykiewicz O. 1988. Uneven pattern of dopamine loss in the striatum of patients with idiopathic Parkinson's disease: Pathophysiologic and clinical implications. N Engl J Med 319:370–371.

18. Kawamoto JC, Barrett JN. 1986. Cyropreservation of primary neurons for tissue culture. Brain Res 384:84–93.

19. Fahn S, Elton RL, and members of the UPDRS Development Committee. 1987. Unified Parkinson Disease Rating Scale. *In* Recent Developments in Parkinson's Disease II. S Fahn, CD Marsden, M Goldstein, et al. (eds). Macmillan, New York, pp 153–163.

20. O'Rahilly R, Muller F. 1987. Developmental Stages in Human Embryos. Carnegie Institution of Washington, Publication 637, Meriden-Steinehour Press, Meriden, Connecticut.

Index